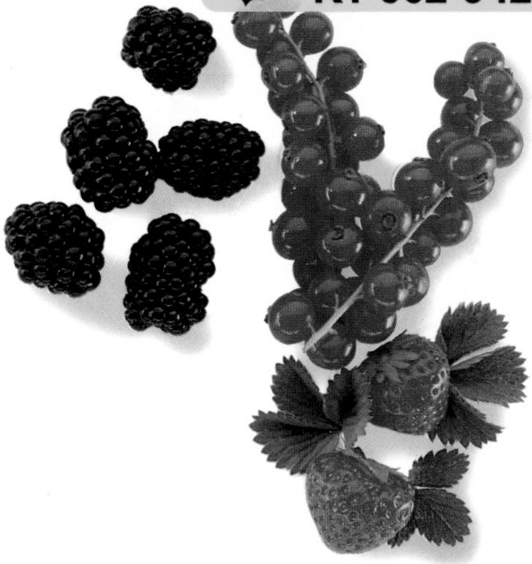

Foods that Harm Foods that Heal

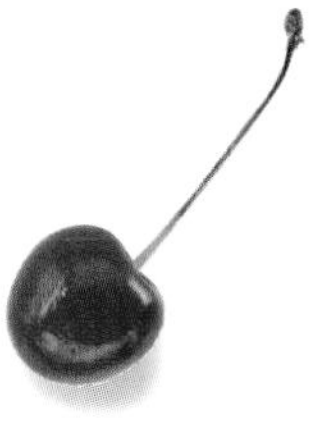

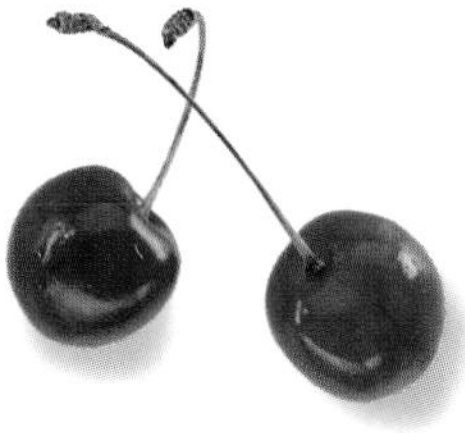

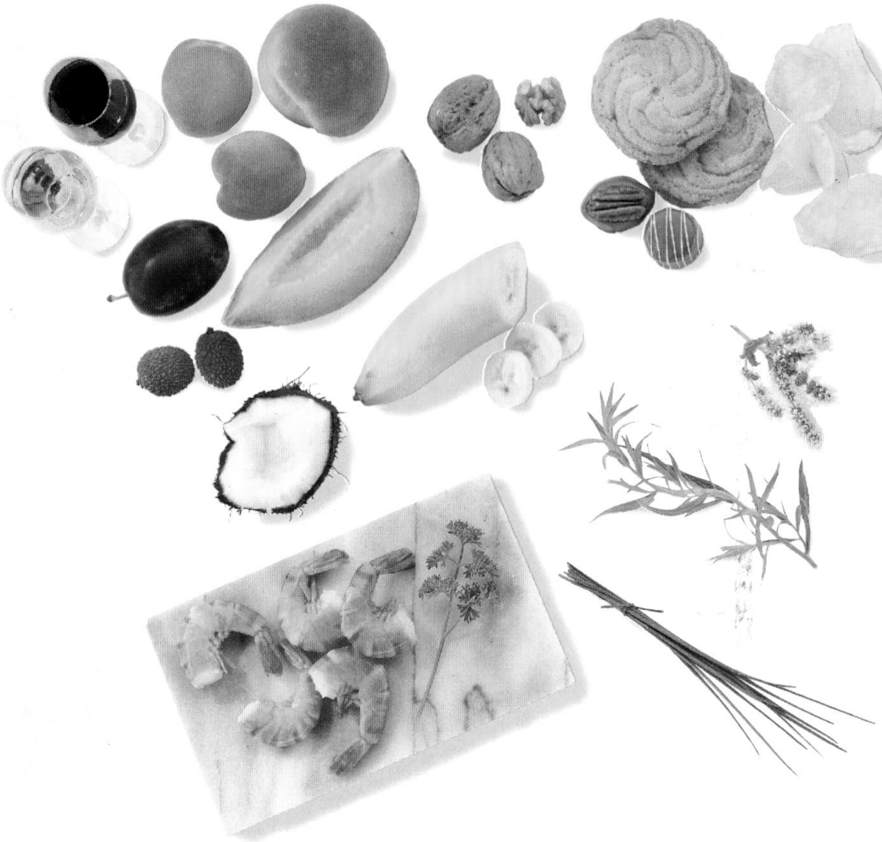

FOODS THAT HARM, FOODS THAT HEAL
was edited and designed by
The Reader's Digest Association Limited, London.

Fourth reprint with amendments 1997

Typeface used in the main text of this book is 10.5 on 12pt Garamond 3.

Printed in Belgium
ISBN 0 276 42193 0

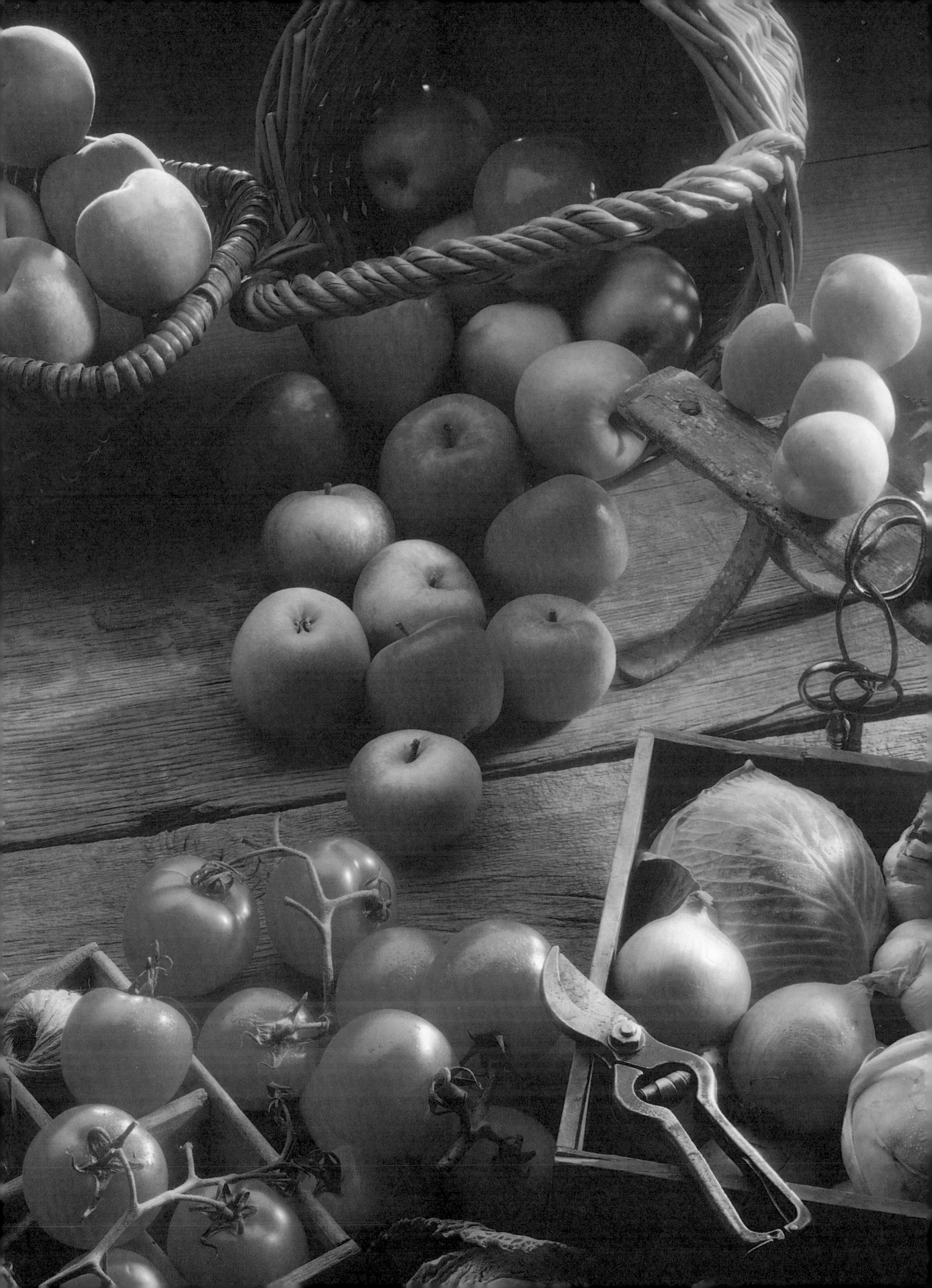

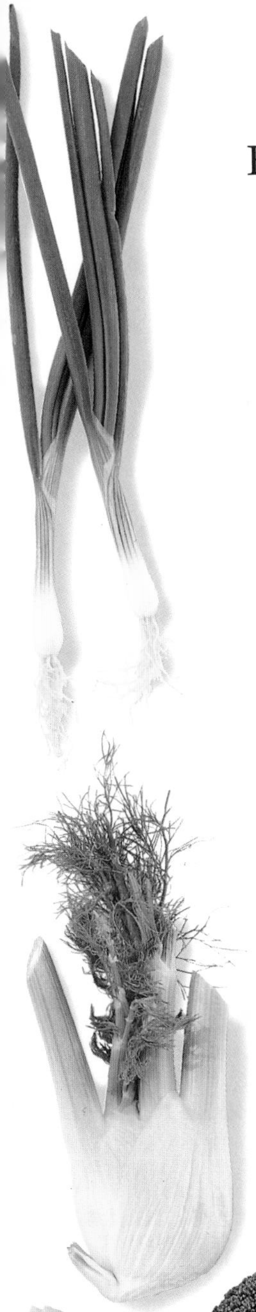

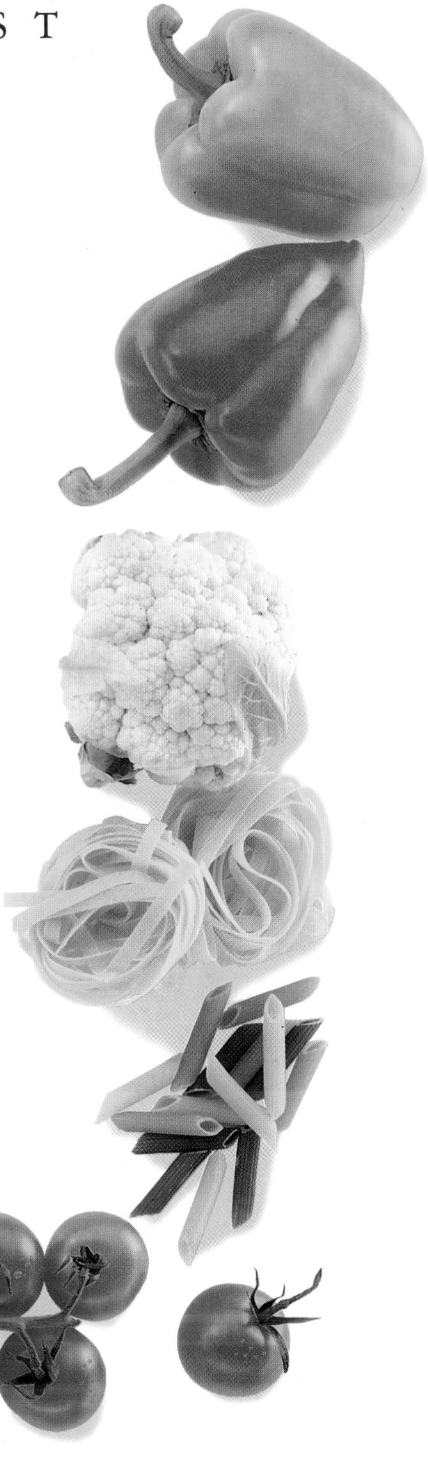

READER'S DIGEST

FOODS THAT HARM FOODS THAT HEAL

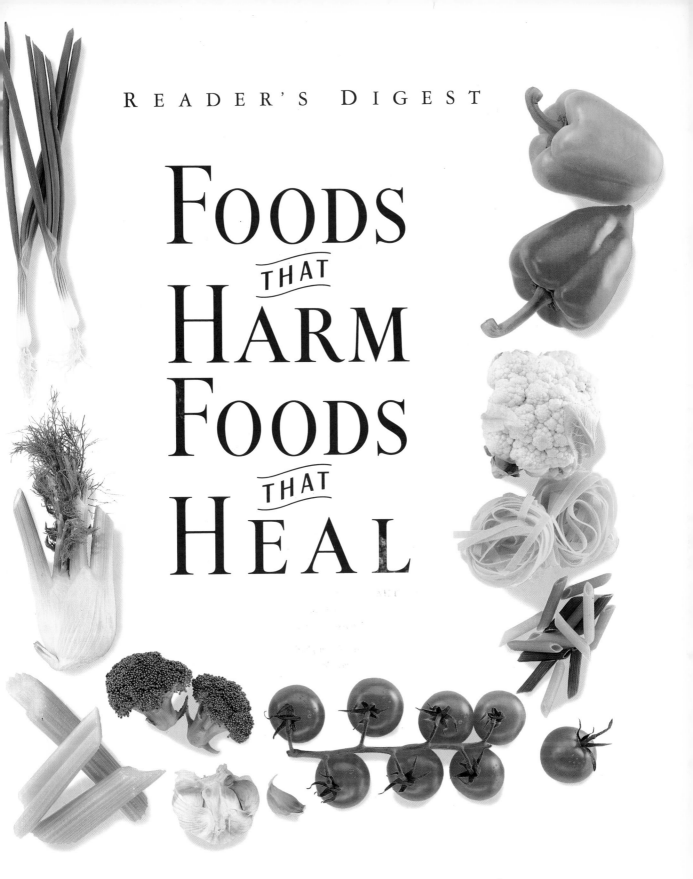

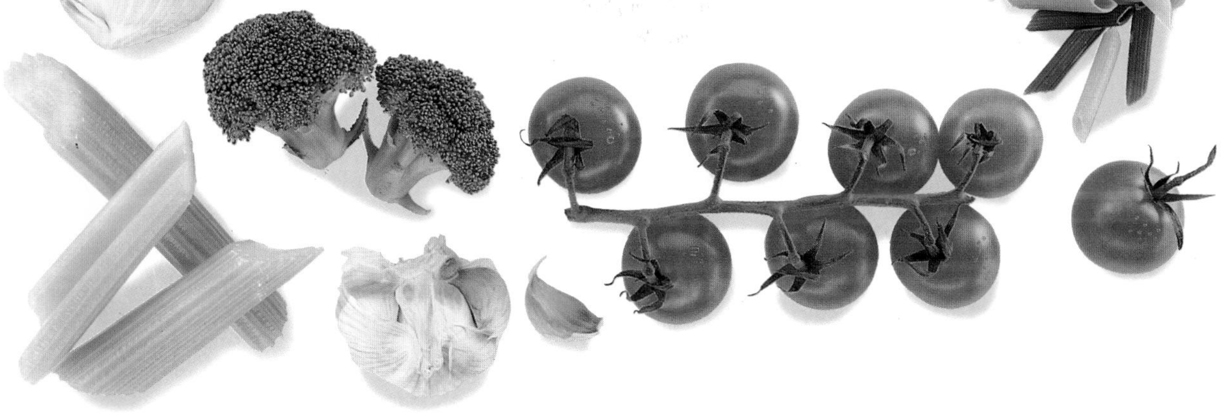

PUBLISHED BY THE READER'S DIGEST ASSOCIATION LIMITED
LONDON • NEW YORK • SYDNEY • CAPE TOWN • MONTREAL

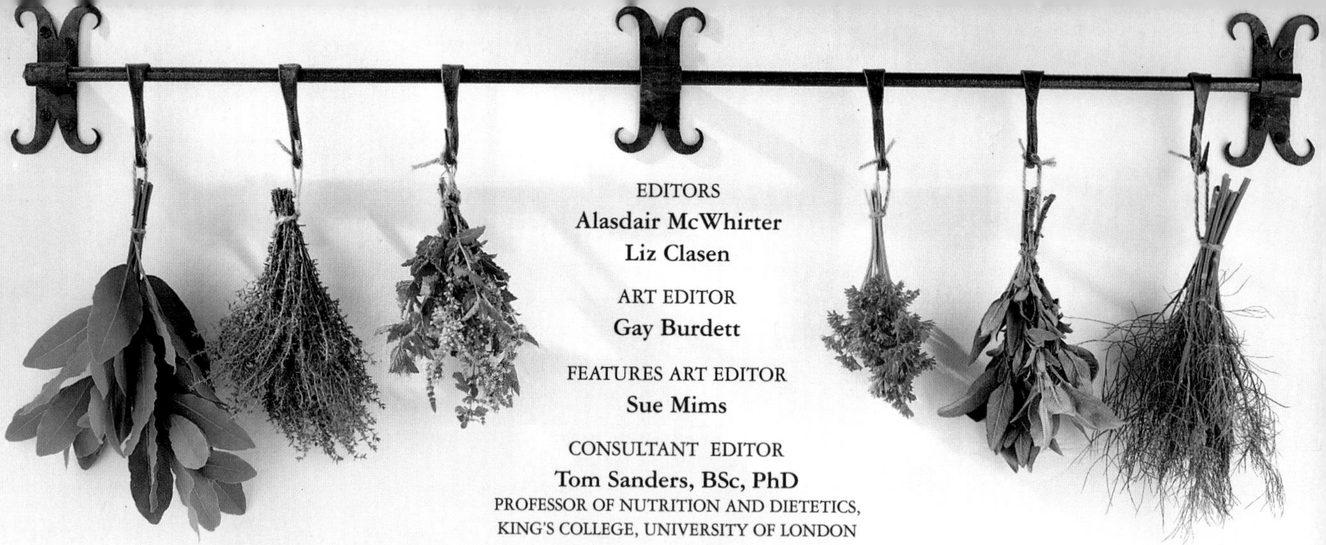

EDITORS
Alasdair McWhirter
Liz Clasen

ART EDITOR
Gay Burdett

FEATURES ART EDITOR
Sue Mims

CONSULTANT EDITOR
Tom Sanders, BSc, PhD
PROFESSOR OF NUTRITION AND DIETETICS,
KING'S COLLEGE, UNIVERSITY OF LONDON

CONTRIBUTORS AND CONSULTANTS

THE PUBLISHERS WOULD LIKE TO THANK THE FOLLOWING PEOPLE FOR THEIR CONTRIBUTIONS TO THIS BOOK

Dr Ann F. Walker, MSc, PhD, MIFST, FRSH, CBiol, MIBiol, MNIMH, MCCPP
SENIOR LECTURER IN NUTRITION, UNIVERSITY OF READING
Dr Alan Lakin, MSc, PhD, CChem, FRSC, FRSH, MIFST
Dr Margaret Ashwell, OBE, PhD, FIFST, FRSH
Anita Bean, BSc
Dr Jonathan Brostoff, MA, DM, DSc, FRCP, FRCPath
Kristen McNutt, PhD, JD
Dr Sheena Meredith, MB, BS
Dr Michèle Sadler, BSc, PhD, FRSH
Christine Steward, MNIMH
Michael A. van Straten, ND, DO, DipAc, MRN, MRO, MB, AcA
Dr Martin Toynbee, BSc, MB, BS, MRCGP
Marianne Vennegoor, SRD
Moya de Wet, BSc, SRD

PHOTOGRAPHERS
Karl Adamson
Gus Filgate
Vernon Morgan
Carol Sharp
Jon Stewart

ILLUSTRATORS
Julia Bigg
Dick Bonson
Glynn Boyd Harte
Hannah Firmin
Clare Melinsky
Francis Scappatricci
Lesli Sternberg
Sam Thompson
Charlotte Wess

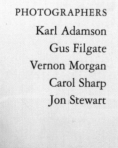

WRITERS
Dr Ursula Arens
Dr Alison Hinds
Susie Orbach
Rose Shepherd
Helen Spence

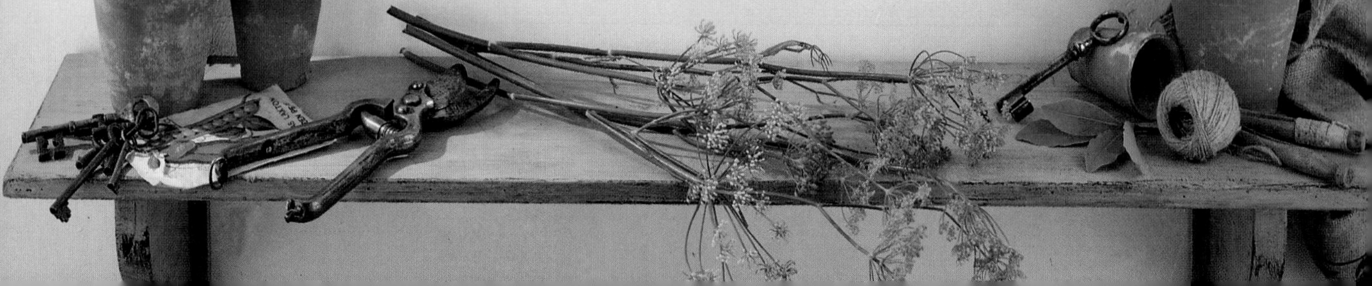

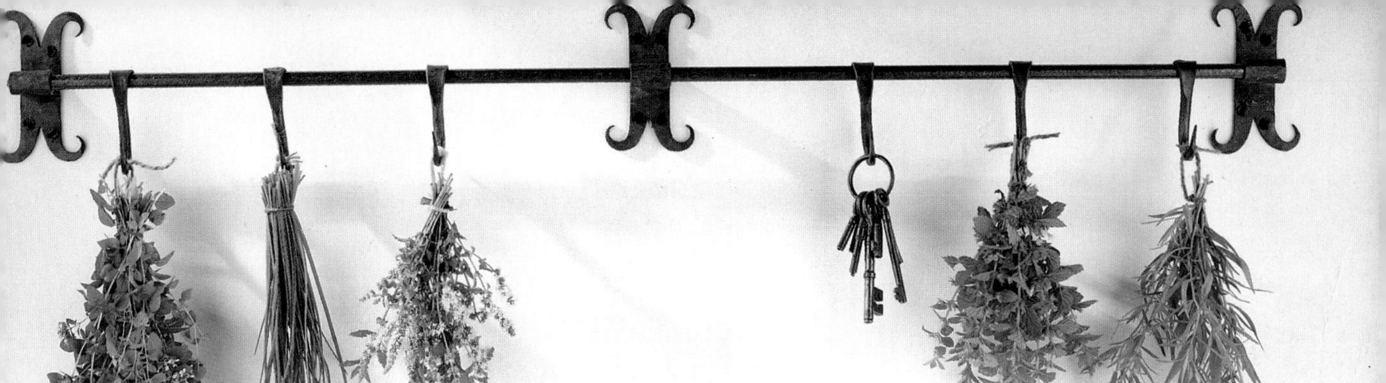

DESIGNERS

Emma Gilbert

Tracey Schmidt

RESEARCHERS

Alistair McDermott

Gisèle Edwards

Emily Pedder

EDITORIAL ASSISTANT

Maria Pufulete

ASSISTANT EDITORS

Celia Coyne • Caroline Johnson • Amanda Rickaby • Peter Schirmer • Helen Spence
Paul Todd • Debbie Voller • Rachel Warren Chadd

READER'S DIGEST GENERAL BOOKS

EDITORIAL DIRECTOR

Robin Hosie

ART DIRECTOR

Bob Hook

EXECUTIVE EDITOR

Michael Davison

MANAGING EDITOR

Paul Middleton

EDITORIAL GROUP HEADS

Julian Browne • Noel Buchanan • Cortina Butler • Jeremy Harwood

RESEARCH EDITOR

Prue Grice

PICTURE RESEARCH EDITOR

Martin Smith

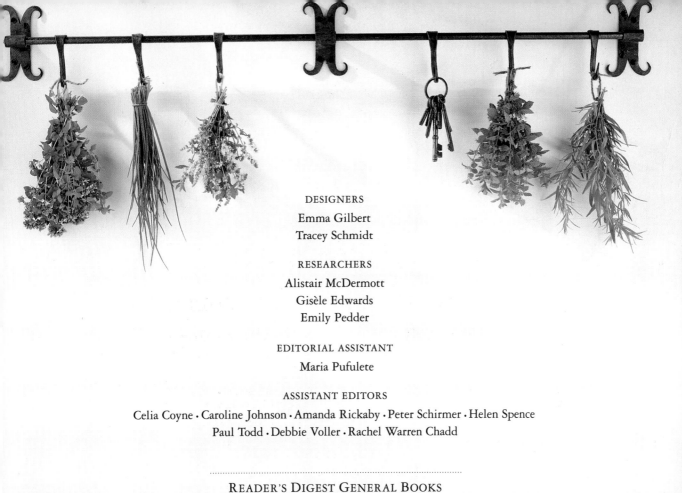

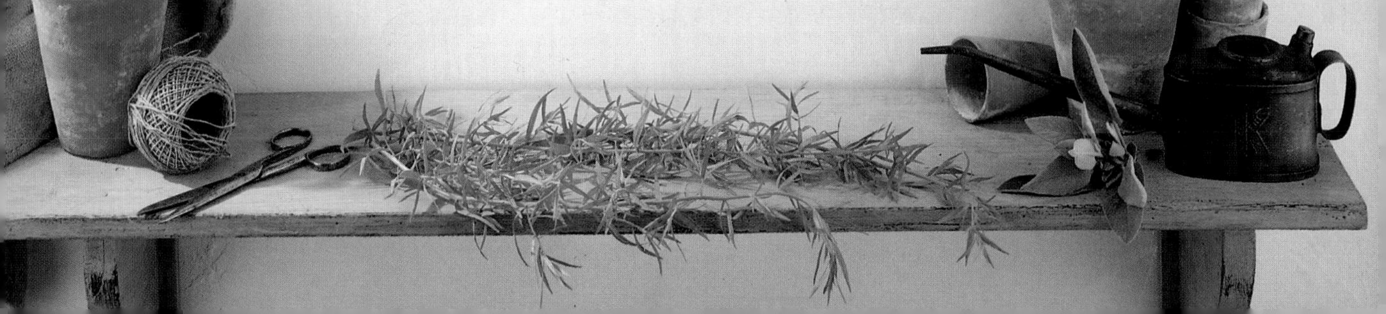

THE FACTS ABOUT FOOD AND HEALTH

Minor changes in your eating habits can lead to major changes in your health: *Foods that Harm, Foods that Heal* explains how. What you eat not only affects your day-to-day health but also helps to determine the quality of your life and even how long you will live. Amid the confusion caused by contradictory claims, scares and reassurances about food and health, this book offers impartial information. It scrutinises the main controversies and presents the facts, supported by scientific evidence. Based on the collective wisdom of more than 300 experts in nutrition as well as in orthodox and natural medicine, *Foods that Harm, Foods that Heal* provides a simple but authoritative A-Z guide to foods and ailments, giving practical advice on how to improve and protect your health. It covers everything from additives and allergies to yoghurt and zinc, and also explains how to ensure that you have a balanced diet.

Nutrition is still a young science, but it is clear that there are few ailments that diet cannot help to prevent, cure or at least make more bearable. As well as having a role in the struggle against

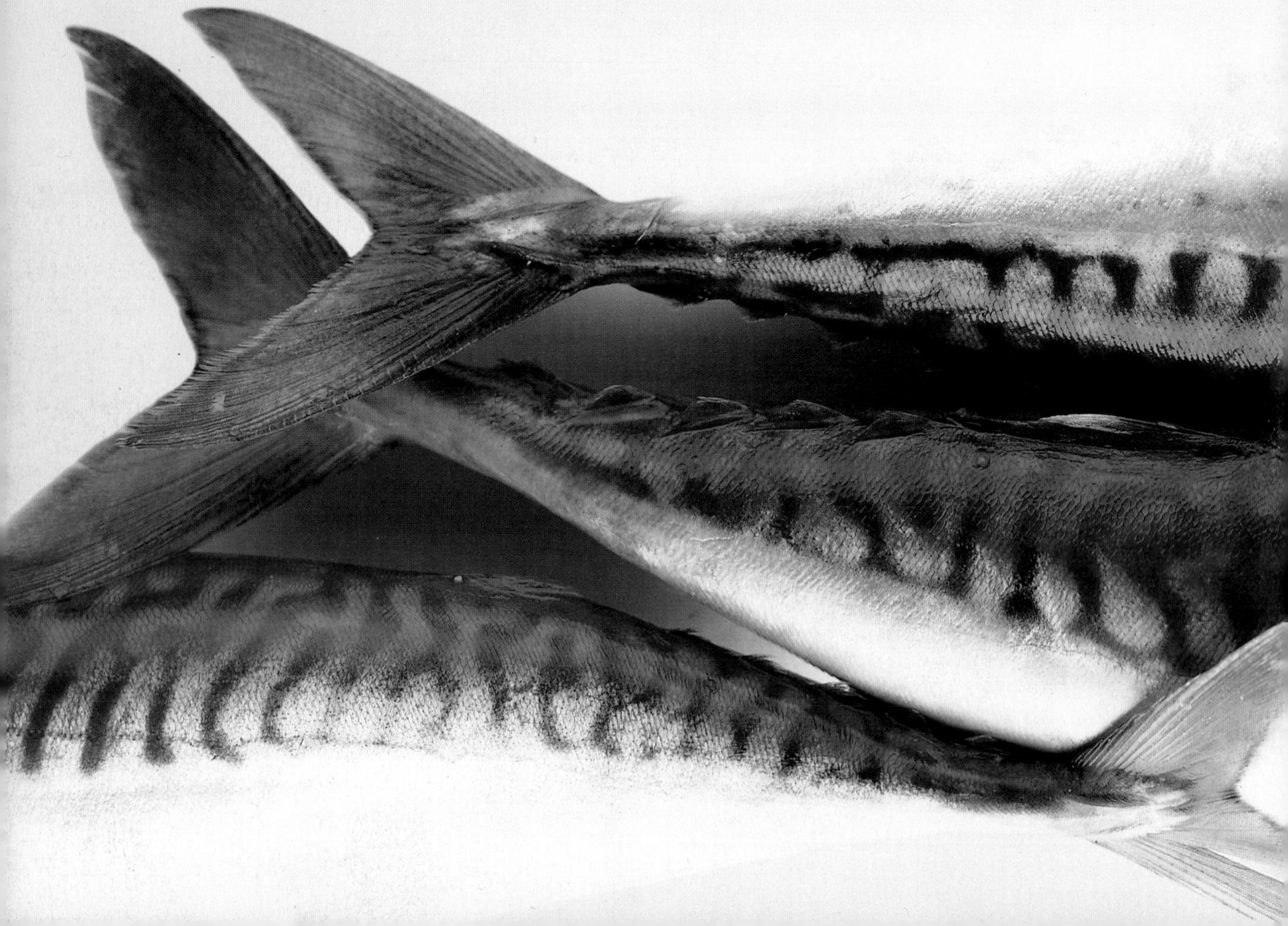

heart disease, cancer and arthritis, diet can also help to conquer stress, insomnia, infertility and low energy levels. This book looks at traditional cures and at natural remedies. It examines statements such as 'feed a cold, starve a fever' and 'chips are bad for you' – and shows that some are based on myth rather than fact.

HOW TO USE THIS BOOK

Many foods in this book are described as being an 'excellent', 'rich', 'good' or 'useful' source of certain nutrients. These terms describe the nutritional value of the food relative to the daily requirement recommended by Department of Health – the Reference Nutrient Intake (RNI). 'Excellent' means that the food provides the entire RNI; 'rich' denotes that it supplies three-quarters of it; 'good' a half; and 'useful' a quarter. A food that is said to 'contain' a nutrient provides at least one-eighth of the RNI. Cross references, printed in SMALL CAPITAL LETTERS, guide you to related entries. At the back of the book, a glossary explains unfamiliar terms, and there are addresses of organisations that can offer helpful advice on specific ailments.

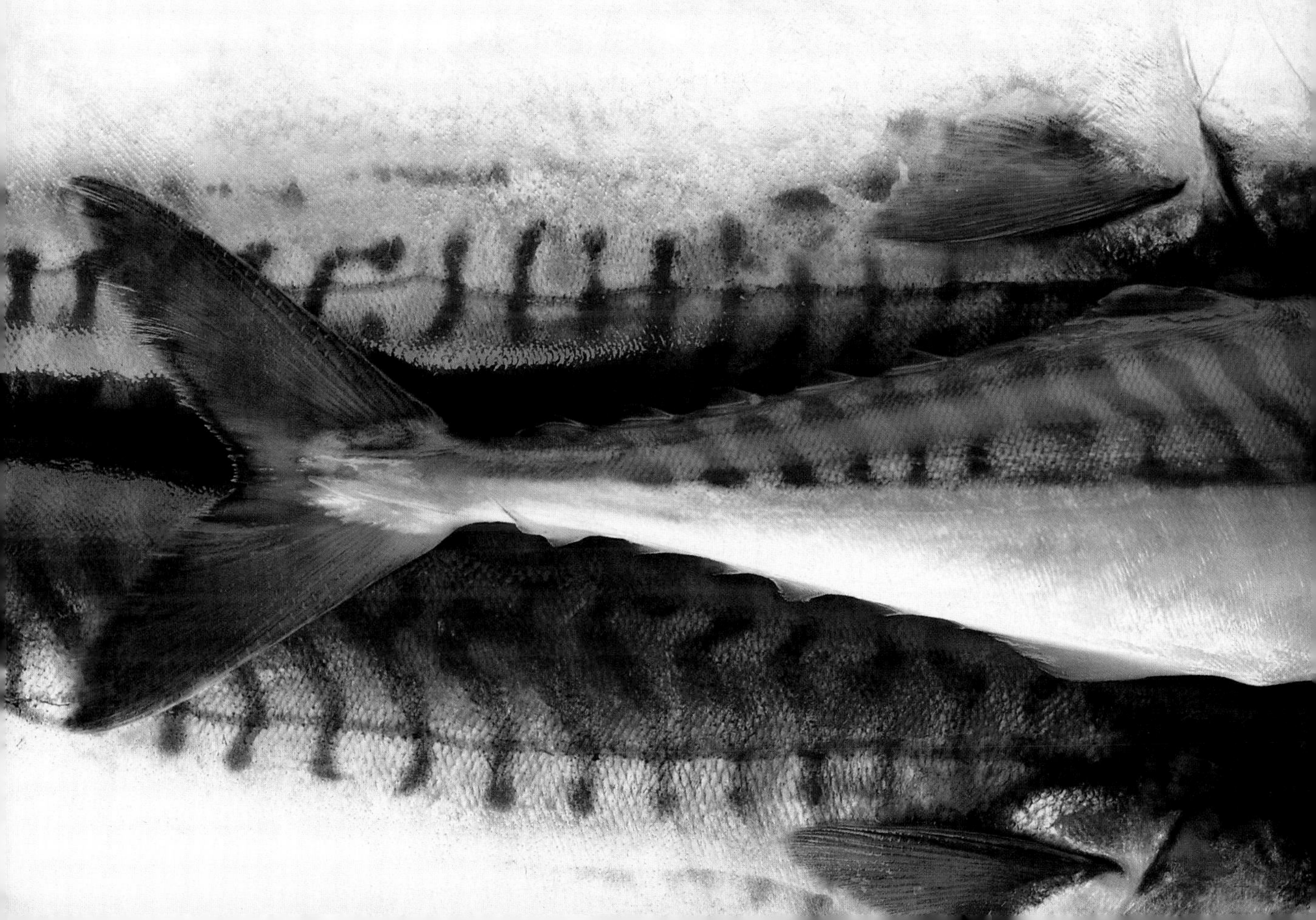

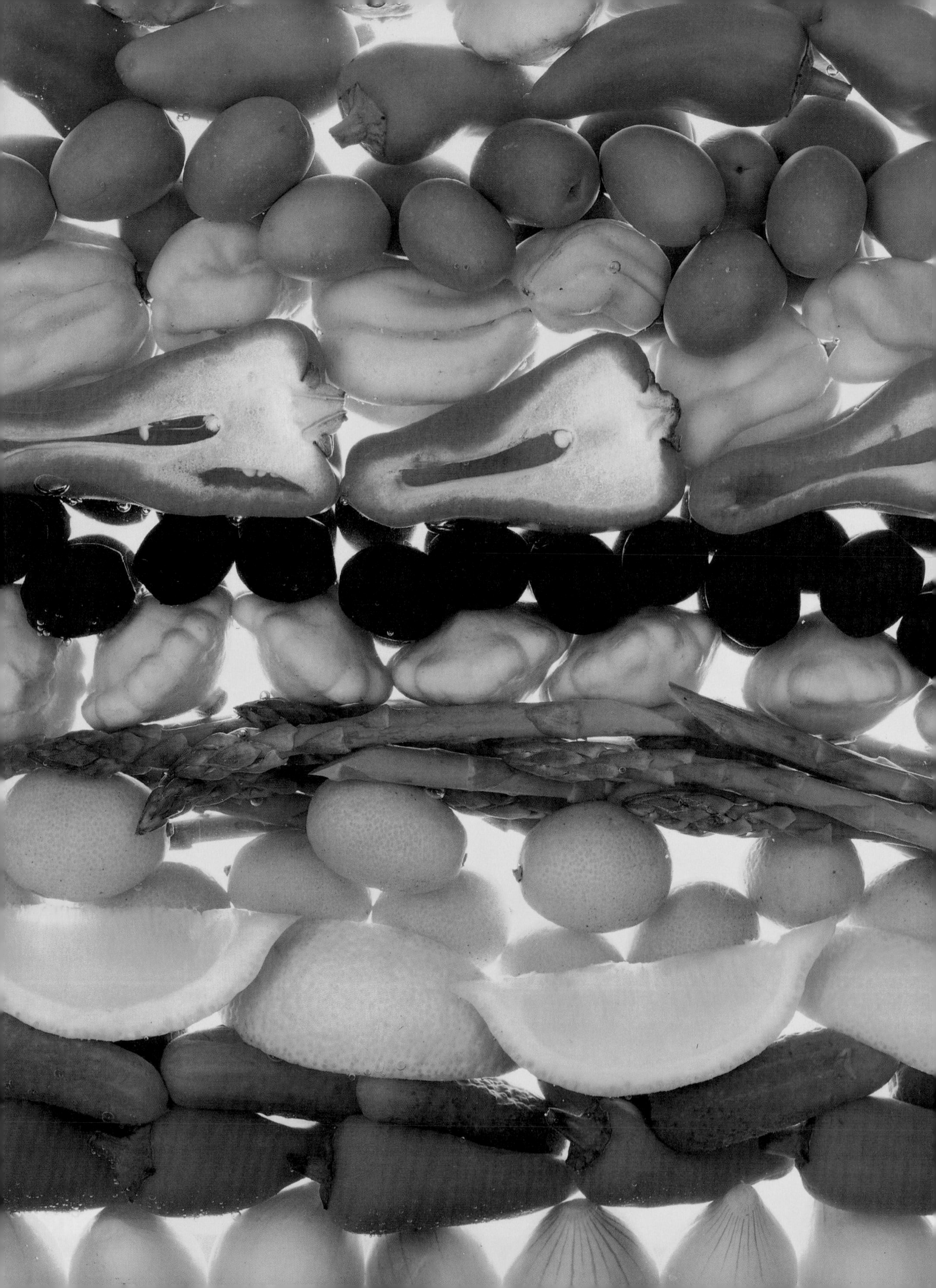

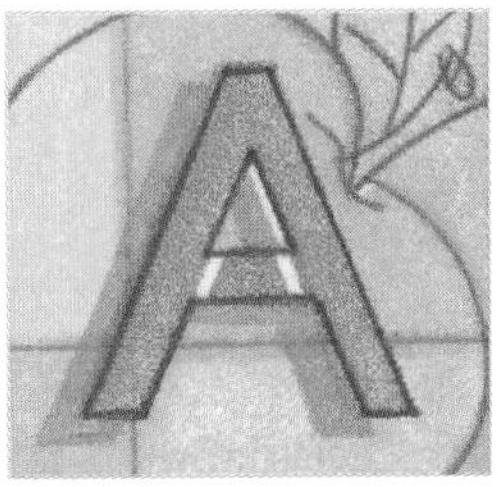

ACNE

EAT PLENTY OF
- *Shellfish, nuts, poultry and lean meat, for zinc*
- *Fresh fruit and vegetables for vitamin C*

CUT DOWN ON
- *Chocolate and sweets*
- *Highly salted snacks*
- *Added sugar*

At some time or other during their teens 85 per cent of young Britons suffer from acne – the unsightly spots which are the bane of growing up. Until recently it was a popular belief – though never proven – that it was the high sugar and fat content in a diet of chips, burgers, chocolates and soft drinks, for example, that caused acne.

Although junk food is still thought to be linked to the problem, the fault may lie less with the prime suspects – sugar and saturated fat – than with iodine-containing chemicals. These are often added to the salt that is used liberally on chips, crisps and many other convenience foods. Equally, a bad complexion or dull-looking skin may have more to do with what you do not eat than with what you do. And a diet based on fast foods, sweets, snacks and alcohol will be low in several vital minerals and vitamins.

Either way, youngsters plagued by pimples should cut down on refined carbohydrates found in sugary foods, fatty and fried foods such as burgers and chips, highly salted snacks, soft drinks and confectionery, in favour of whole grains, fresh fruit and vegetables, lean meat and a moderate intake of polyunsaturated oils.

Acne starts when the sebaceous glands overproduce oil, or sebum, secreted through the pores. Sebum carries dead cell debris away with it, but its overproduction blocks the pores with a sticky mass of oil and dead cells. When this happens, the bacteria normally present in skin convert the mass into compounds that irritate and rupture small glands, causing inflammation and unattractive pustules.

Some people are genetically predisposed to acne, but the most common causes are emotional stress and the increased activity of sex hormones, or androgens. These hormones stimulate the oil glands – typically on the face, shoulders, back and chest – and are especially active during puberty. Boys are more prone to acne than girls because they have higher androgen levels, but many girls also suffer, usually in the week before their period.

Research has suggested that many acne sufferers are deficient in zinc. While burgers and chicken nuggets contain plenty of this mineral, healthier sources include shellfish, nuts, lean meat and skinless poultry. Yoghurt and skimmed milk supply zinc in smaller amounts.

Vitamin A, which helps to maintain a healthy skin, is abundant in liver and eggs, while beta carotene, which the body converts to vitamin A, is found in dark green or orange vegetables such as spinach and carrots, and in orange fruits, including apricots and mangoes.

People with acne should ensure that their diet contains plenty of polyunsaturated fats, which have also been claimed to counteract acne. Several of the B vitamins, normally supplied by a well-balanced diet, are believed to prevent blackheads and leave the skin less greasy, while a lack of vitamin C is known to make people more vulnerable to infection. Vitamin E, found in wheatgerm, eggs, and cold-pressed vegetable oils, helps to heal the skin.

Case study

Robert, an extrovert 15-year-old, had become very withdrawn because of his unsightly acne. He felt unattractive and thought he would never find a girlfriend because of his spotty face. His bedroom began to resemble a pharmacy, as he tried every cream on the market. He had even given up his favourite chocolate in the hope of improving his skin. Then a friend told him about a diet high in zinc that might help. Robert was pessimistic but followed the diet carefully. To his surprise, his acne began to clear up. He had finally found something that worked, and as his complexion improved he regained his confidence.

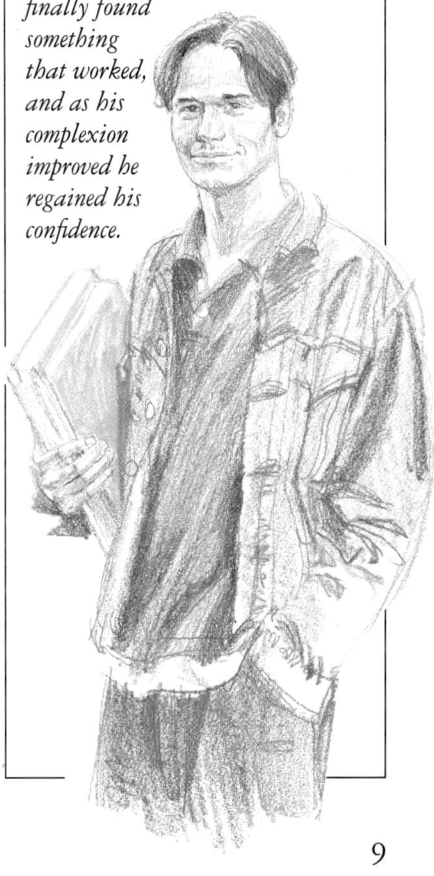

ADDITIVES: USEFUL OR DANGEROUS?

People have been flavouring, preserving and colouring food for centuries. Some additives prevent bacterial contamination; others improve the taste of food. But do any pose a health threat?

BENEFITS

- *Help to prevent food spoiling*
- *Enhance the look and taste of food*
- *Boost nutritional values*

DRAWBACKS

- *Second-rate food can be disguised by colourings and flavourings*
- *A few susceptible people react adversely to additives such as tartrazine and benzoic acid*

Without additives the bread we eat would rapidly become stale, fatty foods would turn rancid and most tinned fruit and vegetables would lose their firmness and colour. Nevertheless, there is evidence that some additives can trigger allergic reactions and even changes in behaviour in susceptible people. There have also been claims that certain additives may be potentially carcinogenic.

Many of the substances added to food during its processing are derived from its natural constituents; others are synthetic chemicals. These can make food safer, improve its quality and facilitate its processing, and may often enhance its taste and appearance.

In Britain, some 3750 substances may be legally added to the food you eat; nearly 3500 of these are flavourings, which need not be specified in anything other than general terms by the manufacturers who use them. Fewer than 10 per cent of all legal additives are synthetic, and natural and synthetic additives represent less than 0.5 per cent of all the food we eat. Medical experts place additives a long way down the list of food hazards, and so far only one person in about 1800 is known to have an adverse reaction to synthetic additives.

Additives serve a range of purposes from colouring food to regulating its acidity. Some perform more than one function. For example, vitamin C (ascorbic acid) is used to prevent tinned fruit and fruit juice from turning brown, as well as to improve the baking quality of wheat, while citric acid is widely used as both a flavouring agent and as an acidity regulator.

Traditional preservatives such as wood smoke, salt and vinegar have always been allowed because of their long history of safe use; but approval of new additives is a lengthy procedure which involves extensive tests.

REPLACING LOST COLOURS

Both processing and storage can result in food losing its natural colour, so manufacturers re-create it – either to make the food look more attractive or because consumers have come to expect foods to be certain colours. Without added colour, tinned peas, for example, would look an unappetising shade of olive green or grey. Critics

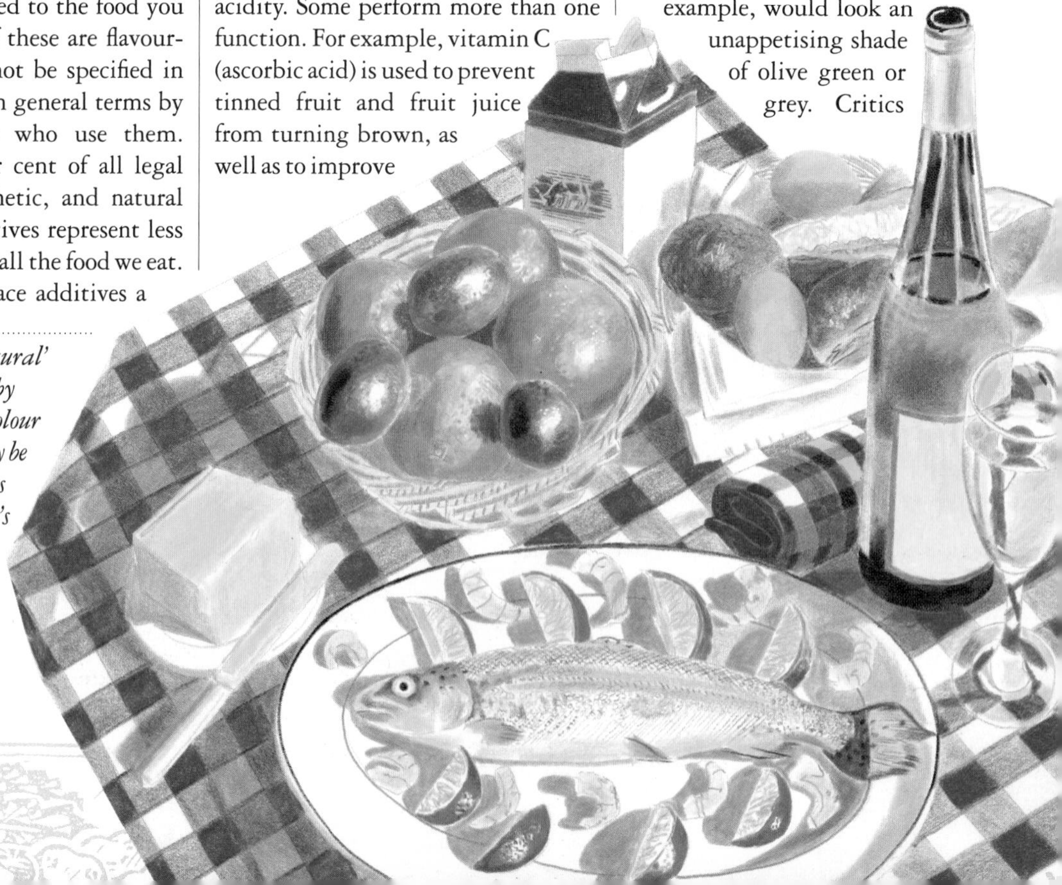

HIDDEN EXTRAS *'Natural' foods may be affected by external factors: the colour of trout or egg yolk may be enhanced by substances in animal feed; butter's yellowness is affected by the beta carotene in grass and feed; wax is used to coat citrus peel; and sulphites destroy surplus yeasts in wine.*

Keeping colourings and preservatives in check

The use of any additive other than an artificial flavouring is controlled by law. All have to be proved to be safe, effective and necessary before they may be used. If an additive has been approved by all the countries in the European Union it is given an E number which must appear on the packaging of foods containing it. Many consumer fears about additives stem from an inability to understand them, but the fact that additives have EU approval should be a reassurance.

ADDITIVES	FOUND IN	WHAT ADDITIVES DO
PRESERVATIVES		
Nitrites and Nitrates (E249-52) Benzoic acid and benzoates (E210-19) Sulphur dioxide and sulphites (E220-28) **Antioxidants** Ascorbic acid/ascorbates (E300-4) BHA/BHT (E320-21)	Processed meats, such as sausages, bacon and ham. Smoked fish. Soft drinks, beer, salad cream. Dried fruit, desiccated coconut, fruit-based pie fillings, relishes. Fruit juices, fruit jams, tinned fruit. Foods where rancidity in fats needs to be prevented, such as crisps, biscuits and fruit pies. 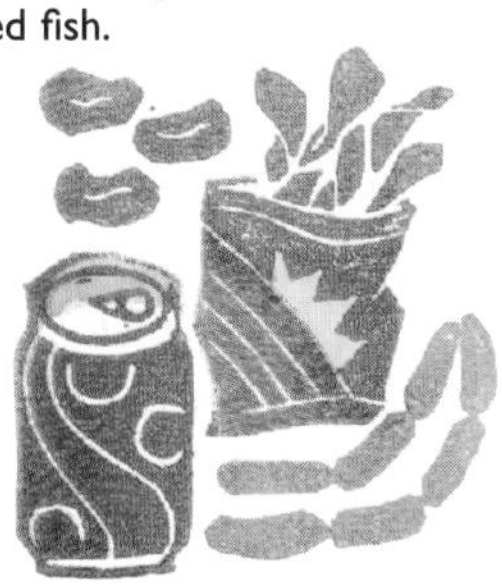	Protect food from fungi and bacteria and extend shelf-life. Nitrites and sulphur dioxide also act as colour preservatives in meats and dried fruits. In rare instances sulphur compounds may trigger allergic reactions, such as asthma. Nitrites convert to potentially carcinogenic nitrosamines. Ascorbic acid prevents fruit juices from turning brown, and fatty foods from becoming rancid. It is also used to improve the baking quality of wheat.
COLOURINGS		
Tartrazine (E102) Quinoline yellow (E104) Sunset yellow (E110) Beetroot red (E162) Caramel (E150)	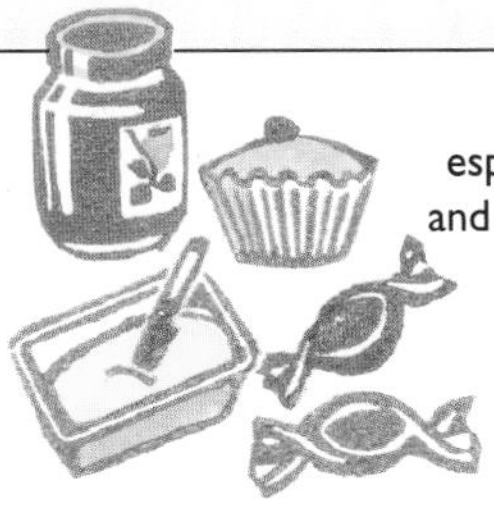 Many processed foods, especially children's sweets and confectionery, squashes and other soft drinks, jams and margarine, biscuits and cakes.	Make food look more appetising and meet expectations of what people expect certain foods to look like. Some may cause allergic reactions such as wheeziness in asthmatics and hyperactivity in sensitive people, especially children.
FLAVOUR ENHANCERS		
Monosodium glutamate, or MSG (621) Monopotassium glutamate (622) Sodium inosinate (631)	Chinese food, gravy powders, stock cubes, packet soups, tinned and processed meats. 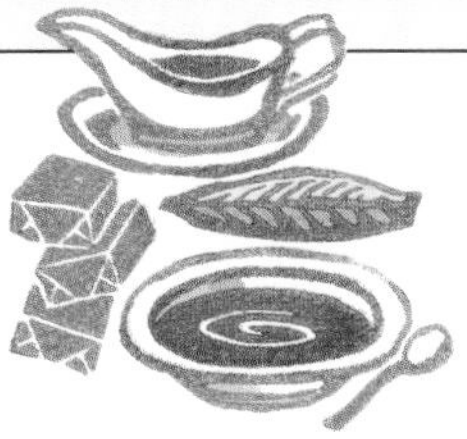	Improve the flavour of many tinned or processed foods. Scientific studies have failed to prove that MSG causes symptoms of food intolerance.
EMULSIFIERS, STABILISERS AND THICKENERS		
Guar gum (E412) Gum arabic (E414) Pectins (E440) Cellulose (E460) Lecithin (E322) Glycerol (E422)	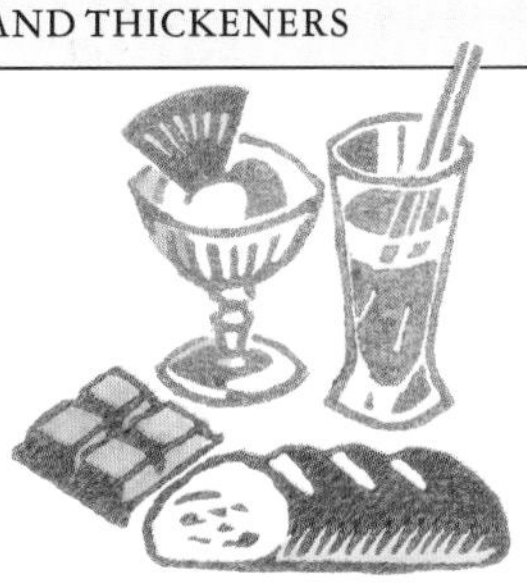 Sauces, soups, breads, biscuits and cakes, frozen desserts, ice cream, margarine and other spreads, jams, chocolate, quick-setting desserts and milk shakes.	Improve texture and consistency, increasing smoothness and creaminess. Stop oil and water from separating out into layers. These additives can make food appear more substantial than it is. Gums can cause flatulence and abdominal pain. Some may trigger adverse reactions in susceptible people.

MONOSODIUM GLUTAMATE

Often used to enhance flavours in processed products, monosodium glutamate (MSG) occurs naturally in many foods, contributing to such strong flavours as those of anchovies and tomatoes.

The purified commercial form is made by fermentation and used like salt in oriental cooking. MSG was blamed for causing Chinese Restaurant Syndrome or CRS. After eating Chinese food, victims experience symptoms of food intolerance, such as swelling of the lips, irritation of the eyes and vomiting. Recent research suggests that substances other than MSG, such as the fermented soya and shellfish sauces widely used in Chinese cookery, are in fact the real culprits.

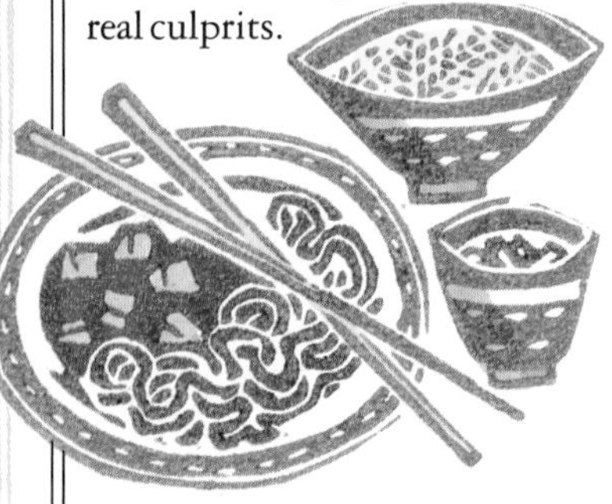

argue that additives disguise the fact that processed foods are not really as nutritious as fresh produce; and that added flavours and colours create a taste for unnaturally strongly flavoured and brightly coloured foods.

In Britain, people like their butter to be bright yellow. This colour comes from beta carotene, which is found in grass and animal feed, and its intensity depends on the cow's ability to metabolise the compound into vitamin A. Jersey cattle, which do not efficiently metabolise beta carotene, produce much yellower butter than Friesians, which do. UK margarine and low-fat spread manufacturers enhance the appearance of their products – which would otherwise appear off-white – and cater for this British preference by adding yellow colouring. Although today's colouring agents are thought to be safe, several of the early coal-tar pigments – now no longer used – were potentially carcinogenic.

Among the more widely used colours, yellow tartrazine (E102) has been found to cause hyperactivity and other adverse reactions in a minority of consumers. Some doctors claim that tartrazine and other nitrogen-based azo dyes – many of which have been banned in Britain – can affect some children's behaviour, making them ill-tempered and disobedient. Others point out that children with adverse reactions to these additives will often react to fruit or other natural foods which contain similar compounds.

Extending the shelf-life

When tinned or even frozen foods deteriorate they can become toxic and, despite increasingly stringent regulations which cover the food processing industry, cases of botulism – a violent form of food poisoning – occasionally occur. Preservatives slow down the deterioration of food – which should be eaten by the 'best before' date. As well as salt, vinegar, alcohol and spices, today's food industry often relies on artificially produced forms of naturally occurring benzoates.

A few people have adverse reactions to benzoic acid; others are allergic to the sulphites and sulphur dioxides which are used to kill the yeasts that cause sugar fermentation in food and alcohol. Inhaling the sulphur dioxide, released when wines are opened and often very pungent, for example, may trigger an asthmatic attack as can drinking wine containing sulphur-based additives. The organic acids, such as acetic acid and propionic acid added to cereal products to prevent the formation of mould, are harmless. Sophisticated modern refrigeration techniques have helped to eliminate the need for some preservatives.

Halting oxidisation

As soon as fruits and fruit juices, or natural fats and oils are exposed to air they react with its oxygen. Many fruits and their juices turn brown, and fats become rancid. To stop these natural processes, producers employ a range of antioxidants. Ascorbic acid (vitamin C) is widely used to stop preserved fruit from losing its colour, and both butylated hydroxytoluene (BHT) and butylated hydroxyanisole (BHA) are used to prevent fats and oils becoming rancid. There has been some controversy over the safety of BHT and BHA as studies of rats which were fed very large amounts of BHT or BHA showed they were more likely to develop cancer. However, other studies have found that rats given smaller amounts lived longer than animals fed on the control diet. Compounds similar to BHT and BHA occur naturally in rosemary and some manufacturers now use extracts of the herb as an alternative antioxidant. Current opinion is that antioxidants are more likely to protect against cancer than cause it.

Replacing lost moisture

Freezing reduces the moisture content of many foods, and to make them palatable again extra water must be added. Polyphosphates help food to retain moisture and are widely used in hams and frozen meats. During the digestive process, polyphosphates are broken down into phosphates which the body absorbs in much the same way that it handles many naturally occurring phosphates. In the past, unscrupulous food manufacturers used polyphosphates to add water to their products, so increasing their weight. The law now demands that the weight or proportion of any added water must be stated on the packaging.

Mixing oil and water

Emulsifiers are used to enable oils to be mixed with water into an emulsion. They are needed to make foods like mayonnaise, margarine and low-fat spreads. Two widely-used emulsifiers, lecithin and monoglycerides, are constituents of such naturally occurring substances as egg yolk and soya.

Non-stick additives

Until recently additives known as mineral hydrocarbons were sprayed on dried fruit to prevent individual pieces sticking together. This was stopped when the government advised manufacturers that these hydrocarbons could gradually accumulate in the body's lymphatic system. However, minuscule quantities are still permitted in chewing gum and the non-edible rinds of some cheeses such as Edam. Because neither chewing gum nor the cheese rinds are meant to be swallowed, they are not regarded as potential health hazards. Mineral hydrocarbons are also still used to stop bread sticking to baking trays.

Sugar substitutes

Substances other than sugar which make food taste sweet fall into two categories: bulk sweeteners and intense sweeteners. Bulk sweeteners – such as sorbitol and xylitol – which have about the same calorific value as sugar, are used in sugar-free sweets, chewing gum and diabetic jam. Intense sweeteners have virtually no calories, so may be used to replace sugar in a calorie-controlled diet. Claims that artificial sweeteners can cause adverse reactions have never been fully substantiated – but many naturopaths still urge people to reduce their intake of SUGAR AND ARTIFICIAL SWEETENERS.

Spot the difference

Many familiar processed foods would be very different were it not for additives. The foods on the top table are complete with all their additives; the lower table suggests how the same foods might look without them.

NOW YOU SEE IT *Here, additives add colour to foods; they also improve its texture and slow down deterioration.*

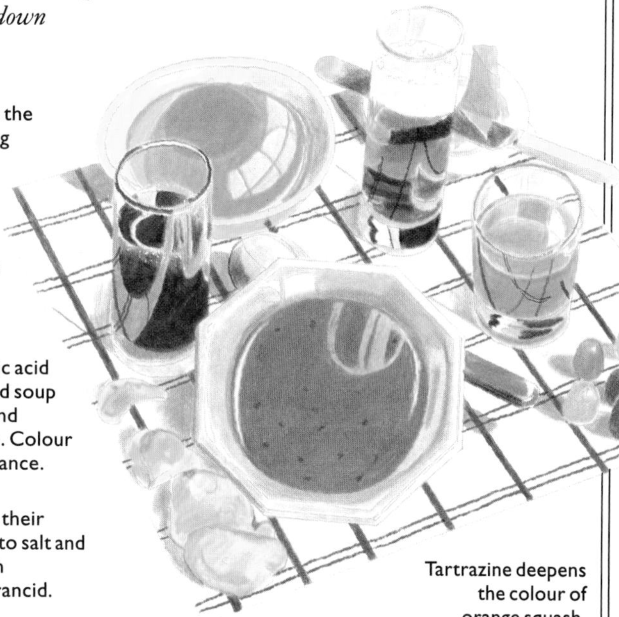
Foam froths on a glass of lager thanks to a 'foam stabiliser'.
Gelatine which sets the jelly, is a quick-acting stabiliser.
Caramel or other colourings give cola drinks their distinctive colour.
Nitrates and benzoic acid help to protect dried soup mix from bacteria and prolong its shelf-life. Colour enhances its appearance.
Potato crisps retain their crunchiness thanks to salt and the stabilisers which prevent fat turning rancid.
Tartrazine deepens the colour of orange squash.

NOW YOU DON'T *Fresh foods need few, if any, additives. But many packaged foods would taste bland and lack any visual appeal without them.*

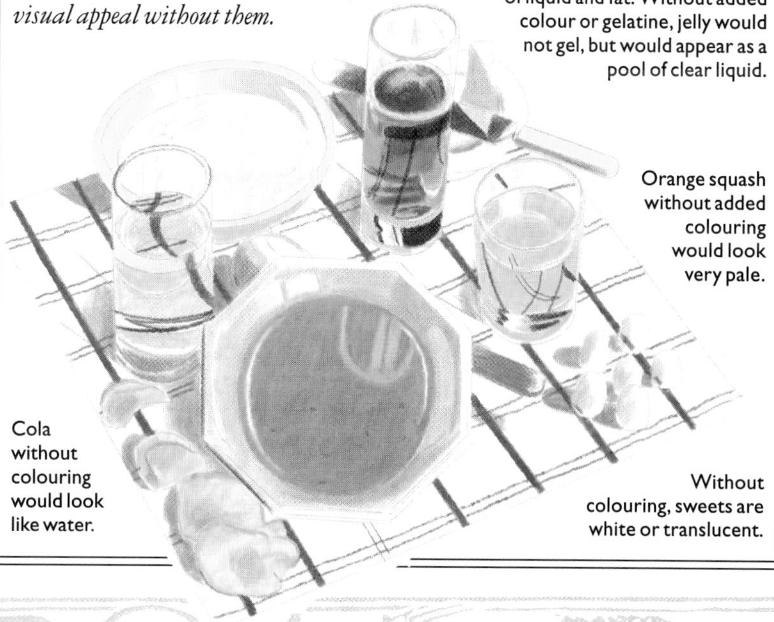
Without colouring or emulsifiers, margarine would be a greyish mix of liquid and fat. Without added colour or gelatine, jelly would not gel, but would appear as a pool of clear liquid.
Orange squash without added colouring would look very pale.
Cola without colouring would look like water.
Without colouring, sweets are white or translucent.

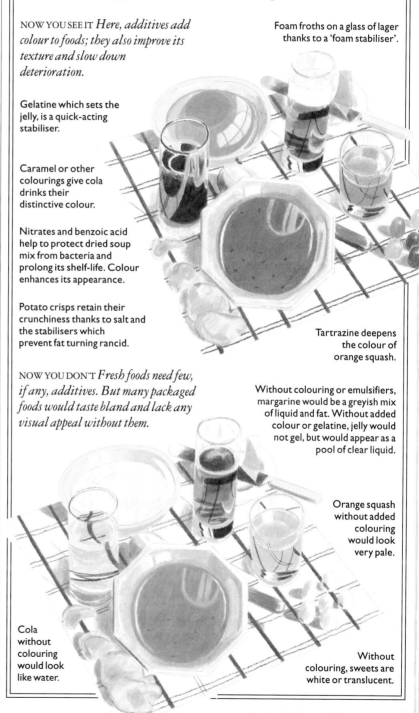

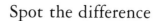

AGGRESSION AND DELINQUENCY

EAT PLENTY OF

- *Wholegrain foods, fruit and vegetables*

CUT DOWN ON

- *White bread, cakes, biscuits and sugar*
- *Tea and coffee*

AVOID

- *Alcohol*

Over the past 20 years, many scientific studies have linked certain elements in food or a lack of key nutrients with antisocial behaviour. Diets high in sugar, refined foods, additives and colourings, for instance, have been cited as possible triggers for aggression, hyperactivity and delinquency.

A series of studies carried out in American detention centres and institutions in the early 1980s reported significant reductions in antisocial behaviour among juvenile prisoners who were fed experimental diets that were low in refined sugar. In the largest study, which involved 3000 young offenders, most snacks and refined foods were also excluded.

One theory is that a diet high in refined foods may be low in chromium. When sugar is refined trace amounts of chromium that are normally present are lost during processing. Chromium is needed to metabolise sugar; without it the body's insulin is less effective at controlling the blood's glucose levels. There may be spells of hypoglycaemia, which may trigger aggressive behaviour as the brain receives less than its usual quota of glucose.

On the other hand, it has been suggested that boosting sugar intake may have a calming effect and can promote sleep in some people. However, a diet that is high in sugar and refined foods can be lacking in important nutrients. Studies have shown, for example, that people with low intakes of thiamin, as a result of following an unbalanced diet, were highly aggressive, impulsive and sensitive to criticism. And in a series of experimental controlled studies among children in hospital, deviant behaviour was closely linked to the absence of well-balanced meals. Excessive amounts of tea, coffee or alcohol can also trigger aggression.

Case study

Alan, a successful young marketing manager, was renowned for his entertaining and informative presentations. Fellow delegates were bemused, however, when one evening, after an important conference, he became aggressive and quite threatening. Over the next few weeks the problem became worse, and when he finally lashed out at a colleague and broke his nose, he decided that the time had come to seek medical help.
The doctor suggested that drinking alcohol suppressed Alan's natural inhibitions, and could radically change his character.
When he was confronted with the fact that even a small amount of alcohol caused him to become aggressive, Alan realised the effect that drinking was having on his career. With exemplary self-discipline, he has now given up alcohol, and his career is flourishing.

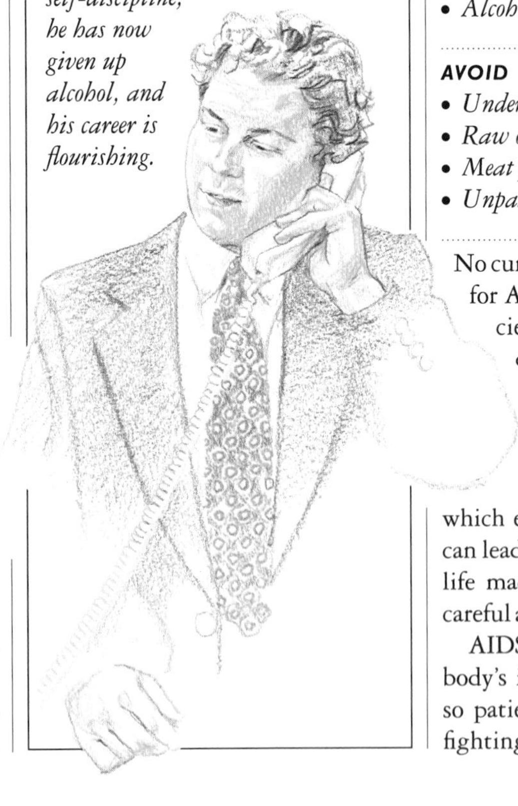

AIDS

EAT PLENTY OF

- *Whole grains*
- *Fruit and vegetables*
- *Nuts and oily fish*
- *Meat, liver and eggs*
- *Pasteurised dairy products*

CUT DOWN ON

- *Tea, coffee and colas*
- *Alcohol*

AVOID

- *Undercooked and unwashed foods*
- *Raw or lightly cooked eggs*
- *Meat pâtés*
- *Unpasteurised dairy products*

No cure or vaccine has yet been found for AIDS (Acquired Immune Deficiency Syndrome), although the quality of life of its sufferers may be improved by the right choice of foods. Similarly, people with HIV (Human Immunodeficiency Virus) which eventually, but not inevitably, can lead to full-blown AIDS, may find life made more bearable if they pay careful attention to what they eat.

AIDS is a disease in which the body's immune system breaks down, so patients are no longer efficient at fighting disease. Signs of the onset of

AIDS are weight loss and general debility. There may also be swollen glands in the groin, neck and armpits; cold sores and other skin disorders; and thrush. As the disease progresses patients may suffer from pneumonia, malnutrition and various cancers. They also run a far greater risk of contracting bacterial infections from food, such as listeriosis from soft-rinded cheese or pâté. Shellfish are also potential sources of infection.

In the later stages, AIDS patients often suffer from serious, potentially irreversible malnutrition. Researchers in Britain and the USA are now focusing increasingly on sound nutrition at the onset of the disease to build up body weight and boost the immune system. The foods to choose are therefore those that do just that; while the foods to avoid are those that could put further strain on an immune system that is already at a low ebb.

Foods to choose

Because treatment involves the use of drugs which may affect – or be affected by – nutrients, people with AIDS or those diagnosed as being HIV-positive should seek the advice of a qualified dietician who will work with medical experts to assess their needs.

Deficiencies in certain nutrients – notably vitamins A, B_6, B_{12} and zinc – are not only known to impair immune function but are often apparent as part of an HIV-positive diagnosis. A diet which typically includes fish, liver, full-fat milk and other dairy products will boost the intake of all of these nutrients. Vitamin B_{12} is found in animal produce and fortified foods, and wholegrain bread and nuts provide both vitamin B_6 and zinc.

Progressive wasting is not an inevitable consequence of AIDS: studies show that weight loss in advanced stages of the disease is largely the result of loss of muscle mass. However, evidence suggests that muscle may in fact help to protect against the onset of AIDS symptoms. Thus, a diet which builds lean, rather than fat tissue, combined with moderate exercise, may be beneficial to HIV sufferers. This means having a diet which is as nutritious as possible and also provides adequate calories. Fats should come mainly from vegetable oils and dairy produce, to ensure adequate supplies of vitamins A, D, E and K.

Wholemeal bread and pasta, rice, barley, potatoes and corn will help to supply the complex carbohydrates vital for energy. Lean meat is a valuable source of protein, but patients should also obtain plenty of protein from dairy produce, nuts and combinations of grains and pulses.

Fighting the virus

Vitamins and minerals are thought to be among the main allies in the fight against the HIV virus. Vitamins B_6, B_{12}, pantothenic acid and folate are vital to immune functions, as is vitamin A (plentiful in liver, egg yolk and many dairy products).

The ANTIOXIDANTS beta carotene (found in dark green leafy vegetables and in orange fruit and vegetables), vitamin C (guavas and citrus fruits are rich sources) and vitamin E (found in cold-pressed oils, nuts and avocados), are important as scavengers of FREE RADICALS. The minerals zinc and iron and the trace element selenium are also thought to be important in the battle against HIV. Some researchers believe selenium may play a key role in delaying the progress of HIV infection.

Until recently, the selenium deficiency which had been noted widely among AIDS sufferers was attributed to the effect of wasting and an increasing inability to digest food. However, there is now some speculation that selenium depletion may promote development to full-blown AIDS.

Rekindling a lost appetite

A poor appetite and nausea are often side effects of AIDS, yet three good meals a day – with plenty of snacks between meals – will help to build up the patient's strength. However, if people with AIDS cannot face three large meals, they should try:
- Eating six smaller meals.
- Taking a high-calorie drink half-an-hour after eating.
- Snacking on nuts and seeds – such as pumpkin seeds – for their calories, vitamins and minerals.

When suffering from nausea, patients should avoid:
- Greasy or spicy foods.
- Acidic drinks.
- Their favourite foods, lest by associating their taste with illness enthusiasm for them is lost.

Many people who are HIV positive or have AIDS turn to a regime of MACROBIOTIC foods. However, such diets may do more harm than good as they tend to be bulky and promote weight loss because they contain too few calories. Since a diminished appetite is part of the nature of the illness, patients are likely to find it hard to eat enough macrobiotic foods. It has been suggested that those who have had AIDS for a long time and who do well on a macrobiotic diet may owe their continuing health to selenium which they get from whole grains, wheatgerm or bran. Selenium may be taken in supplement form, but dietary sources are preferable to supplements; the daily intake from all sources should not exceed 450mcg.

Anyone in the final stages of the illness should be encouraged to eat whatever they like. Eating should never be stressful and any food is better than none at all.

ALCOHOL: MERIT IN MODERATION

The slight benefits to our health offered by moderate drinking are often outweighed by the risk of illness and disease which can follow even small, but frequent excesses.

Today, there is renewed acceptance that alcoholic drinks may have a role in nutrition and health – so long as they are taken in moderation. However, heavy drinking and alcoholism remain major causes of both illness and death.

Ethyl alcohol (ethanol), the main active ingredient of alcoholic drinks, is made by yeast fermentation of starch or sugar. Other substances formed in this process give drinks their particular tastes and aromas. It is these substances, known as congeners, that are responsible for many of the symptoms of a hangover. For example, it is the polyphenols in red wines – and not the alcohol – which give some people migraines. Nevertheless, the main health hazard in beer or any other alcoholic drink is the alcohol itself. Claims that organic wines are much better for you usually have little, if any, scientific foundation.

BENEFITS
- *Moderate consumption is associated with decreased risk of coronary heart disease in older men and women*
- *Can enhance a happy mood*

DRAWBACKS
- *Can deepen an unhappy mood and lead to aggression*
- *Harmful during pregnancy*
- *Harmful if mixed with certain medicines or drugs*
- *May result in a hangover*
- *High intakes linked with an increased risk of certain cancers*
- *Binges may precipitate gout, pancreatitis or a heart attack*
- *Persistent alcohol abuse may cause permanent liver damage*

Red wine may have some medicinal benefits – though not, as is commonly supposed, as an aid in reducing blood cholesterol. Recent research has established that three or four glasses of red wine a day may sustain high levels of blood cholesterol – one of the causes of atherosclerosis. Conversely, drinking three glasses of red wine a day has been claimed to increase the levels of antioxidants in the blood, which may help to prevent the onset of atherosclerosis. Red wine also decreases the tendency for blood to clot.

Alcohol is primarily a source of 'empty' calories, although some drinks do provide micronutrients – particularly WINE and some beers, which contain some minerals and B vitamins. However, because a high alcohol intake makes people feel full, there is a risk that it may displace other more nutritious foods from the diet.

Although it is loaded with calories that supply almost instant energy to the bloodstream, alcohol lacks most essential nutrients and vitamins. Thus people who consistently drink heavily are at risk from nutritional deficiencies. Among the nutrients that heavy drinkers may lack are thiamin, vitamin B, riboflavin, folate, niacin, calcium, magnesium and zinc – although a great deal will depend on the diet of the person concerned and other factors such as their genetic disposition. Heavy drinking also attacks the liver, impairing its ability to store

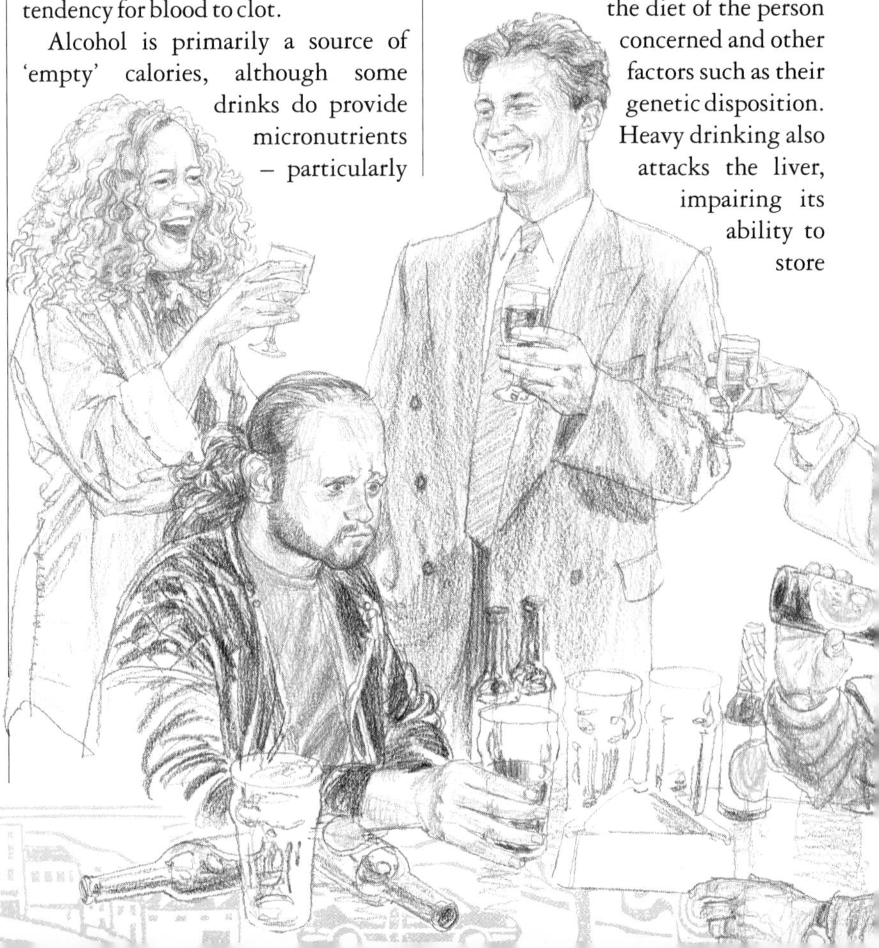

When to call 'time' on your drinking

Use this chart to help you to calculate how many alcoholic drinks you can consume safely each week. A unit of alcohol is the equivalent of a small glass of wine, half a pint of beer or a single whisky or gin. The British Medical Association recommends a limit of 21 units for men and 14 units for women who are not pregnant, spread evenly over a week. However, individuals' tolerance to alcohol varies. 'Saving up' your units and binging is an unhealthy way to drink.

ITEM	ALCOHOL VOLUME	UNITS	MAXIMUM WEEKLY CONSUMPTION		CALORIES
			MEN	WOMEN	
SPIRITS					
Standard bottle (750ml) Single pub measure (25ml)	40%	30 1	⅔ bottle 21 units	½ bottle 14 units	50 per measure
SHERRY OR PORT					
Standard bottle (750ml) Single pub measure (50ml)	20%	15 1	1½ bottles 21 units	1 bottle 14 units	75 per measure
WINE					
Standard bottle (750ml) Single pub glass (125ml)	8-14%	6-10½ 1-2	2-3½ bottles 12-21 units	1⅓-2⅓ bottles 8-14 units	85 per glass Sweet white 100 per glass
ORDINARY BEER, LAGER OR CIDER					
Large can (440ml) Small can (275ml) 1 pint	3.5%	1½ 1 2	14 large cans 21 small cans 10½ pints	9 large cans 14 small cans 7 pints	140 per large can 90 per small can 180 per pint Sweet cider 220 per pint
STRONG BEER OR LAGER					
Large can (440ml) Small can (275ml) 1 pint	7%	3 2 4	7 large cans 10 small cans 5 pints	4½ large cans 7 small cans 3½ pints	280 per large can 170 per small can 350 per pint

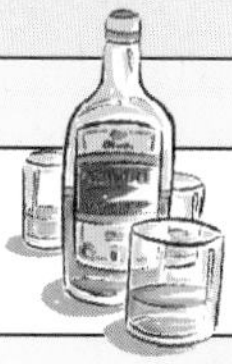
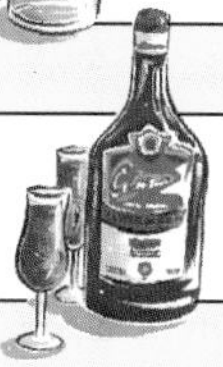
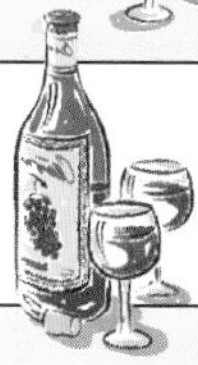
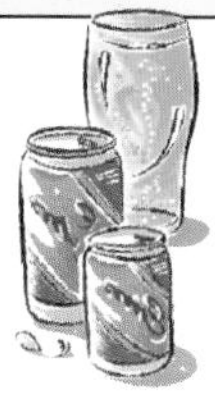
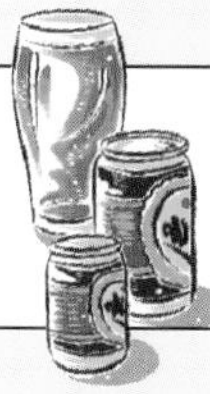

COMPARISON OF UNIT MEASURES

ONE UNIT = **½ pint of beer** = **small glass of wine** = **small glass of sherry** = **small glass of spirits**

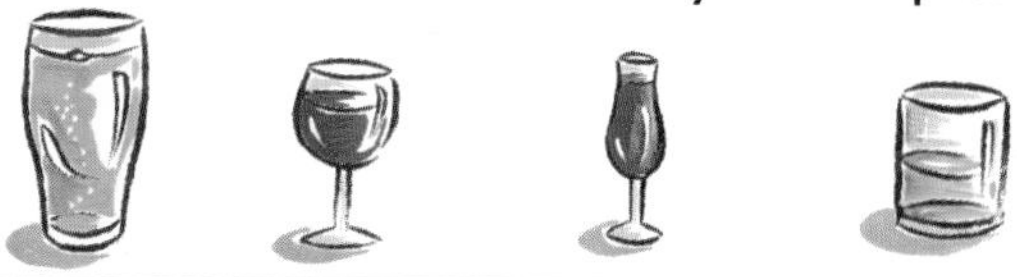

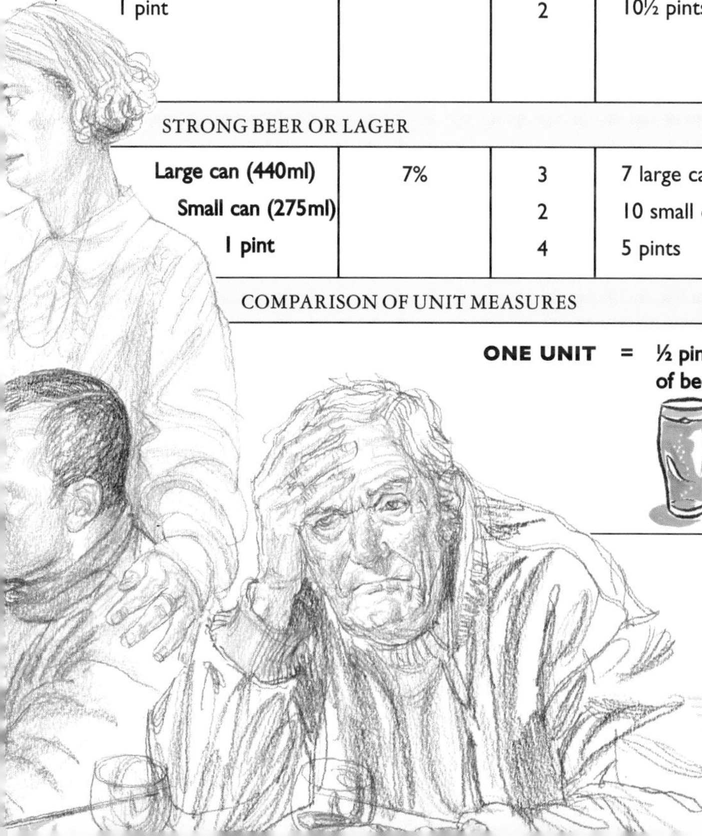

HIGH AND LOW SPIRITS *While some people use alcohol to get themselves into a party spirit, drinking too much can all too easily cause unpleasant changes in mood; from happy to depressed, and from easy-going to aggressive.*

fat-soluble vitamins and to metabolise protein. All alcohol can contribute to obesity, but stouts and beers are particular culprits – hence the typical beer drinker's paunch. Beer actually contains fewer calories than wine or spirits – a half pint of bitter contains less than half the calories in an equivalent volume of wine – but because it is often consumed in larger amounts it can contribute more to the total calorie intake. Stout contains more than twice the calories of most beers.

Spreading your drinking throughout the week puts less of a strain on your liver than spasmodic concentrated bouts of drinking. However, even for moderate drinkers, it is advisable to avoid alcohol altogether for a day or two each week, to let your body cleanse itself. Infrequent 'binge drinking' can also bring on attacks of gout or pancreatitis. Worse still, it can cause abnormalities in heart rhythms, leading – days, or even weeks, later – to alcohol-induced cardiac failure.

When one is too much

Women metabolise alcohol more slowly than men because they tend to have smaller livers and more body fat. There are also racial differences in the rates at which people's enzymes break down alcohol; for example, Oriental people are usually less tolerant of alcohol than Caucasians.

For everyone, there are times when even one or two drinks can be too much – for instance, if you are operating machinery, taking certain drugs, or if you are pregnant.

Heavy daily alcohol consumption of six units or more during pregnancy can damage the foetus, cause birth defects and give rise to the foetal alcohol syndrome, when the baby typically has a low birth weight, learning disabilities, and a characteristically flattened face and cleft palate. Women intending to become pregnant should avoid alcohol altogether, but especially until the twelfth week of pregnancy is over. After that, the occasional alcoholic drink is not considered to be a substantial risk.

DID YOU KNOW?

- That doctors who have questioned patients about their drinking habits believe that most people underestimate their consumption by up to 50 per cent.
- That driving with a hangover may be as dangerous as drinking and driving, because competence may be reduced by as much as 20 per cent, even though the alcohol has left the bloodstream.
- That the hops which give beer its distinctive bitterness and aroma come from a vine which is a relative of cannabis.
- That gin originated as a medicine in Holland. Its name comes from the Dutch word for juniper – *jenever* – which was originally added to the rye distillate for its diuretic properties.

Cause and effect

Absorption of alcohol normally occurs between 15 and 90 minutes after drinking. Alcohol drunk on an empty stomach is absorbed and diffuses more rapidly into all body tissues than when it is taken on a full stomach or with a meal, which can act in the same way as blotting paper and slow down its absorption. Drinks containing 20-30 per cent alcohol by volume are absorbed most quickly; higher concentrations of alcohol irritate the stomach and slow down the rate of absorption. However, all alcohol is absorbed more quickly if taken with a fizzy drink, such as tonic or soda water. These actually 'stir up' the alcohol molecules and allow more of them to come in contact with the gastric cells. This is true of spritzers where the lemonade or fizzy water added to wine speeds up the absorption of alcohol.

Once alcohol has been dissolved in the blood some of it is released into air in the lungs – a physical process on which the Breathalyser test is based. But very little alcohol is actually excreted this way. Most is broken down by the liver; and it is the continual strain placed on the liver's capacity by years of heavy drinking that can lead to cirrhosis.

It takes an hour for the liver to break down each unit of alcohol, so that if you drink six pints of beer or two bottles of wine, even after a night's sleep of eight hours or more, enough alcohol could remain in your bloodstream to be above the legal limit for driving.

People's reactions to alcohol vary, but generally after one or two drinks the heart rate quickens and there is an increased secretion of gastric juices. Intellectual processes function normally, but reactions involving rapid decision making are impaired.

With heavier drinking, coordination becomes markedly worse and the secretion of several hormones is inhibited, leading to dehydration, slurred speech, clumsy movements and a reduced sensitivity to pain. The best safeguard against hangovers – which result from this dehydration and alcohol's congeners – is to drink plenty of water before going to bed.

A regular daily intake of eight or more units by men, or six units by women, leads inexorably to long-term damage. One in five of all heavy drinkers develops cirrhosis of the liver, and about one in five cirrhosis victims dies of liver cancer.

Regular drinking may increase the risk of cancer of the mouth, throat, oesophagus, stomach and liver, and it may also be a factor in the development of cancers of the breast and colon.

ALCOHOLISM

Many alcoholics suffer from malnutrition. The vast majority of their calories come from drink, and their mental state often encourages nutritional neglect. Alcoholism is an addictive illness which some researchers suggest has genetic roots.

Only about five in every hundred heavy drinkers suffer from alcoholism; but unlike other heavy drinkers who can control their intake, alcoholics drink compulsively. A single glass can set them on a binge. However, the effects of prolonged alcohol misuse are identical for both types of drinker. Consuming excessive alcohol decreases the brain's sensitivity to its effect, so intake is increased as more and more is needed to achieve a temporary 'lift'.

Prolonged misuse can lead to socially-destructive personality changes, while both the alcoholic and the heavy drinker tend to disregard their bodies' food requirements.

A poor diet exacerbates the problems caused by alcohol. The resultant low levels of vitamin B_{12} and thiamin, among other micronutrients, cause nerve damage, while severe thiamin deficiency results in disorientation, poor memory and confabulation – inventions to fill the memory gaps. Prolonged abuse of alcohol enlarges the liver and makes it fatty, and one in five of all heavy drinkers develops CIRRHOSIS.

Alcoholic cirrhosis is the most common cause of liver cancer and fatal liver failure. It is most likely to develop when a drinker's diet is low in protein and essential nutrients (particularly fatty acids, vitamins A, C and E, thiamin and zinc) needed to break down alcohol and transport fat out of the liver. Meat, fish and low-fat cheese are all good sources of protein and of zinc, while chicken, lamb's or calves' liver eaten once a week provide vitamin A, thiamin and some vitamin C. Vegetable oils, eggs and wholemeal bread help to replace vitamin E.

Fats are poorly tolerated when the liver is inflamed, so follow a low-fat diet that is high in carbohydrates. Cirrhosis impairs the liver's capacity to store vitamin A and to metabolise some nutrients.

THE SLIPPERY SLOPE

- Drinking to feel at ease, to increase confidence or to try and forget worries.
- Gradually needing more drinks to achieve the same effect.
- Forgetfulness over things that have been done or said when drunk.
- Surreptitious drinking.
- Driving after drinking.
- Frequent hangovers, along with shakes that are 'cured' by another drink – known as a hair of the dog.
- Regularly neglecting meals in favour of alcohol.
- Preferring to drink alone.
- Mood swings that start to cause problems at home and at work.
- Persistent shakes, hallucinations and night sweats.
- Unable to give up, even though warned by a doctor that drinking may prove fatal.

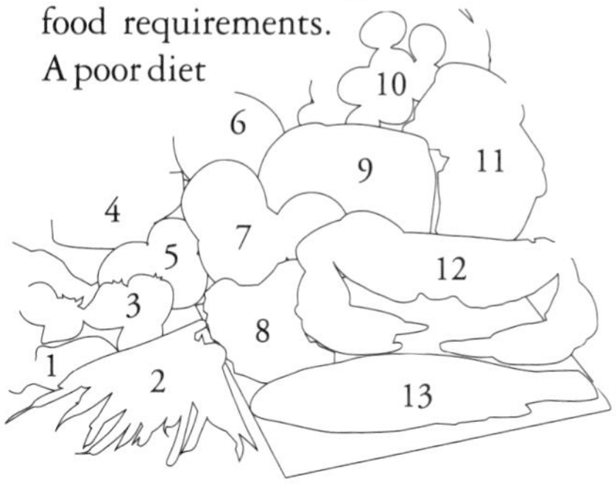

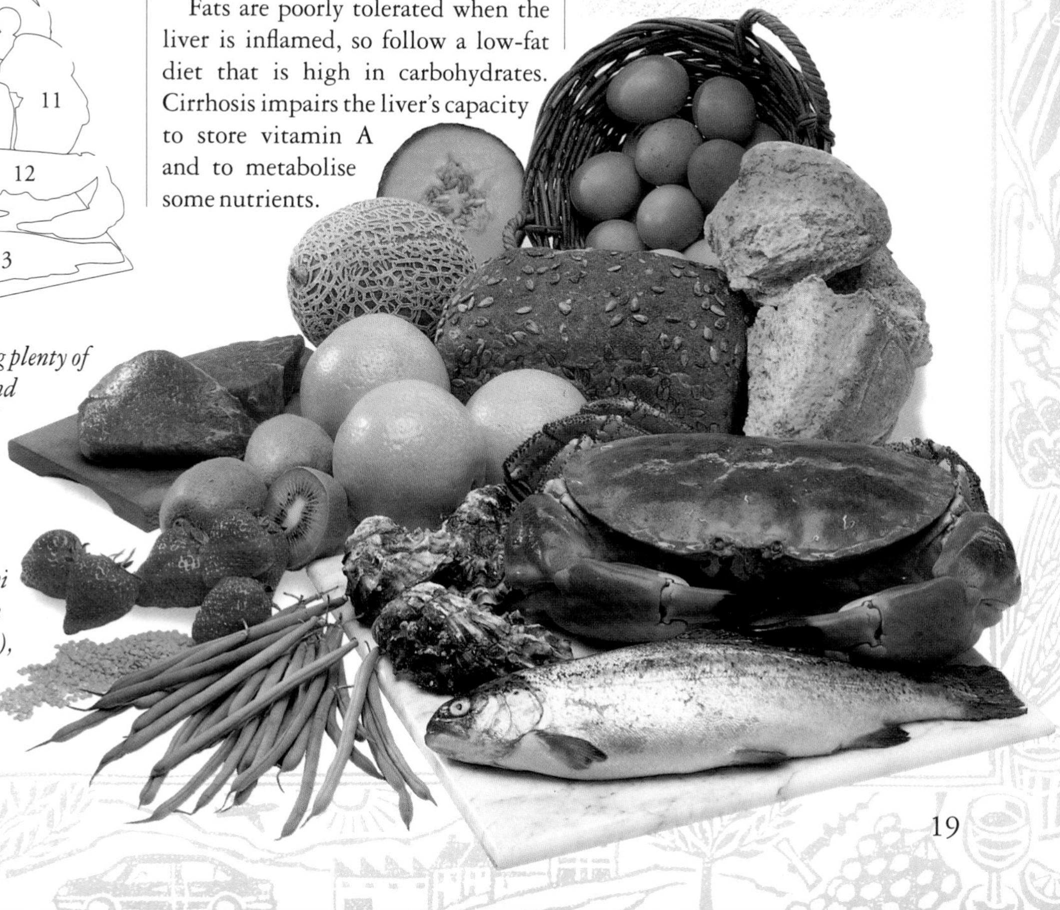

REDUCING THE RISK *Eating plenty of fruit, vegetables, seafood and wholemeal bread as part of a balanced diet will help to guard against cirrhosis. Right: lentils (1), green beans (2), strawberries (3), lean red meat (4), kiwi fruit (5), cantaloupe melon (6), oranges (7), oysters (8), wholemeal bread (9, 11), eggs (10), crab (12), trout (13).*

ALLERGIES

See page 24

ALZHEIMER'S DISEASE

EAT PLENTY OF

- *Potatoes, spinach, offal, soya beans, and green leafy vegetables*

CUT DOWN ON

- *Antacid indigestion tablets*

AVOID

- *Cooking acidic foods, such as some fruits, in aluminium pans*
- *Food additive E541*
- *Too much alcohol*

Tests such as CT (computerised tomography) or other scans are essential in distinguishing Alzheimer's from other diseases of the brain. Alzheimer's disease is a steadily progressive type of dementia, in which nerve cells degenerate and the brain shows signs of wasting.

While it can strike in middle age, Alzheimer's is most often a disease of the elderly. It is characterised by increasing confusion, memory loss, apathy and, often in its initial stages, by deep depression.

What begins as a subtle impairment of mental functions – especially short-term memory – can worsen over an unpredictable period to the stage where the sufferer becomes incapable of self-care. He or she may fail to recognise familiar faces or surroundings, and may forget recent events while vividly recalling those of long ago.

ADVICE FOR HELPERS

For those responsible for the sufferer's care (often elderly partners, or sons and daughters), this is a particularly cruel and frustrating disease that effectively robs them of the person they knew. Often, the carer can only aim to maintain a good quality of life and try to ensure a highly nutritious diet for sufferers. Because the disease saps the appetite and undermines normal self-care, people with the disease often risk nutritional deficiencies. Studies have observed improvements with supplements of vitamins B_{12}, C, D and E, beta carotene and folic acid. There is also some evidence to suggest that low levels of zinc and selenium tend to occur with Alzheimer's disease.

Minor successes have been achieved in treating Alzheimer's patients with supplements of the coenzyme Q10, which has been shown to confer many health benefits on the elderly. So it is worth including foods such as offal, spinach, alfalfa, potatoes, yams and soya beans which are rich in this compound. Remember, too, that as the disease takes greater hold the sufferer may have problems handling cutlery. Where possible, plan meals that can be eaten with a minimum of physical effort and coordination.

POSSIBLE CAUSES

The causes of Alzheimer's are not yet fully understood. Some US researchers believe that genetic factors are only partly responsible.

For more than a decade, scientists have implicated aluminium in a variety of ways; most notably it has been associated with dementia. Although a link has yet to be conclusively proved, aluminium has been found in patches of cell damage, or 'plaques', in the brains of people with Alzheimer's, suggesting that it may have played a part in the development of the disease. It would seem sensible, therefore, to avoid foods and cooking methods that may lead to the ingestion of high levels of this mineral. Do not use aluminium pans for cooking acidic foods such as rhubarb, chutneys, marmalade or tomatoes, as their high acid levels may increase the amount of aluminium these foods take up.

Silicon, in the form of silicic acid, prevents the body from absorbing aluminium. Sources of silicon include kelp and alfalfa, cabbage, lettuce, onions, dark green vegetables and milk. A type of silicon generated from barley during brewing is found in beer, so a pint every day or two may prove to be helpful. However, excessive alcohol intake should be avoided.

ADDITIVES AND ANTACIDS

Read the labels on packet cakes and biscuits. The additive E541, used as a raising agent, is sodium aluminium phosphate, which should be avoided. Nor should certain antacid remedies, high in aluminium hydroxide, be used to treat indigestion as a matter of course; the remedies may offer temporary relief, but a change in dietary habits will often cure the problem.

Foods to fight Alzheimer's

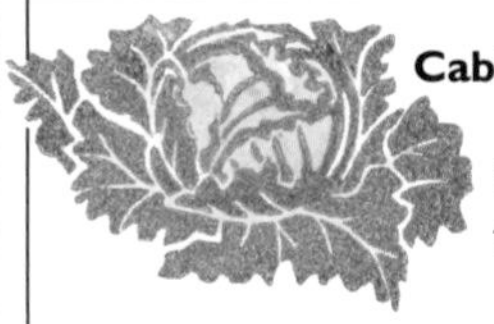

Cabbage Provides silicon which interferes with the absorption of aluminium.

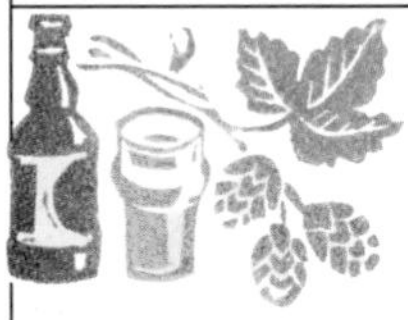

Beer Another source of silicon – the occasional pint may be actively beneficial.

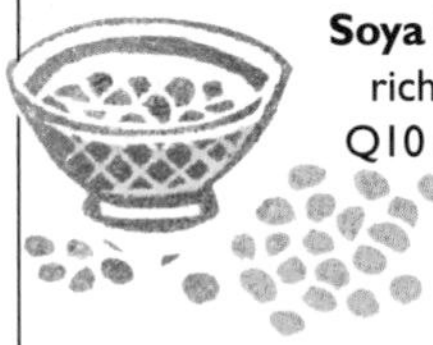

Soya beans These are rich in the coenzyme Q10 as well as being a source of fibre, protein, and carbohydrate.

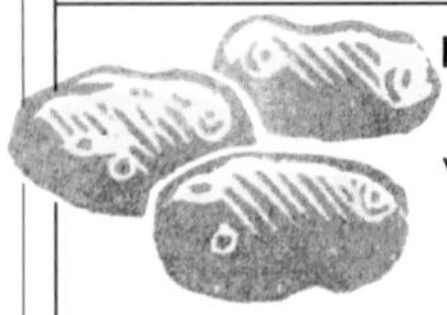

Potatoes Another source of Q10, which also supplies cheap, nutritious carbohydrate.

ANAEMIA

EAT PLENTY OF

- *Meat, poultry and liver*
- *Fortified breakfast cereals*
- *Fresh green vegetables*

AVOID

- *Drinking tea with meals*

When the level of haemoglobin – the vital protein molecule which carries oxygen in the bloodstream – is lowered, or the number of red blood cells falls below normal levels, the supply of oxygen to the tissues is reduced. The anaemia which results may be mild – manifesting itself as tiredness and general weakness – or severe, when symptoms of lethargy are more marked and accompanied by paleness, heart PALPITATIONS, breathlessness, giddiness, swollen feet and leg pains.

THE IMPORTANCE OF DIET

Iron deficiency is the most common cause of anaemia, especially among adolescent girls and women during their reproductive years. Toddlers are also at risk because milk-based diets are often low in iron.

A diet with insufficient red meat and offal, poultry, fish and green vegetables will spark anaemia. Liver is the richest source of iron, but it should be avoided in pregnancy because of the risk of excess vitamin A intake which could result in birth defects. Because iron is not easily absorbed by the body, deficiency can still occur even when a diet is rich in the mineral. Iron absorption can be inhibited by the tannin in tea, so avoid drinking tea with meals. The phytic acid which is present in wheat bran and brown rice can also inhibit iron absorption.

While the body takes in iron more easily from animal sources, such as meat and fish, than from leafy greens, grains and pulses and other plant foods, its absorption from those sources can be improved if meals are accompanied by a source of vitamin C, such as a tomato salad or orange juice taken with the meal. Fortified breakfast cereals are a useful source of iron.

FOUR TYPES OF ANAEMIA

Anaemia can occur for many reasons. A poor diet or loss of blood – through heavy periods or internal bleeding from ulcers or cancer – can cause iron-deficiency anaemia; and when red blood cells break down faster than they can be replaced, such as in sickle-cell disease, the condition is described as haemolytic anaemia. Anaemia may also be due to diseases such as LEUKAEMIA when there is impaired production of new red blood cells; while pernicious anaemia is caused by an inability to absorb vitamin B_{12}.

In some instances, missing haemoglobin can be replaced through careful eating which helps to build up the red blood cells to healthy levels. However, once anaemia has taken hold, supplements of iron and vitamins offer the most effective treatment. Pernicious anaemia is treated by injections of vitamin B_{12}, given every three months.

WOMEN AT RISK

Anaemia resulting from lack of folate or vitamin B_{12} is less common than iron deficiency anaemia. However, vegetarians – and particularly vegans – risk deficiency of vitamin B_{12}, which is not found in foods of plant origin, while pregnant women are at risk of folate deficiency. Once any form of anaemia has been identified, medically supervised supplementation – the provision of extra iron and folate (usually in tablet form), or injections of vitamin B_{12} in the case of pernicious anaemia – is the most effective form of treatment. Eating a well-balanced diet should help to prevent a recurrence.

Case study

Roy, a retired librarian, was experiencing abnormal tiredness. After several weeks he decided to consult his doctor. Roy was given a medical examination and referred for a full blood count, which revealed a low haemoglobin level, suggesting iron-deficiency anaemia. He was prescribed iron tablets, and, over the next two to three months, his haemoglobin levels gradually returned to normal. The district nurse, who visited Roy regularly to take blood for checks, realised that he was not looking after himself properly, and was essentially living on a diet of bread and butter with plenty of tea. Roy explained that he found it difficult to prepare meals, and was worried about the cost. The nurse alerted social services, who have advised Roy about his finances and organised meals-on-wheels. He now eats a varied diet, containing adequate iron, and no longer needs to take iron pills.

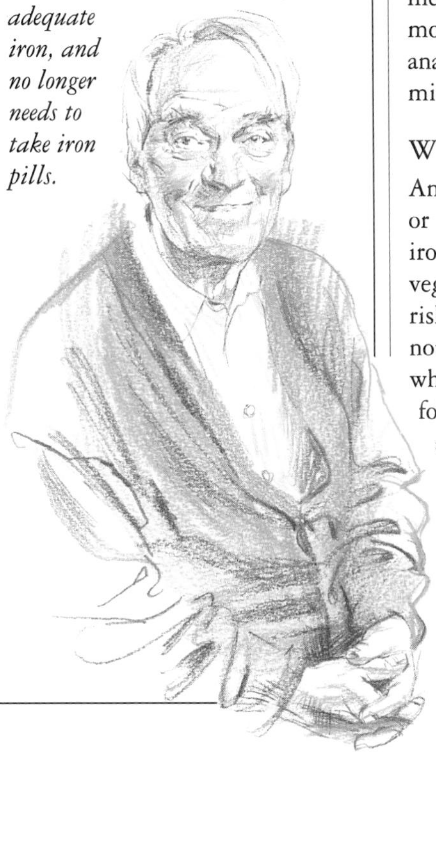

ANOREXIA NERVOSA

Though anorexia nervosa mainly affects teenage girls and young women, about one in ten of all anorexics are boys and young men. This complex psychiatric disorder manifests itself as an obsession to limit food intake and is often spurred by a sense of low self-esteem. An anorexic tries to rise above the appetites and problems of everyday life by pursuing a course of food deprivation – to the point of starvation.

Early signs of anorexia, such as an abnormal concern with weight, growing pickiness at mealtimes and obsessive exercising, often occur before the disorder takes hold. Promoting a balanced diet during puberty is particularly important. The diet should supply plenty of protein, fruit and vegetables and starchy foods such as potatoes and bread. It should also be low in refined starch, sugar and fats, and snacks should not replace main meals.

Anorexics equate extreme slimness with beauty and think that they are overweight when, in fact, they may be dangerously undernourished. When they do eat, they often make themselves vomit or use laxatives to purge the cause of their imagined ugliness.

As dieting becomes increasingly obsessive, the sufferer eats fewer vitamin and mineral-rich foods. A lack of zinc is particularly serious, as it further erodes the appetite and the sense of taste, leading to a 'starvation spiral'. Treatment usually involves careful nutrition and pyschotherapy or counselling; admission to hospital will be necessary for the majority of patients.

The sufferer needs to be brought back into touch with the mechanism of hunger and its satisfaction, which most of us take for granted. This is a delicate but rewarding process, though it may take some time before a normal eating pattern can be achieved. An element of rebelliousness can often colour the anorexic's thinking and can affect the approach to treatment.

Although it is obviously preferable for an anorexic to eat nutritious foods, eating any food should be encouraged. While burgers, crisps, sweets, chocolate and ice cream may not provide a well-balanced diet, these foods still provide vital energy.

ANTIOXIDANTS

Without antioxidants, many of us would be prey to numerous infections and possibly even cancer within a few months. Although our bodies produce their own antioxidants, we also need to boost our defences by eating foods that contain them. Just how important these dietary antioxidants are is a matter of great debate. All too often claims for dietary antioxidants – particularly for supplements – have been exaggerated, but recent research suggests that they may offer protection against certain cancers and heart disease, and may also help to prevent premature ageing.

Antioxidants protect against FREE RADICALS, chemicals which are formed in the body as part of its metabolism

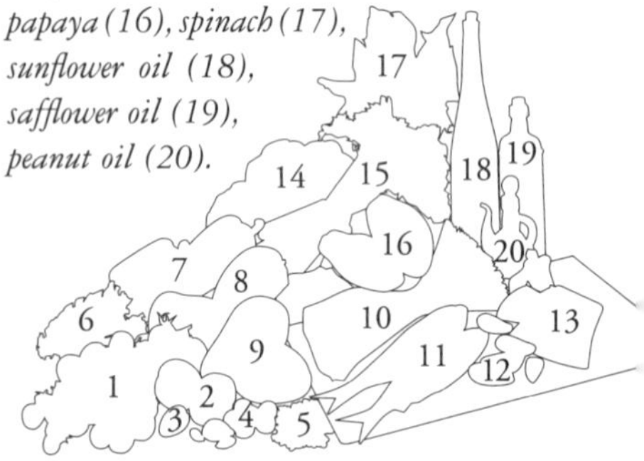

ANTIOXIDANT LARDER *Seafood supplies selenium; oils, vitamin E; and vegetables and fruit, vitamin C and beta carotene. Below: tomatoes (1), apricots (2), almonds (3), hazelnuts (4), sunflower seeds (5), kale (6), red peppers (7), mangoes (8), avocado (9), cod (10), herring (11), mussels (12), cod fillets (13), broccoli (14), carrots (15), papaya (16), spinach (17), sunflower oil (18), safflower oil (19), peanut oil (20).*

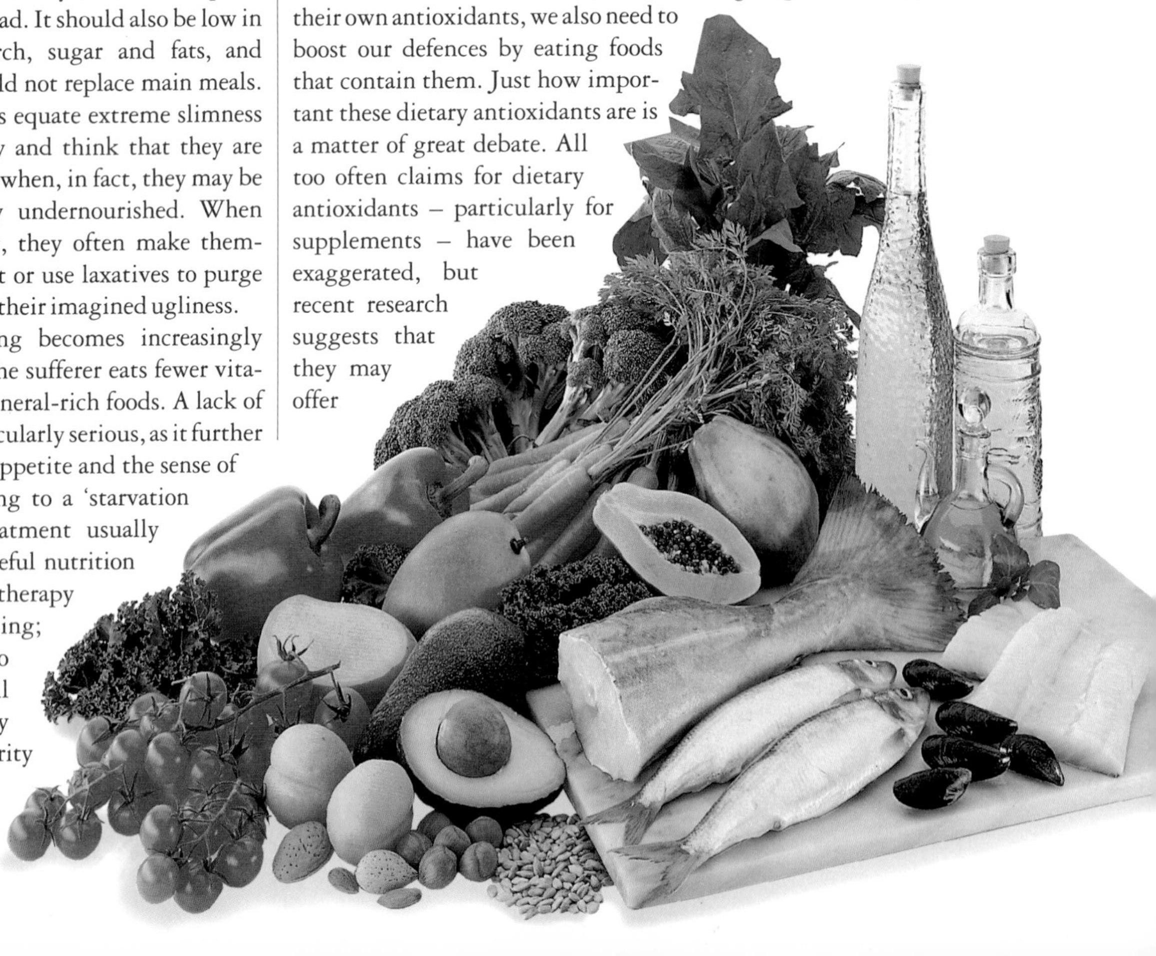

and defence against bacteria. Certain factors, such as excessive exposure to environmental pollution or ultraviolet light, illness and cigarette smoke, can cause the body to increase its production of free radicals. Left unchecked, these unstable and potentially harmful chemicals create conditions that may precipitate heart disease and cancer.

To cope with these free radicals, the body needs more antioxidants than it can produce, particularly during times of illness or when exposed to pollutants. Fortunately, many foods provide antioxidants that help to protect the body against their threat.

Vitamins E and C and beta carotene, the plant form of vitamin A, help to neutralise free radicals, as do minerals such as selenium (found in shellfish and avocados), copper (in nuts, seeds and shellfish) and zinc (in shellfish). Bioflavonoids, found in some fruit and vegetables, including citrus fruits and grapes, also have antioxidant properties. Artificial antioxidants are added to margarine and oils to stop them becoming rancid, and to retain the natural colourings of processed foods.

PREVENTING DISEASE

More research is needed into the role of antioxidants in disease prevention. However, it is thought that free radicals may start the damage that causes fatty cholesterol deposits in the arteries, which can eventually lead to heart disease or a stroke. High levels of antioxidant vitamins and minerals may help to prevent this harmful process, as well as damage to DNA (the genetic material in body cells) that could lead to certain cancers.

SUPPLEMENTS of particular antioxidant vitamins or minerals need to be taken in the correct balance and, even then, too many can be harmful. To obtain an adequate intake of antioxidants, it is safer to eat plenty of fresh fruit and vegetables. Citrus fruit provides vitamin C, and brightly coloured fruit and vegetables supply beta carotene. The vitamin E found in nuts, avocados and vegetable oils may also help to protect against disease.

ANXIETY

TAKE PLENTY OF

- *Meat, eggs, cheese, nuts and green leafy vegetables which are good sources of various B vitamins*
- *Citrus fruits for their vitamin C*
- *Sweet milky drinks*

CUT DOWN ON

- *Tea, coffee and colas, which contain caffeine*
- *Cocoa and chocolate*
- *Alcohol*

Everyone experiences spells of worry and dread at some time or other, but when anxiety is chronic it becomes a medical problem and a doctor should be consulted. Though it is a psychological state, anxiety manifests itself in physical symptoms, and a growing body of medical opinion argues that diet can help to ease, and may even eliminate, some of these.

Physical symptoms include a dry mouth, sweating, breathlessness, a thudding heart, dizziness, chest pains, diarrhoea and fatigue. Anxiety may also undermine the immune system.

A loss of appetite and skipped meals may disturb normal eating patterns. As a result, low food intake can lead to a loss of weight as well as inadequate nutrition. Consequent deficiencies may be aggravated by the further depletions anxiety itself can cause. There is evidence that a lack of magnesium and of vitamin B_6 is associated with anxiety and, when under stress, the body rapidly uses up reserves of vitamin C; those suffering from chronic anxiety will often benefit from an increased intake. So it is crucial to have a balanced diet and eat regularly. Avoiding food can lead not only to increased anxiety, but to the risk of other problems developing, particularly those such as heartburn which are linked to digestion.

Caffeine – found in coffee, tea and some cola drinks, as well as in plain, dark chocolate – is a stimulant. In small doses it can enhance both mental and physical performance, but in larger amounts it can lead to agitation, particularly among people who are sensitive to caffeine.

People suffering from anxiety often reach for a drink, but this is likely to make them feel worse, not better. Many people think that ALCOHOL is a tranquilliser or stimulant, in fact it is a depressant. Indeed, during the withdrawal phase, which occurs 6 to 12 hours after drinking, when blood sugar levels are low, people are particularly susceptible to anxiety attacks.

Sweetened milk is calming

Sweet milky drinks really can help people to overcome anxiety. They contain an amino acid present in milk, called tryptophan, and carbohydrates in the form of sugar. Tryptophan stimulates the production of another chemical – serotonin – which calms the mind and helps to induce sleep.

Sugar has an indirect role in the calming process. When you eat sugar, insulin is released which ties up other amino acids, thereby giving tryptophan easier access to the brain. This causes more serotonin to be released, promoting a more relaxed state of mind.

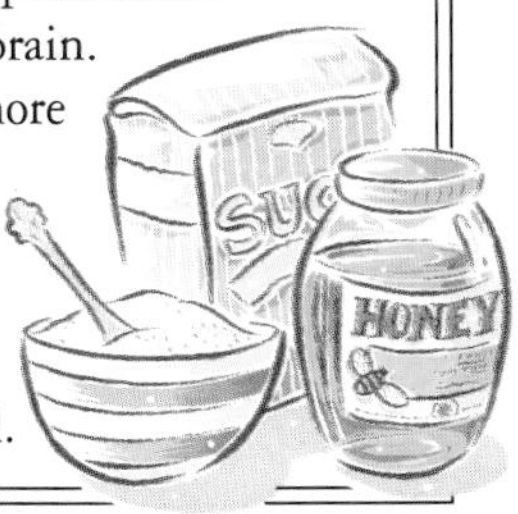

ALLERGIES AND FOOD INTOLERANCE

Substances in foods, house dust and pollen can cause anything from sniffles to migraine, and even sudden death. Allergies are becoming increasingly common, but they are still not fully understood.

Allergens, the substances that give rise to all allergies, are minute particles of matter, found in the environment or in food, which the body regards as alien and potentially harmful. It responds to their threat with an armoury of antibodies released into the bloodstream or tissues.

Individual reactions to these clashes vary in intensity – from sniffles and sneezes accompanying mild hay fever, to the potentially fatal reactions suffered by people who are allergic to peanuts. Similar symptoms and illnesses can be triggered by different allergens, so that hay fever may be sparked by pollen, dust, feathers or animal fur. Equally, the same allergen may cause entirely different reactions in different people. The issue is further clouded by the confusion between an allergy and an intolerance.

ALLERGY OR INTOLERANCE?

Allergic reactions to food can affect almost any part of the body, causing eczema, asthma, urticaria (HIVES) and other health problems. Anyone allergic to peanuts may, for example, swiftly develop swelling of the tongue and throat or a severe ASTHMA attack. In the most acute cases, nibbling only a tiny piece of peanut or eating a biscuit which incorporates peanut oil may even be fatal. The victims of these extreme allergies, or anaphylaxes, have an abnormal extreme reaction to a particular antigen. This can usually be countered with immediate administration of adrenaline by injection. Avoiding the culprit food is the only way to prevent such reactions.

Where there is an adverse reaction to food, but tests for allergy are negative, the phrase food 'intolerance', rather than allergy, is used to describe the condition. Although the immune system may be involved, it is not a major factor in causing the symptoms of reactions to particular foods.

Food intolerance is a highly controversial subject. In many cases, the cause of an intolerance remains a mystery, although it is known that allergic antibodies are not responsible. In some instances, it is the result of an identifiable problem. For example, people with lactose intolerance lack the ability to produce an enzyme called lactase which is needed to digest milk properly; and people with gluten intolerance (see COELIAC DISEASE) suffer from impaired nutrient absorption because gluten damages the lining of their small intestine.

HOW MANY PEOPLE SUFFER?

Allergy-related illnesses seem to be increasing rapidly. Around one in three children now exhibits symptoms of asthma, eczema or hay fever – before the age of eleven.

About 10 per cent of adults suffer from eczema and a similar proportion from migraine, while as many as one in five get hay fever.

Many of these conditions can be triggered by reactions to food. Some experts argue that as many as three in every ten Britons are, to some degree, allergic or intolerant to certain foods. Government figures are extraordinarily conservative, putting the figure no higher than 2 per cent.

Allergies can strike at any age. As people grow older their susceptibility and response to certain allergens will often change – particularly where these stem from diet. Both children and adults may outgrow an allergy without any change in diet; on the other hand, where an allergen has been identified and eliminated from a diet,

Case study

Sharon, a 27-year-old, suffered from what she assumed were cold sores. Occasionally, her lips and tongue tingled when she was eating, and moments later would actually swell, becoming painful and tender to the touch. One summer, the problem became very severe, and Sharon's doctor asked her about her diet. It emerged that her father had grown a bumper tomato crop, and that Sharon was eating several of them with almost every meal. By following the doctor's advice to cut tomatoes from her diet, Sharon has now successfully cured herself.

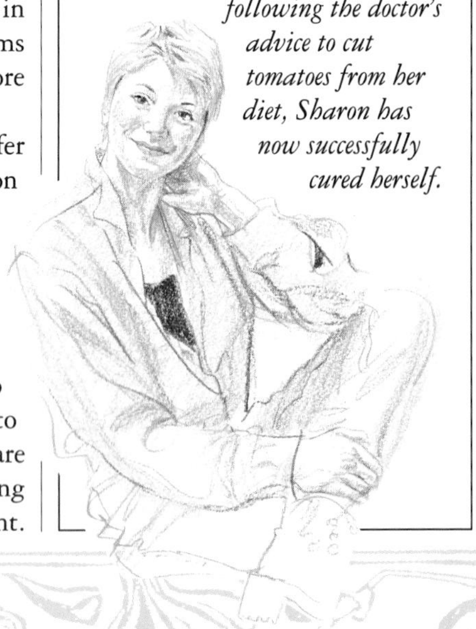

new allergies may surface – sometimes months, or even years later – and cause similar or new symptoms. If a particular allergy is suspected, it can often be diagnosed either by skin testing or by excluding suspect foods from the diet. Both methods are simple and reasonably accurate. However, when there are no clues, identifying an allergy can be as frustrating as looking for a needle in a haystack.

HYPERACTIVE HISTAMINES

The skin and mucous membranes, or linings of the mouth, nose, intestines and some other parts of the body are able to produce a chemical called histamine. One of its functions is to stimulate the production of gastric juices after a meal. It also enlarges the capillaries (tiny blood vessels) to increase the blood flow. When food allergens enter the body or come into contact with the skin, the body reacts by releasing large amounts of histamine and other chemicals. It is the 'histamine explosion' that creates most of the symptoms of the allergic reaction. These may include itchy watering eyes, sneezing, wheezing, the appearance of a rash and diarrhoea.

In mild instances, the tongue or mouth may tingle – after eating raw apples, stone fruits or tomatoes, for example. This type of allergy is often experienced by the same people whose hay fever is sparked by early flowering trees such as silver birch.

SYMPTOMS – SWIFT OR SLOW

Allergens can produce reactions anywhere in the body – in the nose, lungs, skin and even brain. When an allergic reaction appears swiftly after eating a particular food, the cause is often obvious and likely to point to a true food allergy. However, in some cases of asthma, glue ear and chronic rhinitis (characterised by a constantly congested nose), the food allergen may

The most common culprits and their symptoms

Surprisingly, there are no established figures on how many people suffer from a particular food allergy or intolerance. This chart lists the most common culprits in descending order; milk, closely followed by gluten, are the biggest offenders.

FOOD TYPES	DANGER FOODS	SYMPTOMS
Milk 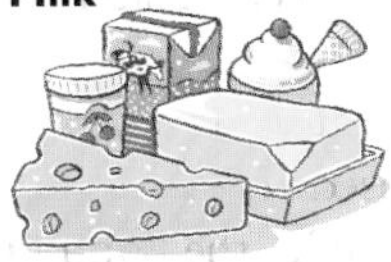	Dairy produce such as milk, butter, cream, ice cream, different types of cheese and yoghurt.	Constipation, diarrhoea, wind; migraine (cheese). Babies may suffer from wind, colic, catarrh and later, eczema.
Gluten 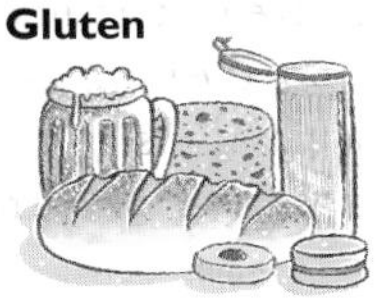	Flour, bread, biscuits, barley, rye, oats, beer, tinned soups, stock cubes; any processed foods containing 'rusk' or hydrolysed vegetable protein.	Migraine, coeliac disease (characterised by diarrhoea and also weight loss).
Eggs 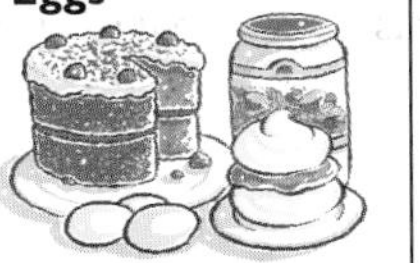	Usually egg white. Cakes, desserts, meringues, mayonnaise, mousses, ice cream and Caesar salad.	Rashes, swelling and stomach upsets. Can cause asthma as well as eczema.
Fish 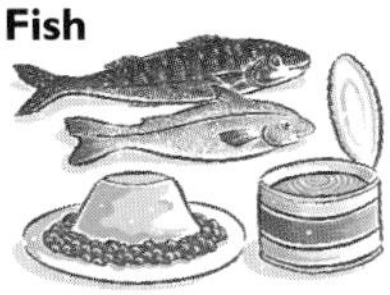	Smoked fish such as kippers, smoked salmon, mackerel and haddock. Fresh fish such as cod and sole.	Migraine, nausea, skin rashes, swelling and stomach upsets.
Shellfish 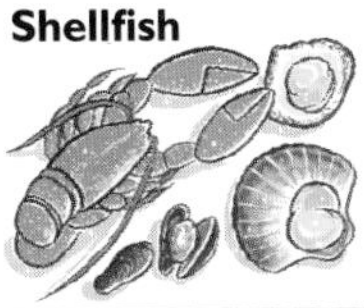	Both crustaceans (lobster, langoustine, prawn, crab) and molluscs (clams, oysters, mussels, scallops).	Prolonged stomach upsets, migraine and nausea.
Nuts 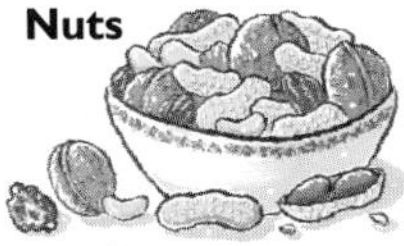	Peanuts (also called ground nuts), walnuts, cashews and pecans. Nut-flavoured bread, biscuits, ice cream and oils.	Rashes, swelling, asthma and eczema. In severe cases, potentially fatal anaphylactic shock.
Soya beans 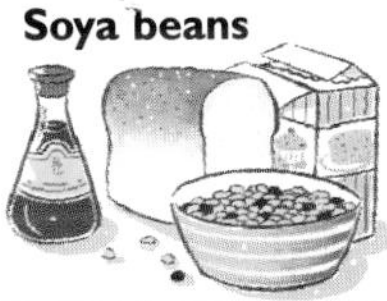	Soy sauce, soya flour, soya milk and tofu, soya oil, cake and pancake mixes, canned condensed soup.	Headaches, indigestion.
Additives 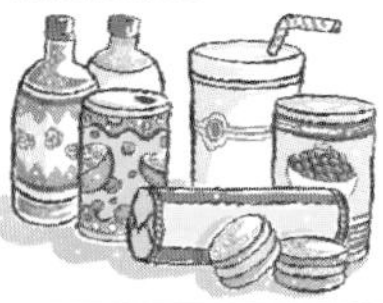	Some packaged, processed or takeaway foods and drinks. Tartrazine, the colouring agent, and the preservative benzoic acid.	Hyperactivity and other behavioural changes have been attributed to ingestion of some additives.

take many hours, or even several days, to produce the symptoms. A person may eat a particular food daily without realising it is causing a mild allergy. Only after avoiding it for two to three weeks will all the symptoms it has caused clear up. If the culprit food is included in the diet once again, all the original problems will reappear.

Migraine triggers

There are various foods that are commonly cited by MIGRAINE sufferers as triggers for their attacks. Cheese, chocolate, citrus and coffee – known as the 'Four Cs' – are the classic culprits. Others are alcohol, in particular red wine, sherry and port; meat extracts and stock cubes; nitrates, in processed meats; and miscellaneous foods ranging from milk to pulses.

Excessive tiredness

Drowsiness can sometimes be due to a food intolerance. While it is natural to feel sleepy after a meal – resting ensures an adequate blood supply to the intestine as opposed to the muscles – some people experience almost continual lethargy. In many instances, these people are found to be sensitive to grains – particularly wheat. The process of digesting wheat can have the effect of releasing chemicals in the brain, inducing excessive sleepiness. Excluding wheat from the diets of such people can improve their general health and boost energy levels.

COULD A CRAVING BE A CLUE?

There is no accurate 'hit list' of the foods or conditions responsible for reactions classed as intolerance. Individual diets, the victim's age and any illness generated by the intolerance all play a part. But a reasonably reliable rule of thumb is that the more a person craves a particular food, the more likely it is that he or she will have a sensitivity to that food.

Why milk causes problems

Nine out of ten of the world's adults are deficient in lactase, an enzyme in the lining of the intestine that breaks down lactose, the sugar present in milk and most dairy products. The enzyme is present in appreciable quantities only while babies are breastfeeding, and usually disappears after weaning when milk is no longer a staple food – its absence leads to lactose intolerance which in turn may cause diarrhoea. However, in Western Europe about 95 per cent of all adults whose diet includes milk, cheese and other dairy products have retained the enzyme and so have few difficulties.

Infant reactions

Food intolerance usually becomes apparent when babies are weaned from breast milk to formula, because the most common food intolerance in the West is to cow's milk. Milk and eggs are frequently the cause of childhood eczema (atopic eczema). Some infants will react very quickly, crying inconsolably, or exhibiting symptoms of colic, diarrhoea or eczema. In others the reaction to foodstuffs may be delayed for hours or by as much as a day. Symptoms are usually relieved once the foods are excluded.

Some breastfed babies react to milk which contains very small amounts of the components from food that the mother has eaten, but such instances are rare. A protective immune protein present in breast milk helps the baby to adjust to new foods which might otherwise provoke an allergic reaction.

Elimination diets

Most doctors now accept that food intolerances can sometimes be the root cause of chronic diseases, including arthritis, Crohn's disease, IRRITABLE BOWEL SYNDROME and hyperactivity. Yet these are only a few of the conditions which are claimed to have responded to elimination diets. Such diets are based on a systematic method of discovering whether a particular food is causing symptoms simply by eliminating it from the diet and seeing what happens. It is a tedious approach and sometimes the results are not clear-cut, but it is the most reliable diagnostic procedure available.

Because a huge range of symptoms may respond to the removal of specific foods from the diet, patients who feel better after starting such a regime may be tempted to expand the range of foods they exclude. But unintentionally eliminating or upsetting the balance of necessary vitamins and minerals can be dangerous; it is wise to consult your doctor or a qualified nutritionist before eliminating any foods from the diet.

How diet can help

One of the most common digestive disorders is IRRITABLE BOWEL SYNDROME with its many accompanying symptoms. These include wind, bloated abdomen and irregular bowel habits which may often alternate between diarrhoea and constipation. At least half of the people with this condition suffer from food intolerance, with wheat grain being the most common culprit. Many people have found that a change in their diet helps to relieve the symptoms. Half of all

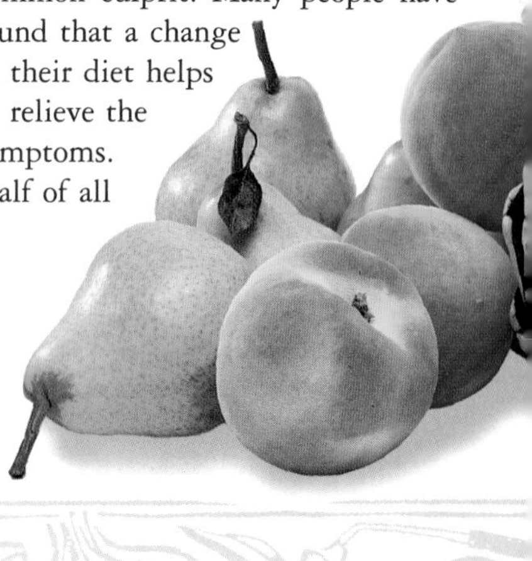

people who are known to suffer from gastrointestinal complaints are sensitive to wheat, according to reports in some medical journals. Careful attention to diet would relieve the symptoms of almost all these patients.

Three out of ten rheumatoid arthritis patients can also be helped to some extent by diet. People with chronic migraine can also respond well. The health of more than half the patients with Crohn's disease can be improved by an elimination diet, while trials in various countries suggest that delinquent behaviour in children can be improved by changes in their diet.

THE EFFECTS OF DRUGS

Certain medication and drugs predispose some people to food intolerance. For example, teenagers may develop digestive disorders after long-term use of tetracycline antibiotics for acne; some people develop irritable bowel syndrome after treatment with antibiotics, and others experience allergic reactions after taking steroids or oral contraceptives. Several mechanisms can therefore produce the same symptoms, making diagnosis even more difficult.

How the elimination diet works

Any restricted diet puts health at risk and any long-term removal of major foods should be carried out only under professional guidance.

Pinpointing culprit foods is difficult since only a few people are sensitive to one single allergen. Eliminating only one food from the diet is rarely effective. All the suspect foods have to be cut out simultaneously for at least a fortnight for any improvements to be observed. 'Testing' the effects of individual foods by returning them piecemeal to the daily regimen is futile unless all symptoms have gone.

The following foods should not be eaten during the first two weeks of the exclusion diet: preserved meats, bacon and sausages; smoked fish and shellfish; citrus fruit; wheat, oats, barley, rye and corn; potatoes, onions and sweetcorn; nuts; corn oil and most vegetable oils; dairy produce; all cheese; most margarines, and eggs. Tap water, tea (other than herbal tea), coffee, alcohol, fruit squashes and fresh citrus juices should also be omitted from the diet, as should vinegar, yeast, chocolate and all foods containing chemical preservatives.

After 14 days introduce foods in this order: tap water, potatoes, cow's milk, yeast, tea, rye, butter, onions, eggs, oats, coffee, chocolate, barley, citrus fruit, corn, cheese, white wine, shellfish, yoghurt, vinegar, wheat and nuts.

Try only one new food every two days and if there is a reaction, do not try it again for at least a month. Continue to add new foods again when symptoms have stopped.

Keep a record of the foods you return to your meals and you can soon build a list of foods your body tolerates – and those which should be eliminated. There is no reason to avoid foods which do not cause problems when returned to the diet.

Though every doctor's approach to the elimination diet differs, overall results are remarkably consistent. Initially, affected by withdrawal, the patient often feels worse, but after six or seven days there is an improvement as the symptoms disappear.

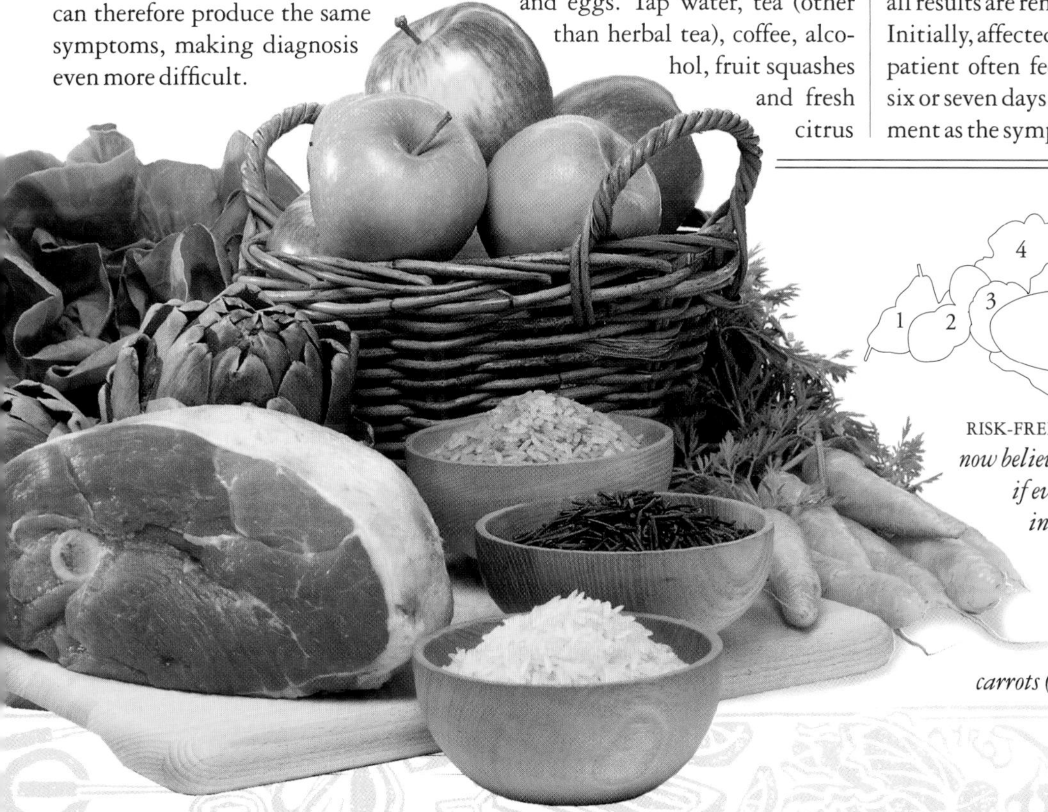

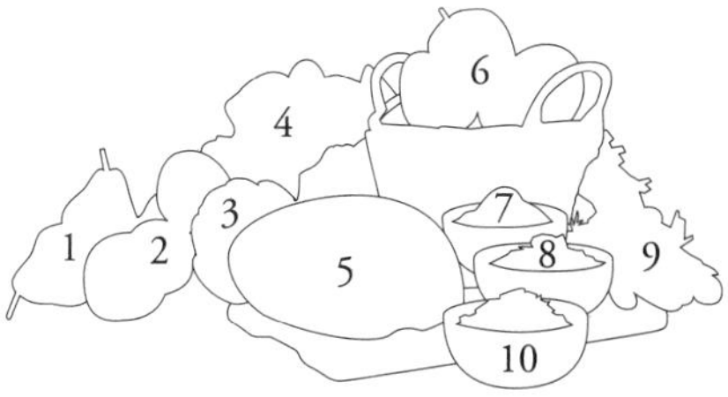

RISK-FREE FOODS *Medical experts now believe that some foods seldom if ever set off reactions. They include: pears (1), peaches (2), artichokes (3), lettuce (4), lamb (5), apples (6), brown rice (7), wild rice (8), carrots (9) and white rice (10).*

Appetite loss

EAT PLENTY OF
- *Fresh fruit and vegetables*
- *Oysters, lean meat and poultry*
- *Nuts, seeds and whole grains*

CUT DOWN ON
- *Bran, which inhibits mineral absorption*
- *Alcohol*
- *Salt*
- *Tea and coffee, which can cause loss of potassium and zinc*

When a normally healthy appetite goes wrong it can be due to a number of causes, ranging from travel sickness to the common cold, from depression to eating the wrong kind of food. If the appetite loss continues for longer than seven days, see a doctor.

When appetite loss is associated with a fairly trivial disorder such as a hangover or indigestion, the appetite will return once the condition has cleared up. If you eat a lot of snacks, which upset your eating patterns, try to tempt your appetite back with fruit, especially bananas, and with the other foods recommended above.

Appetite is regulated by the appestat, a sensory area of the brain which gauges hunger and sends out hormones that tell the body it is time to eat. When the appestat malfunctions – perhaps due to an unbalanced diet, poor general health or a hormone imbalance – the wrong messages are transmitted to the body, with the result that a well-fed person may feel hungry or somebody who is undernourished may have no appetite at all.

Vitamins and minerals

Deficiencies of minerals can inhibit the smooth functioning of the appestat and reduce the desire to eat. Diets with too little zinc, which is found in oysters, crab, lobster, lean meat, poultry and pumpkin seeds, for example, can diminish the senses of both smell and taste and therefore undermine the appetite. Zinc absorption may also be inhibited by eating a lot of bran, taking iron supplements or by drinking too much alcohol. Zinc reserves are also depleted by physical exercise, stress and the periods of rapid growth during puberty.

Elderly people or those undergoing diuretic therapy can be subject to a lack of potassium, a known cause of appetite loss. Bananas and potatoes are particularly rich in this mineral, although plenty of other fruits and vegetables will also compensate for any deficiency, particularly if salt intakes are reduced.

Appetite loss can also be caused by an excessive intake of vitamin D. However, this is unlikely to occur unless the vitamin is taken in tablet form (as prescribed for rickets or osteoporosis) or as fish oil supplements.

Apples

BENEFITS
- *Good source of vitamin C, depending on the variety*
- *May help in the treatment of constipation and diarrhoea*

A fresh apple is the ideal, healthy snack – easy to carry, filling, juicy and refreshing. Some varieties are a good source of vitamin C, which is an antioxidant and helps to maintain the immune system. Apples are also relatively low in calories and contain a high proportion of fructose. This simple sugar, which is sweeter than sucrose – the main component of sugar cane – is metabolised slowly, and so helps to control blood sugar levels.

In herbal medicine, ripe, uncooked apples have traditionally been given to treat constipation, while the stewed

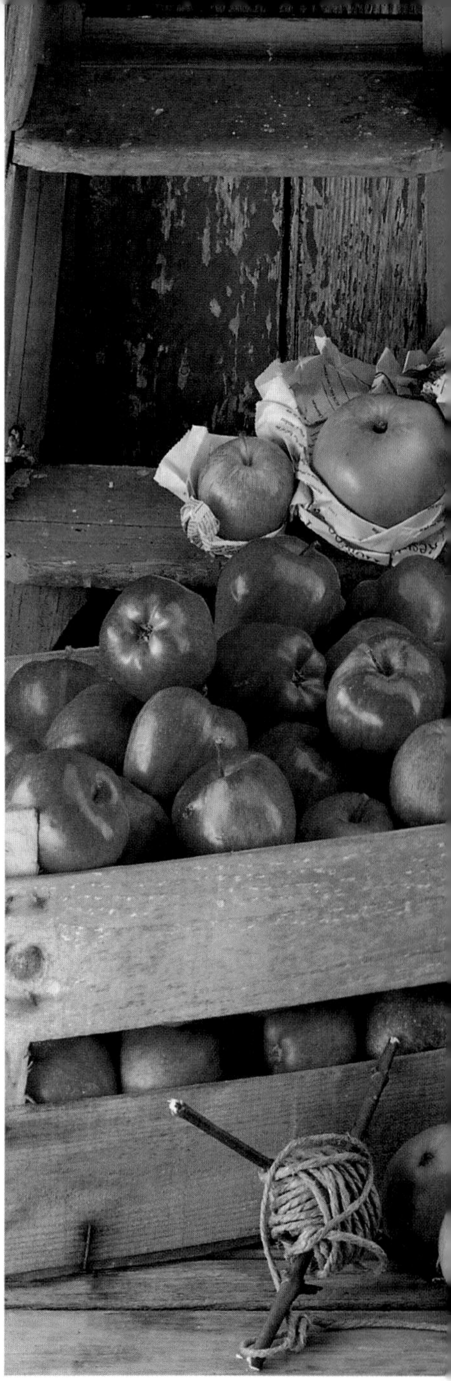

fruit can be eaten for diarrhoea and gastroenteritis. Apples are also used in poultices for skin inflammations.

Choosing apples

Look for apples that are firm to the touch, with no brown bruises. Large apples are more likely to be overripe than smaller ones. Local fruits are at their best – in flavour, scent and texture – when they ripen in the autumn.

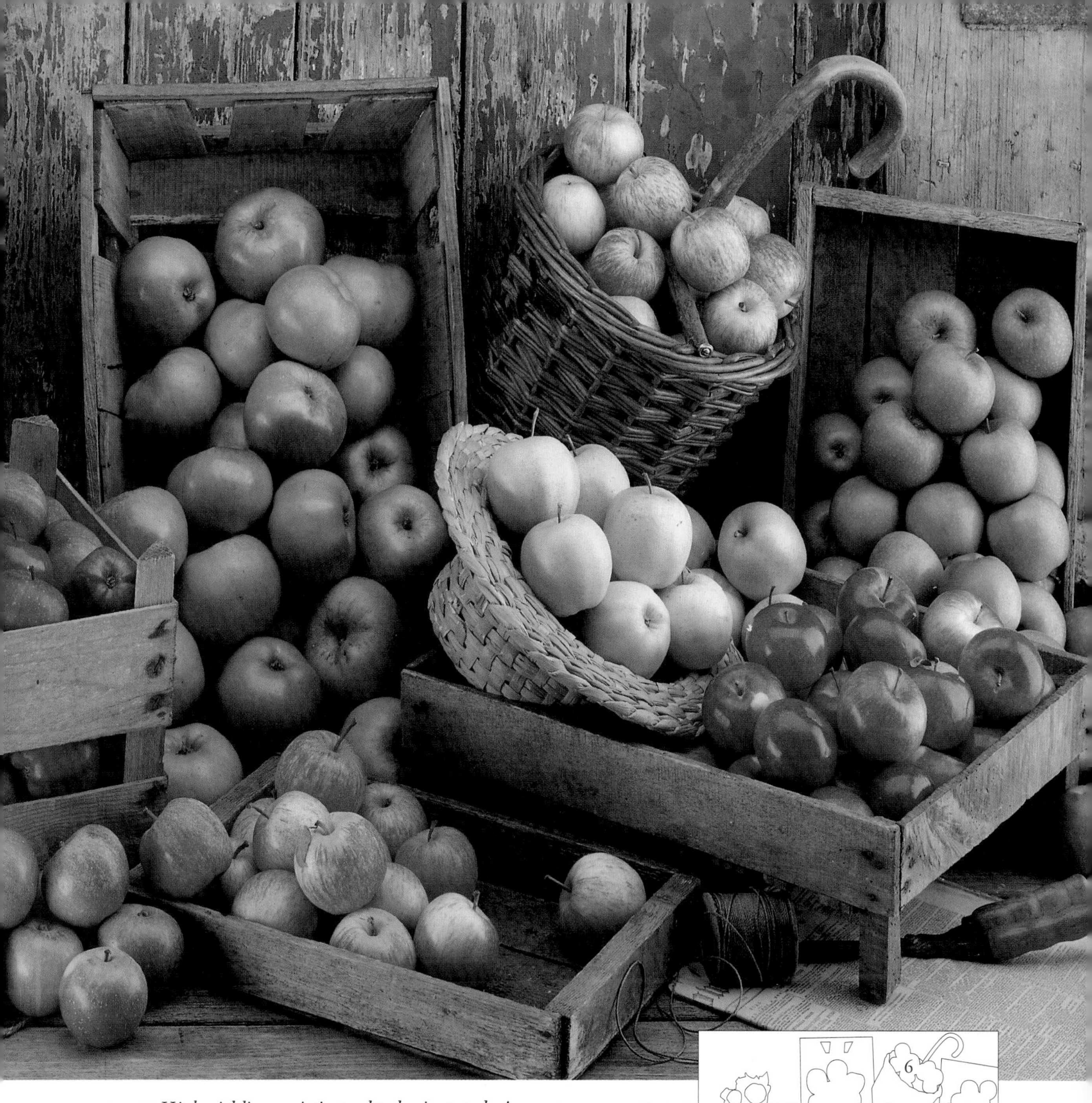

APPLE HARVEST *High-yielding varieties tend to dominate today's greengrocery counters.*

There are thousands of varieties of apple, including some 50 or so grown commercially in Britain, but only a tiny proportion of these are widely available. However, it is worth seeking out the old-fashioned, aromatic types such as Lord Lambourne, Newton Wonder and also Egremont Russet. They may be less regular in size and shape than Granny Smiths and Golden Delicious, neither of which are of British origin, but their flavours and texture will reward the effort.

Unless they have been imported, apples bought out of season will have been stored in a cool environment where the oxygen balance has been chemically lowered. This halts the

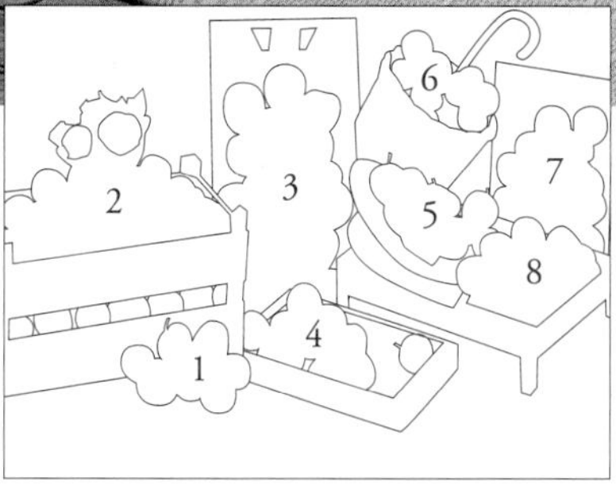

Apples that are widely available include Cox (1), Red Delicious (2), Bramley (3), Royal Gala (4, 6), Golden Delicious (5), Granny Smith (7), Empire (8).

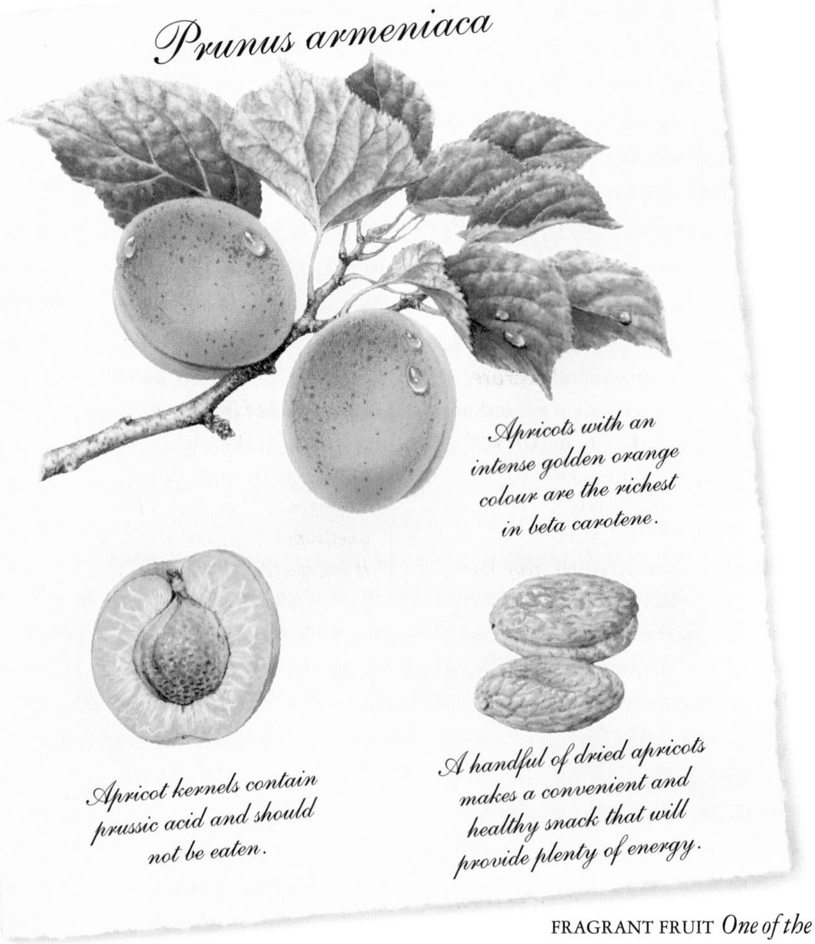
Prunus armeniaca
Apricots with an intense golden orange colour are the richest in beta carotene.
Apricot kernels contain prussic acid and should not be eaten.
A handful of dried apricots makes a convenient and healthy snack that will provide plenty of energy.

FRAGRANT FRUIT *One of the first fruits of summer, apricots are best eaten warm, straight from the tree.*

natural maturing processes, so they can be kept for several months without going soft. When the fruit is again exposed to normal temperatures and oxygen levels – on a greengrocer's or a supermarket's shelves – it continues to mature and may quickly go soft.

In 1989 there was widespread concern in the USA and Britain over the possible carcinogenic effects of Alar, a chemical used to make apple trees more productive. Although not considered a hazard by some scientists, consumer pressure has led Alar to be withdrawn worldwide.

DRIED APPLES

People have eaten fresh and dried apples since the Stone Age, and they were popular with the Egyptians as long ago as the 12th century BC. Valuing the fruit for its durability, the Pilgrim Fathers planted apples as one of their first crops in the New World.

Drying is one of the oldest forms of fruit preservation. The medieval housewife would hang strings of apple rings from the rafters, but today the slices are exposed to the fumes of burning sulphur to prevent them from browning, and then dried in the sun on wire trays. As moisture is lost, natural sugars become concentrated, which is why athletes value dried apples as a source of carbohydrate that is quickly converted to energy. Weight for weight, however, dried apples contain six times more calories than fresh ones. The soft, leathery rings are high in fibre and are a moderate source of iron. However, dried apples lose all their vitamin C during the drying process.

APRICOTS

BENEFITS
- *Fresh and dried apricots are good sources of beta carotene*
- *Dried apricots are a useful source of iron, a good source of fibre and an excellent source of potassium*

DRAWBACK
- *Preservatives in some dried apricots may trigger an asthma attack in susceptible people*

Fresh, ripe apricots are high in fibre and low in calories. They are a good source of beta carotene, the plant form of vitamin A. Beta carotene is one of the ANTIOXIDANT nutrients that current research indicates may help to prevent degenerative illnesses such as cancer and heart disease.

Apricots canned in natural juice have less than half the amount of beta carotene of fresh or dried apricots, but the juice provides a useful source of vitamin C.

DRIED APRICOTS

Although dried apricots are higher in calories than fresh, they are considered to be one of the great health foods because they are a compact and convenient source of nutrients; they even formed part of the diet of American astronauts during some of their space flights. The drying process increases the concentration of beta carotene, potassium and iron. Consumption of potassium is associated with a decline in BLOOD PRESSURE – when it is caused by salt sensitivity. This is because potassium is a natural diuretic that encourages the body to excrete water and sodium.

Many food companies treat apricots with sulphur dioxide (E220) before drying them in order to preserve their rich orange colour. This treatment produces substances that may trigger an asthma attack in susceptible people. Unless dried apricots are known to be sulphite-free, they are best avoided by asthmatics.

ARTHRITIS

EAT PLENTY OF

- *Wholegrain cereals, fresh fruit and vegetables, for osteoarthritis*
- *Soya beans and tofu, if the problem is rheumatoid arthritis*
- *Sardines, salmon, cod and halibut, for rheumatoid arthritis*

CUT DOWN ON

- *Highly refined foods, saturated fats, sugar and salt, for osteoarthritis*

There are around 200 kinds of arthritis, the two most common being osteoarthritis and rheumatoid arthritis. People with osteoarthritis should improve their diet by cutting down on highly refined and processed foods, saturated animal fats, sugar and salt, and by eating more wholegrain cereals and fresh fruit and vegetables. A healthy diet boosts the immune system and provides the sufferer with extra energy to fight the disease.

THE WEIGHT FACTOR

Obesity increases the risk of developing osteoarthritis by putting undue stress on the joints – knees and hips, for example, will not cause as much discomfort when they have less weight to carry. Some form of gentle exercise, such as swimming, cycling or walking, together with a sensible, low-fat diet (see DIETS AND SLIMMING) will therefore help to prevent osteoarthritis, or minimise symptoms if you already have the condition.

Furthermore, regular exercise can play a vital role in the prevention and treatment of all forms of arthritis. It strengthens the muscles responsible for protecting the joints, and helps to prevent stiffness. But you also need to respect your body's limitations in order for exercise to be beneficial.

ALLERGIES OR INTOLERANCES

For some people who develop rheumatoid arthritis, an allergy or intolerance to particular foods may be a contributing factor. Pinpointing the culprit foods can be difficult, but common suspects include dairy products, eggs and cereals. One of the best ways to identify problem foods is to follow an exclusion diet, but this should only be done under medical supervision.

FISH OILS

Scientific evidence has now emerged to show that fish oils can prove helpful to people who suffer from rheumatoid arthritis. Salmon, trout, herring, mackerel, sardines, cod and halibut all contain polyunsaturated

Exercise and arthritis

- Regular exercise can help to reduce joint pain. Try walking or swimming every day for 5 or 10 minutes, gradually increasing the amount of time you exercise.
- Try stretching exercises such as yoga for movement and posture.
- Wear shoes that fit well and are designed specifically for the activity you are taking part in; well-cushioned soles reduce stress on weight-bearing joints.
- Don't push yourself too hard. Too much exercise – particularly anything that jars the knees, hips or other joints – can lead directly to osteoarthritis.
- If you experience extra pain, you may be overexerting yourself and should cut back or change to a less physically demanding activity.

Case study

Fred, a 28-year-old mechanic, was finding it increasingly difficult to manipulate the tools he used in his work. His joints became more and more painful until eventually he was finding it so hard to work that he consulted his doctor. When conventional drug treatment failed to ease Fred's symptoms, his doctor began to suspect a food allergy. He questioned Fred about his diet, and it emerged that he ate about half a loaf of bread each day. Because allergies or intolerances to certain foods, such as cereals, are thought to be a factor in the development of some people's arthritic symptoms, Fred's doctor suggested he should try excluding all wheat products from his diet. This meant cutting out bread, pasta and numerous other foods made with wheat flour. Within weeks, Fred's joint pain had subsided and the swelling had gone down. He is now able to work normally, and maintains his strict wheat-free regime.

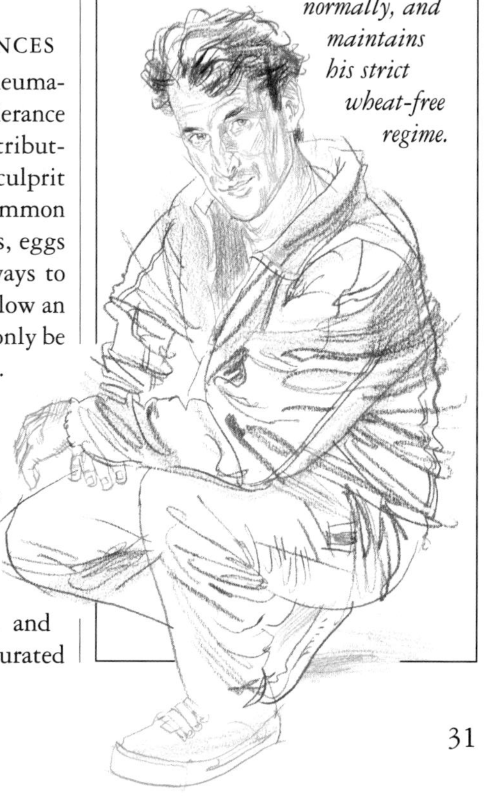

fats called omega-3 fatty acids, which can have an anti-inflammatory effect on the joints of some arthritis sufferers. Inflammation is the body's natural reaction to arthritic diseases, causing pain, swelling, redness and heat.

People with rheumatoid arthritis can try eating fresh oily fish two or three times a week, or they can take fish oils in capsule or liquid form if this is more manageable – keeping to the recommended daily dose. Tinned oily fish (except tuna) also contains these beneficial omega-3 fatty acids, but not in such large quantities. Signs of improvement are normally seen after a period of two to three months.

People who need to take anti-inflammatory drugs may be able to reduce their dosage (with their doctor's permission) by about one-third if they eat oily fish regularly. This reduces the risk of the drugs having any unpleasant side effects.

Evening primrose oil has also been found to have anti-inflammatory effects, and is therefore particularly useful for anyone who does not eat fish. Vegetarians can get omega-3 fatty acids by including plenty of soya beans and tofu in their diet. In fact, several studies have found that a VEGETARIAN DIET helps to relieve some of the symptoms of rheumatoid arthritis.

COPPER BRACELETS

Many people who suffer from rheumatoid arthritis claim that wearing a copper bracelet reduces their discomfort. However, research into this controversial area has come up with no scientific explanation. It is thought that if wearers believe in the power of such bracelets to help them, then this belief may trigger some form of self-healing.

CAUSES AND SYMPTOMS

Osteoarthritis is believed to be a degenerative disease that develops as a result of wear and tear of the cartilage in a joint. Cartilage or 'gristle' provides a smooth surface for bones to slide against, allowing painless and easy movement. When the cartilage is worn away or damaged, the bones rub together causing pain and stiffness, especially during damp weather or the morning after strenuous activity.

Rheumatoid arthritis is a mysterious inflammatory disease in which the immune system turns on itself and starts to attack the joints. Although this progressive condition can strike at any age, it most commonly starts in the joints of the fingers and feet of people aged between 25 and 55. It is three times more likely to affect women than men. Rheumatoid arthritis often lasts for many years with alternating attacks and remissions.

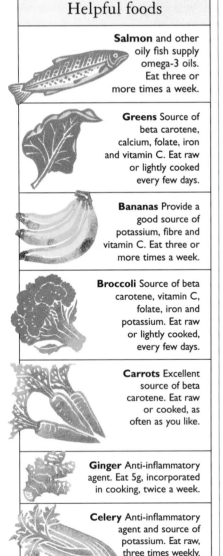

Helpful foods

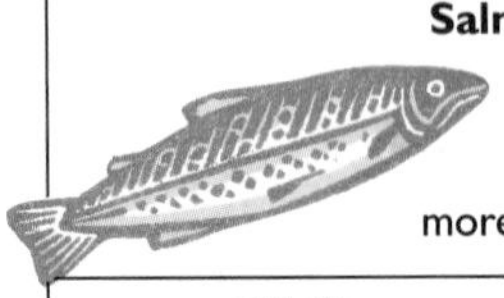

Salmon and other oily fish supply omega-3 oils. Eat three or more times a week.

Greens Source of beta carotene, calcium, folate, iron and vitamin C. Eat raw or lightly cooked every few days.

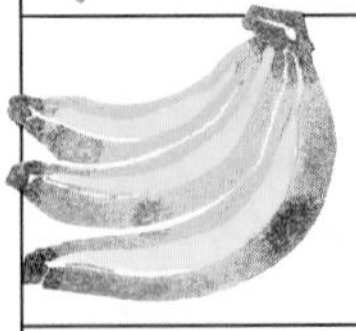

Bananas Provide a good source of potassium, fibre and vitamin C. Eat three or more times a week.

Broccoli Source of beta carotene, vitamin C, folate, iron and potassium. Eat raw or lightly cooked, every few days.

Carrots Excellent source of beta carotene. Eat raw or cooked, as often as you like.

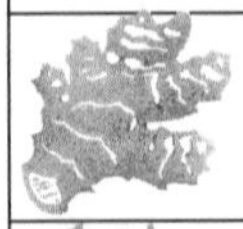

Ginger Anti-inflammatory agent. Eat 5g, incorporated in cooking, twice a week.

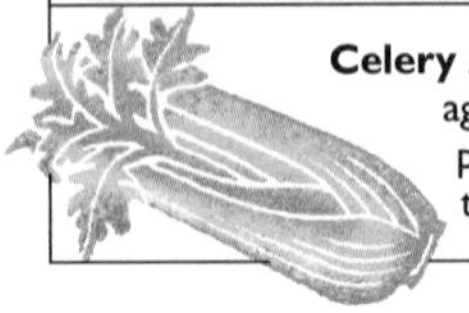

Celery Anti-inflammatory agent and source of potassium. Eat raw, three times weekly.

ARTICHOKES (GLOBE)

BENEFITS

- *Good source of folate and potassium*
- *May help to control cholesterol levels*
- *May improve liver function*

Served hot or cold, with its leaves or stripped down to the heart, the globe artichoke is both a delicacy and a good source of folate and potassium.

Many practitioners of herbal medicine also believe that the vegetable may have healing powers. Researchers in this field have conducted a number of studies on extracts of artichoke and, in particular, a substance called cynarin which is found in the edible base of the vegetable's leaves. Results suggest that cynarin or related compounds in the artichoke may help to control cholesterol levels, improve liver function and have a lasting beneficial effect on gallstone disease.

At least one study, carried out at Freiburg University in Germany in 1979, supports the contention that cynarin can reduce cholesterol levels, although there appears to be little other substantiating scientific evidence. However, many herbalists and health-food shops in Britain supply cynarin-containing preparations based on artichokes. These purport to have a range of medicinal properties, including giving a boost to a sluggish liver.

EDIBLE THISTLE *Globe artichokes (right) are no relation of the Jerusalem artichoke.*

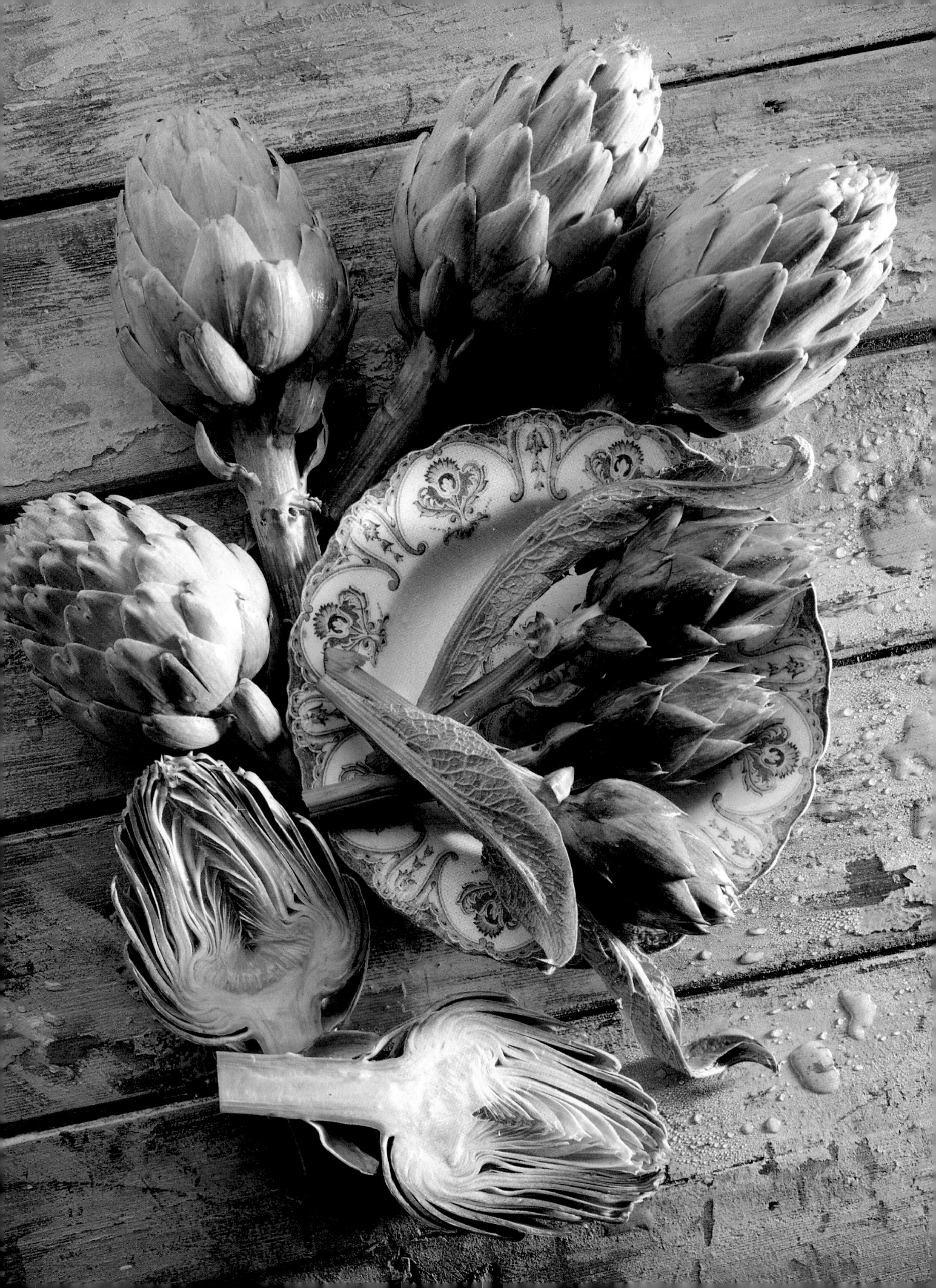

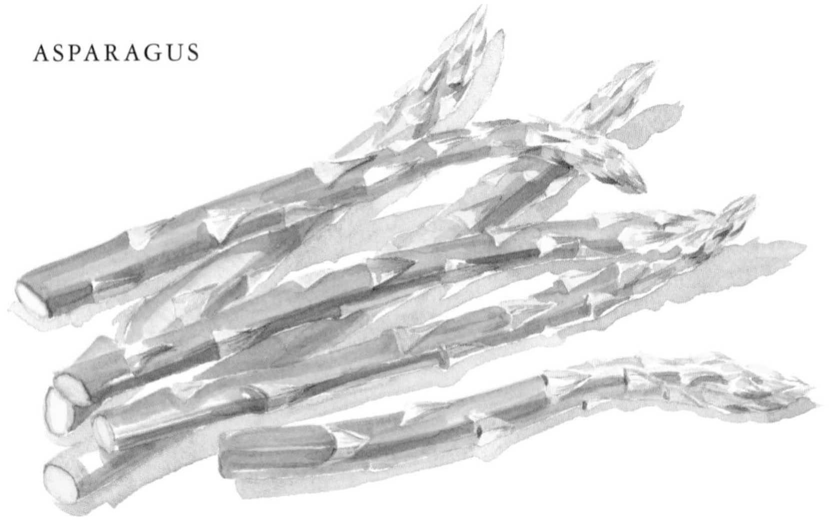

Asparagus

BENEFITS
- *Rich source of folate*
- *Useful source of beta carotene, vitamin C and vitamin E*
- *Diuretic and mild laxative*

DRAWBACK
- *Can make urine smell*

The tender spears of lightly boiled or steamed asparagus are a delicacy with both nutritional and medicinal properties. A 100g (3½oz) portion supplies three-quarters of the folate and a quarter of the vitamin C required each day, as well as vitamin E and beta carotene, which the body converts to vitamin A.

Asparagus is both mildly laxative and a diuretic. It also contains certain sulphur-producing elements which in some people can give urine a distinctive smell. In traditional folk medicine, asparagus has been used as a tonic and a sedative and also to treat neuritis, rheumatism and, less understandably, complaints as diverse as poor eyesight and toothache.

Asparagus spoils rapidly in storage and is therefore best consumed fresh. Sufferers of GOUT should also be aware that it is one of the few vegetables high in purines. A high intake of purines is linked to the gradual build-up of uric acid salts in the joints, which can aggravate this painful condition.

Asthma

EAT PLENTY OF
- *Foods rich in the B vitamins such as green leafy vegetables and pulses*
- *Good sources of magnesium such as sunflower seeds and dried figs*

AVOID

Foods that trigger attacks (according to your susceptibility), such as:
- *Foods containing the additives benzoates (E210-19), sulphites (E220-8) or gallates (E310-12)*
- *Cider, wine and beer*
- *Foods containing yeast or mould, such as bread and blue cheeses*
- *Foods, drinks and snacks containing colourings E102, E104 and E110*
- *Cow's milk, cereals, eggs, fish and nuts (especially peanuts)*

Asthma is a chronic, potentially serious respiratory condition that kills around 2000 people in Britain every year. Some experts divide asthma into two broad groups: extrinsic and intrinsic. The vast majority of cases are extrinsic. This form of asthma tends to run in families along with other allergic conditions such as eczema and hay fever, and to appear first in childhood. Symptoms may be produced by a variety of triggers, such as anxiety, physical stress, infection, environmental pollution, pollen, dust mites and animal hair. Food allergies may also prompt attacks or make them worse, especially among children who have eczema. Intrinsic asthma appears to begin in adult life; external factors do not cause it, but they can trigger attacks. However, many health professionals now believe that there is little difference between the two types, and that all asthma may in fact be extrinsic.

An asthma attack, which can last for minutes or days, makes breathing difficult, and may cause wheezing and coughing, along with a sense of tightness in the chest due to the swelling of inflamed bronchial passages.

Potential triggers

Because an allergy is a highly individual condition, it is not possible to give a definitive list of 'good' and 'bad' foods. Those who suspect that foods are triggering their asthmatic attacks should keep a food diary and seek expert medical help.

Common foods that may trigger asthma in susceptible individuals, however, include cow's milk, wheat and other cereals, yeast and foods containing mould, such as blue cheeses. Nuts (especially peanuts), fish and eggs can produce the most immediate and dangerous reactions.

Certain food additives may also be potential triggers in some people. In the United States, sulphites, once widely used as preservatives on raw fruit and vegetables, have been implicated in the deaths of a very small number of asthmatics. Their use on fresh fruit and vegetables was banned in America in 1986.

In the European Union, sulphites are not allowed to be used on fresh produce. However, they may be used in low levels in burger meat, British sausages, dried fruit, jams, vinegar, processed and frozen vegetables and preserved shellfish. The presence of sulphites must, by law, be indicated on the label of packaged foods, but it is

Case study

Jean was 34 when she developed mild asthma. She did not wheeze all the time, nor did she have severe attacks, but she tended to cough and wheeze on Sunday mornings. Jean assumed that her asthma was triggered by the smoky atmosphere in the wine bar she went to on Saturday nights. One weekend she was invited to a wine-tasting evening of red Bordeaux. No one smoked at the tasting, yet the following morning Jean became particularly wheezy, and realised that smoke could not be to blame. Jean experimented with various wines, and discovered that her wheezing was triggered by red varieties only. She stopped drinking red wine, and no longer suffers from 'Sunday-morning asthma'.

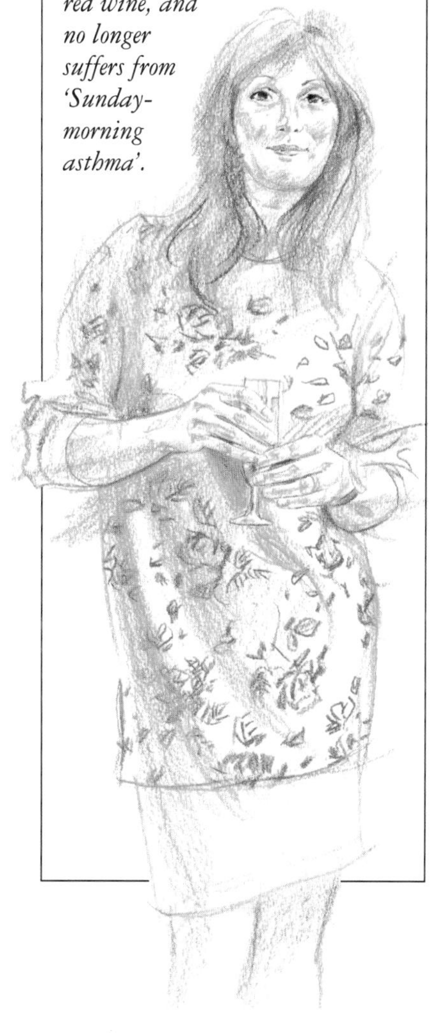

not obvious when such foods are served in delicatessens or restaurants, where of course they do not have any labels.

Sulphites are used in cider, beers and wines, but in Britain no labelling is required. These products may pose a risk for susceptible asthmatics when, for instance, they inhale the bouquet of a wine. Perhaps as a result of bacterial activity during production, some wines also contain levels of histamine that may occasionally prompt asthmatic reactions in susceptible people.

Benzoate preservatives, which are present in a range of products from soft drinks and reduced-calorie jams to chewing gum and fish roe, may bring on asthmatic attacks. Other potential triggers include the less common antioxidant additives – the gallates (E310-12), butylated hydroxyanisole (BHA or E320), and also butylated hydroxytoluene (BHT or E321) – which are used in certain fats and oils, as well as in some breakfast cereals.

In susceptible people, the food colourings E102 (tartrazine, yellow), E104 (quinoline yellow) and E110 (sunset yellow) may also trigger asthma. Under EU legislation the presence of all these additives must be indicated on food labels.

Did you know?

- There are now 200 million asthma sufferers throughout the world, including more than 2 million adults in the UK. One in seven British schoolchildren is asthmatic.
- According to two long-term Australian surveys published in 1994, two-thirds of asthmatic children outgrew the disease by adulthood, especially those with milder symptoms.
- Rates of asthma are five times higher in the developed world than in developing countries. Reasons given by the World Health Organisation are increased exposure to dust mites, which thrive in centrally heated environments, and car exhaust fumes: minute particles, known as pm10s, which are concentrated in diesel exhausts, are inhaled and lodge deep in the lungs where they irritate the sensitive lining.
- Recent research is now beginning to suggest that a high intake of polyunsaturated oils – found in margarines, for example – may predispose some people to asthma.

HELPFUL FOODS

Foods containing the B vitamins, for example leafy green vegetables and pulses, may help asthmatics whose attacks are provoked by stress. There is also some evidence that asthmatics may have a tendency to be deficient in niacin and vitamins B_6 and C.

Antioxidants – which include vitamin A from foods such as liver; beta carotene from brightly-coloured fruit and vegetables such as apricots, carrots and red or yellow peppers, and dark green leafy vegetables such as spinach; vitamin C from citrus fruits; and vitamin E from soya beans and olive oil – may strengthen the lungs' defences by mopping up FREE RADICALS. These potentially harmful substances are generated as part of an asthmatic's inflammatory response to air pollution or allergens.

Magnesium, found in fish, green vegetables, sunflower seeds and dried figs, may help by relaxing the airways. A British study carried out at the University of Nottingham in 1994 suggested that people with low levels of magnesium were more susceptible to asthma attacks.

Current research also suggests that fatty fish such as salmon, mackerel, herring, sardines and cod may help to protect against asthma. They are a rich source of the omega-3 fatty acids, which are thought to have an anti-inflammatory effect.

Before the appropriate drugs were available, asthmatics sometimes took coffee to reduce the effects of attacks. Caffeine is chemically similar to theophylline, used in some medications to dilate the bronchial tubes and assist breathing. In emergencies, two cups of strong coffee should bring relief within 2 hours, with the effects lasting for up to 6 hours. However, coffee, tea and caffeine-containing cola drinks should be avoided by those taking theophylline as the combined effect can be toxic. A high intake of caffeine is also inadvisable if your attacks are triggered by anxiety.

ATHEROSCLEROSIS

EAT PLENTY OF

- *Fruit and vegetables*
- *Oily fish such as herring, mackerel, sardines and salmon*

CUT DOWN ON

- *Saturated fats*
- *Boiled and percolated coffee*
- *Eggs*

AVOID

- *Obesity*
- *Physical inactivity*
- *Smoking*

As we age, our arteries become furred up and harden, a process known as atherosclerosis. This nodular hardening of the arteries is associated with a fatty deposit called atheroma (the Greek for porridge) on the walls of the arteries. It takes hold slowly over many decades, but occurs more quickly among smokers and people with high CHOLESTEROL levels. By the time they have reached their late forties, most men in the industrial West are affected by atherosclerosis. Women are relatively free during their reproductive years when oestrogen keeps their blood cholesterol levels low. However, after the menopause atherosclerosis can often develop quite rapidly.

CAUSES AND SYMPTOMS

Because hardened arteries are less elastic and do not distend easily, blood pressure within them increases and as a result the flow of blood to the tissues is impaired. If the coronary arteries are badly affected, chest pains associated with angina and other forms of HEART DISEASE may develop.

Most heart attacks and strokes among the elderly are caused by atherosclerosis. This results from the accumulation of low density lipoprotein (LDL) – the lipoprotein that carries cholesterol in the blood – in cells called macrophages in the artery wall. Macrophages are cells that mop up cellular debris. Normally they do not take up LDL, but if LDL is oxidised they gobble it up and become so engorged with cholesterol that they form fatty streaks on the artery wall.

Most of these fatty streaks disappear with time, but some of them change into fibrous growths or plaques. This is often caused by the death of macrophages in the fatty streaks. The dying macrophages send out chemical signals that result in scars forming.

Whereas high blood levels of LDL accelerate fatty-streak formation, high blood levels of high density lipoprotein (HDL) will retard it. HDL helps to remove cholesterol from fatty streaks and take it back to the liver.

KEEPING ARTERIES HEALTHY

Giving up smoking and avoiding foods that raise blood LDL levels helps to prevent atherosclerosis. It is important to limit saturated fats, such as dairy products and fatty meats, and foods such as eggs, which are high in dietary cholesterol. Drinking a lot of coffee should also be avoided because it can contribute to high cholesterol levels. This was previously thought to be due to the caffeine content, but is now linked to kahweol and cafestol, two substances found in coffee oil which are now known to increase cholesterol levels substantially. However, they are found only in coffee that has been percolated or left to stand, so that filter and instant coffee can be safely drunk, even by people suffering from coronary problems.

The adoption of a diet that is low in saturated fats and high in polyunsaturated and monounsaturated fats, fresh fruit and vegetables can lead to some regression of atherosclerosis. One theory proposes that the natural antioxidants which are present in fruit and vegetables can help to protect against the disease because they prevent the oxidation of LDL. Although more impressive results have been obtained from drugs that lower cholesterol, these may cause side effects, including depression and, in rare cases, even suicidal tendencies.

Another theory suggests that eating plenty of oily fish, such as mackerel, herring, salmon, sardines, trout and fresh tuna, is beneficial because the omega-3 fatty acids they contain prevent the thickening of the artery walls. There are also studies showing that the consumption of foods high in omega-3 fatty acids increases the elasticity of the arteries, thereby allowing them to distend.

Although excessive alcohol consumption should be avoided, drinking an occasional glass of wine or spirits can be beneficial. It will increase the level of HDL in the blood and as a consequence probably help to protect against the development of atherosclerosis. However, taking regular exercise offers the best protection of all.

AUBERGINE (EGGPLANT)

BENEFIT

- *Low in calories (if baked)*

DRAWBACK

- *Large amounts of fat may be absorbed during preparation and cooking*

The glossy purple aubergine is a familiar component of Indian curries, Greek moussakas and French ratatouille. The raw vegetable contains 15 Calories per 100g (3½oz), but its calorific value rises steeply when it is fried: the same portion cooked in oil contains more than 300 Calories because of the extraordinary amounts of fat absorbed.

The tastiest aubergines are young and firm – about 5-8cm (2-3in) in diameter, with a shiny smooth skin and a fresh green stem and cap. Larger, older specimens can sometimes be woody and bitter. Miniature, white and mauve varieties are also available.

Although young, sweet aubergines may not require it, some recipes call for salting the aubergine before cooking to draw out the bitter juices and reduce the moisture. This makes the flesh more dense so that less fat is absorbed during cooking.

When preparing aubergines, slice or cube them with a stainless-steel knife (carbon steel will blacken the flesh) and then sprinkle with salt. Leave for 30 minutes to draw out the juices. Carefully rinse off all the salt, squeeze or pat dry the slices with kitchen paper and cook as soon as possible before the flesh discolours.

Oriental origins

The aubergine is native to India, but was also a common food in China as long ago as 600 BC, when it was called the Malayan purple melon. Chinese ladies of the time used it as a beauty aid, staining their teeth black with a dye made from its skin. The first varieties that English-speakers came across probably bore egg-shaped fruits – hence its other name of eggplant.

UNCHARTED POWERS?

The aubergine was both prized and feared when it was introduced to Spain by Arab traders during the Middle Ages. For centuries it was valued only as an exotic ornament in Europe because eating it was thought to provoke bad breath, madness, leprosy and even cancer.

In African folk medicine, however, the aubergine has long been used to treat epilepsy and convulsions. In South-east Asia it is still used to treat measles and stomach cancer, although there is no scientific evidence that supports its use as a cancer treatment.

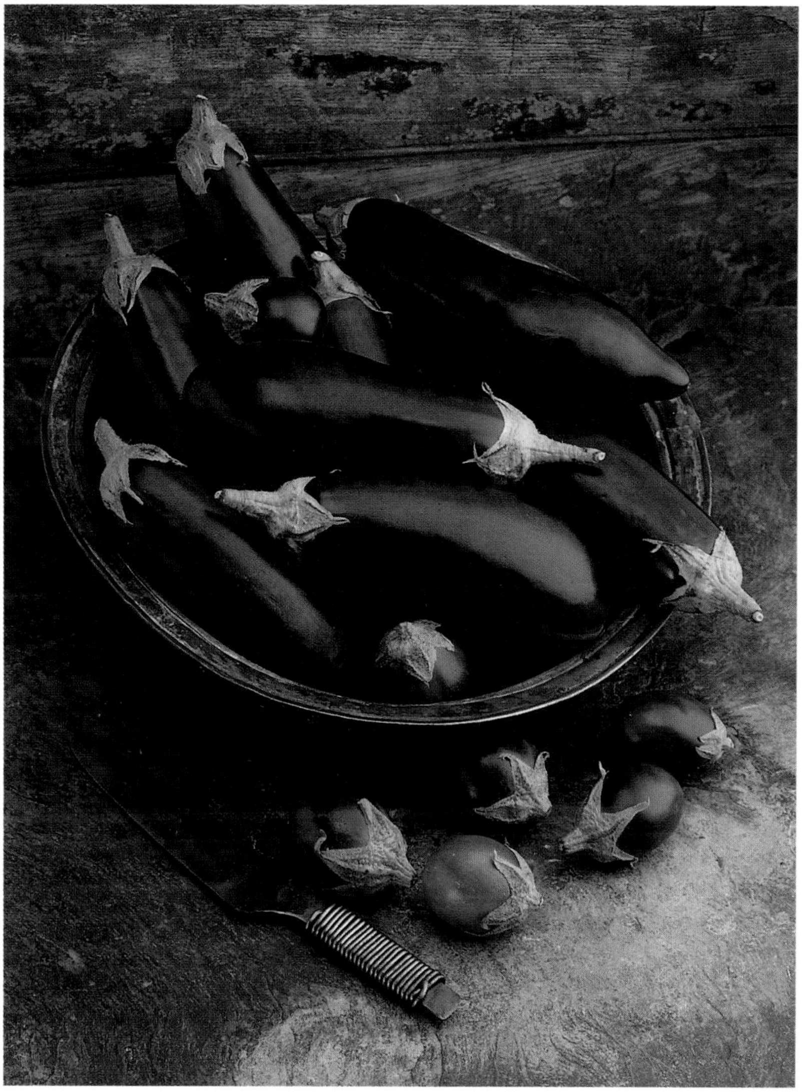

EASTERN PROMISE *Long and pear-shaped, oval or round, glossy purple aubergines are widely used in Asian, Middle Eastern and Mediterranean cuisines.*

AUTISM

EAT PLENTY OF

- *Foods that make up a balanced diet, including fruit, vegetables, poultry, fish, beans, pulses and nuts*

This fairly common – but not always recognised – developmental disorder affects up to 1 in 2500 people. It should become apparent in the first three years of life. Autism is a perplexing, life-long mental disability that is believed to be caused by brain damage rather than by emotional trauma. The condition impairs a child's natural instinct to communicate and form relationships, and the child usually withdraws into an isolated world of his or her own. There is either a lack of language development, or a loss of speech skills that have already developed.

There is no definite proof that diet plays a role in causing autism, or that any diet can cure it. Some autistic children and adults have abnormal diets because of faddy eating patterns, but surveys show that autistic people are not usually undernourished.

Although it has been found that most children with behaviour problems are not particularly affected by diet, some parents may notice that a particular food or drink does make their child's behaviour worse. A normal diet contains several things that can affect brain chemistry. Caffeine, for example, found in tea, coffee and certain soft drinks, has an effect upon the behaviour of many children, and tends to worsen irritability and restlessness.

If you suspect that a particular food upsets your child (according to the National Autistic Society, apples, oranges and tomatoes are frequently cited by parents as causing marked behaviour problems), keep a diary of your child's diet. Make a note of whether he or she has had any of the suspect food, then remove it from the diet, checking ingredient lists to see whether it is included in any processed foods. If after a month the diet has had no effect, the food can be given again. Be aware, however, that restricting the intake of certain foods can also exacerbate the condition.

The most important dietary consideration for children with autism is that they should have a balanced intake of different kinds of food (see BALANCING YOUR DIET).

DIETARY EXPERIMENTS

Recent experiments with vitamin therapy have shown that high doses of certain vitamins – particularly vitamin B_6 – can have a helpful effect on behaviour. However, vitamin therapy should never be undertaken without medical supervision, and it cannot be fully recommended until there have been controlled clinical trials.

AVOCADOS

BENEFITS

- *A rich source of vitamin E*
- *Good source of potassium*
- *High in monounsaturated fats*

DRAWBACK

- *High in calories*

The flesh of a ripe avocado is as good for you as it tastes. It is a rich source of vitamin E, and a good source of potassium. It has useful amounts of vitamin B_6, and also supplies vitamin C, riboflavin and manganese. Vitamins C and E are both ANTIOXIDANTS and can therefore help to prevent the free radical damage that might lead to certain cancers.

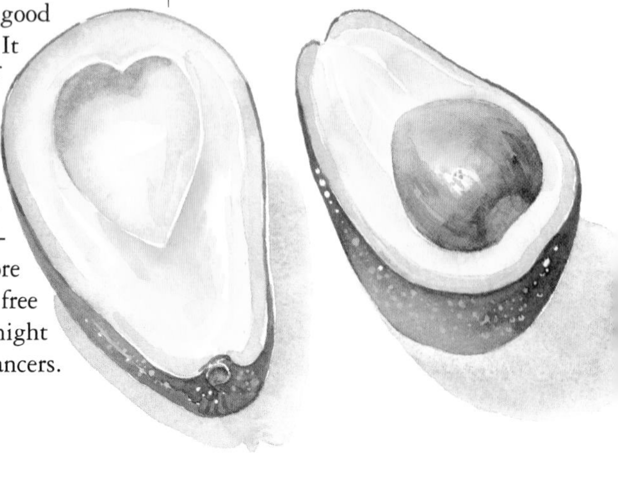

Did you know?

- The avocado has the highest protein content of any fruit. However, some Californian varieties derive more than 80 per cent of their calories from fat.
- Although the Spanish noted the existence of the avocado as early as 1519, it was dismissed as tasteless until it began to become popular in 20th-century America.
- Avocados can be round or pear-shaped, no bigger than a hen's egg or weighing several pounds. They also come in a range of colours, from dark green and crimson to yellow or almost black.
- Unlike most fruits, avocados start to ripen only when they have been cut from the tree. If you buy an unripe fruit, store it at room temperature for a few days.

Potassium helps to control blood pressure as well as maintain a regular heartbeat and a healthy nervous system. Vitamin B_6 is important for the normal functioning of the nervous system. Low levels of B_6 may also be associated with morning sickness.

Like olive oil, avocados have a high content of monounsaturated fatty acids, which are thought to lower blood cholesterol levels. But weight watchers should beware: avocados may contain up to 400 Calories per fruit.

B

BABIES AND FOOD

See page 40

BACKACHE

EAT PLENTY OF
- *Oily fish*
- *Cabbage, guava, papaya and kiwi fruit for their vitamin C*

CUT DOWN ON
- *Coffee, tea and other drinks containing caffeine*
- *Fat and sugar if you are overweight*

Damage to spinal discs, pressure on nerves, misalignment or inflammation of joints, damaged ligaments, or diseased vertebrae can all lead to backache. Other common causes include pregnancy, a bad sitting posture, a bed which does not support your body correctly, a job which involves lifting heavy objects, or suddenly taking up a new sporting activity. A good chiropractor or osteopath should be able to cure most forms of backache, but in the long term a healthy diet may prevent it occurring in the first place.

There are no nutritional 'cures' for backache, though the increased strain that OBESITY puts on the spine may contribute to the problem and a sensible programme of diet and exercise to lose weight may help to ease the pain.

By ensuring that your diet contains all the nutrients needed for healthy bones and muscles you can also reduce the risks of developing back problems. Protein helps to build up the strong muscle tissue that your back needs, while B vitamins, particularly niacin, strengthen and nourish nerve tissues.

Liver and oily fish, such as sardines, mackerel and salmon, are good sources of niacin and vitamin D, which aids the body's absorption of calcium and is important in developing and maintaining healthy bones and nerves. A twice weekly 100g (3½ oz) helping of any oily fish will provide you with the equivalent of the recommended weekly intake of both these vitamins, while the fatty acids that the fish contain can help to suppress inflammation, and so reduce pains in the joints.

Cabbage, guavas, papaya and kiwi fruit are all excellent sources of vitamin C, needed for the development and maintenance of strong bones and a healthy nervous system. The daily recommended intake of vitamin C for an adult is 40mg – this is about as much as you would get from eating two portions of cabbage, a mango, a small papaya or half a guava. However, smokers need twice this amount.

If you are suffering from backache it is wise to cut down on coffee and tea and any other drink containing caffeine as this relatively mild stimulant narrows the smallest blood vessels at the tip of the arteries. This reduces the flow of blood and nutrients carried in the blood to the spinal tendons, which may slow the healing process.

Joints need to keep moving to stay healthy. So whether you want to relieve back pain now or help to prevent it in the future, one of the best things you can do is to keep active.

Persistent backache is a common problem, especially with increasing age. But it is important to consult your doctor for a proper diagnosis, as the pain could be the symptom of a more serious disorder, such as osteoporosis or, in rare cases, cancer.

Case study

Claud, a 55-year-old newsagent, had been suffering persistent pain in his lower back. Recently the pain had begun to spread down his right leg and it was made worse by bending forwards. An examination by his doctor identified the main causes as Claud's weight problem and the awkward way in which he lifted heavy bundles of newspapers at work. Claud's doctor advised him to cut out alcohol and to stick to three meals a day, but to eat smaller portions. He also advised Claud take some exercise – just enough to work up a slight sweat – for 20 minutes three times a week. Claud has lost about 12kg (2 stone) in nine months. He has also been shown how to lift heavy objects properly, keeping his back straight and knees bent – to allow his legs to take the strain. Claud has nearly reached his target weight and his backache has almost gone.

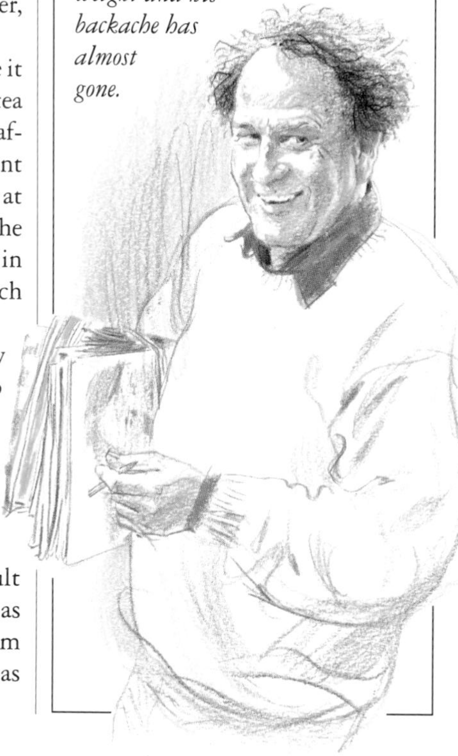

BABIES AND FOOD

First-class nourishment is the best start any parent can give a baby. Nutrients absorbed in the first few months help to ensure healthy development and set the pattern for future well-being.

A mother's milk is the natural nourishment for her newborn baby. Even if the baby is bottle-fed later on, there are great advantages in breastfeeding for the first few days and, if possible, for the first four months. Colostrum, the relatively clear, thin pre-milk secreted just after a mother gives birth, is rich in antibodies which increase a baby's immunity to disease. The mother's breasts then produce thicker mature milk which can supply the baby's complete nutritional needs for up to six months and further boost resistance to infection.

Breast milk is composed of fine digestible globules and contains all the proteins, vitamins and minerals that babies require. It also provides essential polyunsaturated fatty acids which are important components of the human brain and nervous system.

While formula milks can largely replicate these nutrients, natural breast milk does have a unique built-in meal format. As the baby starts suckling, the milk is high in water and protein but as suckling continues, the balance alters: protein and water decrease, and fat content increases. So first the baby's thirst is quenched and then the appetite is satisfied.

For those who can and wish to breastfeed, breast milk is a free, portable and hygienic baby food. There is no need for special equipment or to mix and warm feeds in the middle of the night. Medical evidence also suggests that women who have breastfed have a slightly lower chance of developing breast cancer, especially if they are under 30 years old.

WHY BREASTFEED?

- Breastfed babies suffer fewer respiratory and gastrointestinal diseases than bottle-fed babies.
- They are less prone to allergies, asthma, eczema and colic.
- Breast milk is always at the right temperature.
- According to recent studies, women who breastfeed have a slightly lower risk of developing premenopausal breast cancer.

NOURISH THE MOTHER

A nursing mother must continue to eat the high quality foods recommended during PREGNANCY in order to establish lactation and to maintain an adequate supply of her breast milk.

A deficient diet will not normally upset the nutrient content of her milk but it can reduce the quantity of milk produced, and may affect the mother's health. This is because the body draws on the mother's own reserves of nutrients to achieve the proper breast milk composition if her diet does not supply them.

Current government recommendations suggest that a nursing mother should increase the vitamin and mineral content in her daily diet to a substantial degree.

For instance, women who are not breastfeeding require about 700mg of calcium per day. To ensure that the growing baby has healthy bones and teeth, and to maintain her own calcium supply, the nursing mother requires a daily

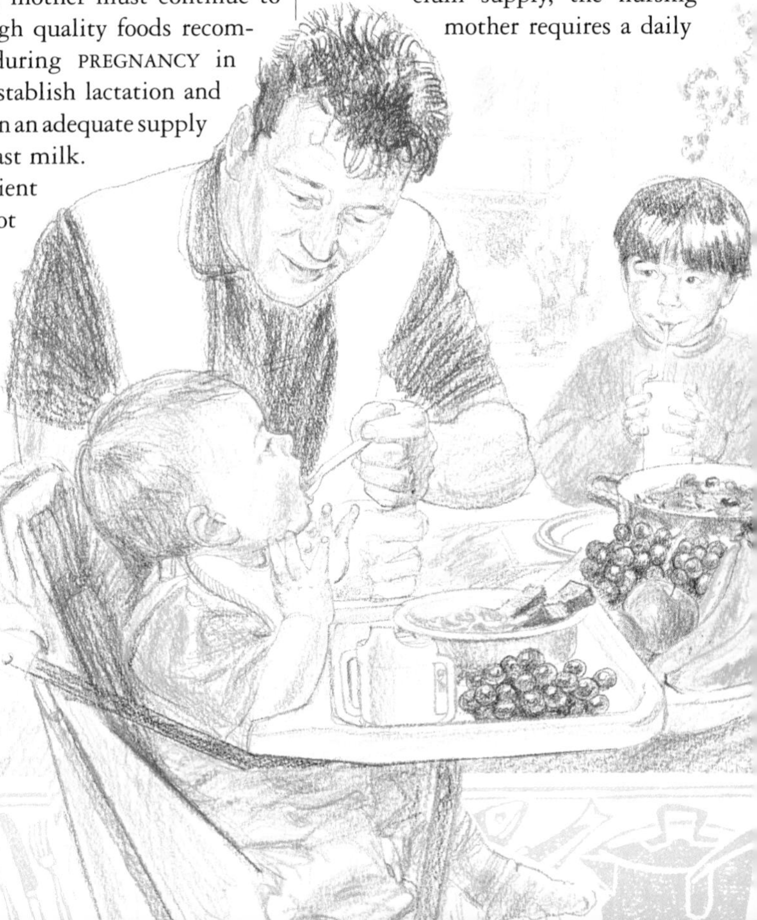

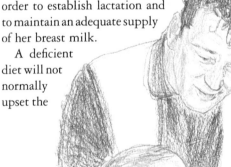

intake of about 1250mg – equivalent to 1.2 litres (2 pints) of milk or about 170g (6oz) of Cheddar cheese.

A diet which includes plenty of fresh fruit and vegetables, dairy products, oily fish, lean meat, pulses, nuts and whole grains such as wholemeal bread and brown rice should supply all the extra vitamins, minerals, protein and energy required.

A breastfeeding mother produces around 500ml (⅞ pint) of milk a day in the early months and up to 800ml (1⅓ pints) in later lactation and therefore needs to drink plenty of fluids – around 2.3 litres (4 pints) is suggested – preferably water, milk and diluted fruit juices.

Bottle-feeding

Mothers choose to bottle-feed, rather than breastfeed, for a variety of reasons. They may need to return to work soon after the birth, or they may be taking essential medication which is dangerous to breastfeeding infants. For both partners, it can often prove a highly positive choice, giving the mother a break and the father a chance to interact with his child.

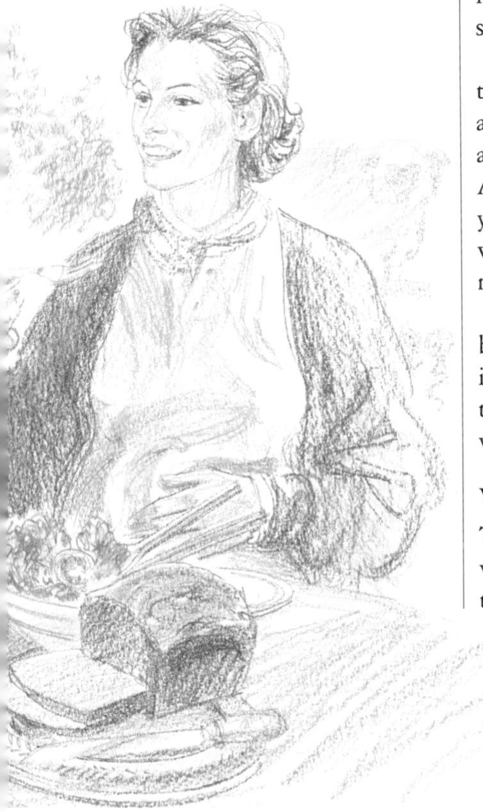

FIRST MOUTHFULS *Family mealtimes around the table give a newly weaned infant the opportunity to experience a variety of new tastes and food textures.*

Manufactured formula milk is designed to provide all the nutrients, vitamins and minerals that babies need. Like breast milk, it should be given for at least six months and preferably for the first year. Most formula milks contain the same basic nutrients; in Britain, the composition of all brands is standardised under Department of Health and European Union regulations.

When preparing formula, follow the manufacturer's instructions precisely. Do not be tempted to pacify a hungry baby by adding an extra scoop of formula, cereals or rusk to make the milk more concentrated as this raises the sodium content in the feed which increases the baby's thirst and could, in some cases, also cause dehydration.

Be meticulous about sterilising bottles and teats. If you mix formula in advance, keep it in the refrigerator, and then for no longer than 24 hours. Always examine it before you feed your baby; formula milk smells sour when it goes off and stale formula does not mix when shaken.

If the baby does not drink the entire bottle, throw away what is left; this is important because air blown back through the teat contains bacteria which can contaminate the milk.

Weaning

Today, most paediatricians advocate weaning at four to six months old, and then introducing new foods gradually – one by one – over the following year. Infants who are weaned too early may suffer dietary deficiencies as the milk is displaced by weaning foods; they may also be more prone to allergies. Initially, the nutritional balance of the solid foods a baby starts to eat is not particularly important as breast or formula milk still supplies the bulk of the nourishment required.

First helpings

The first solids fed to a baby must be easy to digest and unlikely to provoke an allergic reaction. Most mothers start with baby rice softened with breast milk or formula milk and fed

BREASTFEEDING ADVICE

Breast milk can be adversely affected by what a nursing mother eats and drinks.

- Alcohol passes into breast milk and can make a baby sleepy and unable to suckle efficiently; an occasional drink, however, may help to relax a mother and will not harm the baby.
- Caffeine in tea, coffee and cola may affect breast milk; it may make babies nervous and irritable, and upset their sleep pattern. Its diuretic effect can also drain the mother's body just when she needs extra fluid for milk production.
- Most drugs, including nicotine, reach babies through breast milk; ideally a nursing mother should not smoke or take any drugs. She should always consult her doctor before taking any medication.

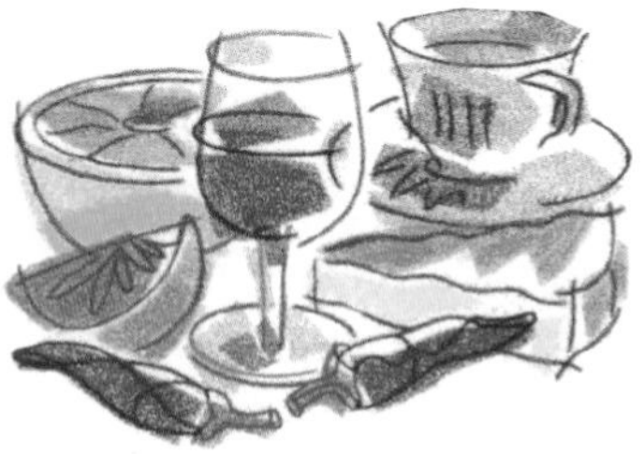

from a spoon. This can be followed by the gradual introduction of sieved or puréed fruits and vegetables. (Spinach, turnip and beetroot should be avoided, however, until the baby is at least six months old as these contain nitrates which can, in rare instances, cause a form of anaemia in very young babies.)

Cooked pulses, such as lentils or soya beans, that are put through a sieve (not a blender, which will not remove the potentially harmful husks) can then be added to the diet, followed by puréed meat such as chicken. Salt should never be added to baby food; an excess can cause dehydration.

Eggs (which should be well cooked), wheat-based cereals, bread, fish and cheese may be introduced between six and nine months to increase both the amount and variety of foods in the diet. It is best to avoid spicy foods, as these can irritate the digestive tract and cause diarrhoea. It may be worthwhile keeping a weaning diary to record each food the baby eats and to monitor any adverse effects which may indicate a food intolerance. Stomach upsets or a sneezy cold may regularly follow the times the baby ate eggs or bananas, for example.

It is also recommended that babies should not drink cow's milk until they are 12 months old, mainly because it is low in iron. As an alternative to breast milk, after the age of four months, a 'follow-on' formula is preferred. Young children should not be given skimmed and semi-skimmed milk because they lack vitamins A and D and contain too few calories.

Weaning heralds the appearance of teeth which is traditionally the time for giving rusks although these are by no means essential. Rusks are usually made of wheat flour which may provoke a food intolerance, and even so-called 'low-sugar' rusks are highly sweetened and contain salt. Chewing on solid foods does help the teething process; some parents give chunks of raw apple or peeled carrot, for instance. Never let children eat unattended in case they choke.

A wide range of plastic teething aids is also available; the liquid-filled versions which can be chilled in the refrigerator are very soothing and have the added advantage of not coating new teeth with sugar and starch.

At this time, it is important not to give a child habit-forming sugary drinks – they contain few useful nutrients and can lead to tooth decay. Sugar appears on labels in many guises: as glucose, fructose, honey, dextrose or sucrose. Avoid artificially sweetened sugar-free drinks: there is no need to restrict the calorie intake of a young child or encourage a sweet tooth; the diet should be as free of additives as possible. The best drink to quench a child's thirst is water – preferably boiled; babies drink it quite happily if it is given regularly from an early age.

COMMERCIAL BABY FOODS

Manufactured baby foods are quick and easy to prepare although many people prefer to feed their babies with home-cooked food. Manufacturers offer gluten-free foods, pure fruit purées and baby juices; most contain no salt and little or no sugar. Commercial baby foods are prepared under carefully controlled conditions to ensure that they are perfectly safe.

- Do not use an opened stored jar of food if it looks watery or smells odd, and transfer canned foods into covered dishes before storing.
- Never feed your baby straight from the jar and then store any remaining food, as saliva on the spoon will encourage bacterial growth on the leftovers.

Case study

When three-month-old Simon was weaned from breastfeeding to a cow's milk formula, he developed diarrhoea and dermatitis. Switching his feed to a soya milk formula seemed to help. However, at the age of eight months, cow's milk was reintroduced into Simon's diet, and the baby again developed diarrhoea so his parents assumed that this was the culprit food. Simon was referred to a consultant paediatrician who was not convinced that Simon had an allergy. He suggested that after a few weeks back on the soya milk formula, the baby should be fed a teaspoonful of cow's milk and if he suffered no further adverse symptoms, cow's milk should be added gradually to his diet. By the time he celebrated his first birthday, Simon was enjoying a diet which included cow's milk – with no ill effects.

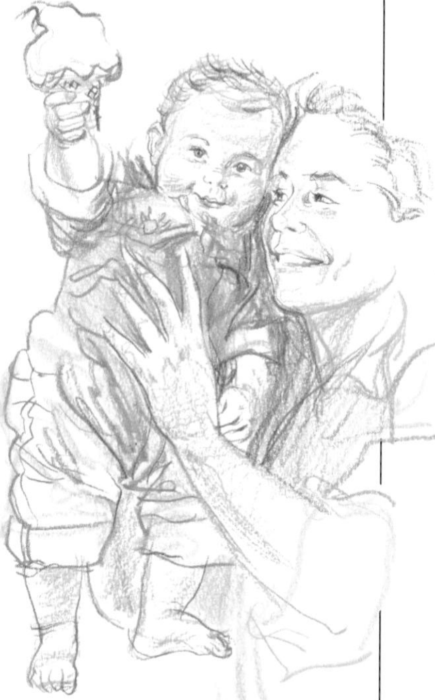

Weaning: introducing new foods in the first year

The Department of Health advises that the majority of infants should not be given solid foods before the age of four months, and a mixed diet should be offered by the age of six months. It is vitally important to supervise infants' mealtimes, because of the risk of choking, or of falling out of a high-chair. Semi-solid foods should be fed from a spoon, and not mixed with milk or any other drink fed from a bottle or feeder cup. Try to introduce a cup from about six months.

MILK AND DAIRY	STARCHY FOODS	VEGETABLES AND FRUIT	MEAT AND MEAT ALTERNATIVES	OCCASIONAL FOODS
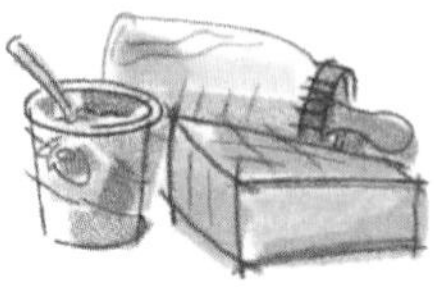		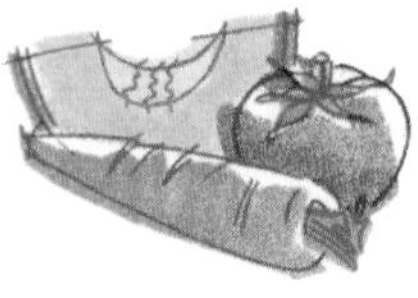	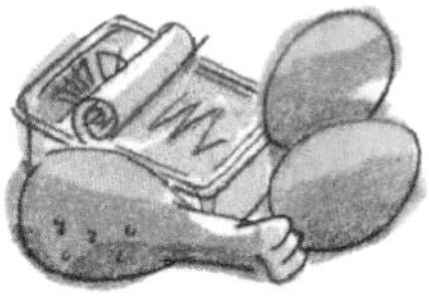	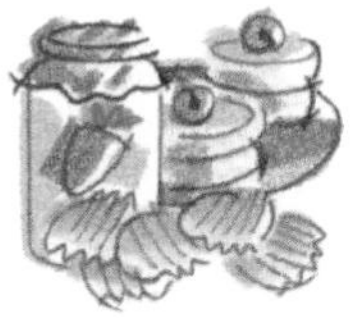
4-6 MONTHS				
Minimum 600ml (1 pint) breast or infant formula daily Cow's milk products, such as yoghurt, custard and cheese sauce, can be used after 4 months.	**Introduce after 4 months** Smooth cereal mixed with milk; use low-fibre cereals, such as rice based ones. Mash or purée starchy vegetables.	**Introduce after 4 months** Soft-cooked fruit and vegetables sieved into a smooth purée. Blended foods will usually contain indigestible residues.	**Introduce after 4 months** Soft-cooked meat or pulses. Add no salt or sugar to food during or after cooking.	Choose low-sugar desserts; avoid high-salt foods and puddings containing artificial colours or sweeteners. Try fromage frais with puréed fruit.
6-9 MONTHS				
500-600ml (about 1 pint) breast milk, infant formula or follow-on formula daily Also use any milk to mix with solids. Hard cheese, such as Cheddar, can be used as 'finger food'.	**2-3 servings daily** Start to introduce some wholemeal bread and cereals. Foods can have a more solid, 'lumpier' texture. Begin to give 'finger foods', such as toast.	**2 servings daily** Raw soft fruit and vegetables, such as banana, melon and tomato, may be used as 'finger foods'. Cooked vegetables and fruit can be a coarser, mashed texture.	**1 serving daily** Soft-cooked minced or puréed chicken, or meat, fish or pulses. Chopped hard-boiled egg can be used as a 'finger food'.	Encourage savoury foods rather than sweet ones. Fruit juices are not necessary – try to restrict them to mealtimes; they can be diluted with four parts boiled water; or just offer water.
9-12 MONTHS				
500-600ml (about 1 pint) breast milk or infant milks daily Also use any milk to mix with solids but do not give cow's milk on its own as a drink to children under 12 months – it will not provide them with enough iron.	**3-4 servings daily** Encourage wholemeal products; discourage foods with added sugar, such as biscuits and cakes. Starchy foods such as pasta can be of normal adult texture.	**3-4 servings daily** Encourage lightly cooked or raw foods. Chopped or 'finger foods' are most suitable. Offer unsweetened diluted orange juice with meals, especially if the diet is meat-free, to aid iron absorption.	**Minimum 1 serving daily from animal source or 2 from vegetable sources** In a vegetarian diet, use a mixture of different vegetable and starchy foods (macaroni cheese, dhal and rice).	May use moderate amounts of butter (preferably unsalted) and small amounts of jam on bread. Try to limit salty foods or any other food or drink that contains a lot of additives.

Bad breath

TAKE PLENTY OF

- *Raw vegetables and apples to help to protect the gums*
- *Ginger, cinnamon, mustard and horseradish for the sinuses*
- *Wholegrain cereals and water to avoid constipation*
- *Carrots, broccoli, spinach and citrus fruit for beta carotene and vitamin C*

CUT DOWN ON

- *Sugar, sweets, sweet drinks, cakes and biscuits to protect the teeth and gums and reduce plaque*

AVOID

- *Garlic, onions and curry*
- *Alcohol and all tobacco products*

Unless it is caused by illness, halitosis can usually be eliminated by sensible eating habits and thorough oral hygiene. Bad breath is usually a trivial complaint, and it is often caused by curry, garlic, alcohol or cigarettes.

DIGESTIVE DISORDERS and CONSTIPATION can also cause halitosis, and here again a healthy sensible diet can often help. However, it is important to seek professional dental or medical advice if the cause of halitosis is not easily identified or remedied.

Food odours can be avoided by chewing a few dill seeds or a couple of coffee beans after a meal. Caraway and cardamom seeds are also effective, while chewing a sprig of fresh parsley is claimed to rid the breath of garlic and alcohol odours. Regular brushing with a good toothbrush, and eating plenty of fibre-rich foods such as raw vegetables, apples and pears help to massage the gums and keep them healthy. Reduce plaque formation by cutting down on sugary drinks and foods – particularly foods that stick to the teeth – and brush and floss your teeth as regularly as possible.

Breath as a health indicator

Sometimes breath odour can be a key to medical diagnosis – the acetone smell of a diabetic coma, the ammonia smell of uraemia or the fishy smell of liver failure.

But the most common cause of bad breath can usually be found in the mouth – a bad tooth or abscess, a build up of tartar, inflamed and infected gums or rotting food in crevices or mouth ulcers.

A gargle and mouthwash made by adding 30 drops of tincture of myrrh (available from most chemists) to a glass of warm water will help to keep your breath sweet. Patent antiseptic mouthwashes can kill helpful as well as harmful bacteria.

Problems in the mouth, the nose and sinuses, the lungs or the stomach and digestive tract can all lead to bad breath; so can use of the sedative paraldehyde. To relieve sinus problems and catarrh, try reducing your intake of dairy products and eat decongestant spices such as ginger, cinnamon, mustard and horseradish. It may also help to add 5 or 6 drops of eucalyptus oil to a bowl of hot water then inhale the pungent steam.

Chronic chest infections require medical attention, but you can help yourself to avoid them by not smoking and by eating plenty of carrots, broccoli, spinach and citrus fruits for their beta carotene and vitamin C, which help to protect lung tissue.

Constipation, ulcers and indigestion can provoke halitosis. Sucking peppermints or chewing gum may hide it, but it is best to deal with the cause by increasing your fibre and fluid consumption. Try eating wholemeal bread instead of white, eating plenty of fruit and vegetables and drinking a couple of extra glasses of water a day.

Balancing your diet

See page 48

Bananas

BENEFIT

- *High in potassium*

DRAWBACK

- *Cause intestinal wind if unripe*

Healthy, filling and conveniently wrapped, bananas are one of nature's ideal snacks. Bananas are grown in most of the world's tropical areas. They are harvested when still green, and begin to ripen during transportation. Most are still not fully ripe when sold and they should be stored at room temperature until they are ripe. They will then keep in a refrigerator for four or five days if they are wrapped in newspaper. Although the skin may turn dark brown, the flesh should stay fresh, firm and cream-coloured.

Unripe bananas contain 'resistant' starch – so called because it cannot be digested in the small intestine – which then ferments in the large intestine, often causing wind. Because most of the starch content turns to sugar as the fruit ripens, bananas are not only sweeter when ripe, but can also be much more easily digested.

Because ripe bananas are so easy to digest, and rarely cause allergic reactions (though they can trigger migraines in a few adults), they are a popular solid food for babies.

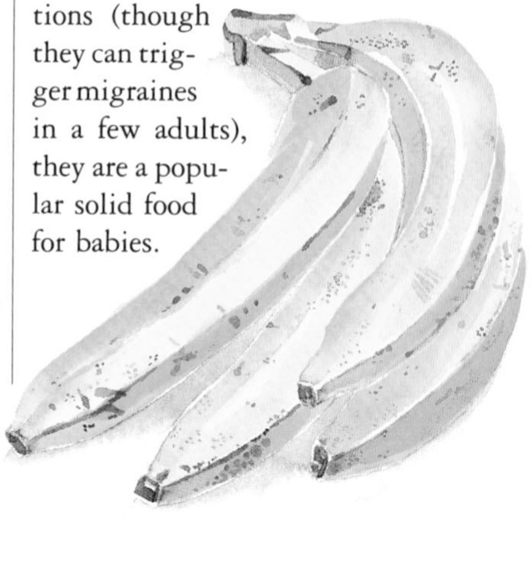

Did you know?

- Weight for weight dried bananas contain about five times more calories than fresh.
- India produces more bananas than any other nation.
- Linford Christie, the Olympic gold-medallist sprinter, includes fried plantain in his breakfast before competing or training.
- In east Africa bananas are fermented to make beer.

They are also good for treating childhood stomach upsets; in the USA, children with diarrhoea are often fed the 'brat' diet – comprising bananas, rice, apple-sauce and toast.

Perhaps the banana's blandness is the reason why many sufferers of stomach ulcers report that it is a soothing food. Several attempts have been made to investigate the medicinal impact of bananas and plantains on stomach ulcers and there have been claims that bananas may stimulate cell and mucus production in the stomach lining; by thickening the stomach walls and sealing its surface, they may help to heal existing ulcers and stave off new ones. However, there is as yet very little evidence to support these claims.

Bananas are a good source of potassium, which is a vital mineral for muscle and nerve function. Potassium also helps to regulate blood pressure.

They also contain a high level of natural sugar in both their fresh and dried form, which they release quickly into the bloodstream. This explains why many athletes, especially tennis players, often eat bananas before, or even during, a competition.

'GREEN BANANAS'

Plantains, which are colloquially known as 'green bananas', are indigestible and unpalatable when eaten raw. Because they are rich in tannin, they can taste bitter, though some of this flavour disappears in cooking.

Plantains contain more starch than bananas because they are eaten before they are fully ripe. Some research has linked low incidence of stomach and bowel cancer with a diet high in indigestible starch. More research is being carried out to investigate this apparent link and to establish whether starch is as important as fibre in helping to ward off cancer of the bowel.

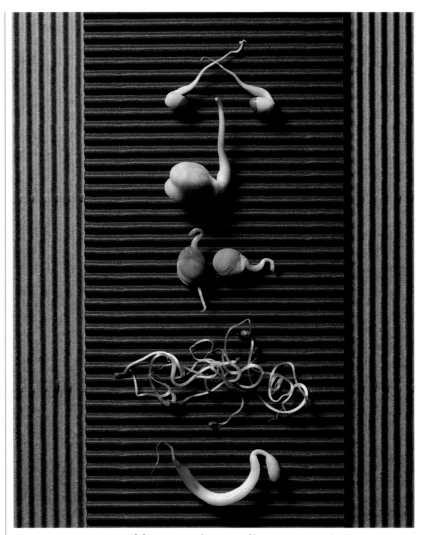

SPROUTING BEANS *Five of the most popular types of bean sprout are (from top to bottom) mung bean, chickpea, green lentil, alfalfa and soya bean.*

BEAN SPROUTS

BENEFITS

- *Good source of vitamin C*
- *Useful source of B complex vitamins*
- *Low in calories*
- *Provide easy-to-digest protein*

DRAWBACK

- *May provoke allergic reactions in some people, particularly those suffering from lupus*

Anyone who enjoys Chinese food is probably familiar with mung sprouts, the most commonly sprouted bean. The translucent white shoots are about 5cm (2in) long with a tapering root and a pale green pod.

Alfalfa (which produce fine, pale green spindly shoots), lentils, aduki beans, chickpeas and soya beans are also used for sprouting. Soya sprouts should be cooked first to destroy the toxic proteins that they contain, and chickpeas must be cooked before they become tender enough to eat.

Unlike most other vegetables, which start to lose their vitamin content as soon as they are picked, bean sprouts continue to grow and to form nutrients. As soon as the bean germinates, all the starches, oils and other nutrients packed into it – to nourish the tiny new plant – begin to turn into vitamins, enzymes and other forms of proteins, minerals and sugars. The vitamin C content of a bean increases a phenomenal 600 times when it starts sprouting. A single helping of fresh-sprouted mung beans contains about three-quarters of the adult daily requirement of vitamin C. Sprouting also substantially increases some of the B vitamins present in the bean, including thiamin, folate, B_6 and biotin.

Germination also uses up the indigestible sugars in the seeds, so bean sprouts produce less intestinal wind than beans which have not sprouted. However, bean sprouts may sometimes produce an allergic reaction in people suffering from lupus.

HOME-GROWN BEAN SPROUTS

As well as being low in calories and packed with vitamins, bean sprouts are easy and cheap to grow at home. Commercial bean-sprouters are available, but jam jars are just as effective.

Pick over the beans to remove any damaged or discoloured ones, then soak the remainder in tepid water overnight or for about 12 hours. Drain, rinse and place them in the jam jars, allowing room for the sprouts to grow. Cover the jars with muslin or cotton tops held in place by elastic bands and leave them somewhere warm and dark (sprouting beans do not flourish in extreme temperatures, and sunlight makes them taste bitter).

Rinse the bean sprouts gently in tepid water two to four times a day. They will be pale green, fresh and ready for eating in two to six days.

> **Can diet help you to stop smoking?**
>
> If you are trying to stop smoking, a diet that is rich in alkaline food may help. Researchers have discovered that while acidic urine rapidly depletes a smoker's nicotine reserves, the urine produced after eating alkaline food – such as bean sprouts, peas or milk – takes less nicotine with it, thus delaying the craving for tobacco.

BEEF

BENEFITS

- *Contains a wide range of nutrients, including valuable minerals, particularly iron and zinc*

DRAWBACKS

- *High intakes are linked to cancer of the colon*
- *Too much beef fat can contribute to heart disease*

Current trends towards vegetarianism, concern about 'mad cow disease' and the possible links between eating red meat and heart disease have led to white meats gradually replacing beef as the major source of animal protein in both Britain and the USA. Nevertheless, the nutritional benefits of beef should not be ignored. With the exception of fibre, beef contains most of the nutrients our bodies need, though some, such as calcium, vitamin C and folate, are present only in small amounts. It is also a valuable source of essential minerals such as iodine, manganese, zinc, selenium, chromium, fluoride and silicon – though the quantities of these can vary substantially, depending on the soil which supported the animal's grazing or on the components of the manufactured feed it consumed.

Due to modern breeding techniques and popular demand, beef is much leaner than it used to be. Lean beef contains less than 5 per cent fat, less than half of which is saturated fat, so that the risk of beef raising cholesterol levels has fallen. Nevertheless, there remains an apparent link between the incidence of cancer of the colon and people whose diets include large amounts of red meat.

The nutritional composition of different sorts of beef varies widely – for example 100g (3½oz) of corned beef contains 950mg of sodium, compared to 320mg in stewed mince, and only 56mg in grilled lean rump steak. The total fat in 100g (3½oz) of corned beef is 12.1g, in mince 15.2g but only 3g in lean rump steak.

THE IMPACT OF COOKING

How beef is prepared and cooked will substantially affect the nutrients that it contains. By simply trimming off excessive visible fat before cooking you can reduce the total fat in the finished dish, which is especially important in stews and casseroles.

Joints should be roasted, raised up on a rack or trivet, so that the fat drips into the pan and can be removed before the residual juices are used to make gravy. You can cook steaks and chops in the same way, grill them or use a frying pan with ridges in the bottom to dry-fry them. Take care when barbecuing beef, too. Overcooking meat on the barbecue often chars or burns bits of the food, forming substances which have been shown to produce mutations in bacteria and may encourage the production of carcinogens. This is particularly so in beef products with a high fat-to-meat ratio such as most sausages and burgers.

BEEFBURGERS AND BACTERIA

The ubiquitous beefburger unfortunately occupies a fairly lowly rung on the nutritional ladder. Commercially produced burgers are often high in fat, additives and preservatives; and many tend to be made with low-quality beef – but a lot depends on the brand.

If a burger is undercooked it can also harbour harmful bacteria. At least one strain of the bacterium *E. coli* can invade meat during slaughtering. This bacterium is a source of many gastric disorders, including bloody diarrhoea which may be accompanied by a high fever that can last anything from one to eight days. When infected meat is minced the bacteria are distributed throughout the finished product and if the resulting burger is cooked rare some of the bacteria may survive. This particular strain of *E. coli* temporarily affects the health of more than 20 000 Americans each year and kills about 50 people a year in Britain. The old, young and weak are particularly at risk from FOOD POISONING.

OFFAL

Ox liver (which was formerly a popular prescription to treat patients suffering from pernicious anaemia) and calves' liver are rich sources of easily absorbed iron and vitamins A and B_{12}.

Kidneys are also an extremely rich source of vitamin B_{12}; a typical serving can provide about 20 times the adult daily requirement. Although liver and kidneys are low in fats, they do contain very high levels of cholesterol; however, these are likely to affect only people whose blood cholesterol levels are already high.

Pregnant women, or those planning to become pregnant, are advised not to eat liver or any liver products such as pâté because the level of vitamin A in liver is so high – between 12230 micrograms and 31700 micrograms per 100g (3½oz). Such huge quantities of vitamin A can adversely affect the baby in the womb and may cause birth defects.

SCARES AND CHEMICALS

A number of scares regarding beef have hit the headlines in recent years. BSE (bovine spongiform encephalitis) otherwise known as 'mad cow disease' is only one of the worries about beef. Another major concern is the illegal use of chemicals in beef farming.

Antibiotics have long been banned as additives to animal feed. And the use of growth-promoting hormones on beef cattle to produce larger amounts of lean meat per animal was banned by the European Union in 1988. However, researchers have found signs that hormones are still being used widely and illegally in many parts of Europe.

Hormones shorten the time that it takes to get animals ready for slaughter. Some of the substances are the same as the drugs used illegally by athletes to increase muscle strength. Animals being fed hormones quickly gain more weight, but with less fat, than untreated animals. Some growth-promoting hormones are still used legally in the USA. However, the ban was introduced in Europe because no one really knows the effect that these hormones have on the health of the animal during its lifetime or on the health of humans who regularly eat meat containing these hormones.

Putting 'mad cow disease' into perspective

BSE (bovine spongiform encephalopathy) or 'mad cow disease', is a slow, ultimately fatal illness that affects cattle, which are usually between three and five years old. First identified in Britain in 1986, BSE is believed to have started when cattle were fed processed offal from sheep suffering from a similar condition called scrapie.

A similar illness affecting the human central nervous system, Creutzfeldt-Jakob disease, kills about 50 people in Britain each year. The illness, which can take 20 years to develop, was present in Britain long before the recent BSE epidemic and there is little evidence that its incidence is increasing. Nevertheless, official assurances that it is impossible for humans to catch BSE have failed to convince many medical experts.

BSE is believed to be passed on only through infected offal, especially the brain and spinal cord. It is now illegal to include these parts of the cow in any food product.

A report on BSE in Britain commissioned by the European Parliament has criticised both modern intensive farming practices and methods of cattle feed manufacture. Feed was being produced not only from normal abattoir waste, but also from sheep carcasses infected with scrapie.

Amazingly, before 1988, the carcasses of cows which had died from BSE were also processed and put back into the food chain as cattle feed. Fortunately the number of cases has fallen rapidly since this practice was banned.

BALANCING YOUR DIET

The athlete who burns up lots of calories and the pensioner enjoying a leisurely retirement are poles apart in their energy requirements, but both need a balanced intake of nutrients to remain healthy.

Three main rules should govern what we eat: food should nourish; it should help to safeguard health and – when necessary – play a role in fighting ailments or disease. It should also look and taste good.

There are no 'good' or 'bad' foods – only good or bad diets. If, for example, you have eaten only fruit and salad all day, a burger with all its trimmings or a large helping of fish and chips may be exactly what your body needs. All foods contain different levels of nutrients, but no single food can provide all the vitamins and minerals our bodies need, in the right amounts.

To maintain health and function efficiently, our bodies need 13 vitamins and 16 minerals as well as fats, carbohydrates and protein. And, although it is not a nutrient, our bodies also need plenty of WATER. By eating a variety of foods in sensible proportions we can obtain optimum levels of every nutrient needed to maintain good health.

HEALTHY PROPORTIONS *For a varied, well-balanced diet choose foods from each level in the same ratio as they appear in the food pyramid.*

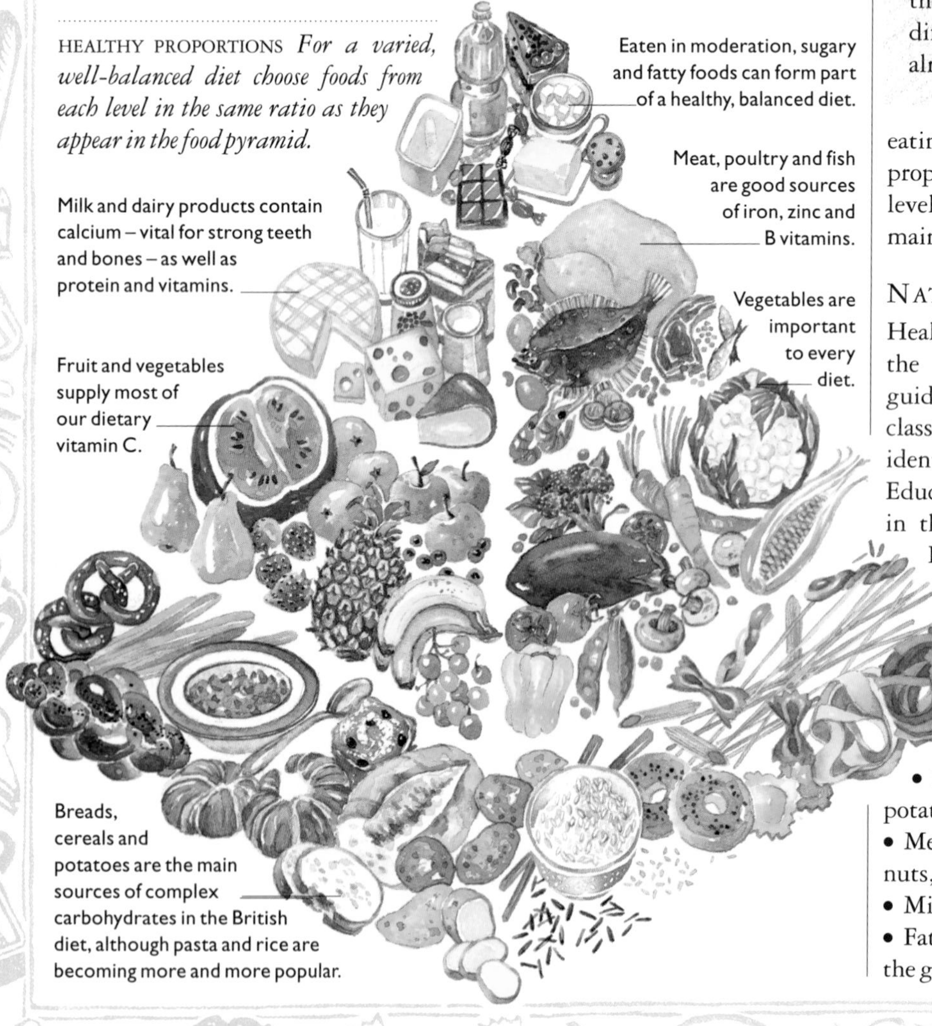
Eaten in moderation, sugary and fatty foods can form part of a healthy, balanced diet.
Meat, poultry and fish are good sources of iron, zinc and B vitamins.
Milk and dairy products contain calcium – vital for strong teeth and bones – as well as protein and vitamins.
Vegetables are important to every diet.
Fruit and vegetables supply most of our dietary vitamin C.
Breads, cereals and potatoes are the main sources of complex carbohydrates in the British diet, although pasta and rice are becoming more and more popular.

THE NUTRIENTS PEOPLE NEED

Nutritional needs vary individually, depending on a variety of factors including age, sex, level of physical activity, metabolic rate and state of health. However, whether a person needs a low daily intake of 1500 Calories or a high intake – around 3000 Calories – the proportions of food from the different food groups should almost always remain the same.

NATIONAL GUIDELINES

Health authorities in both Britain and the United States have drawn up guidelines for healthy eating. These classify foods in groups – five bands are identified by the British Health Education Authority, and six appear in the four-tier US 'food pyramid'. However, the American pyramid differs from the British model only in that it places fruit and vegetables into separate categories. The other four groups – shared by both health authorities – are:

- Bread, cereals such as rice, and potatoes (complex carbohydrates).
- Meat, fish and alternatives such as nuts, pulses and eggs (proteins).
- Milk and dairy foods.
- Fatty and sugary foods (which form the group of simple carbohydrates).

The food groups: finding the path to healthier eating

The ratio of foods which supply our daily needs should reflect the groups in the food pyramid. A balanced diet will include six daily servings of complex carbohydrates; five servings of fruit or vegetables; two servings of milk or yoghurt (including calcium-enriched soya milk); two servings of protein; and 15-25g (½-1oz) of fats and oils.

FOOD GROUPS AND THEIR NUTRIENTS	TRY TO	TRY NOT TO
CARBOHYDRATES		
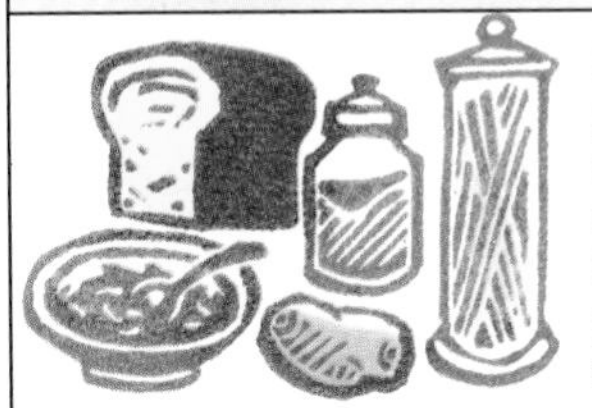 In Britain, bread, cereals and potatoes are the principal sources of nutritious complex carbohydrates (starch), fibre (non-starch polysaccharides), calcium and iron, and the B vitamins.	Choose wholemeal, brown or high-fibre breads, increasing your intake by making sandwiches with thicker slices. Eat bread with your main meals and have a larger helping of potatoes, rice or pasta rather than higher-fat foods.	Fry any of the foods in this group; spread butter or margarine thickly on bread, as this provides unnecessary fat; or add rich, creamy sauces or oily dressings to these foods.
FRUIT		
This group includes fresh, frozen and canned fruits, fruit juice and dried fruit, and provides vitamin C, carotenes, folates and fibre as well as some simple carbohydrates. 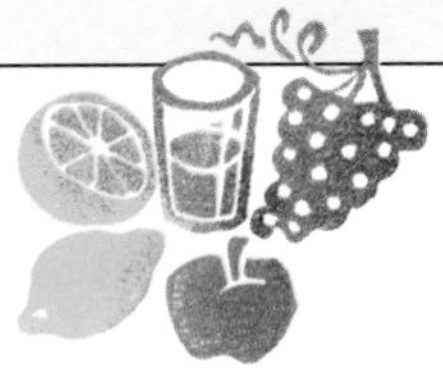	Select a wide variety of fruits, eating more by having fruit for dessert, as a snack, or even accompanied with meat or cheese, as part of a sandwich.	Eat excessive amounts of fruit in one sitting: it may lead to indigestion or an upset stomach, particularly if the fruit is unripe.
VEGETABLES		
These are the backbone of most diets – whether vegetarian or not. They are vital in providing not only vitamins and minerals, but fibre and carbohydrates. 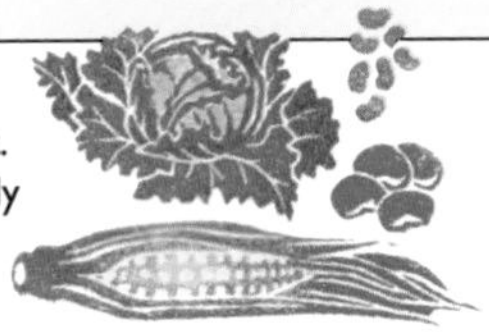	Use tomatoes and other vegetables – fresh or frozen – in sauces, or serve them either as traditional side dishes or with meat or pasta.	Deep-fry vegetables which tend to soak up substantial amounts of fat; stir-frying in a little oil is much healthier.
MILK AND DAIRY PRODUCTS, EXCLUDING BUTTER AND CREAM		
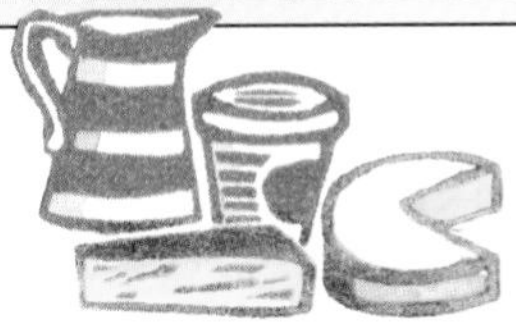 The main nutrients obtained from this group are calcium, magnesium, protein, riboflavin and vitamins B_{12} and A.	Eat moderate amounts of these dairy products, choosing reduced-fat versions – such as semi-skimmed milk or low-fat yoghurt – most of the time.	Consume large amounts of full-fat varieties of cream, milk, cheese and butter. Skimmed milk is as good a source of calcium as whole milk.
MEAT, POULTRY, FISH AND ALTERNATIVES SUCH AS DRIED BEANS, EGGS AND NUTS		
These foods are important sources of the minerals iron and zinc, of protein, and of the B vitamins, especially vitamin B_{12}. 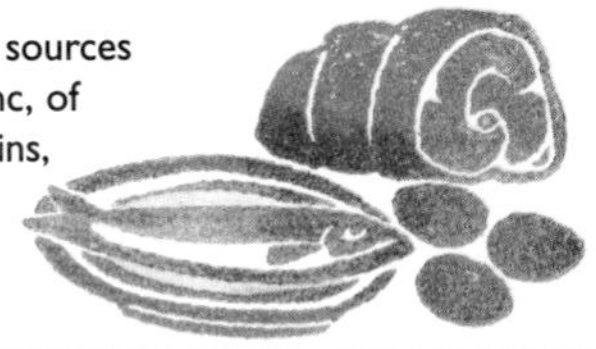	Eat moderate amounts of these foods, choosing lean meat and trimming all visible fat from it. Eat fish at least twice a week, and include a portion of oily fish such as mackerel or salmon.	Fry meat or fish, or add fat to those which are already rich in oils. Grilling, poaching, steaming, stir-frying and oven roasting are all healthier options.
FATTY AND SUGARY FOODS		
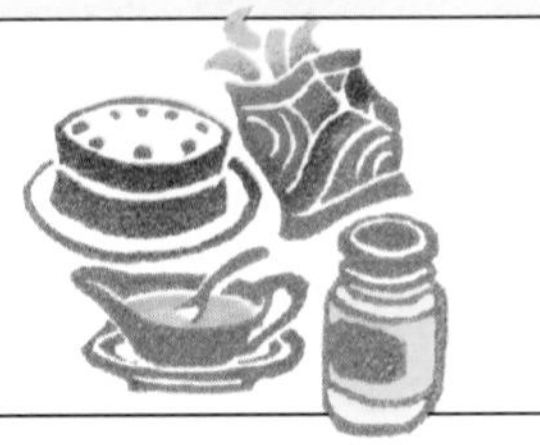 Margarine, butter, other spreading fats, cooking oils, cream, chocolate, crisps, biscuits, pastries, cakes, ice cream, sweets and sugar are part of this group.	Choose lower fat and lower sugar alternatives, eating only small amounts and using spreads and oils sparingly. Skim fat from meat juices when making gravy.	Be tempted to eat more chocolate and other sweet foods at festive times, or fill yourself up with between-meal snacks from this group too often.

Most people who adapt their diets to 'fit' the food pyramid will find that they increase their average intake of complex carbohydrate and cut down on fats, especially saturated fats, and sugar. These simple dietary modifications will help to reduce the risk of heart disease and other diet-related conditions such as diabetes mellitus and some forms of cancer.

ADOPTING THE GUIDELINES

Interpreting official guidelines is not as daunting as it might at first appear. You do not need to apply the recommended balance to every meal or even to every day's meals. You could, for example, achieve it over a period of one or two weeks.

When a food comprises a complete dish or meal – whether pizza, curry, or quiche – its main ingredients determine its place in the pyramid or guide. Quiche, for example, is made mainly from eggs so it falls in the protein category – although the pastry, being a mixture of fat and flour, fits into both the fat and the carbohydrate groups. Pizza is mostly bread dough, so it falls mainly under the carbohydrates grouping; but the toppings – say cheese and tomato – are classified as dairy and vegetable respectively. Beef curry and rice would be grouped under protein and carbohydrate. The failing of all of these 'complete' meals is their lack of vegetables or fruits; accompanying such meals with a mixed salad, peas or broccoli, say, and eating a piece of fresh fruit to follow, would provide a meal with a balance of foods as shown in both the pyramid and the chart.

HOW TO ACHIEVE THE BALANCE

Both the British and the American health authorities offer a range of recommendations for achieving a well-balanced, healthy diet. For most of us, this means a change towards more vegetables, fruit, bread, breakfast cereals, potatoes, rice and pasta.

- Eat regularly and enjoy your meals and snacks.
- Eat a wide variety of foods.
- Eat enough food to maintain a healthy weight.
- Eat plenty of foods rich in starch and fibre.
- Don't eat too much fat.
- Use the pyramid to plan your meals.
- Do not eat sugary foods too frequently.
- Ensure you get plenty of vitamins and minerals in your food.
- If you drink alcohol, keep within sensible limits.
- Use only moderate amounts of salt in cooking.
- Avoid adding salt to food at the table or during preparation.
- Remember that both snacks and meals count towards the balance.

MALNUTRITION CAN AFFECT THE OVERWEIGHT

Even when people eat large amounts of food, they are still likely to suffer from malnutrition if they have an unbalanced diet. And eating too much, as well as throwing the diet out of balance, can cause OBESITY and therefore increase the risk of serious conditions such as high BLOOD PRESSURE, angina, heart disease, diabetes and ARTHRITIS. Britons generally eat more saturated fats and sugar, and less starch and fibre than they should, which has resulted in the United Kingdom having one of the highest rates of coronary heart disease (CHD) in the world.

THE MEDITERRANEAN DIET

Relatively high levels of fish, olive oil, vegetables and fruit help to make the Mediterranean diet so healthy. The Italians, Spaniards and Greeks also eat less meat than the average Briton. Furthermore, they eat less saturated fat and sugar, and more complex carbohydrates such as bread, pasta, rice and potatoes. Extensive research supports the view that the lower death rates from coronary heart disease and some cancers in the Mediterranean region are, at least in part, related to the local diet. The imbalances which

HOW MUCH LIQUID WE NEED

British nutritionists suggest each of us should drink 1.5-2 litres (3-4 pints) of fluid daily to maintain healthy kidneys and prevent urinary infections. The body needs extra liquids when energy expenditure is high, and also in hot weather.

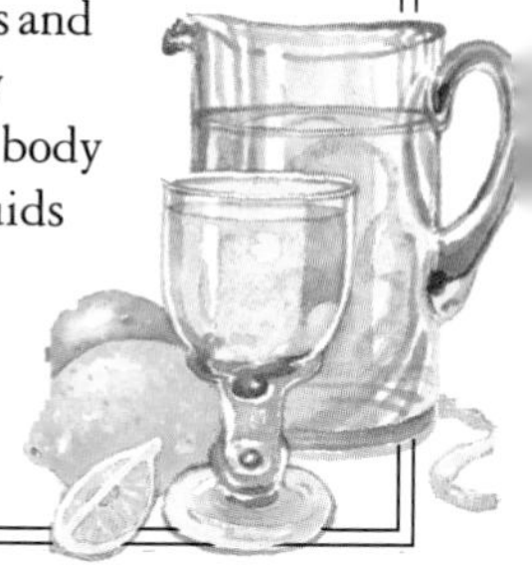

DELICIOUS AND NUTRITIOUS *Eating sensibly need not be dull. These colourful and appetising meals offer the correct balance of nutrients needed for good health.*

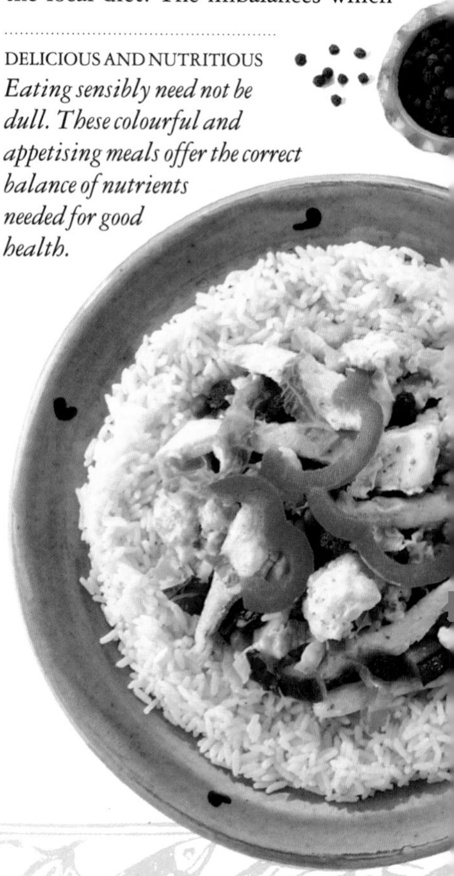

exist in the typical British diet can be rectified, however, simply by following the guidelines on required proportions of basic food groups.

A DIET FOR EVERYONE?

Although the recommended balance of foods applies to most people, including vegetarians, people of all ethnic origins, and those who are overweight, it is not appropriate for everyone. Infants under two, for example, should always be given milk or dairy produce which has not had the fat content reduced, and they also need more dairy foods than adults; but between the ages of two and five – as children make a gradual transition onto family foods – the guidelines begin to apply.

People with special dietary needs and those under medical supervision should check with their doctor to see if this balance of foods is suited to them.

WHAT ABOUT SUPPLEMENTS?

Vitamin and mineral supplements are no substitute for good eating habits, and the majority of people will meet all their nutritional requirements by following the basic guidelines outlined in the chart and food pyramid. A few people do need supplements, however. Women who are planning to conceive or who are already pregnant (see PREGNANCY) need folic acid to protect the embryo from neural tube defects, and may need extra iron; the elderly might require vitamin D and iron; and people with OSTEOPOROSIS are sometimes prescribed supplementary calcium.

Consult a doctor or dietician if you think you need extra vitamins or minerals.

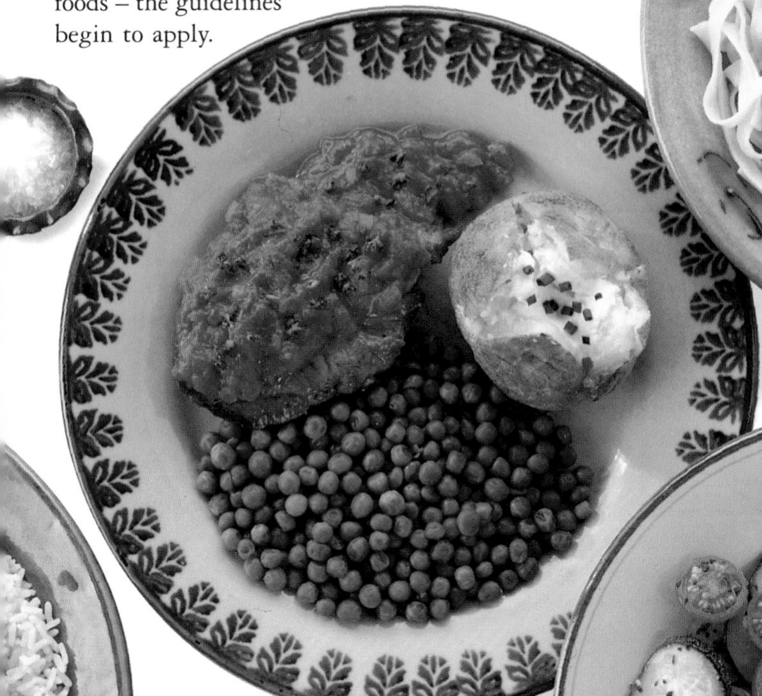

A pork chop in spicy tomato sauce, jacket potato with yoghurt and peas is a filling yet low-fat meal.

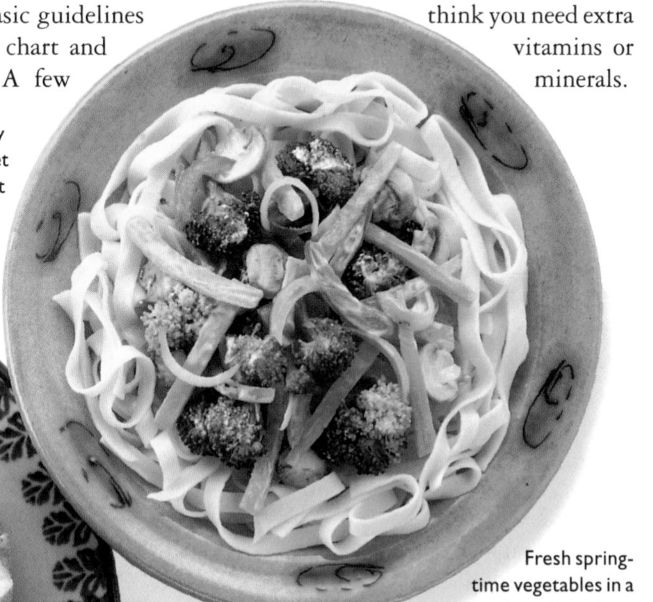

Fresh springtime vegetables in a light olive oil, yoghurt and cheese sauce are served on a nest of fettucine to make a perfectly balanced vegetarian meal.

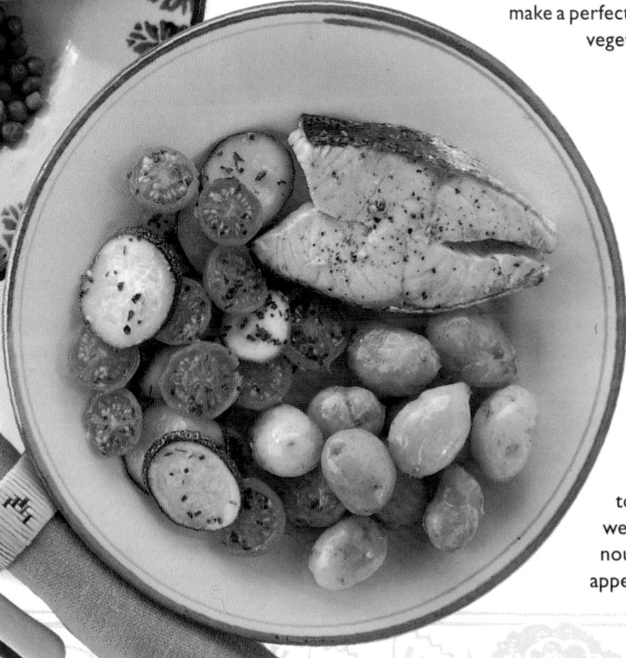

Grilled salmon steak with new potatoes, courgettes, and cherry tomatoes – a well-balanced, nourishing and appetising meal.

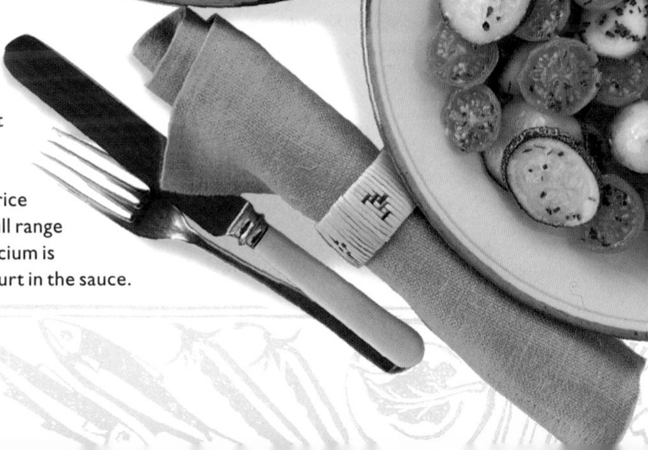

Fragrant chicken and vegetables with rice supplies the full range of nutrients. Calcium is provided by yoghurt in the sauce.

BEETROOT

BENEFITS

- *Good source of folate*
- *Rich in potassium*
- *Contains some vitamin C*
- *Leafy tops are rich in beta carotene, calcium and iron*

Although beetroot has a reputation for stimulating the immune system and is thought to be rich in natural cancer-fighting compounds, the long-held belief of central European folk medicine that the popular root vegetable combats cancer has yet to be proved.

Beetroot has edible leafy tops, which contain beta carotene, calcium and iron; these may be cooked in exactly the same way as spinach. In ancient civilisations only the leaves were eaten, the root being used purely medicinally – to treat ailments such as headaches and toothaches.

Today, only the root is usually eaten – raw, ready-boiled, pickled in vinegar or canned. Beetroot has one of the highest sugar contents of any vegetable, containing the equivalent of a teaspoonful of natural sugars per 100g (3½oz) portion. It is a relative of sugar beet (once used only as an animal feed, but today harvested for sucrose).

What is unusual about beetroot is that the taste and texture of the processed vegetable remain quite faithful to those of the fresh original. Vinegar gives pickled beetroot an added piquancy. However, pickling beetroot does reduce the levels of all its nutrients – both vitamins and minerals.

Nutritionally, freshly boiled beetroot is a good if not better source of nutrients than the raw vegetable. It has higher levels of most minerals, including potassium (which regulates the heartbeat, and maintains normal blood pressure and nerve function). Most of the vitamin levels remain the same, including vitamin C, and there is only a slight loss of folate. Some people do eat beetroot raw, grated in a salad, but most prefer it cooked.

Leaving the beet unpeeled during boiling will stop the colour caused by the strong red pigment betacyanin bleeding out and staining cooking utensils. Commercially, betacyanin pigment is extracted from beetroot to create a food colouring called, not surprisingly, beetroot red. It is used in food processing to add colour to anything from oxtail soup to ice cream, and bacon burgers to liquorice.

PINK URINE?

There is no cause for alarm if, after eating beetroot, urine or stools appear pink. Parents who feed their babies beetroot purée are often distressed by the resulting pink nappies. All that this indicates is a genetically inherited inability to metabolise betacyanin, the red pigment. The harmless compound simply passes straight through the digestive system.

BEETROOT'S BENEFITS

Apart from the various anti-carcinogens that beetroot (either raw or boiled) is thought to contain, it is also a good source of folate – an essential vitamin for healthy cells (deficiency of which is associated with ANAEMIA).

Fresh raw beetroot juice is such a concentrated source of vitamins and minerals that it has few rivals as a tonic for convalescents. For anyone who dislikes the taste, they can try diluting it with carrot juice.

BISCUITS

BENEFITS

- *Convenient snack foods*
- *Some biscuits are high in fibre*
- *Good source of carbohydrates*

DRAWBACKS

- *Sugary types may cause tooth decay*
- *Many are high in fat*
- *Poor source of nutrients*

Whether sweet or 'plain', biscuits provide a handy snack and a quick source of carbohydrate to keep hunger at bay. Crispbreads and crackers can also make an alternative to

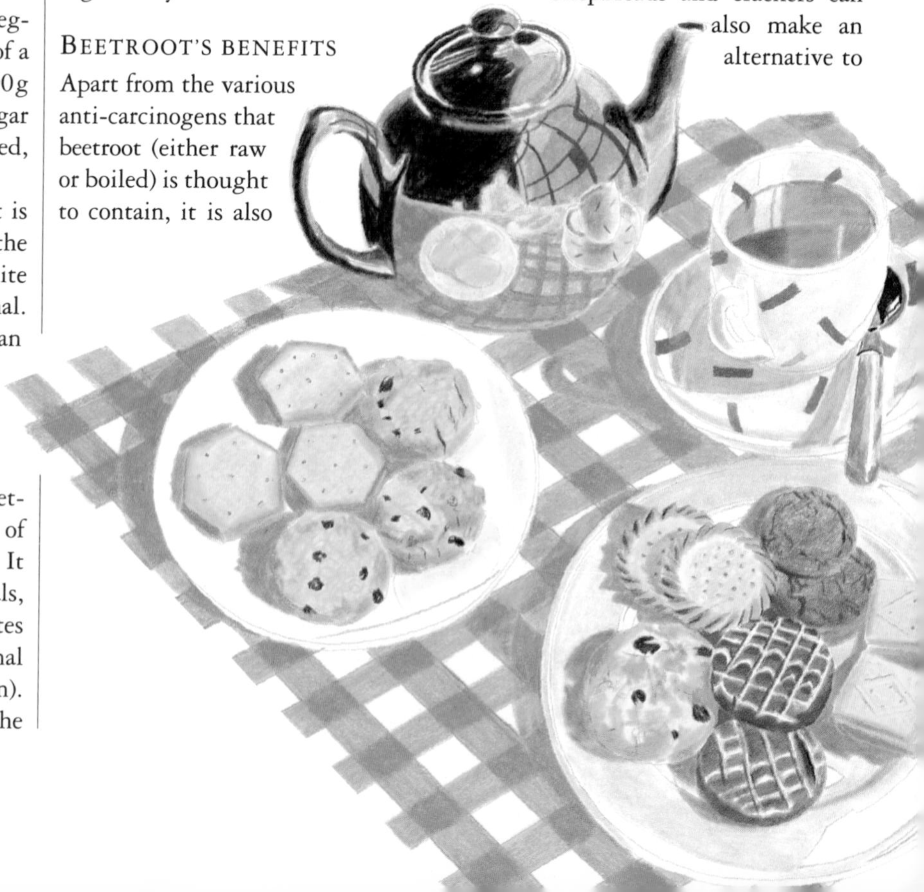

bread. But, while most varieties are high in fat, few biscuits actually offer more than a token in terms of nutritional value. Nevertheless, Britons munch their way through nearly 600000 tonnes of biscuits every year.

PLAIN BISCUITS

The low calorie count of crispbreads has made them particularly popular in the West among slimmers, and the high fibre content is an added benefit. Two pieces of crispbread provide about 60 Calories, the equivalent of a slice of wholewheat bread.

Most crispbreads are baked from wheat, rye flour or a mixture of the two. But while wholemeal rye flour contains less protein, less niacin and more riboflavin (vitamin B_2) than wheat flour, the nutritional differences are minuscule within the context of a balanced diet.

Cracker biscuits have a similarly low nutrient value and calorie count. Made of highly refined white flour, their fibre content is negligible.

SWEET BISCUITS

While sweet biscuits are a convenient form of readily available energy, the refined sugar in them has no nutritional value; it is a source of 'empty' calories, and is potentially harmful to the teeth. Sweet biscuits are not only rich in sugar, but are usually made from 'patent' flour which is even more refined than white 'baking' flour. This retains little of the wheat grain, and has been stripped of virtually all its dietary fibre. Biscuits that are made with bran, and which claim to have a higher fibre content, appear to be a healthier option, but they are also high in fat and rich in sugar. If eaten frequently, they too may encourage tooth decay.

Biscuits are generally made from the least healthy types of fat. Animal fats, butter, hydrogenated fats or palm oil are commonly used, all of which are high in saturated FATS or trans fatty acids; high intakes of both types of fat have been linked to coronary heart disease. These solid fats are needed as most other vegetable oils tend to make poor quality biscuits.

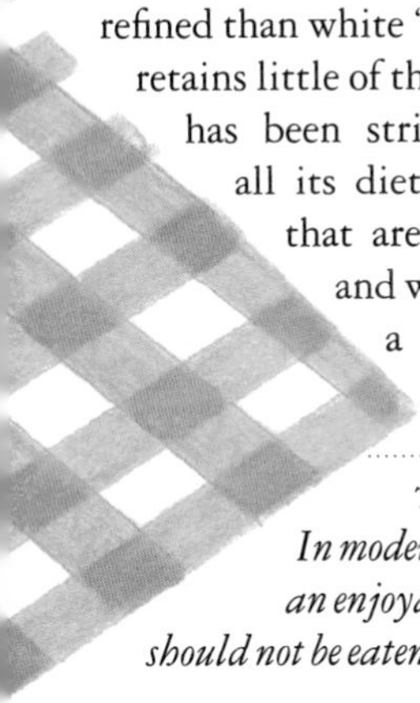

TAKING THE BISCUIT
In moderation, biscuits make an enjoyable treat – but they should not be eaten in large quantities.

BLACKBERRIES

BENEFITS

- *Useful source of vitamin C*
- *Contain fibre and folate*

DRAWBACK

- *Contain salicylates (natural aspirin); anyone intolerant to aspirin may also react to blackberries*

Blackberries are a useful source of vitamin C, which helps to fight infection and boost the immune system. Fresh blackberry juice makes an excellent all-round tonic because it provides carbohydrates for energy, it is rich in bioflavonoids and it also contains fibre as well as folate.

Most blackberries are now commercially cultivated and are larger than their wild counterparts. Wild berries have a more concentrated flavour, but may be contaminated by lead from exhaust fumes or polluted by pesticides if picked from roadsides or hedgerows alongside cultivated land.

Anyone who is intolerant to aspirin may find that they experience a similar reaction after eating blackberries. This is because blackberries contain salicylate, a natural aspirin-like compound which has been known to trigger HYPERACTIVITY in susceptible people.

Blackberry leaf tea

In herbal medicine, blackberry leaf tea is used as a remedy for diarrhoea, as a decongestant and a stomach tonic. Mrs Grieve in *A Modern Herbal* (1931) suggests adding 25g (1oz) dried leaves to 600ml (1 pint) boiling water.

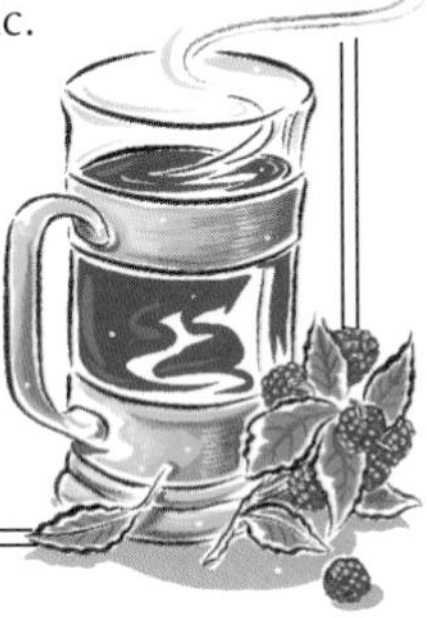

BLACKCURRANTS

BENEFITS

- *Excellent source of vitamin C*
- *Soothe sore throats*
- *Combat bacterial stomach infections*

Blackcurrants are high in vitamin C, which is vital in improving iron absorption for vegetarians. Weight for weight, they have four times as much vitamin C as an orange. One 15g (½oz) tablespoonful supplies 30mg of the vitamin – three-quarters of the UK recommended daily intake. Studies show that the vitamin C in blackcurrants is particularly stable; a syrup of blackcurrants will lose only 15 per cent of its vitamin content in a year.

Blackcurrant skins contain pigments called anthocyanins, which are known to inhibit bacteria such as *E. coli* – a common cause of stomach upsets. In Scandinavia, the dried, powdered skins are used to treat diarrhoea. Anthocyanins are also anti-inflammatory, which is why a blackcurrant drink soothes sore throats.

WARNING

Blackcurrant cordial must be well diluted. Even ready-mixed blackcurrant drinks should be further diluted as they can cause severe dental caries.

Blood pressure

To help reduce hypertension

EAT PLENTY OF

- *Fresh fruit and vegetables*
- *Oily fish*

AVOID

- *Salty foods and added salt*
- *Pickled foods*
- *Fats, especially saturated fats*
- *Excessive amounts of alcohol*

There is little doubt that good nutrition and healthy growth in childhood help to prevent high blood pressure (or hypertension) as an adult. Research suggests that diet may be especially important during pregnancy and the first few years of life. Even in middle age, when it is normal for blood pressure to increase as part of the natural ageing process, the wrong kind of diet is still believed to contribute to unhealthily high blood pressure levels. Aside from diet, other influences include emotional problems, anxiety and stress – but sometimes the cause is unknown.

The silent killer

Widely known as the 'silent killer', because its outward symptoms are so difficult to detect, high blood pressure affects between 15 and 30 per cent of the adult population of most Western countries. It often comes on in middle age, and is likely to affect more men than pre-menopausal women because of hormonal differences.

As people age, their hearts have to work harder to pump blood around the body. Hypertension occurs as a result of increased resistance to blood flow of the small blood vessels (arterioles), which have muscular walls. Most types of high blood pressure are caused by the arterioles losing their ability to relax normally. Drugs can be used to dilate them, so lowering their resistance to the blood flow. However, these may have side effects and they can also interfere with the body's effective use of nutrients.

Case study

Samuel is a 56-year-old coach driver with a fairly sedentary lifestyle. Following an annual medical check-up, he was dismayed to learn that he had high blood pressure. Samuel's doctor prescribed a thiazide diuretic drug – the first line of treatment for hypertension – and advised him to lose weight. His doctor recommended that Samuel should stick to a well-balanced diet, stop adding salt to his food, and cut out second helpings. He also prescribed a brisk 20-minute walk three times a week. After about six months, Samuel had lost 9.5 kg (1½ stone) and brought his blood pressure under control. Fortunately, his condition was treated before it caused any damage to his kidneys or heart. His doctor still monitors his blood pressure, but has now taken Samuel off his medication.

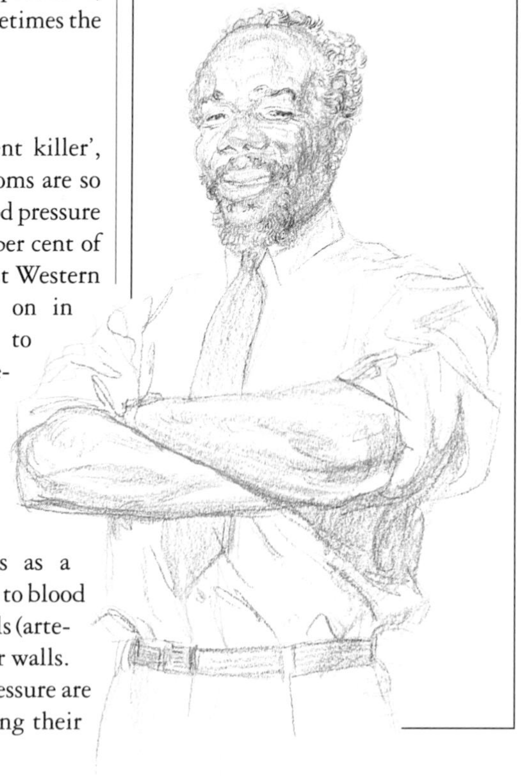

Not all the ramifications of high blood pressure are fully understood. However, it is a recognised factor in strokes and it is also known to increase the risk of heart and kidney disease.

High blood pressure increases the risk of suffering a stroke because of the narrowing, or chance rupturing, of some of the delicate blood vessels in the brain. It may thicken or burst the tiny blood vessels in the back of the eye, resulting in blurred vision or blindness. It can also damage the kidneys and lead to renal failure.

When combined with a high blood-cholesterol level, hypertension will often accelerate the development of ATHEROSCLEROSIS, a nodular hardening of the arteries.

Common causes

Hypertension can be caused by kidney problems or hormonal imbalances, especially adrenal gland malfunctions. Sometimes pregnancy or the birth-control pill can cause a temporary hypertension. But most people who suffer from high blood pressure have what is termed essential hypertension. Although its cause is not completely understood, genetic factors are implicated as problems with high blood pressure tend to run in families.

Environmental factors, such as STRESS and noise, often appear to be involved as well.

Why diet is crucial

Aside from medication, a change to a healthy well-balanced diet (which is low in fat) coupled with a reduction in alcohol intake are often top of the list on a doctor's recommendations for high blood pressure. Indeed OBESITY and excessive ALCOHOL consumption are both important causes of hypertension. Avoiding alcohol leads to a prompt fall in blood pressure in some heavy drinkers, and overweight people suffering from high blood pressure usually show a similar drop, as long as they lose weight gradually. Rapid weight loss followed by weight regain may increase the risk of hypertension.

CUTTING DOWN ON SALT

Statistics show that hypertension is at last becoming less prevalent in both Britain and the United States, which some research studies are attributing to the drop in the consumption of table SALT. Even where hypertension is treated with drugs, it is possible to achieve further reductions in blood pressure through modest reductions in salt intake. Much of the salt we eat is added at the table or during cooking, but many everyday processed foods such as bread, cheese and breakfast cereals contain significant amounts of 'hidden' salt. Although it is impractical to cut out all processed foods, you should be able to achieve a noticeable reduction in blood pressure by avoiding pickled, smoked and salted foods, and not adding extra salt at the table.

Eating at least five daily portions of fruit and vegetables (especially garlic and celery) also helps to lower blood pressure. Potassium, supplied mainly by fruit and vegetables, is thought to counteract some of the effects of a high salt intake. However, any hypertensive patients with KIDNEY DISEASE should avoid a high intake of potassium as it puts an excessive load on the kidneys. Eating oily fish (provided it is not pickled, smoked or salted) may also reduce blood pressure. Hypertensive patients may be prescribed DIURETICS, which reduce salt levels in the body.

EXERCISE: GENTLY DOES IT

Regular exercise has an effect in lowering blood pressure. However, someone with undiagnosed severe hypertension who starts taking rigorous exercise is at risk of having a heart attack. Anyone wanting to get fit should start with a gentle routine, gradually increasing its rate, severity and duration. If you have high blood pressure, consult your doctor first. Exercise can also have a role in helping people to deal with stress, a known influence on hypertension. Learning how to relax and reduce stress levels can be surprisingly effective in lowering blood pressure.

THE GLOBAL PICTURE

Worldwide there has been a fall in the number of hypertension sufferers, but nowhere has this been more dramatic than in Japan – and this is partially attributed to the decline in salt intake because of refrigeration and freezing replacing salting and pickling as methods of food preservation. Another theory points to the increased stature of recent generations of adults in all developed countries. A short physique is generally associated with an increased risk of hypertension, and this may go some way towards explaining why it is less common not just in Japan but also in the West.

Understanding blood-pressure measurements

When measuring blood pressure – expressed in millimetres of mercury – two readings are taken. One, the systolic, is the pressure when the heart contracts. The other, the diastolic, is the pressure when the heart relaxes. Systolic pressure is given first; a reading of 120/80 (an average reading for a fit young person) means a systolic pressure of 120mm and a diastolic pressure of 80mm. A fit middle-aged person might have a reading of 135/90. Between 140/90 and 160/110 indicates mild hypertension. Readings above this point to severe hypertension. Depending on an individual's medical history, a blood pressure reading as low as 95/60 can still be seen as healthy.

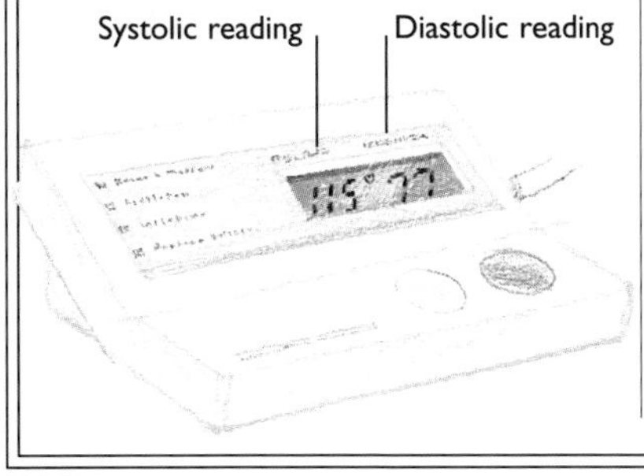

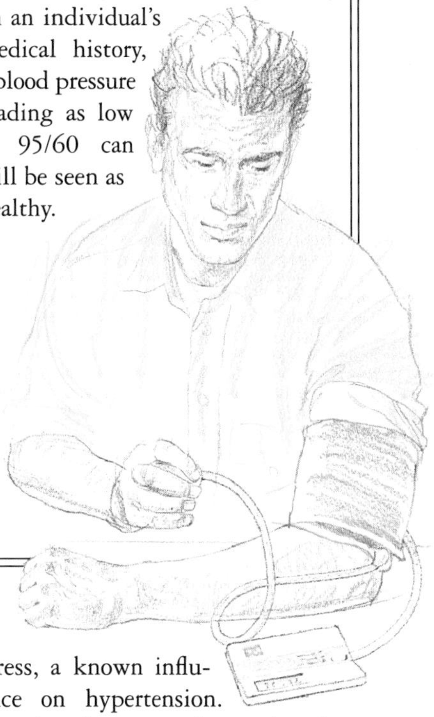

Check it out

Adults should have their blood pressure checked at least every five years. Anyone over 40 should be checked out every two years, especially if there is a family history of high blood pressure.

If you do have a blood pressure problem, follow your doctor's advice, adopt the general dietary advice given here, and try to reduce your STRESS levels.

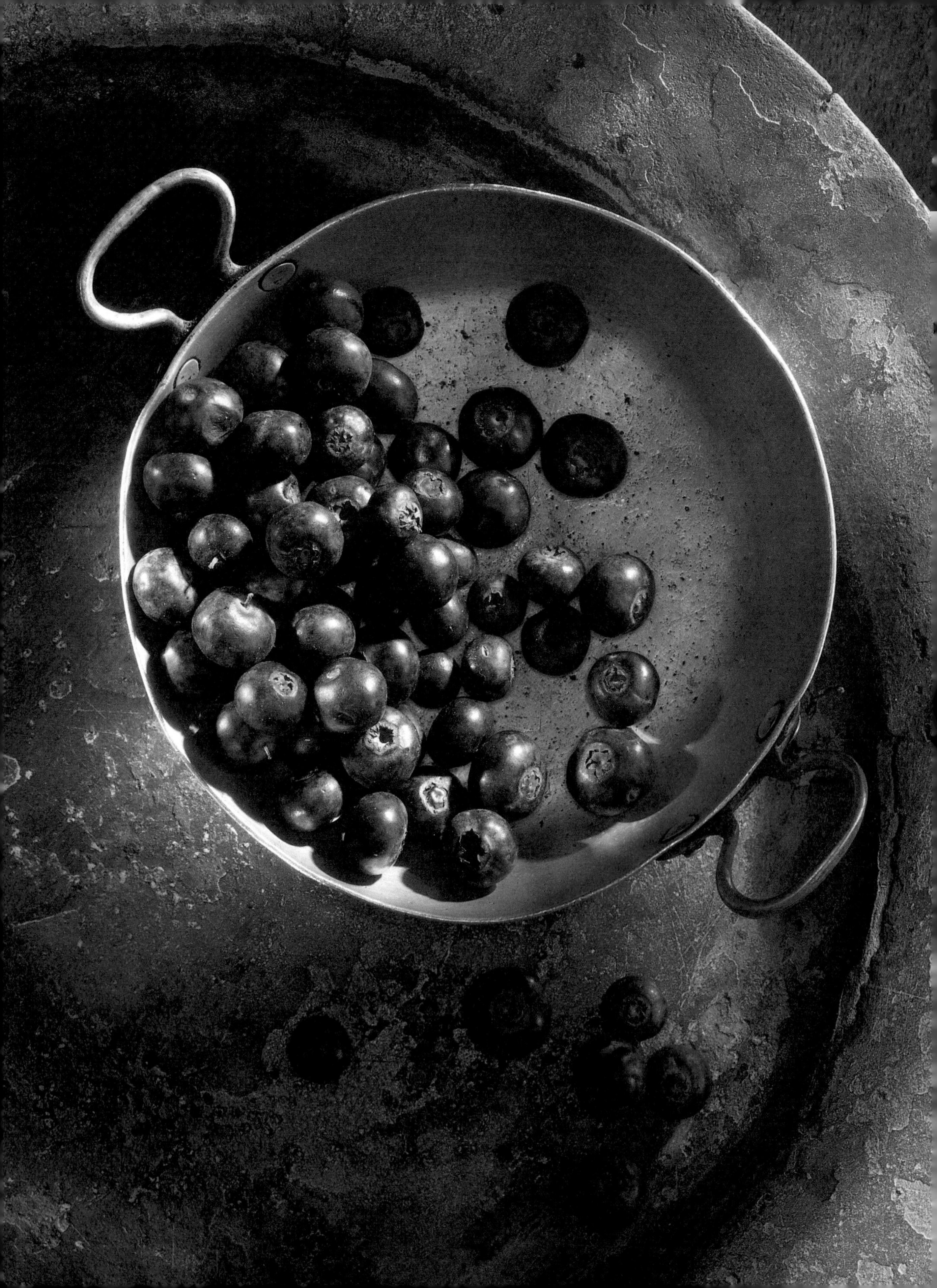

BLOOD SUGAR LEVELS

EAT PLENTY OF
- *Fruit and vegetables*
- *Starchy foods, in several small but regular meals*

AVOID
- *Obesity*

Almost all foods of plant origin contain carbohydrates which are broken down into sugars – mainly into glucose – during the digestive process. Absorbed in the gut, glucose is a major source of fuel for the body. Some can be stored in the liver and muscles in the form of glycogen which can be broken down to release glucose when energy reserves are low.

About one in five of all middle-aged Britons have impaired glucose tolerance – their blood sugar levels are slow to return to normal after a meal high in carbohydrates. The disorder is often a precursor of DIABETES and is associated with increased risk of a heart attack.

WHEN EXERCISE HELPS

Glucose tolerance is improved by spreading carbohydrate intake over several small, rather than a few larger meals. Regular physical exercise, which helps to remove glucose from the bloodstream to the muscles, also boosts glucose tolerance, as does a reduction in weight if you are particularly overweight. Starchy foods as well as fruit and vegetables help to slow down the rate of glucose absorption.

Blood glucose levels are regulated by hormones, particularly insulin, and following a meal high in carbohydrate, their levels rise. In response to these rising levels of glucose, the pancreas secretes insulin, which stimulates the removal of glucose from the bloodstream into the liver and muscles. When too much insulin is secreted, blood sugar levels rebound and this can cause temporary symptoms of HYPOGLYCAEMIA (low blood sugar) such as cold sweats and irritability. Hypoglycaemia is treated by eating small amounts of glucose or sucrose.

Glucose is also the major source of fuel for the brain, which cannot store glucose and so depends on a steady supply from the blood. A sudden drop in blood glucose levels can trigger mood changes, irritability, and coma or even death. However, the brain can adapt, to some extent, by using ketone bodies as an alternative fuel – produced by the liver's metabolism of fat when the body's supply of carbohydrate is low. These ketone bodies, with an odour similar to nail varnish, can be detected on the breath.

Escaping the 'sugar trap'

Because any form of sugar reaches the bloodstream very quickly its metabolism is also rapid, so that within 20 to 30 minutes the blood sugar levels have often tumbled to well below their original levels, inevitably triggering a craving for another sugary snack. This creates a self-perpetuating cycle known as the 'sugar trap'.

Regular snacks of chocolate bars, biscuits or gooey cake may temporarily satisfy this craving for sugar, but are equally likely to prompt a desire for more of the same. A snack of wholemeal bread or crispbread with hummous and cucumber is much healthier – providing as much energy and more nutrients than a small bar of chocolate or a slice of iced cake.

BERRIES TO BEAT BUGS *Blueberries have natural antibacterial properties which can help to guard against an upset stomach.*

BLUEBERRIES

BENEFITS
- *May help to combat cystitis*
- *Have antibacterial properties*
- *Ease digestive upsets*

DRAWBACK
- *May trigger allergies*

Unlike many berries which are so sour they have to be cooked with sugar to make them palatable, blueberries are naturally sweet and can be eaten raw, so preserving their vitamin C. Though they are a good source of the vitamin, you would need to eat almost 300g (10½oz) of fresh berries to meet the average adult's daily requirement.

Traditionally, the berries were dried and used to cure diarrhoea and food poisoning. Medical research now offers a scientific basis for such remedies for they contain antibacterial compounds (called anthocyanins) which are particularly effective against some forms of *E. coli*, the main culprits in many gastrointestinal disorders.

Because the berries inhibit bacteria such as *E. coli* (which can spread up the urinary tract to the bladder), they are a valuable aid against recurrent urinary tract infections such as cystitis. At the same time (like cranberries) blueberries contain a substance which can prevent infectious bacteria from clinging to the mucous membranes of the bladder and urethra.

Recent US studies suggest that the berries may improve sight and provide protection against worsening vision, glaucoma, cataracts and similar disorders; however, more research will be needed before these claims for the fruit can be finally proved or disproved.

Like many other berry fruits blueberries are potential causes of allergic reactions, the most common symptoms of which are swelling of the lips and eyelids, and an itchy swollen rash.

Boils

EAT PLENTY OF

- *Poultry and seafood, particularly oysters, to provide zinc*
- *Oily fish and liver for vitamin A*
- *Garlic for its antibacterial properties*
- *Fresh fruit and vegetables for vitamin C*
- *Wholemeal bread, nuts and seeds for vitamin E*

The red, painful, pus-filled swellings known as boils are caused by bacterial infection of the skin. More extensive boils are called carbuncles. They are most likely to occur when the body's resistance to bacterial infection is low, either following illness or because of an unbalanced, unhealthy diet.

If you are suffering from boils, try to give your immune system the best chance of fighting the infection. Zinc, in particular, has been found to boost the immune system. The normal daily intake should be about 8mg – the amount contained in 150g (5½oz) of minced beef, for example. If suffering from boils, you can increase your zinc intake to 30mg for a week or two but, if using supplements, ensure that they also contain copper as increasing zinc intake can interfere with the way copper is metabolised in the body.

Although useful amounts of zinc can be found in poultry, cereals and fish, the only food that will provide 30mg – if eaten in normal amounts – is oysters. Half a dozen oysters will provide around 35mg of zinc.

Eat plenty of raw garlic, which has natural antibacterial properties, and to help to improve the general health of the skin, make sure you have an adequate intake of vitamins A, C and E. Vitamin A is found in oily fish, liver and dairy products; vitamin C is found in almost all fresh fruit and vegetables; and vitamin E is found in wholemeal bread, cereals, nuts and seeds.

Bran

BENEFITS

- *May reduce the risk of bowel cancer*
- *Oat bran contributes to lower blood cholesterol*
- *Helps to prevent constipation*
- *May help to prevent piles and diverticulitis*

DRAWBACKS

- *Too much can cause irritable bowel syndrome, abdominal bloating, and can also reduce absorption of calcium and iron*

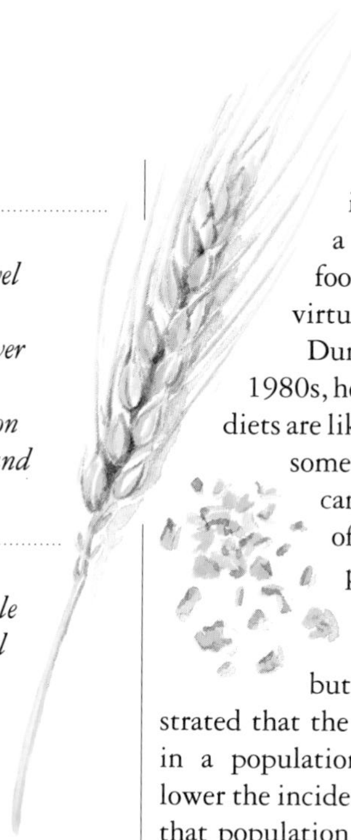

As one of the richest sources of dietary FIBRE, bran (the outer husk of wheat, rice or oat grains) enjoyed a vogue in the 1980s and early 1990s. A tablespoon of bran – a third of which by weight is fibre – will provide a third of the daily requirement of 18g (⅔oz) and may help to reduce the risk of cancer of the bowel as well as helping to prevent constipation, diverticulitis and piles.

Oat bran also contains soluble fibre which can help to reduce blood CHOLESTEROL levels. When fats are digested, soluble fibre can bind to cholesterol causing it to be excreted as waste rather than reabsorbed.

However, early enthusiasts for high-fibre diets who used bran to treat constipation, digestive problems and obesity were not aware of the potential dangers of an excessive intake of insoluble fibre which often aggravated the condition or caused new problems including irritable bowel syndrome and mineral deficiencies.

Fibre's role in the smooth functioning of the large bowel and its relation to the reduced risk of bowel cancer was observed in the late 1960s by Dr Dennis Burkitt, a Briton who was for many years a medical officer in Africa. He noted that where indigenous people had a diet rich in fibrous food, bowel cancer was virtually unknown.

During the 1970s and 1980s, he wrote that high-fibre diets are likely to protect against some of the most common cancers in the West – of the bowel, breast, prostate and uterus. Experts do not accept all of these claims but research has demonstrated that the more fibre contained in a population's normal diet, the lower the incidence of bowel cancer in that population. Dr Burkitt was also the first to suggest that constipation and diverticulitis (a form of colonic inflammation) were a direct result of insufficient bran fibre in the diet; these claims are now largely confirmed.

However, during the 1980s and early 1990s, when bran's benefits were first widely publicised, the potential dangers of adding three, four or even more tablespoons of uncooked bran to the daily diet were not understood. Raw bran is now known to aggravate certain conditions and may cause new problems. The phytic acid it contains can also inhibit the body's absorption of minerals such as calcium, iron, zinc and magnesium. During baking, however, enzymes in the yeast destroy much of the phytic acid so that wholemeal bread is a far healthier source of fibre than uncooked bran. Four slices of wholemeal bread provide the equivalent fibre of three tablespoons of bran.

Heat during processing destroys most of the phytic acid in high bran breakfast cereals, making them a safer source of roughage, but the large amounts of salt and sugar that many of these breakfast foods contain make them a less healthy option than unsweetened muesli or porridge oats.

BREAD

See page 60

BREAKFAST CEREALS

BENEFITS

- *High-fibre varieties are a good source of insoluble fibre, which aids bowel function, and soluble fibre which helps to lower blood cholesterol levels*
- *Generally low in fat*
- *Most brands have added vitamins and minerals as well as providing a slow, steady release of energy*

DRAWBACKS

- *Many brands contain large amounts of hidden sugar and salt*

The popularity of commercially produced breakfast cereals stems from Dr John Harvey Kellogg, who invented cornflakes in 1899. His aim was to provide patients at his sanatorium in Michigan, USA, with a healthier alternative to the traditional cooked breakfast. Today, cornflakes and other variations on natural cereals, whether they are based on corn, wheat, oats, rice or bran, still share his aim of providing a high-fibre, low-fat start to the day.

In fact, a simple dish of cooked oats offered these benefits centuries earlier: the Roman historian Pliny described how, in the 1st century AD, Germanic tribes ate porridge made from oats. Because the starch in oats is digested and absorbed slowly, porridge provides a slow and steady release of energy that lasts for several hours.

Oats are an important ingredient in muesli, which the Swiss pioneer of the natural health movement, Dr Max Bircher-Benner, discovered when he joined a shepherd to share a porridge-like dish common to the peasants of that area. The traditional mix is 30 per cent rolled oats, 30 per cent wheat flakes, 10 per cent sultanas, 10 per cent hazelnuts and 20 per cent fresh apple or some other seasonal fruit. Oats are also a rich source of both soluble and insoluble FIBRE and this combination makes them an ideal food for maintaining proper bowel function by helping to guard against constipation. Soluble fibre also helps to lower blood cholesterol levels, so reducing the risk of heart disease and stroke.

BRAN is another source of fibre, but because too much of it may interfere with mineral absorption and can cause digestive problems, processed bran cereals may be preferred to raw bran because they contain lower levels of insoluble fibre and are more palatable. However, processed bran cereals may be high in added salt and sugar.

Most commercial breakfast cereals contain added nutrients in the form of vitamins and minerals, particularly the B vitamins and iron. However, they are usually high in added sugar, particularly those brands aimed at the children's market.

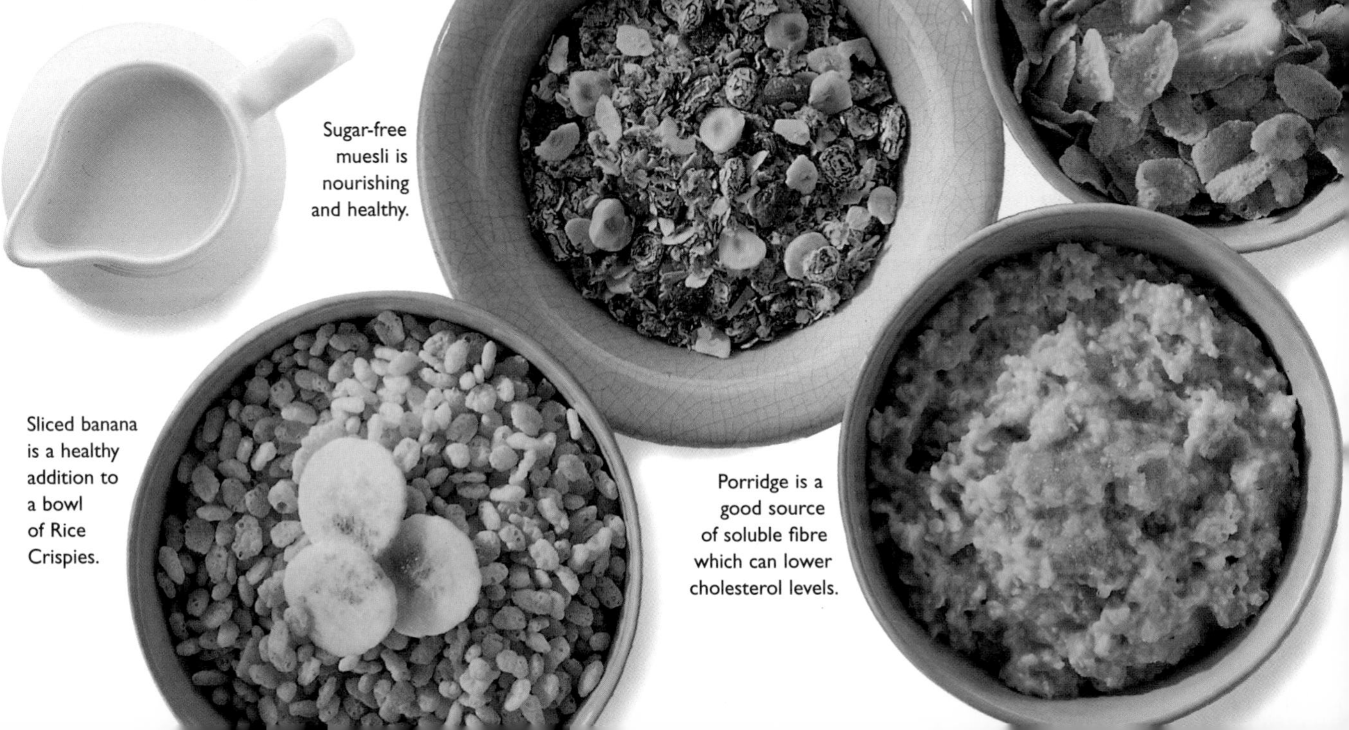

HIGH IN FIBRE, LOW IN FAT *Commercial breakfast cereals contain added vitamins and minerals. Their nutritional value can be boosted with fresh fruit.*

Strawberries will add vitamin C to a bowl of cornflakes.

Sugar-free muesli is nourishing and healthy.

Sliced banana is a healthy addition to a bowl of Rice Crispies.

Porridge is a good source of soluble fibre which can lower cholesterol levels.

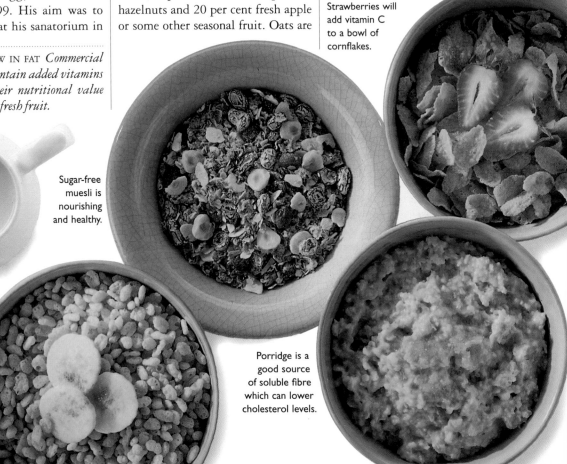

BREAD: A HEALTHY SOURCE OF ENERGY

The growing range of exotic breads has revitalised the loaf's traditional image. Today bread is recognised as an important part of our diet, but we are still not eating enough of it.

In recent years the poor public image of bread as a fattening, stodgy and unappealing source of food has changed dramatically. In Britain, people are being urged by the Department of Health to eat at least five slices daily. This dietary U-turn – prompted by a better understanding of the nutritional importance of starch and fibre – has been helped by the expanding range of breads available in bakeries and supermarkets.

Today bread is seen as being both healthy and full of flavour. Its high fibre content makes it a useful weapon in helping to prevent and treat intestinal disorders; it may even ward off some types of cancers. A recent report by the World Health Organisation argues that bread's complex carbohydrates reduce cholesterol levels in the blood and help to manage diabetes.

Rich in iron and vitamins, especially the B complex group, bread is also a valuable source of calcium, the mineral vital for forming and maintaining healthy bones and teeth. Domestic consumption of bread in Britain has more than halved in the past 40 years. However, it remains a staple in many homes and each person eats an average of three slices daily. This amount of white bread – which must by law be fortified – provides just under one-sixth of an adult's daily calcium needs.

Two popular misconceptions are that bread is fattening (it is not – what is fattening is what is spread on it) and that white bread is poor quality food. While white bread does not contain all the fibre and natural goodness of its wholemeal cousin, it is still nutritionally valuable, particularly when, as in Britain, it is enriched with specific minerals and vitamins.

WHEAT INTOLERANCE

One person in every thousand in Britain and 1 in 300 in Ireland is intolerant or sensitive to gluten, one of the proteins in wheat flours. In anyone suffering from COELIAC DISEASE – a disorder of the bowel – gluten damages hair-like projections in the small intestine. This prevents the proper absorption of nutrients and can cause poor growth and digestive upsets in children and a wide range of symptoms in adults.

GIVING DOUGH A LIFT

The yeast used in bread-making to raise the dough is a harmless single-celled organism which multiplies rapidly in warm, damp conditions.

Breads made with wheat flour rise best because, when the flour is kneaded with liquid, the gluten proteins in wheat absorb water to form an elastic dough. This traps gas from the fermenting yeast, forming bubbles of carbon dioxide to give the bread a light texture. Flours with a high gluten content are described as being 'strong'

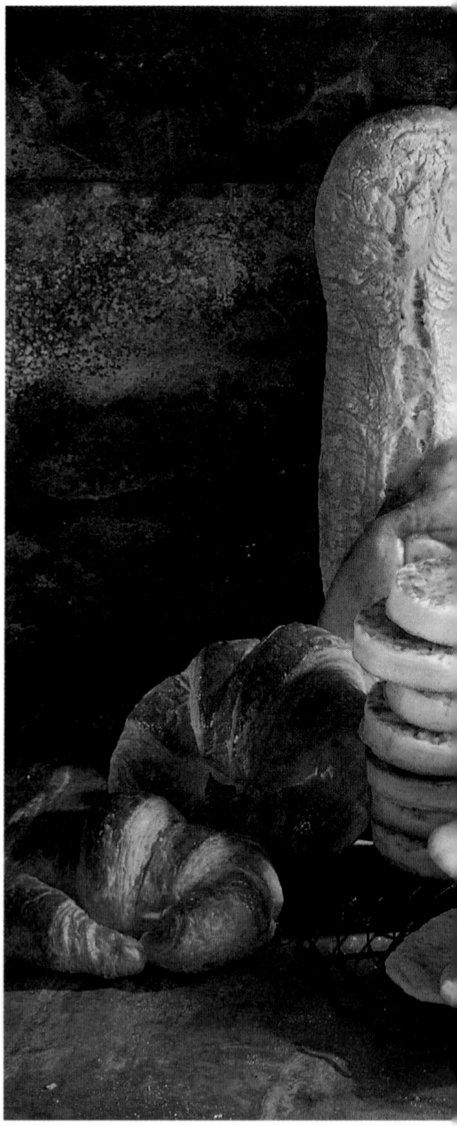

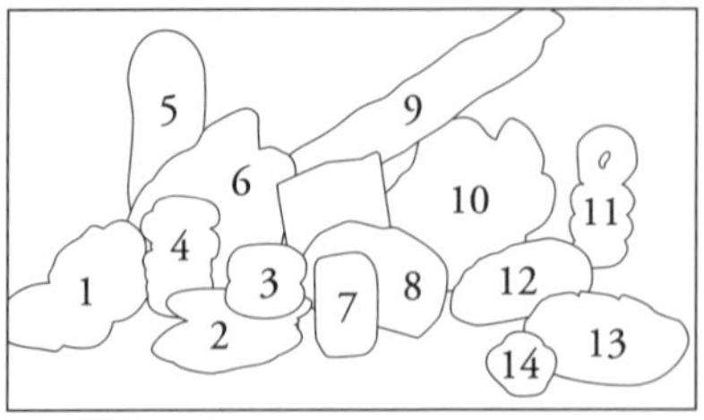

OUR DAILY BREAD *Many different breads are available, including: croissant (1), pitta bread (2), muffin (3), crumpet (4), ciabatta (5), naan (6), malt loaf (7), wholemeal (8), baguette (9), crusty wholemeal (10), bagel (11), poppy-seed (12), pain de campagne (13), brioche (14).*

flours. Other grains, such as rye, can be ground to produce 'soft' flours. They contain less gluten than wheat, so that fewer gas bubbles are trapped in the dough. The resulting breads, such as German pumpernickel, are heavier and more dense.

The liquid in raised, or leavened, breads is usually water, milk or a mixture of the two. It dissolves and disperses the yeast through the flour.

Today most bread in the Western world is mass-produced and, apart from flour, liquid and yeast, it contains additives including fat, preservative, salt, emulsifiers and, in some white breads, flour bleaches.

Salt is added for flavour and to strengthen gluten, which makes the dough more malleable. The relatively high level of salt in most manufactured breads (the equivalent of 350 mg a slice or approximately 1½ teaspoons in a typical loaf) is the other potential nutritional drawback.

In Britain, all flours other than wholewheat flours are required by law to contain the added nutrients thiamin, niacin, calcium and iron. According to nutrition experts the fats used in bread-making pose no risk to

BENEFITS
- *Good source of starch and protein*
- *High fibre content*
- *Contains B complex vitamins*
- *Contains iron and calcium*

DRAWBACKS
- *High salt content*
- *Some people are gluten intolerant*

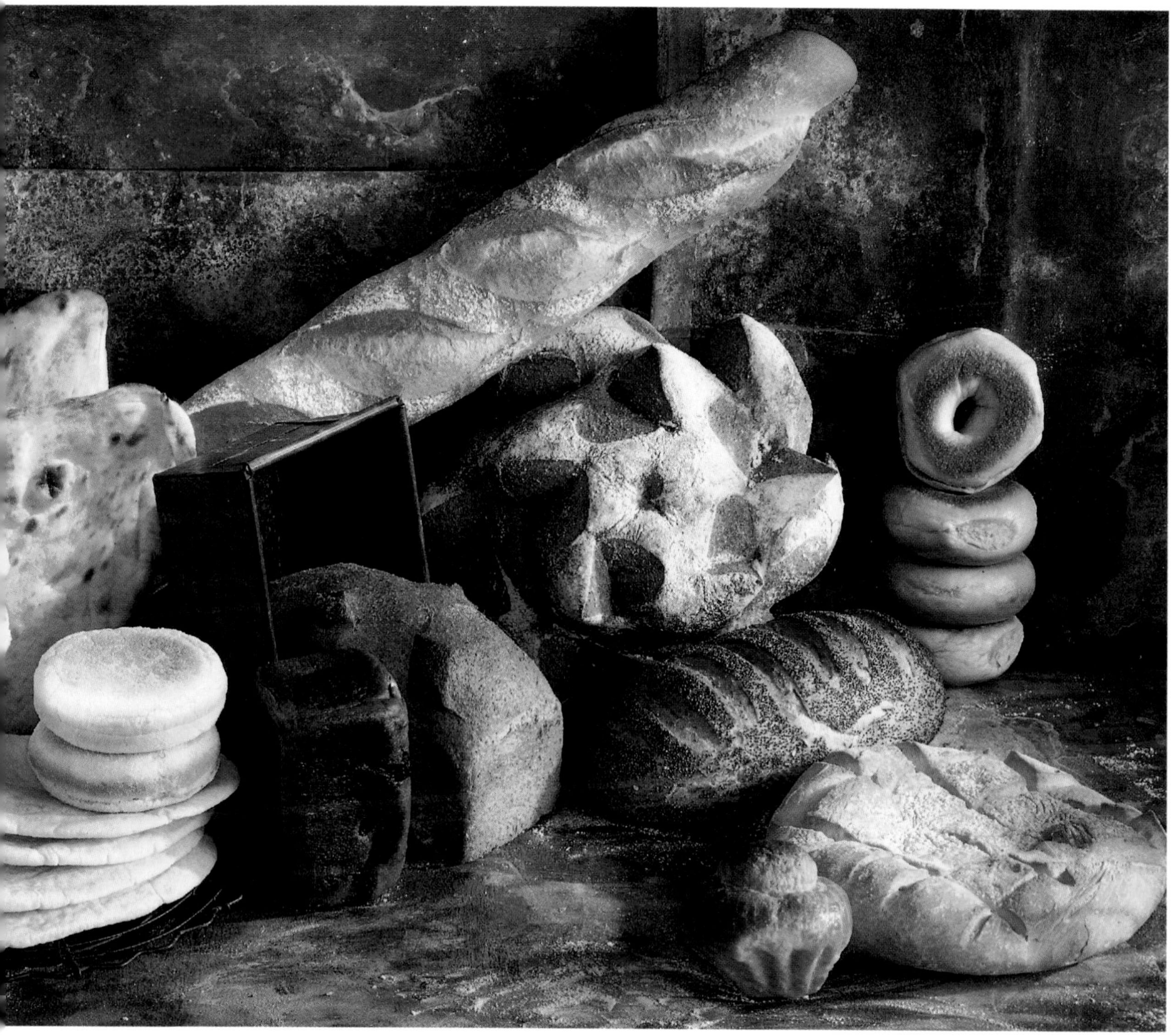

health because such small amounts are used. Vegetable oils are usually used because they make the dough more elastic, which allows it to hold more bubbles – so increasing the loaf's size and lightness.

THE WORLD'S BREADBASKET

There is a wide range of international breads now available in local supermarkets. The most common include:

Bagel Eastern European and Jewish roll with a hole, boiled and then baked from proved yeast dough, often sprinkled with caraway or poppy seeds or coarse salt. Normally made with white flour but wholemeal, rye and onion-flavoured versions are available.

Brioche Light, yeast-leavened roll or loaf originating in France, somewhere between cake and bread in texture and taste. Usually made with white flour and enriched with butter and eggs, making it higher in fat, protein and calories than almost all other breads.

Chapatti Indian flat disc of bread which can be leavened or unleavened. Normally made with wholemeal wheat flour, it is a source of protein, fibre, iron, magnesium and thiamin.

Ciabatta Also known as 'olive bread', this Italian bread is made from white or brown flour bound with olive oil. It is chewy and often flavoured with herbs – added to the dough or sprinkled on the crust before baking.

Croissant Rich, flaky breakfast roll shaped as a crescent. It is high in fat (especially when made with butter).

Crumpet Circular yeasted bread baked on one side with a honeycomb texture. It has a salty taste.

Focaccia Italian yeasted dough bread, similar to pizza, usually baked as a large disc and flavoured with olive oil, coarse salt, herbs and garlic.

Fruit breads Usually made from malted or white bread dough to which some sugar and raisins or other dried fruit or rind has been added.

The language of bread

Descriptions of bread vary widely. However, there are some rule-of-thumb guidelines:

- White bread is made with flour milled from the inner part of the wheat grain after the husk has been removed. It also contains water and yeast along with various additives, preservatives and emulsifiers. The flour is often bleached.

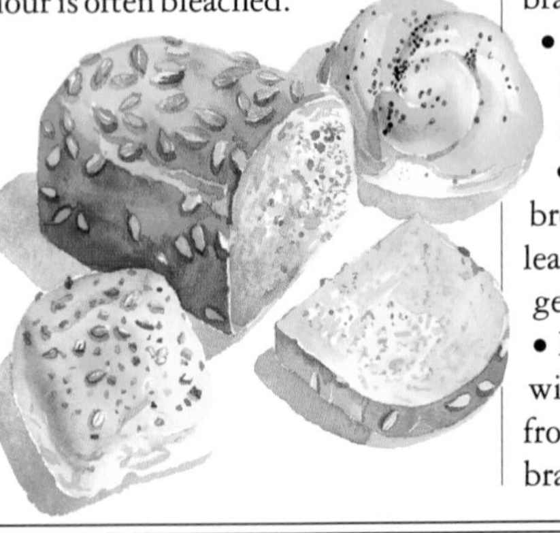

- Brown bread is made from wheat flour with some of the bran removed. Its colour often comes not only from the brown part of the wheat grain but also from added colouring such as caramel.
- Wholemeal bread (also known as 'wholewheat') is made with either wholegrain flour or white flour with bran and wheatgerm added.
- Granary bread is made with brown flour to which malted flour and wheat kernels are added.
- Wheatgerm bread is made with brown or white flour to which at least 10 per cent processed wheatgerm has been added.
- High-fibre white bread is made with white flour with added fibre from non-wheat sources such as rice bran or soya hulls.

THE 'ACCIDENT' OF SOURDOUGH

The first raised or leavened bread seems to have been accidental – when airborne wild yeasts found their way into plain wheat dough, expanding it and giving a lighter-textured bread. The Egyptians kept this process going by using a piece of uncooked dough from one batch to start another. Spread by the Romans, this technique led to what is today called sourdough.

Matzo Traditional Jewish unleavened bread similar to a cracker, made with wheat flour and water, and sometimes salt. True matzos should be baked under the supervision of a rabbi.

Muffin English, round, yeast-proved roll with a mildly sour flavour and a chewy crust. White and wholemeal versions are available, as well as cheese, chocolate and fruit varieties.

Naan A flat, teardrop-shaped yeast-leavened bread from India, baked on the hot side of a tandoori oven. It is a source of thiamin and niacin.

Pitta Middle Eastern flat bread which is sometimes split to form a pocket into which a variety of fillings are placed. White and wholemeal versions are available.

Pumpernickel A heavy, dark brown rye bread originating in Germany. It is steamed and baked for many hours and has a slightly sour, rich flavour.

Rye breads Popular in the Scandinavian countries, Germany and Russia, these are made with rye flour (or a high proportion of rye mixed with wheat flour) and are slightly sour. The low gluten in rye flour makes the breads heavier and more dense.

Tortilla Of Mexican origin, these round, unleavened breads are made by mixing corn or wheat flour with salt and water and baking the flattened dough on a hot griddle.

The nutrients in different types of bread

While the basic principles of bread-making are universal, regional and national variations – in baking methods, as well as in types of flour and other ingredients – now provide a wide choice. There can be large differences in the calories and levels of nutrients found in various types. The contents of 100g (3½oz) – three smallish slices – are shown below.

TYPE OF BREAD	CALORIES	FIBRE (g)	CARBOHYDRATE (g)	PROTEIN (g)	FAT (g)	VITAMINS AND MINERALS
WHITE						
Made with refined flour which may be bleached.	235	1.5	49.3	8.4	1.9	Contains twice as much calcium as wholemeal bread. White flour is fortified with calcium, niacin, iron and thiamin.
BROWN						
Made from wheat flour with some of the bran removed, may contain added colour, such as caramel.	218	3.5	44.3	8.5	2.0	Calcium content is similar to that of white bread.
WHOLEMEAL						
Also known as wholewheat.	215	5.8	41.6	9.2	2.5	Contains 40 per cent more iron than white bread and three times more zinc. Levels of phosphorus, magnesium and manganese are significantly higher. Has higher levels of B vitamins than white or brown bread, and contains vitamin E.
OTHER						
Chapatti	328	2.5	48.3	8.1	12.8	Naan bread contains more vitamin E per 100g (3½oz) than wholemeal bread, and 30 per cent more calcium than white bread.
Croissant	360	1.6	38.3	8.3	20.3	
Malt bread	268	2.3	56.8	8.3	2.4	
Matzo	384	3.0	86.6	10.5	1.9	
Naan bread	336	1.9	50.1	8.9	12.5	Rye bread also contains high levels of vitamin E.
Pitta (white)	265	2.2	57.9	9.2	1.2	
Rye bread	219	4.4	45.8	8.3	1.7	

White: Three slices of white bread provide about one sixth of the daily calcium requirement.

Chromium is removed from white flour during processing. People with diabetes often have a chromium deficiency.

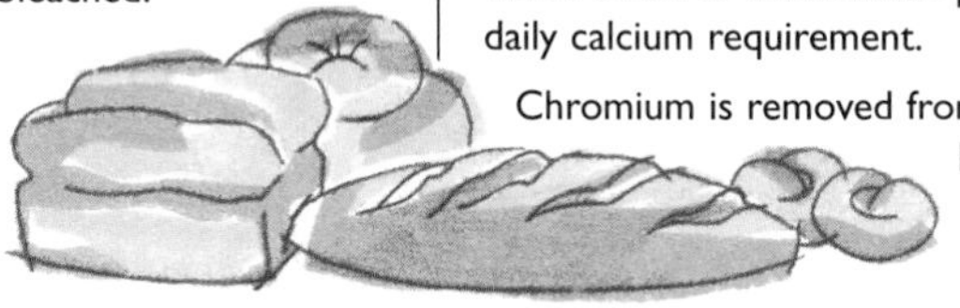

Brown: Soya protein is added to most commercial breads.

Wheatgerm bread is made with brown or white flour with at least 10 per cent processed wheatgerm. It contains as much calcium as white bread, while levels of other nutrients are slightly lower than those in wholemeal bread.

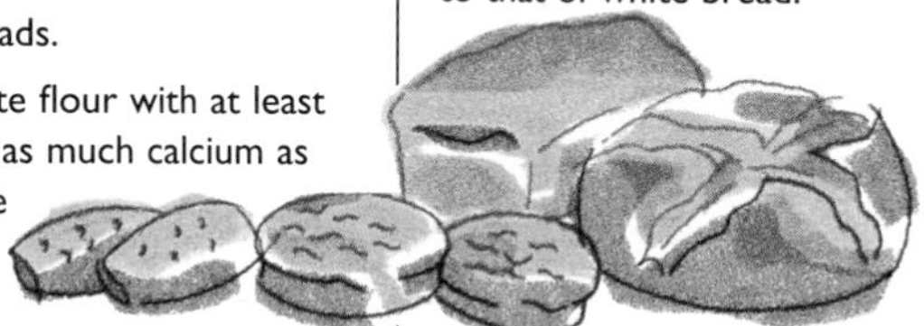

Wholemeal: Granary bread which has added malt flour and wheat kernels contains higher levels of most nutrients than regular brown bread.

Four slices of wholemeal bread provide more than 25 per cent of the daily iron requirement for a woman and 40 per cent of that for a man.

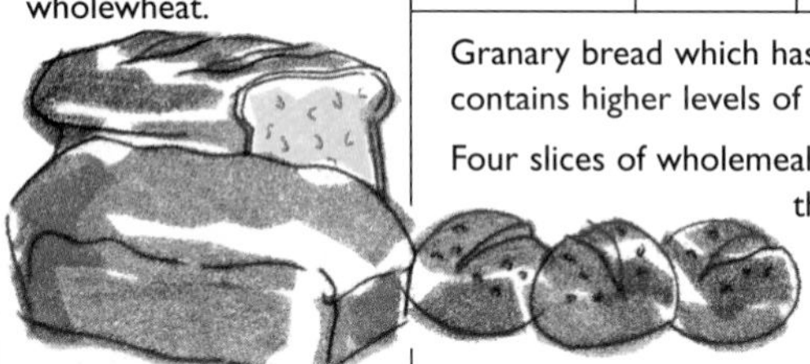

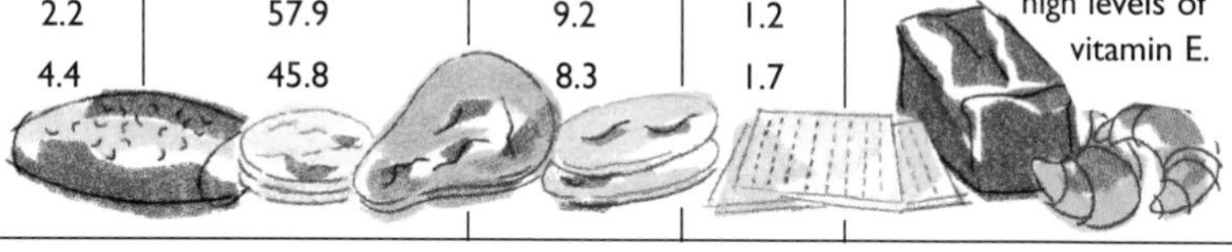

BROAD BEANS

BENEFITS
- *Supply protein*
- *High in soluble fibre*

DRAWBACKS
- *May cause flatulence*
- *May react with certain antidepressant drugs to produce high blood pressure*
- *Can trigger favism, a severe inherited disorder*

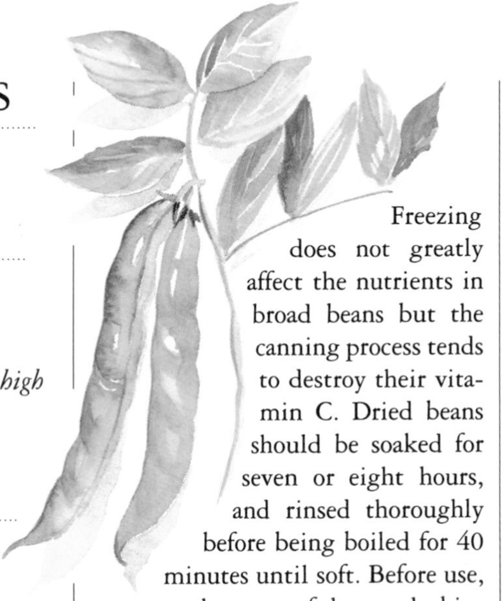

Broad beans are nutritious, filling, inexpensive and can be a useful low-fat, high-fibre component of any balanced diet. The shelled beans provide beta carotene which the body converts to vitamin A, and also contain some iron, niacin, vitamin C and vitamin E. A small (100 g, 3½ oz) portion supplies more than a quarter of the daily requirement of phosphorus which, among other functions, helps to maintain healthy bones and teeth. The beans are also high in soluble FIBRE which can help to lower blood cholesterol levels.

Like other pulses, broad beans are a source of protein and, when combined with cereal foods such as pasta and rice, the quality of the protein supplied is equivalent to that from animal sources such as meat or eggs.

Fresh beans which are pale green or creamy white are at their best in late spring and early summer. Their pods should be crisp and bright green; brown patches indicate rot. Young beans, no thicker than a finger, with pods around 7.5 cm (3 in) long are the most delicious and can be cooked and eaten in their entirety. Mature broad beans with pods up to 30cm (12in) long must be shelled before cooking.

The beans may be eaten hot or cold; puréed broad beans, with their outer tough skin removed, make an enriching thickener for soups and stews. Freezing does not greatly affect the nutrients in broad beans but the canning process tends to destroy their vitamin C. Dried beans should be soaked for seven or eight hours, and rinsed thoroughly before being boiled for 40 minutes until soft. Before use, pop them out of the tough skins by squeezing them gently between your thumb and forefinger. Long cooking reduces the content of indigestible sugars in dried broad beans, and therefore minimises flatulence; seasonings such as ginger, fennel, bay or cumin also help to prevent intestinal wind.

WARNING

Susceptibility to favism is a genetically inherited enzyme deficiency quite common in Mediterranean countries. It makes some people develop a severe anaemic reaction to vicine, a toxic substance found in broad beans.

People who are taking any of a group of antidepressant drugs known as monoamine oxidase inhibitors (MAOIs) are warned by their doctors to exclude broad beans from their diet as the combination of beans and these drugs can produce a dramatic rise in BLOOD PRESSURE called a hypertensive crisis.

Other foods which can produce the same reaction include yeast extracts, cheese, bananas, pickled herring, and also wine.

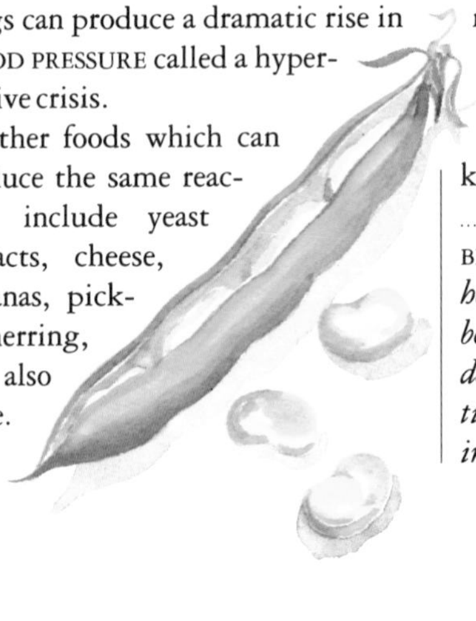

BROCCOLI

BENEFITS
- *Excellent source of vitamin C*
- *Useful source of beta carotene*
- *Contains folate, iron and potassium*
- *May help to protect against cancer*

One portion of boiled broccoli (100 g, 3½oz) provides just over half the recommended daily intake of vitamin C, useful amounts of beta carotene, which the body converts into vitamin A, and some folate, iron and potassium. The darker the florets – whether purple, green or deep blue-green – the higher the amounts of both vitamin C and beta carotene.

Like cauliflower, Brussels sprouts and cabbage, broccoli is a member of the crucifer family of vegetables. Cruciferous plants contain a number of beneficial phytochemicals (see VEGETABLES), including indoles – nitrogen compounds which may offer some protection against cancer because they help to prevent carcinogens from damaging DNA, the substance which holds a cell's genetic material. Phytochemicals retain their powers whether the vegetable is fresh, frozen, raw or cooked. Boiling broccoli, however, almost halves its vitamin C content. Light steaming, microwaving or stir-frying is preferable.

Broccoli is believed to have originated in the Mediterranean – its name derives from the Latin *bracchium*, meaning 'branch'. Since the 16th or 17th century, a popular variety has been cultivated in the Italian province of Calabria where it is known as calabrese.

BROCCOLI HARVEST *The tender flower heads, or florets, of broccoli are richer in beta carotene than the stalks, and the deeper the colour, the higher their nutritional value. The freshness of broccoli is indicated by crisp, easily snapped stalks.*

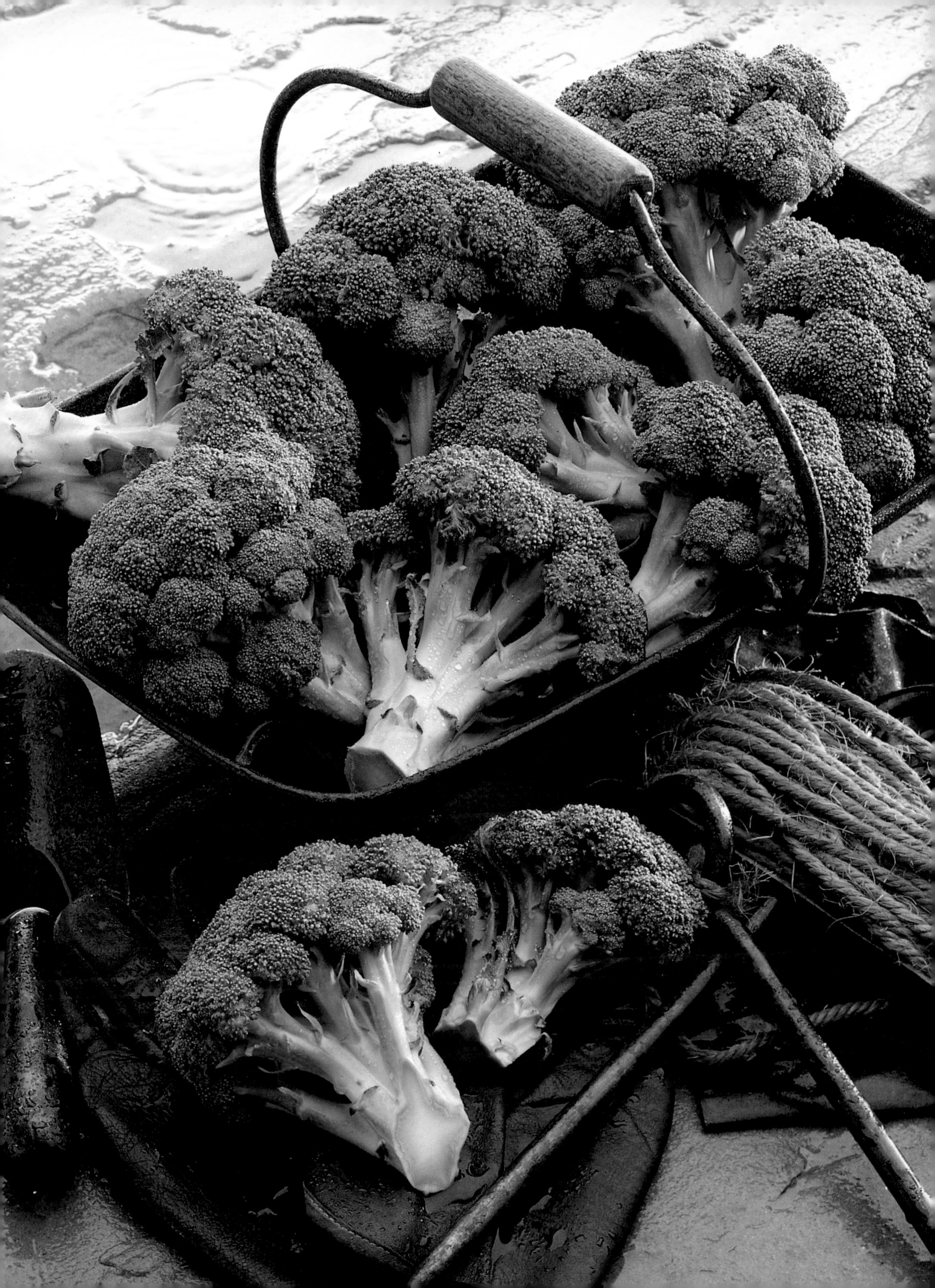

BUTTER OR MARGARINE: WHICH IS BETTER?

Butter has had a bad reputation, but margarine shares some of its drawbacks and relies on additives to make it palatable. Both butter and margarine should be used in moderation.

The debate over whether butter or margarine is healthier has raged for years. Most nutritionists now say butter is better – as long as it is eaten in moderation. Butter is certainly a more natural product than margarine which relies heavily on colourings and other additives to turn it from a greyish, unappealing spread into the more familiar finished product. Usually butter and margarine have the same total fat content and provide the same amount of energy (typically 81 per cent fat and 740 Calories per 100g or 3½oz), although some margarine manufacturers have lowered the fat in their product to 70 per cent (635 Calories per 100g).

Margarine was invented by a French chemist as a cheap butter substitute in the 1860s, when it was made with beef suet and skimmed milk. Today's margarine is far more sophisticated and highly processed. Vegetable oils are used either on their own or combined with animal fats or fish oils. Margarine also usually contains water, whey, emulsifiers to bind the oil and liquids, salt, colouring and flavouring agents.

By law margarine must be fortified with vitamins A and D – which occur naturally in butter. Vitamin A plays a vital role in good vision and healthy skin and is an important antioxidant,

Comparison of various spreads (values per 100g, 3½oz)

CALORIES	FATS	VITAMINS	DID YOU KNOW?
BUTTER			
740	**Total 81g** of which saturated 54g, monounsaturated 20g, polyunsaturated 3g, trans fats 4-8g	A 887μg D 0.76μg E 2mg	'Spreadable' butters contain less salt than standard butters. The natural trans fats in butter do not raise blood cholesterol in the same way as the artificial trans fats in margarine.
MARGARINE, HARD			
740	**Total 81g** of which saturated 36g, monounsaturated 33g, polyunsaturated 9g, trans fats 9-14g	A 790μg D 7.94μg E 8mg	Margarine is fortified with vitamins A and D; the vitamin E content varies according to the oil used and whether it has been added as an ingredient. Beta carotene is also added to give margarine its golden colour.
MARGARINE, POLYUNSATURATED			
740	**Total 81g** of which saturated 16g, monounsaturated 21g, polyunsaturated 41g, trans fats 0.7-6g	A 900μg D 7.94μg E 8mg	This has a similar nutritional profile to hard margarine. Sunflower and safflower margarines have the highest vitamin E content. Like butter, margarine is 16 per cent water.
LOW-FAT SPREAD			
390	**Total 40g** of which saturated 11g, monounsaturated 18g, polyunsaturated 10g, trans fats 0.4-7g	A 1084μg D 8μg E 6.33mg	Low-fat spreads are 50 per cent water. They contain 6 per cent protein (compared to 0.4 per cent in butter and margarines) which produces a 'creamy' feeling in the mouth.
VERY LOW-FAT SPREAD			
270	**Total 25g** of which saturated 7g, monounsaturated 11g, polyunsaturated 4g, trans fats 0.2-3.5g	A 820μg D 8μg E 6.7mg	These spreads have a higher salt content than butter, margarine and low-fat spreads. Very low-fat spreads are more than 60 per cent water and about 6 per cent protein.

BENEFITS

- *Both make food more palatable*
- *Generally good sources of vitamins A and D*
- *Polyunsaturated margarine is an important source of vitamin E and essential fatty acids*

DRAWBACKS

- *High in calories (unless it is a low-fat spread)*
- *Margarine contains potentially harmful trans fatty acids*
- *Butter and hard margarines are high in saturated fat*

while vitamin D helps the body to absorb calcium, which is needed for healthy bones and teeth.

TRANS FATTY ACIDS

In the manufacture of margarine, liquid oils are converted into a solid spread by a chemical process called hydrogenation. As well as hardening the oils, the process changes their chemical structure, turning some of the unsaturated fatty acids into trans fatty acids – a less healthy form of polyunsaturates that have much the same effect on the body as saturated fats. They raise the levels of cholesterol and research now indicates that trans fats are linked to heart disease.

Some margarine companies have reformulated their products in order to reduce their trans fat content. Soft margarines labelled 'high in polyunsaturates' contain considerably less saturated fats and trans fatty acids than other types of margarine and butter and are good sources of vitamin E. However, recent research is beginning to suggest that high intakes of polyunsaturated oils may predispose some people to asthma.

Low-fat spreads are made mainly from water and whipped butter or vegetable oils; the proportions of saturated fats vary, so check the labels carefully. Low-fat spreads usually contain 40 per cent fat and around 390 Calories per 100g (3½oz), and very low-fat spreads contain about 25 per cent fat and 270 Calories per 100g. Some spreads are as low as 5 per cent fat. These are made with fat substitutes, such as whey protein, that imitate the texture of fat. Their high water content makes them unsuitable for cooking and they often contain gelatine, and so are unsuitable for vegetarians.

Many people prefer the taste of butter to other spreads, but have been discouraged from buying it because it is high in saturated fat and cholesterol. However, many nutritionists believe that, as long as it is not eaten to excess, butter can be preferable to margarine as it is a relatively natural product.

Generally, all yellow spreads should be used in moderation. If you buy speciality breads that taste interesting in their own right, you can dispense with spreads altogether.

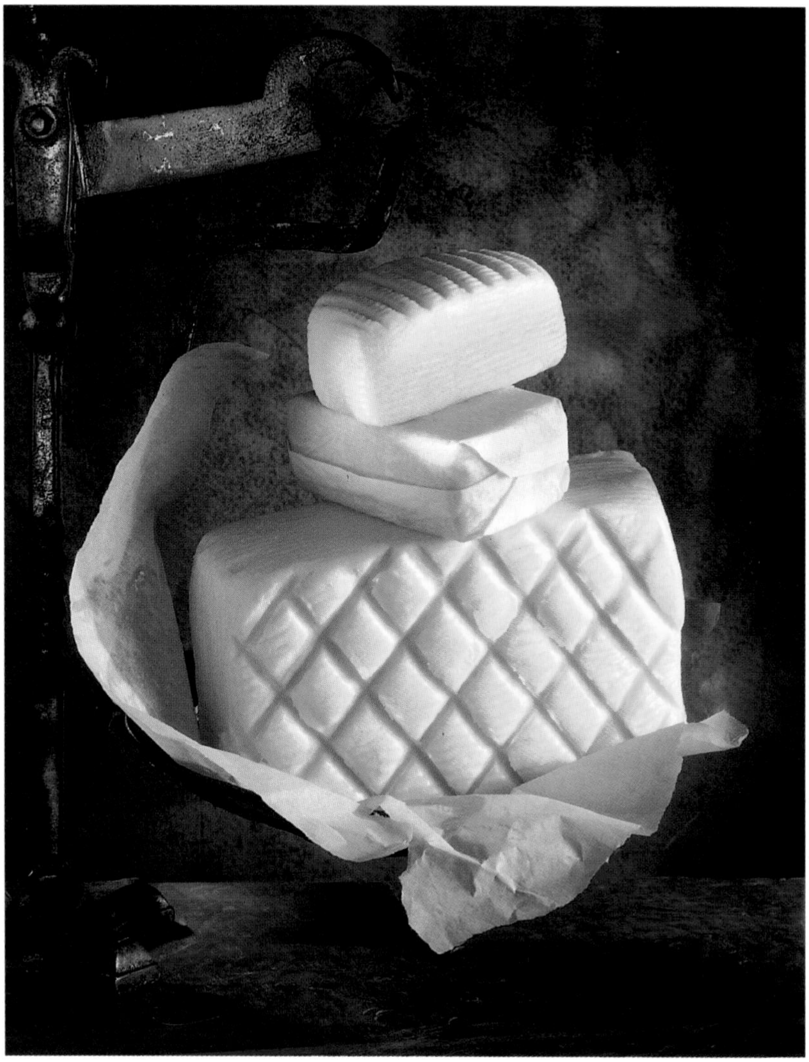

THE APPEAL OF BUTTER *Though it is high in saturated fats and cholesterol, butter is gaining popularity once more because it is a much more natural product than highly processed margarines.*

Bronchitis

EAT PLENTY OF
- *Fresh fruit and vegetables*
- *Oily fish such as mackerel or sardines*
- *Lean meat and pumpkin seeds*

CUT DOWN ON
- *Alcohol and caffeine*

AVOID
- *Smoking, which is particularly harmful to people with bronchitis*

There are two forms of bronchitis – chronic and acute. The chronic form is more common in Britain than anywhere else in the world and is often the result of smoking. In the UK it is the second most frequent cause of lost working days – 30 million are lost each year. Yet it is known that the condition can be alleviated by giving up smoking and adopting a sensible diet.

Invading a weak system

Acute bronchitis is almost always a secondary infection; bacteria invade when someone is already weakened by a cold or flu virus. Asthma sufferers and others with lung problems, the elderly, very small children and babies, and also smokers, are its most likely victims. The resulting persistent cough, wheezing and shortness of breath, together with green or yellow phlegm are common symptoms of acute bronchitis. If this is not treated, it may develop into PNEUMONIA.

Bouts of chronic bronchitis often recur year after year; some of its symptoms can be experienced almost daily. Sufferers endure repeated fits of coughing and may also produce copious amounts of phlegm.

A healthy diet will help to strengthen the body's natural resistance. Adequate intakes of vitamins A and C as well as zinc are needed for the proper functioning of the immune system. Carrots, spinach, spring onions, leeks and cantaloupe melon provide plenty of beta carotene (the plant form of vitamin A), which is also known to help lung conditions. A small portion of liver each week is another good source of vitamin A (but should not be eaten during pregnancy). Fresh fruit and vegetables are vital for vitamin C. Shellfish (particularly oysters), pumpkin seeds and lean beef all supply dietary zinc. Oily fish are thought to have an anti-inflammatory effect in the lungs.

Case study

Andy, a factory worker, discovered that he had mild bronchitis when his company offered him a medical consultation as part of his pre-retirement course. He had worked in the factory since leaving school and could remember the dust and fumes of those days, although conditions were excellent now. He also smoked, and the doctor warned him that unless he gave up the habit and improved his diet, he could end up an invalid with chronic bronchitis like his father and grandfather before him. Andy was advised to eat more fresh fruit and vegetables, and oily fish such as mackerel and sardines which may help to reduce inflammation in the lungs. He has given it a try; his breathing is easier and the bronchitis does not seem to be any worse.

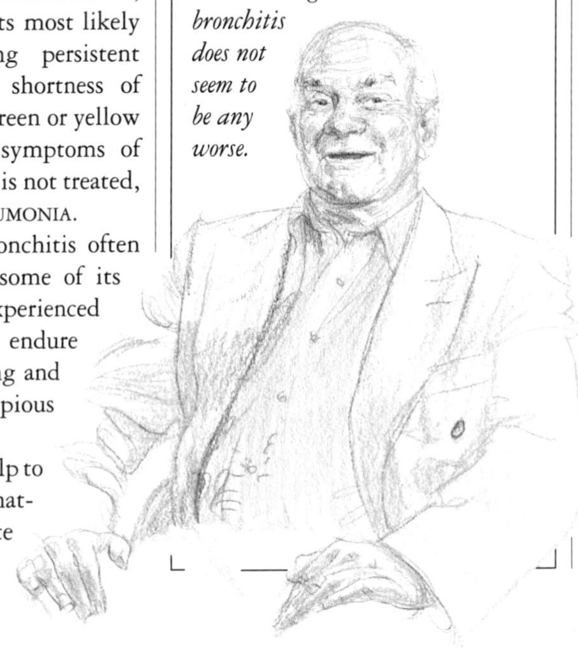

High intakes of fats and sugars should be avoided because they tend to displace more nourishing foods that contain the micronutrients needed to support the immune system. Too much alcohol or coffee will also inhibit the immune system since, to cleanse their toxins from the blood, the liver has to draw on extra micronutrients, thus depleting the body's reserves.

The immune system can be damaged by exposure to heavy metals such as lead and cadmium. It is therefore important to avoid food which may come from areas affected by traffic pollution. Foods that are high in cadmium include commercially produced mushrooms grown in manure, kidneys from mature animals, and shellfish caught in waters that have been exposed to industrial pollution.

To breathe more freely

As a fragrant alternative to the many chemical decongestants now available, aromatherapy can offer natural inhalants such as the essential oils of eucalyptus, hyssop and sandalwood.

Eucalyptus oil is particularly good for relieving congestion and clearing the head. Hyssop is also a decongestant and sandalwood is a relaxant that helps to ease muscular or nervous tension.

To inhale, pour a few drops of each onto a paper towel, or add them to a bowl of hot (but not boiling) water using the following proportions: three of eucalyptus to two of hyssop and two of sandalwood.

As a massage, apply the oils in the ratio of 15:10:5. Other helpful oils include cajuput, niaouli and pine.

BRUSSELS SPROUTS

BENEFITS
- *May help to reduce the risk of cancer of the colon and stomach*
- *Good source of folate and indoles, which may help to prevent certain types of cancer*
- *Useful source of dietary fibre*

DRAWBACK
- *Renowned for their ability to produce intestinal wind*

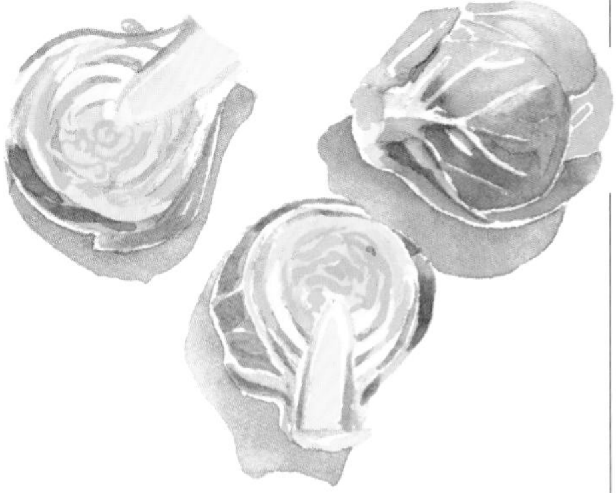

Like the cabbages which they resemble in miniature, Brussels sprouts and other cruciferous vegetables contain nitrogen compounds called indoles which are thought to reduce the risk of certain cancers. Brussels sprouts are also rich in vitamin C and beta carotene, which is converted into vitamin A by the body.

Their only potential drawback is that – like the cabbage – they may produce unpleasant intestinal wind.

THE CANCER FACTOR

Brussels sprouts may help to protect against some types of breast cancer which are linked to high levels of the hormone oestrogen. The indoles contained in Brussels sprouts stimulate the liver which in turn breaks down the hormone. Experiments in the USA suggest that by accelerating oestrogen's metabolism and speeding its elimination from the body, less of the hormone is available to feed the dependent malignancy.

Women who metabolise oestrogen rapidly are thought to be less likely to contract cancers of the breast or uterus; and where these cancers already exist, it is possible – though not yet proven – that vegetable indoles may inhibit their spread to other parts of the body. However, as over-cooking may leach indoles into the cooking water and reduces the effectiveness of many vitamins, Brussels sprouts are best eaten lightly cooked.

Because prevention and treatment of colon and stomach cancer involves eating plenty of starchy foods, fibre and vegetables, there is speculation that cruciferous vegetables – which contain both fibre and indoles – may also help to prevent this form of cancer.

Research in the USA suggests that low blood levels of folate (of which Brussels sprouts are a good source) may predispose people to lung cancer by making the lung cells more vulnerable to tumour formation. Thus eating Brussels sprouts, which are a good source of this nutrient, may also offer some protection against lung cancer.

Sprouts at their best

Choose small, bright green, firm sprouts with tightly packed leaves and no patches of yellow. If they are old and loosely packed they will have an unpleasant sulphurous smell and, when cooked, will be spongy and taste bitter. Sprouts will keep in the refrigerator for a few days without rotting as long as they are left unwashed and their outer leaves are removed. Rinse them and, to ensure that they are evenly cooked rather than soft on the outside and hard in the middle, cut a small cross into their base. Sprouts should be cooked as quickly as possible in fast-boiling water in an uncovered saucepan; sulphurous gases can build up if the pan is covered with a lid.

BULIMIA NERVOSA

Diet plays an important role in the management of bulimia. Victims of this psychiatric disorder are trapped in a cycle of starving, bingeing and vomiting, and need to regain control of their eating habits. Treatment in hospital or a clinic focuses on the establishment of three regular, balanced meals a day, avoiding in-between snacks and the high-fat, high-sugar fast foods often eaten during binges. Bulimics may also need reassuring that a healthy appetite is normal.

Self-induced vomiting, and the excessive use of diuretics and laxatives associated with bulimia, disturb the body's serum electrolyte level (the ions including sodium and potassium which circulate in the blood). This may lead to serious dehydration and produce a potassium deficiency which can cause poor kidney function, weak muscles and irregular heartbeat. Early treatment often entails a diet to restore a normal balance. Eating foods that supply plenty of potassium such as dried fruits, nuts, seeds, avocados and bananas, will usually achieve this.

However, the overall goal is to persuade the sufferer to adopt a healthy eating pattern which includes a wide range of foods containing all the essential nutrients in a sensible balance. Anything that might potentially upset that balance or affect the sufferer's state of mind, such as excessive coffee, tea or alcohol, should be discouraged. It is important to include a reasonable amount of carbohydrate foods such as wholemeal bread, pasta and rice but to limit FATS and also the consumption of snack foods such as crisps, biscuits and confectionery.

Balancing fats, carbohydrates and protein in line with the guidelines laid down in DIET AND SLIMMING will help the sufferer to achieve and maintain an optimum stable weight which is essential for recovery.

A diet relatively high in fibre will help the movement of food through the digestive system and cut out dependence on laxatives. This must be introduced gradually, however, to limit the discomfort often experienced by bulimics whose digestive systems, after years of abuse, will probably be unused to the normal passage of food.

CAUSES AND SYMPTOMS

Bulimia nervosa is a severe stress-related eating disorder that affects at least 3 women in 100. It may be difficult to detect because victims are secretive and, unlike those who suffer from the related eating disorder, anorexia nervosa, are often of normal weight rather than noticeably thin.

The majority of sufferers are females aged between 15 and 34. They are often perfectionists in their work but also suffer from low self-esteem and find a focus for their emotional difficulties in attempts to control their eating. The root of the problem may be some emotional disturbance but the actual disorder will start because they imagine that the solution lies in transforming their bodies; they have an obsession with slimness and often a distorted body image.

Although numbers appear to be rising, there are far fewer male sufferers; a review of medical literature between 1966 and 1990 indicates that bulimia affects only about 1 in 500 adolescent boys and young men. This may be because men are less subject to the social pressures to achieve an 'ideal' body shape, and also tend to channel their emotional problems in other ways than through food and diet.

Bulimics often embark on crash diets which tend to create havoc with both appetite and digestion. As a result, they end up bingeing – eating anything from 3000 to 6000 Calories in one sitting. Such binges are followed by guilt, depression which can be severe or even suicidal, and self-induced vomiting. Bulimics tend to make excessive use of laxatives, slimming pills and diuretics in their quest to lose weight. They may also drink large amounts of alcohol as a way of trying to blank out their problems.

Other symptoms include absence of, or irregular, menstrual periods, swollen neck glands, weight fluctuation, and damage to the teeth caused by the action of acidic vomit on dental enamel. Poorly functioning kidneys may result in oedema – swollen feet and ankles. Sufferers may also experience irregular heartbeats, muscle weakness and even epileptic seizures.

Medical treatment, which can take up to three years, may require a short stay in hospital or a residential centre for people with diet-related illnesses, where their diets, attempts to vomit and use of laxatives can all be carefully monitored. Antidepressants may be prescribed. When discharged, outpatient follow-up is essential. Psychotherapy or counselling is a vital part of the treatment and may involve the patient's family.

How bulimia is diagnosed

- Recurrent episodes of bingeing.
- Lack of control over the binges.
- The regular use of self-induced vomiting, laxatives, diuretics, strict dieting, fasting, or vigorous exercise to prevent weight gain.
- A minimum average of two binge-eating episodes per week for at least three months.
- Persistent concern over body shape and weight.

BURNS

TAKE PLENTY OF
- *Water and fruit juices*
- *Protein foods such as lean meat, fish, pulses and grains*
- *Fresh fruit and vegetables rich in vitamin C*

CUT DOWN ON
- *Tea and coffee*

AVOID
- *Alcohol*

Burn victims need a diet which replaces the fluids, protein, sodium, potassium and essential fatty acids that are lost when tissue is destroyed. First-degree burns cause skin to redden; second-degree burns may also include blistering, and third-degree burns can destroy skin cells, exposing the body to bacterial infection, and damage underlying muscle.

People who suffer extensive burns therefore need plenty of calories and high-protein foods to assist tissue repair; in the most severe cases this would be delivered intravenously.

Vitamin C, zinc (found in meat and shellfish), and also the essential fatty acids contained in oily fish and vegetable oils, all play an important part in the healing of wounds and burns.

Tea and coffee consumption should be reduced because both are diuretics; alcohol should be avoided because it dehydrates the body and dries the skin.

BUTTER

See page 66

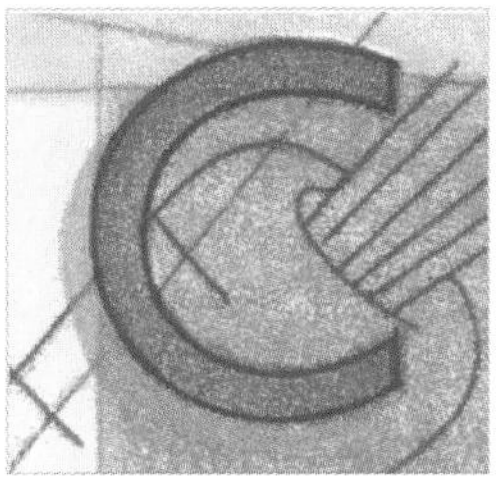

Cabbage

BENEFITS

- *May help to prevent cancer of the colon*
- *Can help to relieve gastric ulcers*
- *Excellent source of vitamin C*

DRAWBACKS

- *Can cause flatulence*
- *May contribute to iron deficiency if eaten in excess*

This much maligned vegetable has a considerable reputation in traditional medicine. Cabbage is a vitamin-rich food which contains only 16 Calories in an average boiled portion.

The green varieties of cabbage are particularly rich in vitamins C and K and are a good source of vitamin E and potassium. Beta carotene, fibre, folate and thiamin are also present.

Cabbage is claimed to help gastric ulcers because it contains a substance called S-Methylmethionine, that is thought to promote healing of ulcers and to relieve pain. The traditional remedy prescribes 1 litre (1¾ pints) of raw cabbage juice per day for at least 8 days for the benefit to be felt. However, if consumed in excess, the juice can inhibit iron absorption which may eventually lead to anaemia. Cabbage can also cause flatulence.

Perhaps most important of all, cabbage contains a wealth of compounds that may help to protect against cancer. Research, done in Japan and the USA, suggests a link between regular consumption of cabbage and the suppression of the growth of precancerous polyps in the colon.

Cabbage also helps to speed up the metabolism of oestrogen in women, which might offer a degree of protection against hormone-related cancers such as cancer of the breast and ovary.

Cabbage needs handling with care if the nutrients are to be preserved. It is an excellent source of vitamin C when raw, but more than half is usually lost into the cooking water when it is boiled. Using a microwave oven to cook cabbage can greatly reduce the vitamin loss. Most of the nutrients are concentrated in the dark, outer leaves.

Sauerkraut gets its flavour from bacterial fermentation. The helpful micro-organisms may help to promote healthy bacteria in the gut which can improve digestion, nutrient absorption and the synthesis of vitamin B.

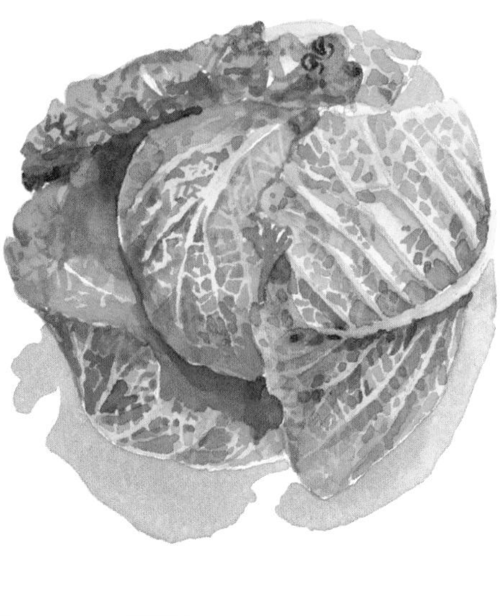

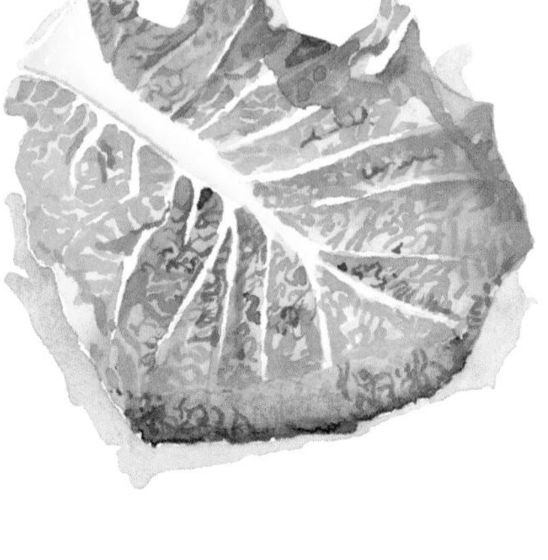

Caffeine

BENEFITS

- *A mild stimulant that can improve mental performance and heighten alertness*

DRAWBACKS

- *Potentially habit-forming and can cause withdrawal symptoms*
- *May cause insomnia*
- *Can accelerate the loss of minerals from bone*
- *May induce migraine in susceptible individuals*
- *Excessive amounts can lead to tremors and palpitations*

The stimulant caffeine is found mainly in coffee and tea but is also present in chocolate, in some colas and in some cold and pain relief tablets.

Caffeine stimulates the heart and central nervous system and can help to enhance mental performance when the brain is sluggish. It also stimulates the output of acid in the stomach, which can aid digestion, and dilates the airways in the lungs.

Though caffeine is relatively nontoxic it can become addictive. Too much coffee, or tea (which contains about two-thirds the amount of caffeine found in instant coffee) may cause tremors, sweating, palpitations, rapid breathing and sleeplessness and may also induce migraine attacks. However, sudden withdrawal should be avoided since this can cause severe headaches, irritability and lethargy.

The caffeine in most colas and in chocolate can cause childhood insomnia. Taken late in the day, even two glasses of cola or half a bar of dark chocolate can prevent a child sleeping.

There is no need to avoid caffeine if you have had a heart attack, but it is advisable to drink coffee or tea only in moderation. Medical advice is that no one should drink more than six cups of

Which has more caffeine?

Coffee is the best-known source of caffeine but tea, chocolate of all sorts, colas and some painkillers also contain it. Compare the caffeine levels in a single 150ml (¼ pint) cup or a 125g (4oz) bar of chocolate.

Ground coffee	115mg
Instant coffee	65mg
Tea	40mg
Cola	18mg
Cocoa	4mg
Drinking chocolate	3mg
Decaffeinated coffee	3mg
Decaffeinated tea	3mg
Dark chocolate	80mg
Milk chocolate	20mg
Two painkiller tablets	60mg

tea or coffee a day. But people with high blood pressure, heart problems or kidney disease should drink less, or gradually cut it out of their diet.

Pregnant women and those breast-feeding should restrict themselves to one cup of ground coffee or two cups of instant coffee a day. Because foetuses absorb caffeine but expel it more slowly than adults, newborn babies can suffer withdrawal symptoms.

Some studies suggest that heavy caffeine consumption may make it more difficult to conceive.

Coffee is a diuretic and increases the rate of excretion of calcium. High caffeine intakes are associated with an increased risk of OSTEOPOROSIS – a disease which weakens the bones, causing them to become brittle.

Cakes and Pastries

DRAWBACKS

- *High in calories and saturated fats*
- *High in dietary cholesterol when made with a lot of eggs, butter or cream*
- *High in sugar and refined carbohydrates*

Flour, sugar, salt, solid fats, eggs and milk or cream are the basic ingredients used to make most cakes and pastries.

Solid fats are more suitable for baking than liquid vegetable oils so most cakes are made with butter or margarine. Both are high in saturated fat and some margarines also contain trans fatty acids. Both of these can increase blood cholesterol levels, and are linked with heart disease. Many manufacturers use 'partially hydrogenated vegetable fats', which are hardened oils, to make pastry. The hardening process changes the oil's chemical structure, forming more saturated and trans fatty acids.

A LITTLE OF WHAT YOU FANCY

As part of a balanced diet, the odd slice of cake will do no harm, but if you get into the habit of eating cakes every day, you will ruin your appetite for nutritious meals and consume a considerable amount of saturated fats and

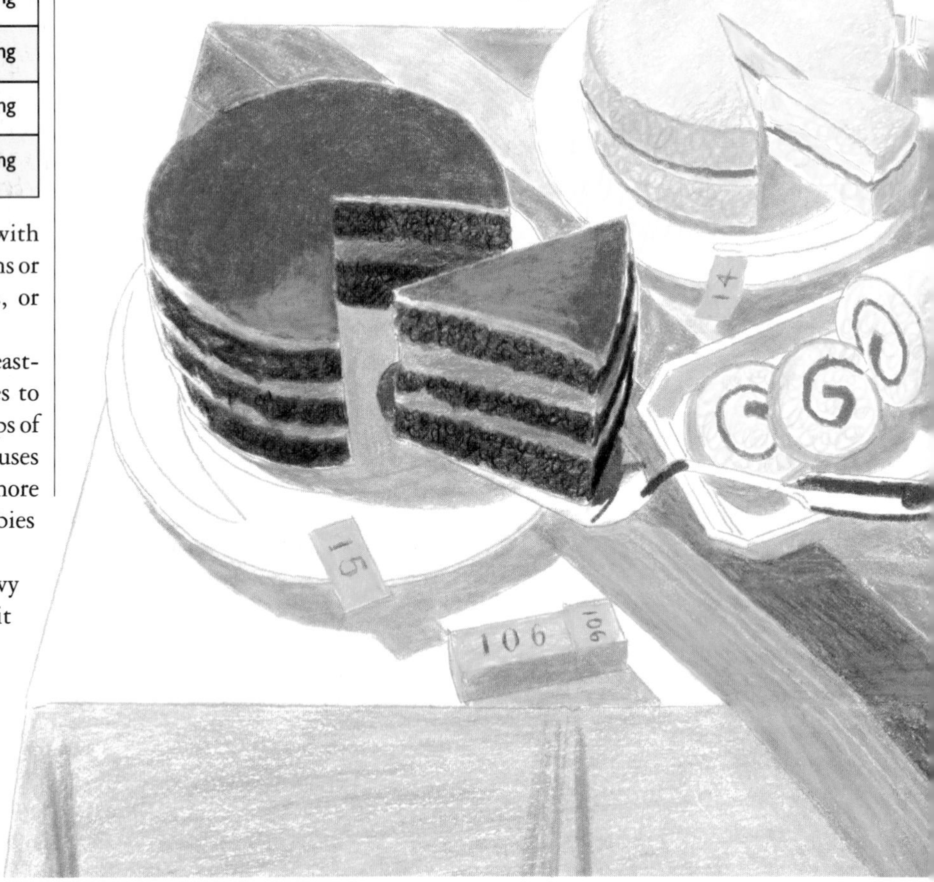

NAUGHTY BUT NICE *Tasty homemade cakes are winners at the village fête but tend to be low in nutrients and high in saturated fats as well as sugar.*

sugar. While sugar icings and jam fillings are not too bad for your waistline, a butter icing will double the fat content of the cake.

Some cakes, such as fruit or carrot cake, have a healthy image, but even these tend to be high in fat. Generally, there are no cakes that can be considered to be good for you from a health point of view. Although there are ways to make cakes with a reduced saturated fat content or an increased fibre content, the taste often suffers as a result.

Some commercially available cakes claim to be virtually fat-free, but they are usually still high in sugar; others claim to be low-sugar. If you have to watch your cholesterol intake, the low-fat cakes are a healthier option.

Cakes and pastries are not such a problem for children because they need plenty of energy. However, it is not a good idea to encourage frequent consumption of these foods as the sugar can cause tooth decay. Even for children, it is probably best to reserve cakes for an occasional treat.

CANCER

See page 76

CARBOHYDRATES

In previous decades, starchy carbohydrates such as bread, pasta, potatoes and rice were considered to be fattening, stodgy and generally unimportant foods. The modern view is, however, that they are an essential part of a balanced diet and we should be eating more of them. Government guidelines suggest that our current carbohydrate intake which, in Britain, is on average about 45 per cent of total calories consumed, should increase to about 50 per cent. The general dietary aim is that an increase in carbohydrates should be matched by a decrease in the amount of fat we eat, in order to help reduce the risk of coronary heart disease.

Carbohydrates are converted by the body into glucose and glycogen (the animal equivalent of starch in plants). During exercise, our muscles are fuelled by glucose in the blood and by glycogen, stored in the liver and in the muscles themselves. Glucose and glycogen are interconvertible; if the body has enough glucose, carbohydrates will be converted into glycogen, and if there is a shortage, glycogen will be turned into glucose. The digestion of carbohydrates helps to maintain the balance between the level of glucose in the blood and stores of glycogen.

There are three main forms of carbohydrate: sugars, starch and fibre. Both starch and fibre are complex carbohydrates. Table sugar and sugars that are added to food and drinks are simple carbohydrates. They are digested and absorbed rapidly – although only glucose is readily available for use by the body. Other simple sugars, such as fructose (from sucrose and fruit) and galactose (from milk sugar – lactose), cannot be used quite as fast since they must first be converted to glucose.

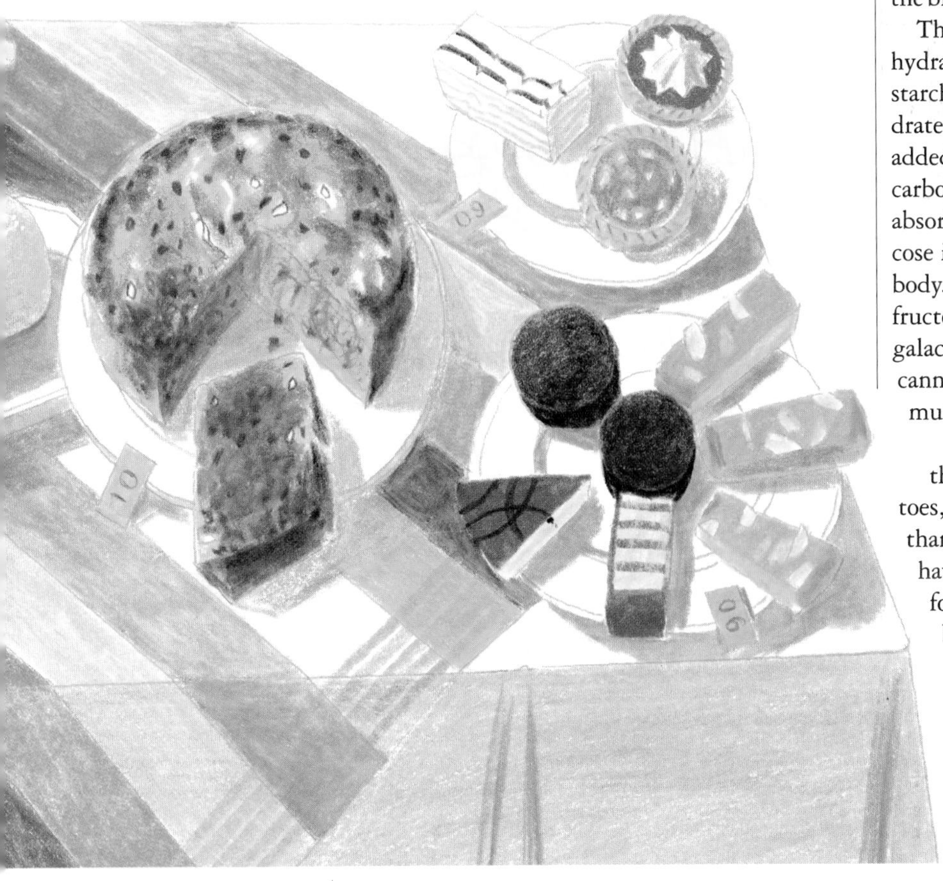

Complex carbohydrates, such as the starch found in bread and potatoes, are broken down more slowly than simple sugars. By the time they have been digested, the body's need for glucose has often been satisfied by simple sugars provided by other foods, and so they tend to be converted into glycogen – ready for future energy needs.

A measure of how quickly the energy from a carbohydrate is made available for use by the body is the glycaemic index.

Generally, foods with a high glycaemic index are quickly broken down into glucose and provide a fast energy fix, while those with a lower index take longer to break down and tend to boost long-term energy stores rather than meet immediate energy needs.

Muscles normally contain enough glycogen to fuel about 90-120 minutes of intense physical activity. Glycogen stores can be boosted in preparation for prolonged periods of physical exercise, such as a climbing weekend, or endurance sports such as long-distance running, by eating a carbohydrate-rich diet – containing about 600g (1lb 5oz) of carbohydrate a day, or around 70 per cent of the daily calorie intake – for about three days beforehand.

After taking a lot of exercise, when glycogen levels are reduced, uptake of glucose by the muscles can be increased by a factor of three or four.

A high-carbohydrate diet composed of sugars and starches replenishes and increases the body's reserves of glycogen, which enhances the capacity for endurance exercise. This is best achieved by eating more fruit and vegetables and more complex carbohydrates, which are found in foods such as potatoes, yams, rice, pasta, bread, pulses (such as peas and beans), breakfast cereals, tortillas, chapattis and starchy root vegetables.

Eating an extra one and a half slices of brown bread, for example, would provide the extra 100 Calories needed to achieve the government's recommended 5 per cent increase in carbohydrates, in a diet of 2000 Calories a day.

Eating more dietary fibre, found in fresh fruit and vegetables – particularly those of the cabbage family – is now thought to help protect the body against various cancers, including cancer of the colon. Some types of carbohydrate, such as resistant starch, are not digestible by the small intestine and pass into the large intestine, or colon. There, along with other forms of dietary fibre, they increase stool weight and speed the passage of food residues through the digestive tract. This is thought to contribute to warding off cancer of the colon.

Although the useful role of most carbohydrates is now widely recognised, SUGAR continues to come under fire – because it has few nutritional benefits and can contribute to tooth decay if it is eaten too frequently. Many experts believe it is best to spread carbohydrate consumption throughout the day as evenly as possible, so that there are not vast swings in blood sugar levels. This is particularly important for people with diabetes. Common sugars (simple carbohydrates) and some of their sources are:

- Glucose, found in honey, fruit, vegetables and some soft drinks.
- Fructose, which is found in fruit and honey.
- Lactose, in milk and dairy products.
- Maltose, which is found in sprouting grains, malted wheat and barley, and malt extract.
- Sucrose, from table sugar, as well as fruit, vegetables and many foods and drinks which contain added sugar.

Did you know?

- Just because you cannot see sugar in the ingredients list on a food packet, does not mean that it is not there. Look out also for sucrose, lactose, maltose, fructose, honey, molasses, glucose, dextrose, corn syrup and invert syrup.
- Lactose is the sugar which is unique to milk – there are no other sources of it.
- Slow-release carbohydrates are those which are absorbed more slowly and release glucose into the bloodstream more slowly. The slowest of them all is fructose.
- The degree of milling can make a difference to how rapidly the body derives glucose from cereals. The bigger the particle size the more difficult it is to digest and the more slowly glucose is released into the bloodstream. Stone-ground wholemeal bread has a larger particle size so it has a lower glycaemic index than roller-milled wholemeal bread.
- White bread and wholemeal bread release glucose into the bloodstream at more or less the same rate, since most commercially produced breads use finely milled flour.
- Carbohydrates make up three-quarters of the living world. The most abundant form of carbohydrate is cellulose, found in plants; it is indigestible to humans.
- Carbohydrates make up about 75 per cent of people's total calorie intake globally. However, in the developed world they comprise only 45 per cent of the diet.
- Fructose (fruit sugar) is about one and a half times as sweet as sucrose (ordinary table sugar) so you need less of it. Lactose (milk sugar) is about half as sweet as sucrose.
- Cotton and starch are almost entirely made up of glucose. But because the glucose units are joined in different ways only starch is digestible.
- Glycogen is the store of carbohydrate in animals and because it has a similar structure to starch it is sometimes referred to as animal starch.
- One gram of carbohydrate (sugar or starch) provides 4 Calories – the same as protein – but much less than either fat, which provides 9 Calories per gram, or pure alcohol, which provides 7 Calories per gram.

Carbohydrates in the daily diet

There are three main types of carbohydrates – sugars (simple), starches and fibre (complex). These are present in varying amounts in different foods. For example, a ripe banana contains about the same amount of carbohydrate as a slice of bread, but it is mostly in the form of sugar. Bread, however, is mainly made of starch.

Carbohydrate should ideally provide about 50 per cent of everyone's total energy intake – mainly in the form of starchy foods such as potatoes, cereals, pasta, rice and bread. If you need 1000 Calories of carbohydrates a day, for example, choose foods that contain all three types of carbohydrate, rather than eating 15 slices of white bread or 17 packets of crisps.

Below are four suggested combinations of food that would supply the recommended daily carbohydrate requirement for an average person in the correct balance. The last group is suitable for a person with gluten intolerance, who cannot eat wheat.

I small bowl (60g/2oz) of cereal
4 large slices of wholemeal bread
175g (6oz) boiled potatoes
I thin slice carrot cake (without the icing)
I pear, I peach and a portion of melon

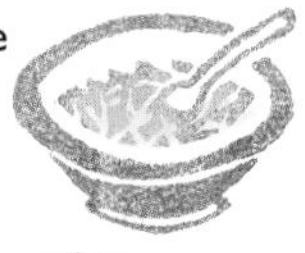

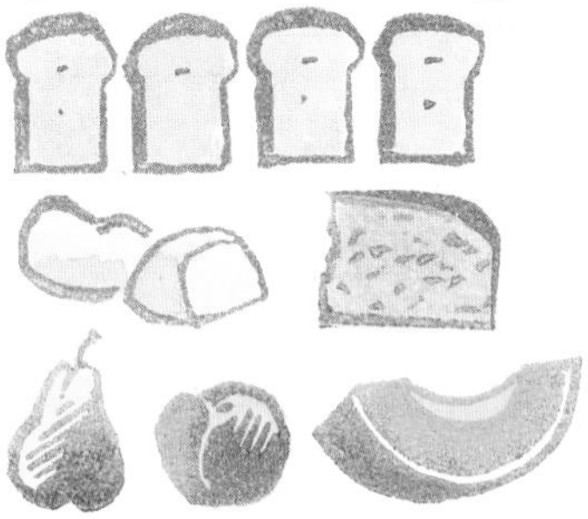

2 slices of toast and I bowl of cereal
I large slice of wholemeal bread
Chickpea, mung bean and red kidney bean salad
I serving of rice (175g/6oz)
I scone
I kiwi fruit, small bunch of grapes, 2 tangerines

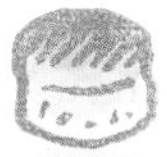

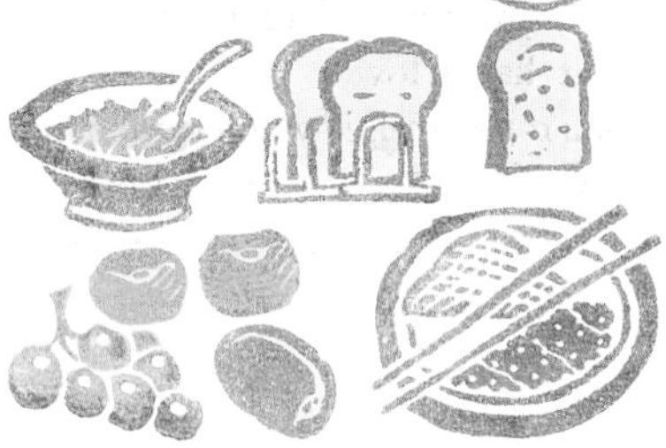

2 large slices of bread
I large jacket potato (175-225g/6-8oz)
I large helping of pasta
I digestive biscuit
I banana, I apple, I orange

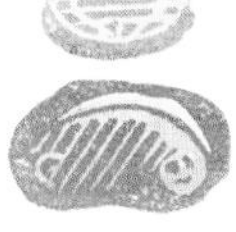

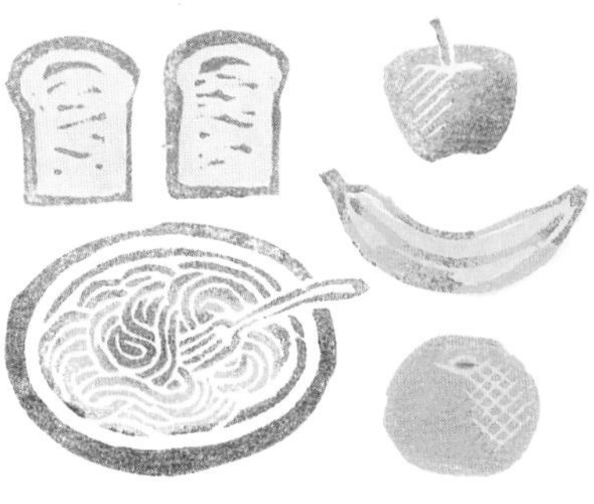

For someone with gluten intolerance
I bowl of cornflakes or Rice Crispies
4 large slices of gluten-free bread
I medium potato
I packet of crisps
175g (6oz) serving of cooked rice
2 bananas, I orange

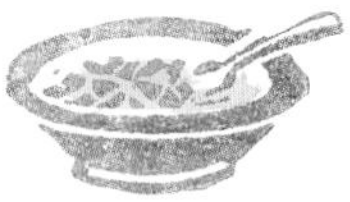

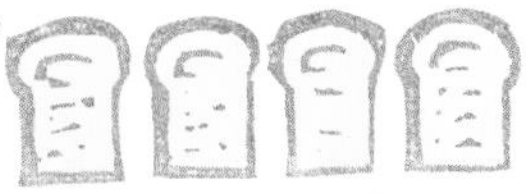

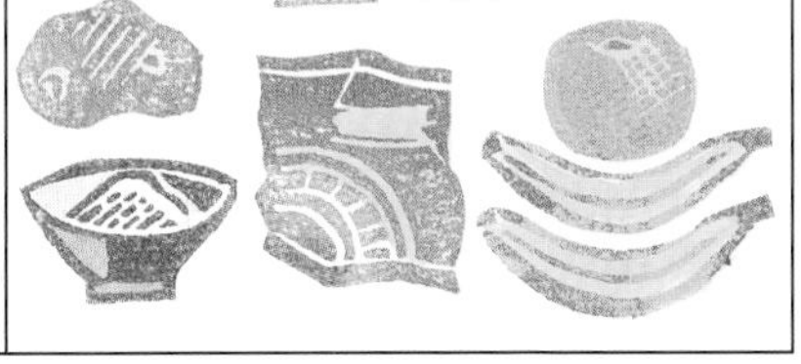

Carpal Tunnel Syndrome

EAT PLENTY OF

- *Yeast extracts, wheatgerm, oats, meat, green leafy vegetables and bananas for their vitamin B_6*

CUT DOWN ON

- *Alcohol, caffeine and smoking*

Carpal tunnel syndrome is caused by pressure on the nerve going from the forearm to the hand, thumb and fingers. It produces pain, numbness and pins and needles in the thumb, index and middle fingers of one or both hands. Women between 40 and 60 years old are most frequently at risk. It may affect women when they start to take the Pill, and those who suffer from PMS. It is also common during pregnancy. Men and women with rheumatoid arthritis are also prone to carpal tunnel syndrome.

The symptoms often disappear without treatment, but changes in diet can hasten this and may avoid the need for more drastic treatment such as cortisone injections or surgery.

One study claimed that within a few weeks of increasing their intake of vitamin B_6, up to 85per cent of sufferers found their condition had improved. Drinking alcohol destroys B_6, so it is wise to cut down. Sufferers are also likely to benefit from eating foods that provide B_6 such as yeast extracts, wheatgerm, oats, meat, offal, green leafy vegetables or bananas. Daily supplements of 50-100mg of vitamin B_6 are safe, but anything more should be taken only on medical advice as high doses taken for prolonged periods can damage the nervous system.

Caffeine and nicotine can interfere with peripheral circulation. Gradually cut down on your caffeine intake and try to give up smoking altogether.

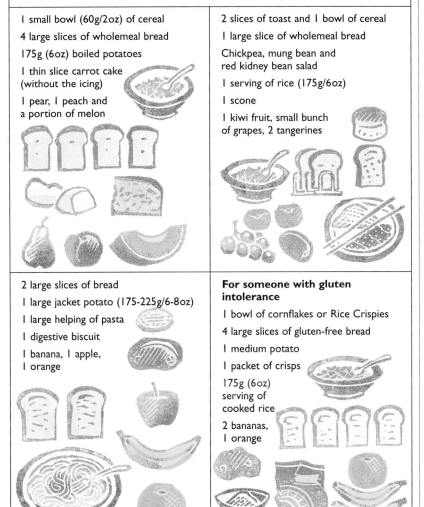

CANCER: HOW DIET CAN HELP

Known and feared from earliest times, cancer remains a major killer. However, some cancers can be cured and experts believe that correct nutrition may help to prevent many forms of the disease.

Cancer causes one in every five deaths in the USA and an estimated one in four in Britain. Lung cancer is the most common form of the disease in Britain, and the highest killer. The second most common is skin cancer, which is seldom fatal if caught early. Indeed, many cancers can now be treated successfully.

There is strong evidence that certain foods can help to protect against cancer; that low intakes of these foods may increase the risk; and that other foods contain cancer-forming agents (carcinogens) which actually promote the growth of tumours. Diet is believed to be linked to the causes of one-third of all cancers; however, because the disease can take up to 30 years to manifest itself clinically, cause and effect are difficult to establish.

GARLIC – A POSSIBLE DEFENCE?

Garlic and onions – for which medicinal properties have long been claimed – may prove powerful allies in the fight against cancer. Scientific studies in China suggest that they may neutralise cancer-causing chemicals and reduce the risk of tumours. A study of 16000 Chinese found that people with the highest intakes of garlic or onions were those least likely to suffer from cancer of the stomach.

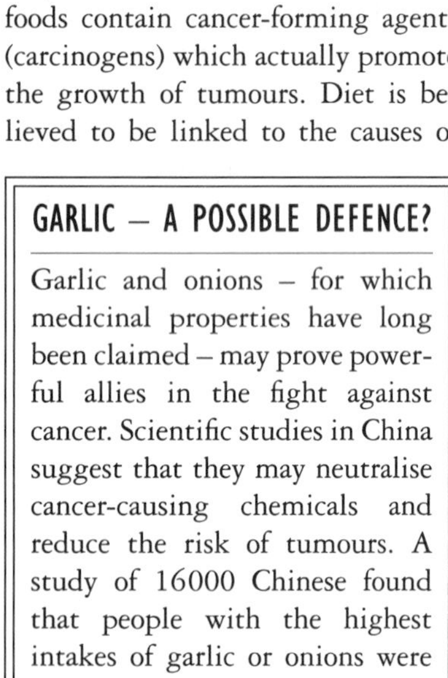

HOW CANCER SPREADS

Normally, body cells grow and reproduce in an orderly way, each cell fulfilling a specific role. By contrast, cancer cells proliferate rapidly and to no set pattern. Cancers are caused by damage to the genetic material in cells. This stage, known as initiation, can be sparked by external factors, the most important being radiation, viral infections and certain chemicals. Cancerous cells fulfil no normal function, invading and destroying neighbouring tissue at random as they develop into abnormal growths. Often they spread from their primary site, carried via the bloodstream and lymph vessels, to distant parts of the body where they cause secondary tumours, or metastases.

FREE-RADICAL DAMAGE

An imbalance of FREE RADICALS encourages conditions that allow some cancers to develop. Free radicals are formed during the body's chemical processes and as part of its natural defence mechanism. Exposure to radiation, pollution or some foods sparks their overproduction, when they can damage healthy cells that may then turn cancerous. Some vitamins and minerals – known as ANTIOXIDANTS and free-radical scavengers – counteract the impact of harmful free radicals.

Diet may trigger the initiation of cancer by supplying carcinogens, but it can also provide agents that block their effects. The immune system should react immediately to mutant cells and help to keep cancer in check, but an immune system impaired by poor diet can allow a cancer to develop. Diet also affects the production of hormones, which can be another influence on a cancer's rate of growth.

While fats are an important source of energy, high intakes have been linked with certain types of cancers. Make sure that fats provide no more than 35 per cent of your daily calorie intake. Saturated fats, most of which are derived from animal sources, are particularly suspect. High intakes of animal fat drive the liver to produce

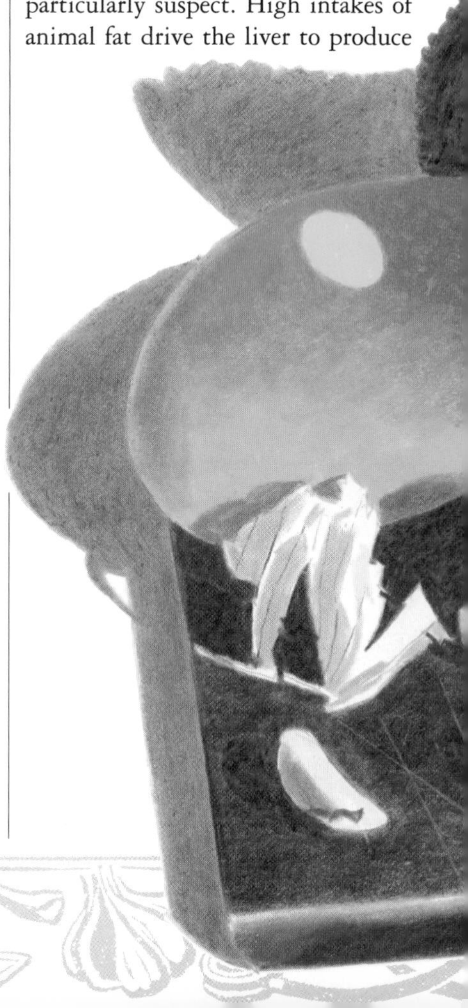

increased quantities of bile, and as bacteria in the gut work on these, small quantities of potential carcinogens are produced. Trimming fat from meat may diminish the risk, but there is an argument for eating no animal products at all since vegans are at less risk from cancer of the colon than meat-eaters or even vegetarians.

A high-fat, low-fibre diet can lead to excess weight, changes in the way the intestines function and constipation, all of which potentially increase the risk of cancer. For instance, cancers of the womb, gall bladder and breast are more common among obese people. Certain cooking methods have also been implicated in encouraging cancer. Charring food when roasting, grilling or barbecuing, for instance, can produce large amounts of potentially carcinogenic substances in the burnt areas. For this reason, the burnt patches should not be eaten. Some moulds are also carcinogenic, so any mouldy food should be discarded.

Products such as delicatessen meats and bacon should be eaten in moderation. Not only do they contain large amounts of sodium, but they are preserved with nitrites and nitrates which react with food constituents called amines to form nitrosamines – substances that have been linked with stomach cancer.

Many other chemicals, such as pesticides, growth hormones, antibiotics, tenderisers, flavourings, preservatives, stabilisers and dyes, are introduced to food during cultivation or processing. While there is no direct evidence that these chemicals have been responsible for causing cancers, you may still want to choose foods that do not contain any artificial substances. There is now a wide range of ORGANIC fruit, vegetables, meat and many other foods.

EAT PLENTY OF
- *Fresh fruit and vegetables for beta carotene and vitamin C*
- *Wholegrain cereals*

CUT DOWN ON
- *Alcohol*
- *Fats, particularly saturated fats*
- *Smoked or salt-preserved foods*
- *Meats, especially processed meats*
- *Charred or barbecued foods*

AVOID
- *Smoking*
- *Sunbathing without protection*

THE ROLE OF VITAMINS

It is important to ensure that your diet provides a healthy supply of vitamins A, C and E. These antioxidant vitamins 'mop up' harmful free

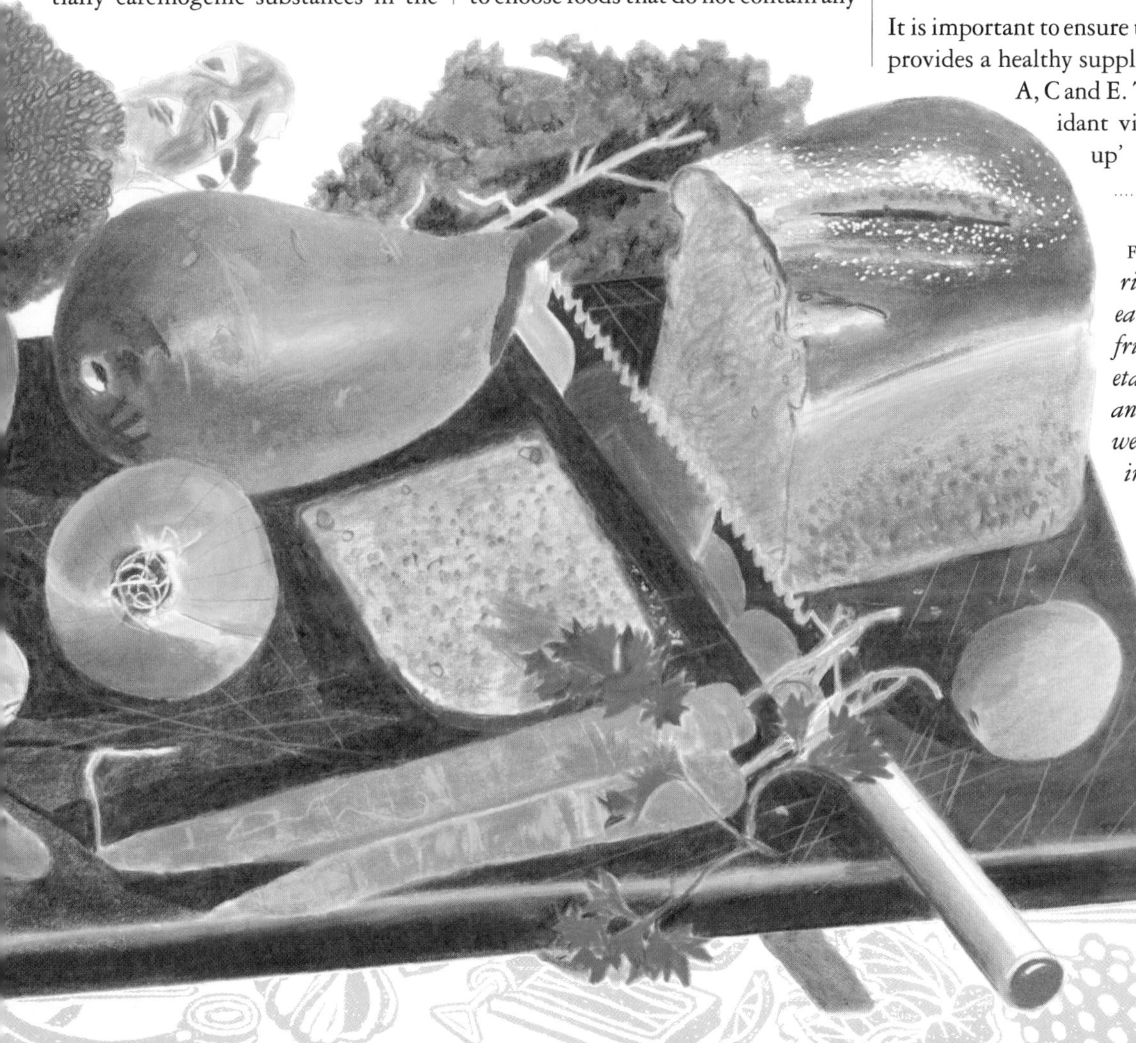

ANTI-CANCER FOODS *Cut the risk of cancer by eating plenty of fruit and vegetables for their antioxidants, as well as foods rich in fibre, such as brown bread.*

radicals. Vitamin A has also been claimed to have specific anti-tumour properties. It is found in offal and fish-liver oils. But for the cancer-conscious it may be better to obtain beta carotene (which the body converts to vitamin A) from brightly coloured fruit and vegetables. Recent studies have linked diets that include plenty of such vegetables with a reduced incidence of cancers of the lung, bladder, breast, cervix and lining of the womb.

Vitamin C, found in fresh fruit and vegetables, is a scavenger and a powerful antioxidant. It also acts to prevent nitrosamines forming in the stomach.

THE LYMPH GLANDS' WORST ENEMY

Hodgkin's disease is the best-known of the lymph cancers. It can occur at any age and takes less time to manifest itself than many other cancers. The incidence is highest among young adults and elderly people. While the cause of the disease remains unknown, there is current research into a suggested link with the Epstein-Barr virus (which causes glandular fever). Symptoms may include enlarged lymph glands, an enlarged spleen, abdominal pains, weight loss and anaemia. Eventually, the bone marrow is affected.

To give a depressed immune system the best possible chance of beating infection, people with Hodgkin's disease should follow the same well-balanced diet as other cancer patients. However, while this will help to maintain the patient's strength, it is no substitute for medical treatment. See a doctor at the first signs of illness: if Hodgkin's disease is diagnosed early, there is an excellent chance of making a full recovery.

Vitamin E protects fatty tissues and cells and helps to maintain a healthy heart. Bioflavonoids, found in some vegetables and fruit, including grapes and the pith of citrus fruits, also have antioxidant properties. Riboflavin (B_2) is thought to have a special role in the prevention of oesophageal tumours; together with vitamin B_6 it helps to break down potential carcinogens. A deficiency of folate is known to increase the risk of cancer of the cervix.

Selenium – a trace element found in eggs, offal, many seafoods and fruit and vegetables grown in soil with a high selenium content – is a potent antioxidant that works in harmony with the vitamins A, C and E. A lack of selenium is associated with an increased risk of certain cancers. This is heightened when there is also a low intake of vitamin E.

FIBRE'S PROTECTIVE ROLE

Foods high in dietary fibre may offer vital protection against cancer of the colon and also against the so-called 'Western' cancers (of the colon, rectum, prostate, uterus and breast) associated with high-fat, low-fibre diets.

Insoluble fibre, found in bran, for example, prevents the accumulation of food residues in the bowel and hence reduces the extent to which the colon wall is exposed to potential carcinogens, including those produced by bacterial action on bile acids. Soluble fibre, found in fruit and vegetables, is also important; in the process of digestion and elimination, it carries toxins and carcinogens out of the body.

A POSSIBLE BREAKTHROUGH

One of the most important areas of current research is the link between breast cancer and plant chemicals known as indoles. By rendering the hormone oestrogen less potent, indoles are thought to reduce the risk of breast cancer. They are found in Brussels sprouts, broccoli, cabbage and other cruciferous vegetables. Researchers are also investigating the possibility that soya beans and soya products, such as tofu, protect against cancer, particularly breast cancer, due to the plant hormones known as phytoestrogens that they contain.

While the protective merits of certain foods (and the potential danger of others) are gradually being accepted by the medical profession, the role of diet in the treatment of cancer remains contentious. The stage of the disease, the type of treatment and whether it is thought the patient will respond to treatment, all influence the argument.

Despite continual progress in the battle against cancer, the illness still claims many lives. Patients with advanced cancer, who have little hope of recovery, should be given whatever foods they feel like eating – regardless of whether the foods are thought to be 'good' or 'bad' for them.

THE DANGERS OF SUNBURN

Skin cancer is the second most common cancer in the UK. The most dangerous form is malignant melanoma, which has one of the fastest increase rates of all cancers in the UK. If diagnosed early it can be treated, but each year it causes more than 1500 deaths. Most at risk are fair-skinned people, especially if they have red hair, and those not usually exposed to the sun except for intense bursts during holidays (see TRAVELLERS' HEALTH). Sunny days with cool winds can still be dangerous, even in Britain. Beta carotene, found in many brightly coloured fruit and vegetables, may help to protect against SUNBURN, but it is no substitute for using good sun creams and other precautions.

The network that links diet with cancer

The advance of medical knowledge, coupled with a growing understanding of the roles of vitamins in both preventing and curing disease, has brought new hope to people with cancer. Non-dietary factors are thought to account for two-thirds of cancers, for example a virus is the principal cause of cervical cancer. Nutritional factors are believed to be linked with the other third of all forms of the disease – either through lack of essential nutrients in the diet or an excess of certain types of food. Low intakes of beta carotene, for instance, may be linked to the development of cancer of the bladder and could increase the risk of cancers of the lung, larynx and oesophagus. Low levels of B vitamins and vitamin C have also been linked to cancers, as have alcohol and smoking – both of which are thought to deplete the body's reserves of these vitamins. Certain additives have been pinpointed and, again, the risks may be reduced by increased vitamin intake. Follow the red leaves below to discover the web of connections between diet and cancer.

Abnormal cervical smears have been linked with a low dietary intake of **vitamin C**. There is thought to be a link between **smoking**, low vitamin C levels, and cervical cancer.

It is widely accepted that **smoking** causes lung cancer. However, it is also related to cancers of the mouth, throat, oesophagus, pancreas, bladder and cervix.

Nitrates and **nitrites**, used to preserve some meats, react with food constituents to form **nitrosamines** in the stomach which have been linked to cancer of the stomach.

Women with cervical cancer may be low in **vitamin B_6**. **Smoking** depletes the body's reserves of B vitamins.

Poor levels of **vitamin C** have been associated with cancer of the oesophagus and larynx. Both **smoking** and **alcohol** consumption deplete the body's reserves of vitamin C.

A good intake of **vitamin C** may inhibit the formation of carcinogenic **nitrosamines**.

Nitrates and **nitrites** are widely used in many smoked and salty foods, such as bacon and cured meats.

Levels of **folate**, a B vitamin, have been found to be low in patients with cervical cancer. The proliferation of pre-cancerous cells can be reduced by folate supplementation. **Alcohol** can destroy some of the B vitamins such as thiamin and folate.

A high intake of **alcohol** has been linked to increased risks of cancers of the mouth, oesophagus, pharynx, larynx and liver.

In countries where the diet is high in smoked, pickled and salty foods, there is a high incidence of stomach cancer. Such a diet is usually also low in **vitamin C**.

High intakes of fruit and vegetables are protective against many forms of cancer.

Low intakes of **beta carotene** have been linked with increased risks of cancer of the larynx, lung, stomach, large bowel and bladder. Excessive **alcohol** can hamper its absorption.

Cancers of the breast, womb and gall bladder are more common among **overweight** people than among their slimmer counterparts.

Vegetarians are less likely to contract cancer of the colon than meat eaters. A vegetarian diet is typically high in **fibre**, low in saturated fat and includes plenty of fruit and vegetables.

Dietary **fibre** may help to protect against all the 'Western' cancers (cancers of the colon, rectum, prostate, uterus and breast).

A diet high in fat is a significant factor in cancers of the colon and rectum. Fats are major factors in **obesity**.

Carrots

BENEFITS
- *Excellent source of beta carotene, the plant form of vitamin A*
- *Contain fibre*

DRAWBACK
- *May contain pesticide residues*

The greatest nutritional benefit of the carrot is that it is an excellent source of beta carotene. Research has linked low beta carotene levels in the blood with increased risk of some cancers. There is also evidence that high intakes of beta carotene may help to protect against damage caused by FREE RADICALS. The body converts beta carotene into vitamin A which is needed for healthy vision as well as the maintenance of mucous membranes.

Seeing in the dark

One of the first symptoms of vitamin A deficiency is 'night blindness', the inability of the eyes to adjust to dim lighting or darkness. Vitamin A combines with the protein opsin in the rods of the retina to form visual purple (rhodopsin), a substance in the eye which is needed for good night vision. If you are deficient in vitamin A, just one carrot a day should be enough to improve your night vision.

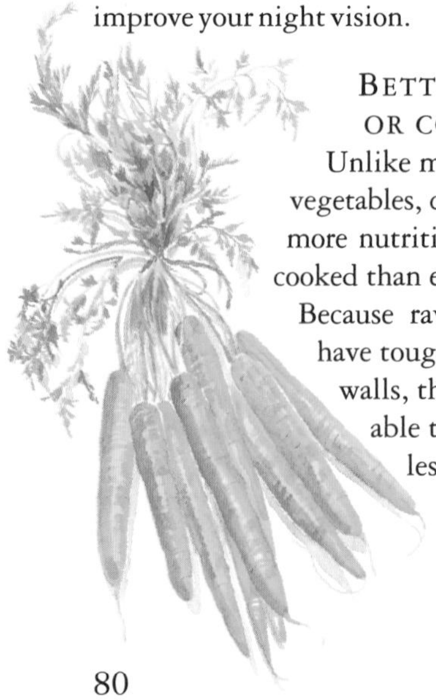

Better raw or cooked?

Unlike most other vegetables, carrots are more nutritious eaten cooked than eaten raw. Because raw carrots have tough cellular walls, the body is able to convert less than 25 per cent of their beta carotene into vitamin A. Cooking, however, breaks down the cell membranes, and as long as the cooked carrots are served as part of a meal that provides some fat the body can absorb more than half of the carotene.

Puréed carrots are good for babies with diarrhoea, providing essential nutrients and natural sugars.

Carrots have been known to contain toxic chemicals: recent routine tests found unacceptably high levels of organophosphorus pesticides (used to kill the carrot fly) in some carrots. Peeling carrots and slicing off their tops removes virtually all of these residues.

Catarrh

EAT PLENTY OF
- *Pungent or spicy foods such as garlic, onions and chilli peppers*

Everyone needs a little watery mucus to protect and lubricate the membranes that line the passages of the throat, nose and lungs. But when the membranes become inflamed or irritated, they produce a thick, excessive mucus known as catarrh. This, combined with the swelling of the mucous membranes, can cause a blocked or runny nose, coughs and earache. If the symptoms last for more than a few days, and if the catarrh is green or yellow, this may point to an infection such as a COLD or flu.

Decongestants

Spicy foods such as chilli peppers, curry spices, ginger, horseradish, mustard seed and black pepper can help to clear the breathing passages. You can feel this happening when you eat hot spicy foods, as they make your eyes water and your nose run.

In herbal medicine, garlic and onions are recommended as natural alternatives to nasal decongestants.

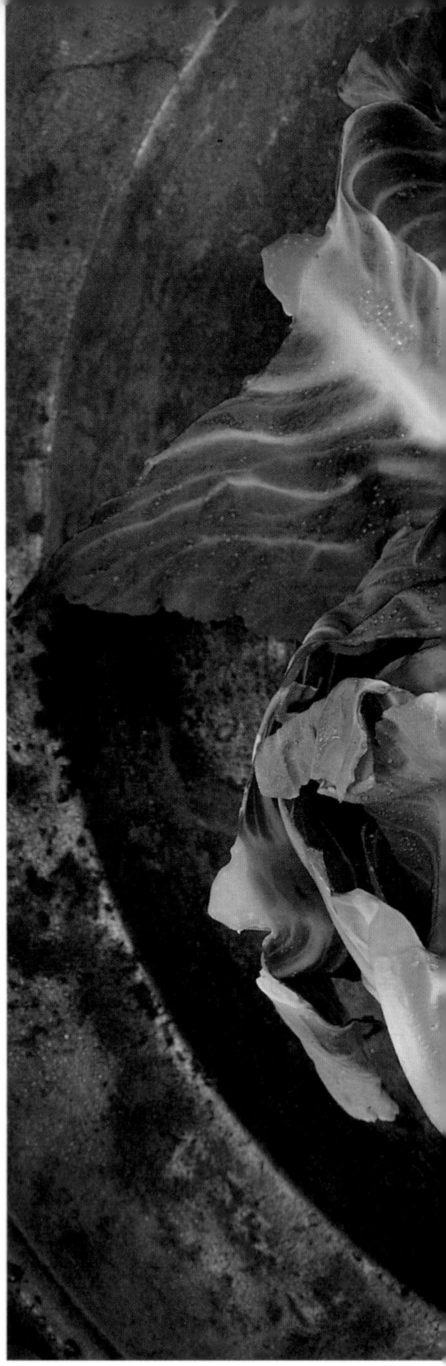

Try eating plenty of both, either raw in salads or added to your cooking. Use fresh garlic rather than garlic powder or pills. After eating garlic you can help to reduce breath odours by rinsing your mouth with water to wash away the pungent oils, and chewing sprigs of fresh parsley.

Commercial decongestant nasal sprays can help to relieve stuffiness, but should not be used for more than a week at a time. There are, however,

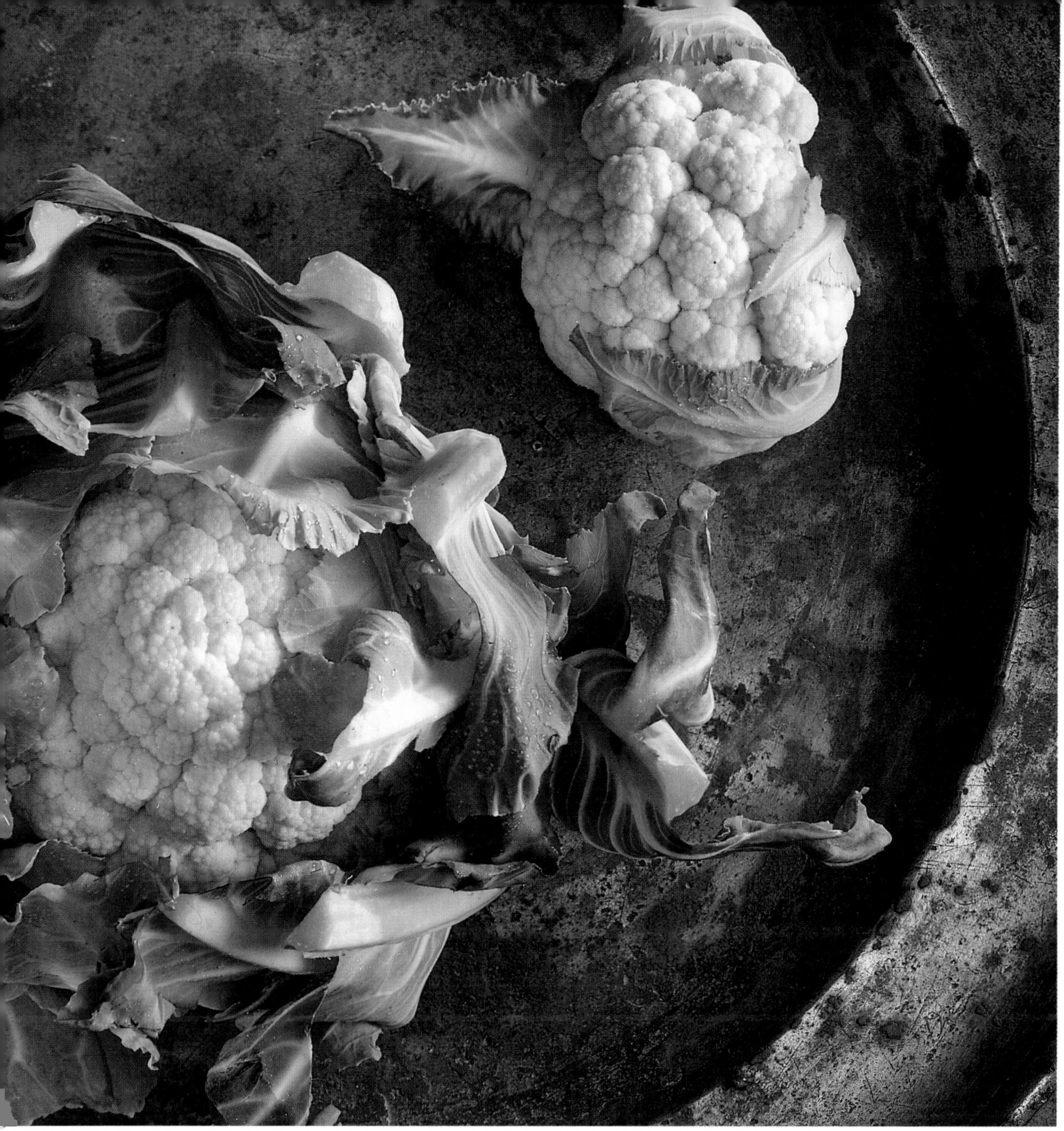

KING OF CABBAGES *Cauliflower is a member of the cancer-fighting cruciferous family, which includes Brussels sprouts and broccoli.*

some essential oils which can be used quite safely as decongestants. Use a mixture of two drops each of basil, thyme and lemon oil in a bowl of hot water, cover your head and the basin with a large towel and inhale the steam for 10 minutes. Eucalyptus oil can also be used as an effective decongestant, either inhaled from a bowl of hot water or added to water in a vaporiser.

CAULIFLOWER

BENEFITS

- *Good source of vitamin C*
- *May help to ward off cancer*

DRAWBACK

- *May cause flatulence*

Like all members of the cruciferous family of vegetables, the cauliflower is a rich source of nutrients, including vitamin C. It also contains sulphurous compounds that may help to protect against various cancers – particularly cancer of the colon. An average helping of raw cauliflower (100g, 3½ oz) supplies more than the recommended daily intake of vitamin C. Even after a portion has been lightly boiled, it will still provide more than half the recommended daily amount.

Because cauliflower contains only 28 Calories per serving, it is a good component of a balanced slimming diet: filling but not fattening (unless topped by a rich cheese sauce).

Like other fibrous vegetables, cauliflower may cause flatulence as the gut breaks down the cellulose. Eating it with spicy accompaniments such as garlic, caraway, ground coriander and cumin will ease digestive discomfort; herbs which help the digestion include tarragon, bay and fennel.

Cooking tip

The sulphur in cauliflower can cause unpleasant smells during cooking. Steaming in a covered pan can create a build up of sulphur and may taint the cauliflower's flavour; fast boiling in an open pan is preferable.

Celeriac (Celery Root)

BENEFITS

- *Good source of potassium*
- *Contains fibre and vitamin C*

This winter root vegetable is related to celery and is sometimes called celery root. After the tough skin has been peeled, it can be eaten cooked as a hot vegetable or made into a classic French salad by slicing into fine matchsticks, parboiling, and tossing in a mustard mayonnaise.

Celeriac is a good source of potassium. When eaten raw, it contains vitamin C as well as soluble fibre, which can lower blood cholesterol.

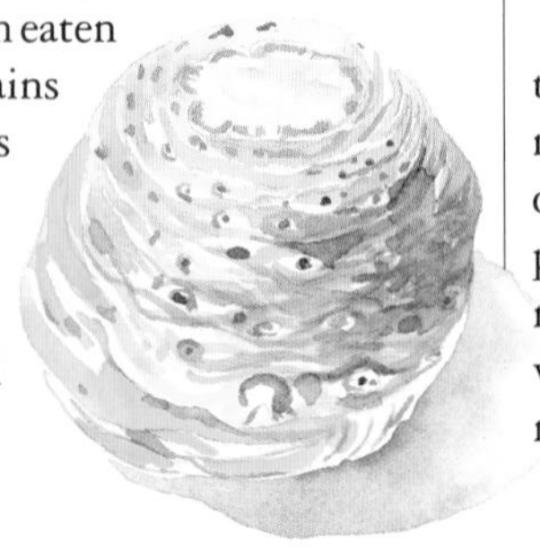

Celery

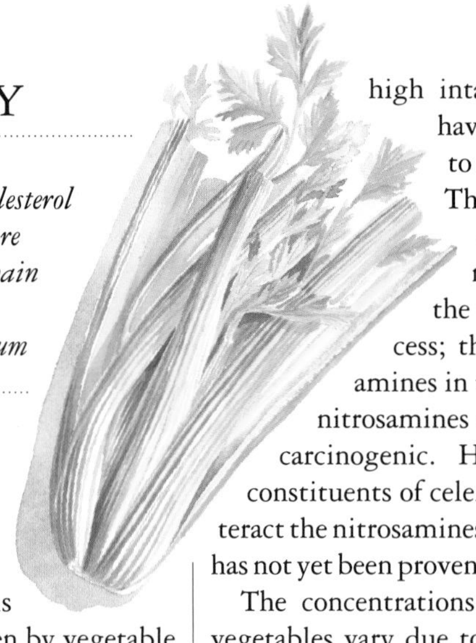

BENEFITS

- *May help to lower cholesterol levels and blood pressure*
- *Helps to relieve joint pain*
- *Low in calories*
- *Good source of potassium*

DRAWBACK

- *May be high in nitrates*

Slimmers tend to eat a lot of celery because it is so low in calories – even by vegetable standards. A 100g (3½oz) portion – about two sticks – contains a mere 7 Calories. It is also a good source of potassium, which helps to maintain healthy blood pressure (as long as no salt is added). Celery also helps the kidneys to function efficiently and so hasten the excretion of wastes.

Celery was used to treat hypertension in traditional Oriental medicine, and recent studies at the University of Chicago Medical Center do suggest that it can help. Scientists found that a compound in celery (called 3 n-butyl phthalide) not only acts as a sedative but can also lower blood pressure.

Celery contains an anti-inflammatory agent which can help to alleviate the painful symptoms of gout, caused by the build-up of uric acid crystals in the joints. Indeed, herbalists often advise people with gout to drink a tea brewed from celery seeds. The seeds, which can be bought at health food shops, also contain an oil which acts as a natural tranquilliser.

Celery belongs to a group of plants that can accumulate high amounts of nitrate. The issue of setting safe levels of nitrates in plants and vegetables, particularly lettuce and spinach, has recently been the subject of discussion within the European Union. The reason for all the concern is because high intakes of nitrate have been found to be harmful. The nitrates are converted into nitrites during the digestive process; these react with amines in the gut to form nitrosamines – which can be carcinogenic. However, other constituents of celery might counteract the nitrosamines' effect but this has not yet been proven.

The concentrations of nitrates in vegetables vary due to many factors, including the individual soil conditions, particular plant species, light intensity and the kind of fertilisers used. Estimates of the average dietary intakes of nitrate by most consumers have been found to be within internationally recognised safe limits. However, while vegetables such as celery, lettuce and spinach can be eaten in moderation, they should not be eaten in large amounts over a long period – as a major part of a slimming diet, for example. Cooking celery by steaming or lightly boiling will help to reduce the nitrate levels.

Cellulite

EAT PLENTY OF

- *Fruit and vegetables*

CUT DOWN ON

- *Fatty foods such as meat, dairy products, ice cream, chips, crisps, biscuits and cakes*

The term 'cellulite' was coined by French doctors for what they believe to be a special kind of lumpy looking fat. It usually affects a woman's thighs, bottom, and sometimes the upper arms and lower part of the abdomen. The term has never been successfully translated; *cellulitis*, an extremely painful inflammation of the tissues, has nothing to do with cellulite.

Many naturopaths, beauticians and manufacturers of various cellulite creams, claim that cellulite is caused by a build-up of toxic waste matter in the body tissues, due to a poor diet that is high in refined and processed foods, and low in fresh fruit and vegetables. The resulting pockets of water, fat and impurities are said to give the skin a dimpled appearance, which is often referred to as the 'orange-peel' effect. This dimpled skin becomes more noticeable if an affected area is bunched up by pinching it around the edge. Naturopaths usually recommend people with cellulite to go on a detoxifying diet that includes plenty of fresh fruit and vegetables, and to cut out tea, coffee and alcohol.

DOES IT REALLY EXIST?

While the word cellulite has been adopted as a simple term for this dimpled skin, the theory that it is a form of 'internal pollution' is not supported by any sound medical evidence, and only serves to provoke unnecessary feelings of guilt and low self-esteem in women. Most doctors and scientists agree that the dimpled fat is just ordinary fat, and that toxins have nothing to do with this entirely natural process.

The reason that so many women – even slim women – get cellulite on their hips and thighs, is because the female hormone oestrogen makes women acquire fat there; and they store more of their fat just under the skin's surface, whereas men store some of their fat internally, underneath muscles. After the menopause, women deposit more fat on the upper parts of their bodies, but this tendency can sometimes be reversed by hormone replacement therapy (HRT). And as women grow older, surface skin becomes thinner and less elastic, and the dimpling becomes more exaggerated. Cellulite is therefore a natural characteristic of the female body and – while it may be distressing for those women who have it – it does not cause any physical harm.

It is worth noting that the dimpling effect may be made worse by sunbathing, since excessive exposure to sunlight is known to cause the skin to lose its elasticity.

Liposuction, injections and electrical treatment are unlikely to have any lasting effect, but massage may sometimes help. Doctors believe that the best ways to improve the appearance of cellulite are to take regular exercise – swimming, cycling, walking and dancing for example – and to go on a low-fat diet that includes plenty of fruit and vegetables. As rapid weight loss can exacerbate the problem, it is best to lose weight slowly.

CEREALS

See page 84

CEREBRAL PALSY

One in every 400 children born in the United Kingdom has cerebral palsy. It is a group of neurological disorders characterised by problems of bodily control – known as motor disability – which begins before the age of three. It ranges from a mild form, where a fairly normal life is possible, to a severe form, where the patient requires total care.

People with cerebral palsy have abnormal muscle tone and function, which can interfere with chewing and swallowing food. Since it is important to ensure the person eats a balanced diet, food preparation and appearance are of great importance.

Puréed foods, and other dishes such as porridge and soup, which are easy to eat, must be palatable and nutritious. Care should be taken to ensure that calorie intake matches demand. People with cerebral palsy find it difficult to consume large quantities of food, so the food should be packed with nutrients and calories, to ensure that an adequate supply can be obtained from a small amount. When devising a suitable diet, it is best to seek the advice of a doctor.

CAUSES OF CEREBRAL PALSY

The disorder results from injury to the brain and can be caused by many factors arising during pregnancy, birth or the early years of childhood. These include illnesses and infections during pregnancy, such as rubella, complications in labour and extreme prematurity or diseases during infancy such as meningitis and jaundice. Cerebral palsy can be hard to detect in infancy, and is often suspected only when a child fails to reach normal 'motor milestones', such as crawling, walking and independent feeding.

Cerebral palsy is not a progressive condition, but it is permanent and, strictly speaking, incurable, although there are some experts, such as the late Dr András Petö of Budapest, Hungary, who would disagree. Petö's philosophy was that a motor disorder is not a medical problem but a learning difficulty which, with the right teaching, can be overcome by stimulating the nerve pathways to 'bypass' damaged areas. The Petö Institute's programme involves exercise to strengthen muscles and a lot of intellectual exercises – reading, drawing and speaking – to stimulate brain cells. The regime is very physical – putting demands on both the person with cerebral palsy and the parents and minders. More mainstream approaches share Petö's goal of 'orthofunction': helping a child to maximise his or her potential and to become independent in movement, self-care and communication.

CEREALS: ARE WHOLE GRAINS HEALTHIER?

Versatile and energy-packed, cereals are found in an enormous range of foods – from rice, bread and breakfast cereals to semolina, whiskey and popcorn.

Wheat and other cereals are at their most nutritious in wholegrain form when they contain greater levels of most B vitamins and fibre. They are excellent sources of carbohydrates and provide protein (which is useful for vegetarians).

Most of the wheat grain's fibre, oil and B vitamins, as well as iron, vitamin E and a quarter of its protein, come from the germ at its base and the layer of starchy tissue which surrounds its core – the endosperm. For most cereals, milling involves the removal of the outer husk, or bran, and the nutrient-rich germ from the endosperm which is then used to make flour.

The separation process increases the storage life of flours because the oils of the germ are susceptible to oxidation and can become rancid within a few weeks. Although cereal bran adds bulk to the diet, an excess can irritate the bowel. Milling often involves complex sifting operations to produce highly refined flours from which almost every trace of bran has been removed. The presence of bran adds substance and texture to refined products.

Many people prefer the softer texture of refined cereal products such as white BREAD and polished white rice. Most manufacturers now compensate for nutritional losses that result from milling by fortifying foods such as BREAKFAST CEREALS with B vitamins and iron. By law, calcium, iron, thiamin and niacin must be added to the white flour used for baking bread.

Though they may be fortified with vitamins, refined products contain less fibre than wholegrain foods. Fibre helps to prevent constipation and may help to reduce the risk of developing bowel disorders including haemorrhoids and bowel cancer.

Barley, oats, rye and wheat contain gluten – a complex mixture of cereal proteins – which have to be avoided by people with COELIAC DISEASE.

THE MOST COMMON CEREALS

Barley is a staple food in the Middle East, but in the West it is used mainly in the form of malt by brewers and distillers, and as animal feed. Pearl barley, which is added to soups and stews, is highly refined, offering plenty of carbohydrate but little in terms of vitamins and fibre.

Maize or corn is gluten-free and is the basis of an extraordinarily wide range of foods including popcorn, cornflour, cornmeal, breakfast cereals, bourbon and other American whiskeys and corn syrup – a sweetener used in many manufactured desserts.

Millet is also gluten-free and therefore a useful cereal for people with gluten intolerance. For the same reason, it cannot be used for raised breads but is made into flat breads in Asia and north Africa where millet is a staple food.

Oats contain gluten and are therefore unsuitable for people with coeliac disease. Because milling removes most of the husk but leaves the germ intact, oatmeal is relatively high in protein and oil. This means that, unless it is steamed before packaging, it also turns rancid more quickly than most other cereals. The soluble fibre in oats is believed to be particularly helpful in lowering blood cholesterol levels.

Rice is the staple food for around half the world's population. Nutritionally, brown rice is a good source of B vitamins. It also contains calcium and phosphorus. Although it contains iron, the phytic acid in the rice bran inhibits its absorption. White rice, which has had its outer layers stripped away, contains mostly carbohydrate and a little protein. It is low in thiamin unless it is parboiled before milling, although some types of white rice are fortified with thiamin. (See also RICE.)

Rye contains enough gluten to make a weak dough, but the bread produced, such as rye bread and pumpernickel, is heavy and moist. A type of American whiskey is distilled from rye, and the grain is also used in crispbreads.

Wheat is classified as hard or soft according to the gluten content of the many different varieties. The hardest, and highest in gluten, is durum which is used to make PASTA. The softer, lower-gluten flours are preferred for biscuits, cakes and pastry.

SEMOLINA consists of coarse particles of wheat endosperm. Finely ground semolina is mixed with water and flour to make pellets which are served steamed in the north African dish couscous. Wholewheat flour, which includes the bran and the germ, is a useful source of dietary fibre and B complex vitamins.

Bulgur or cracked wheat, which has to be soaked before use, contains a similar breakdown of nutrients. It is the basis of the Lebanese dish, tabbouleh.

NATURALLY NOURISHING *Whole grains contain considerably more vitamins, fibre and protein than refined cereals.*

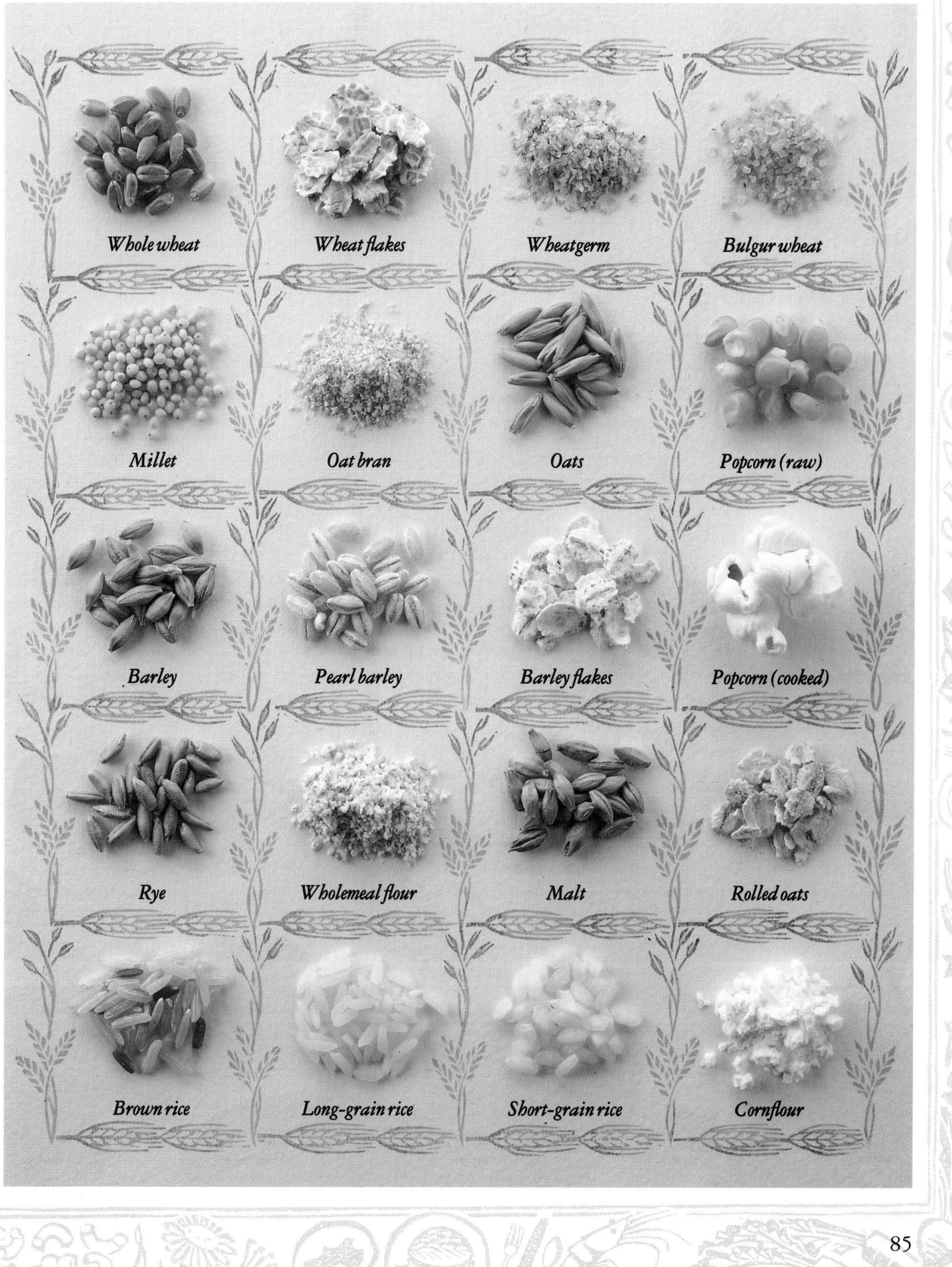
Whole wheat
Wheat flakes
Wheatgerm
Bulgur wheat
Millet
Oat bran
Oats
Popcorn (raw)
Barley
Pearl barley
Barley flakes
Popcorn (cooked)
Rye
Wholemeal flour
Malt
Rolled oats
Brown rice
Long-grain rice
Short-grain rice
Cornflour

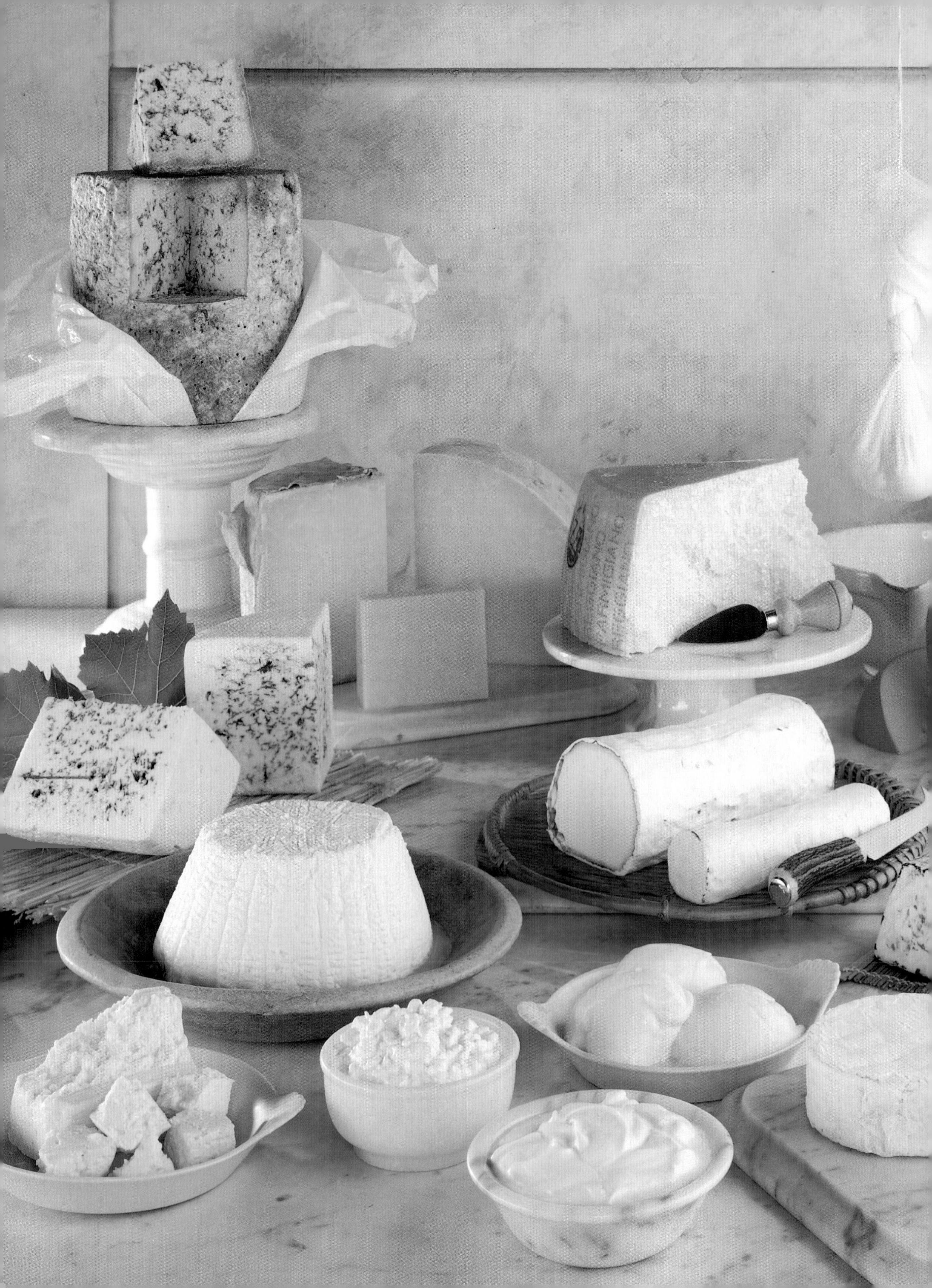
PARMIGIANO REGGIANO

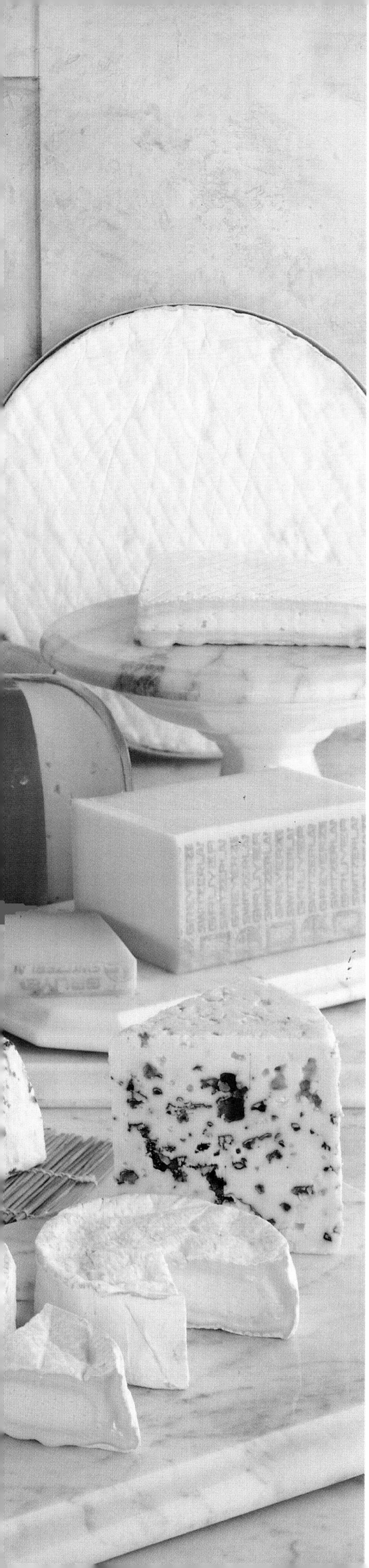

Cheese

BENEFITS
- *Good source of protein and a rich source of calcium*
- *Important source of B_{12} for vegetarians*
- *May help to fight tooth decay*

DRAWBACKS
- *Some cheeses are high in saturated fat and calories*
- *May trigger migraines and other allergic reactions in susceptible people*

A convenient and nutritious snack, cheese should be eaten in moderation. This is because some cheeses are very high in saturated fat. Weight for weight, Cheddar, for example, contains six times as much saturated fat as sirloin steak. However, cheese also provides valuable protein, calcium and vitamin B_{12}. Most people obtain essential vitamin B_{12} from meat, thus cheese can make an important contribution to a vegetarian diet.

The high amount of calcium in cheese may help to reduce the risk of OSTEOPOROSIS. Research has shown that eating plenty of calcium during childhood and adolescence helps to prevent this condition in later life. The calcium contained in cheese and other dairy products can be absorbed by the body much more easily than the calcium in other foods.

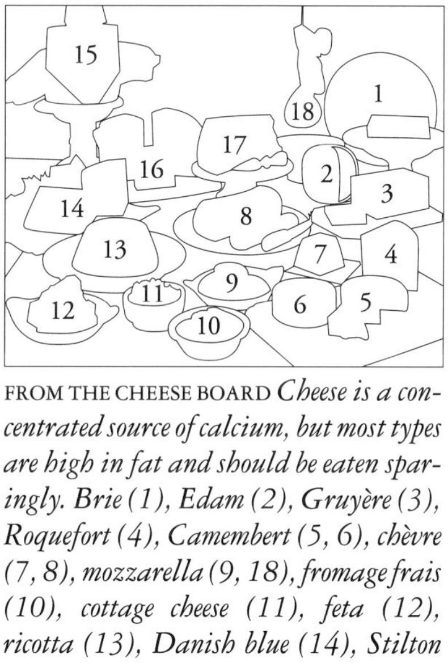

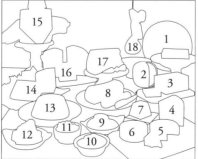

FROM THE CHEESE BOARD *Cheese is a concentrated source of calcium, but most types are high in fat and should be eaten sparingly. Brie (1), Edam (2), Gruyère (3), Roquefort (4), Camembert (5, 6), chèvre (7, 8), mozzarella (9, 18), fromage frais (10), cottage cheese (11), feta (12), ricotta (13), Danish blue (14), Stilton (15), Cheddar (16), Parmesan (17).*

Cheese also helps to fight tooth decay caused by sugary foods. It seems to work by preventing the formation of acids in the mouth which attack the enamel on teeth. Tests demonstrate that eating small amounts of cheese after meals halves the number of cavities caused by sugar. It was discovered that the cheese did not have to be swallowed to have an effect, the protection is derived just from chewing it.

High intakes of saturated fat are known to increase blood cholesterol levels, which in turn can contribute to ATHEROSCLEROSIS – a major factor in heart disease and strokes. Some cheeses have a much lower total fat content than others: hard cheeses such as Cheddar, Parmesan and Stilton contain up to about 35 per cent fat; soft cheeses, including Camembert and Brie, contain on average about 26 per cent fat; while ricotta and cottage cheese can contain as little as 11 and 4 per cent fat, respectively.

Cheese causes an allergic reaction in susceptible people; usually as part of a general sensitivity or intolerance to dairy products. This can contribute to a range of symptoms and diseases, such as ECZEMA, MIGRAINE and ear infections. Fresh goat's and sheep's milk cheeses cause fewer allergic reactions than those made from cow's milk.

Migraine triggers

If you suffer from migraine as a result of eating cheese, the culprit is probably a chemical called tyramine. This sets off nerve and blood-vessel changes in the brain, triggering an attack. Cheeses with the highest tyramine content are blue-veined varieties, such as Stilton and Gorgonzola, as well as mature Cheddar, Gruyère and Parmesan. By contrast, the unripened cheeses, such as cream cheese, cottage cheese and fresh goat's cheese, are less likely to trigger migraines.

THE RISK OF FOOD POISONING

Many cheeses are made from pasteurised milk. The process does not kill all the micro-organisms although it destroys the harmful ones, leaving a pure 'starter liquid'. It is not appropriate to boil milk to sterilise it as this makes the calcium salts within the milk insoluble, and soluble calcium is needed for rennet to solidify the cheese. Cheeses made from unpasteurised milk may contain various micro-organisms, such as salmonella and listeria, which are normally killed during pasteurisation. This is usually no problem, but when the bacteria in the cheeses multiply beyond a certain level, FOOD POISONING may result. Salmonella poisoning induces gastro-intestinal symptoms which can be life-threatening to the very old or very young. Listeria poisoning resembles flu and is particularly hazardous to babies and pregnant women as well as those who are already ill.

Case study

Joshua's mother was being driven to distraction by her little boy's behaviour. The five-year-old was always awake until the early hours, slept poorly and was impossible to discipline. His bad temper and hyperactivity were making him a notorious 'troublemaker' at school, where his teacher was finding it impossible to settle him to any task.

On the advice of a friend, Joshua's mother had removed orange squash and any other products containing tartrazine from his diet, as she knew that this additive could cause hyperactivity in children. But Joshua showed no signs of improvement. Joshua's mother became convinced that her son must have an allergy to some other food he was eating, but was unsure how to go about putting him on an exclusion diet since he was so young. She decided to see a specialist in food allergies.

On the ground that cow's milk is the most common trigger of childhood allergies, the dietician advised her to eliminate all dairy products from Joshua's diet. This she did, but his behaviour still did not alter. Then she discovered that Joshua was regularly raiding the fridge for cheese. His mother stopped buying cheese and after two weeks Joshua had become a much more manageable, sweet-natured little boy.

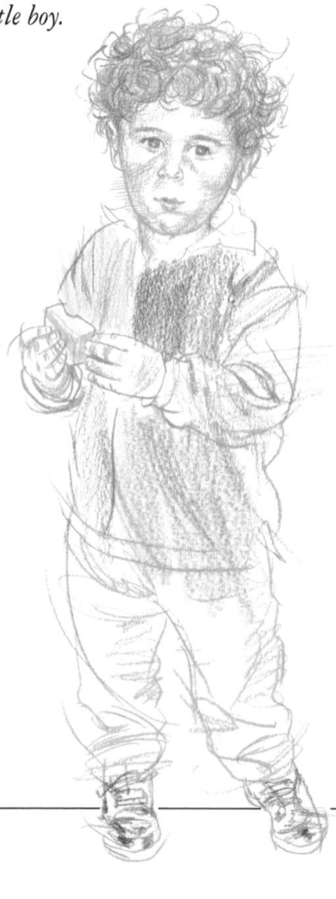

CHERRIES

BENEFITS
- *Good source of potassium*
- *May help to prevent gout*

The raw edible varieties of cherries are a good source of potassium, which helps to stabilise the heartbeat and keep the skin healthy. They also contain useful amounts of vitamin C.

First brought to Britain by the Romans, cherries have been growing here since AD100. They are valued in natural medicine for their cleansing properties – the fruit is believed to remove toxins and fluids and cleanse the kidneys. Their mild laxative action can help to relieve constipation. Eating 225g (8oz) of cherries per day – fresh or canned – will also lower levels of uric acid in the blood, which may help to prevent GOUT.

CHERRY VARIETIES

There are more than 1000 varieties of cherries. The edible varieties can be divided into sour cherries, such as Morello, and sweet cherries, like Napoleon and Bing. The sweet varieties are the best for eating raw, while sour cherries are ideal for using in pies, sorbets and liqueurs. Hybrid cherries, such as Dukes, are good for both eating raw and cooking.

When buying sweet cherries, look for plump, firm fruits with a green stalk to indicate freshness. They are normally pale yellow or dark red but can be purple or almost black, depending on the variety. Sour cherries should be plump, round and are usually scarlet or deep crimson in colour.

CHERRY RIPE *Yellowish Queen Anne cherries (right) are sweet, while scarlet Morello cherries (left) are sour but make delicious pies. Bing cherries (foreground) are best eaten raw, while the versatile Dukes (back) can be cooked or eaten raw.*

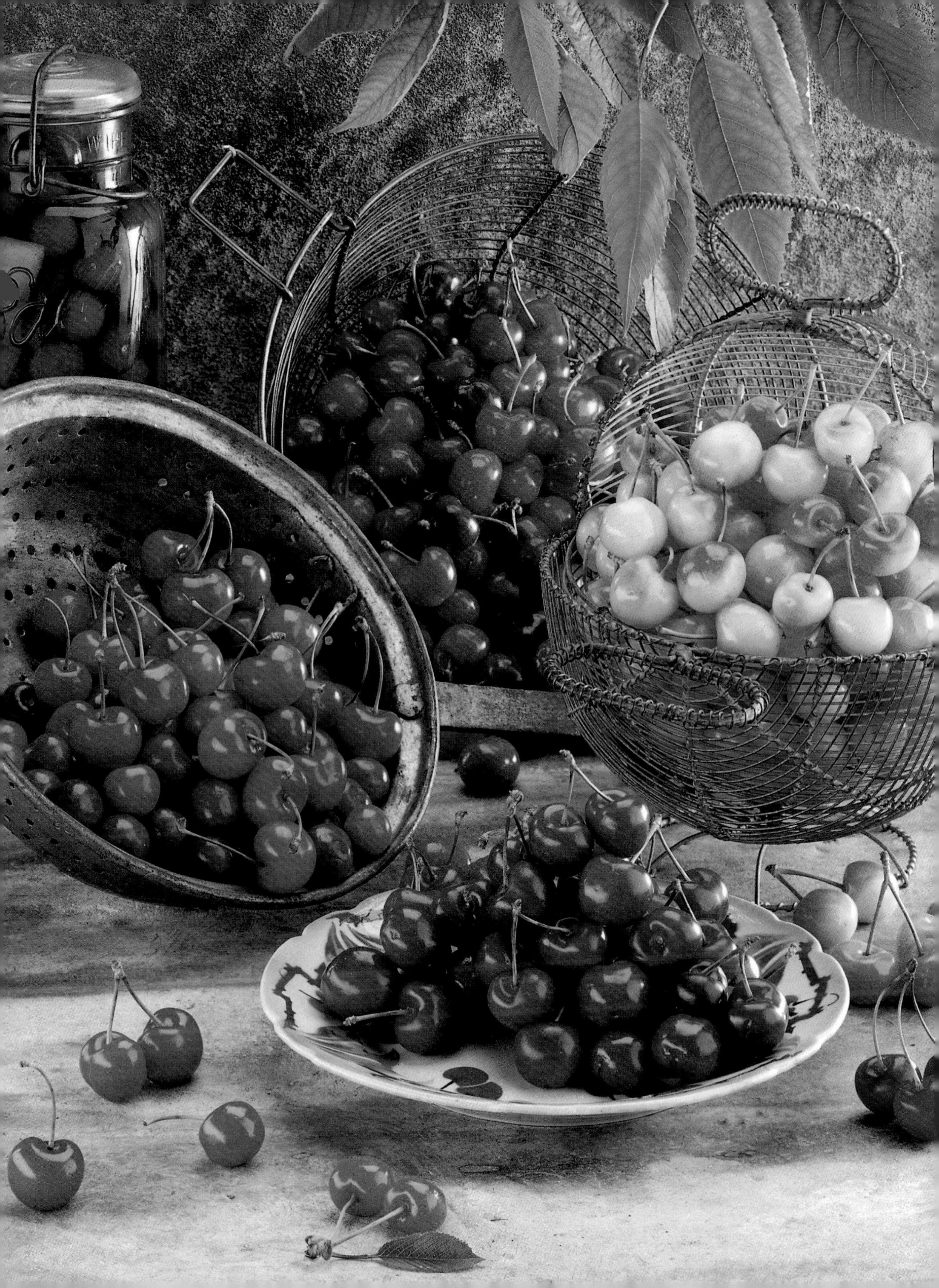

CHILDREN AND DIET

Eating habits are often set in the first few years of life, when it is vital that all the child's nutritional needs are met. How can you make sure that your child grows up to be strong and healthy?

You can encourage your children to adopt healthy eating habits by setting a good example. Taking a positive attitude towards nutritious foods makes you a good role model: by introducing a variety of delicious healthy foods to your children, you will be helping to establish eating patterns that will last for a lifetime.

THE GROWING YEARS

Dramatic changes take place in our bodies between the ages of 1 and 20. Muscles strengthen, bones lengthen, height may more than triple and weight can increase tenfold. Girls have sudden spurts of growth between the ages of 10 and 15, and boys slightly later, between 12 and 19. Children's calorie needs vary; 1200 a day for a one-year-old, 1600 for a five-year-old, 2100 for a 16-year-old girl and 2700 for a boy of the same age. The table of recommended daily intakes (see page 92) is a useful rough guide.

CHANGES IN APPETITE

The amount of food that children need to meet their energy and nutrient requirements varies according to their size, weight, gender and their level of activity. Appetite is usually a reliable guide to food requirements; do not fall into the trap of forcing children to eat more than they want to. Yesterday's notion of 'cleaning your plate' is not only old-fashioned, but also encourages indigestion and obesity, and can lead to lifelong dislikes of certain foods. It is better to serve smaller portions in the first place, or encourage children to serve themselves.

In any event, the appetite decreases around the age of one, and then fluctuates according to whether the child is going through a period of slow or rapid growth. It is perfectly normal for young children to have an enormous appetite one day and little interest in food the next. Eating patterns also change completely when children reach their teens; teenagers usually develop voracious appetites to match their need for extra energy, which they tend to satisfy by eating snacks 'on the run', rather than sitting down to breakfast, lunch

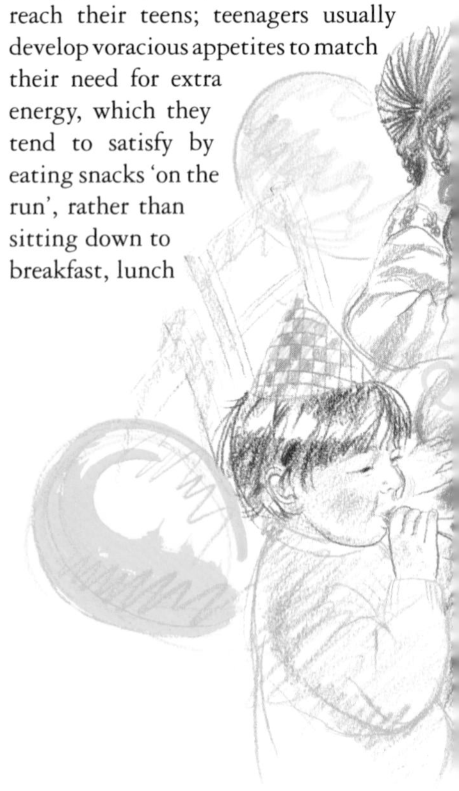

Dos and don'ts: encouraging good eating habits

- Do set the example you want your child to copy with your own eating habits. Share mealtimes and eat the same healthy dishes.
- Do discourage snacking on junk foods. Keep a plentiful supply of healthy foods, such as fruit, raw carrots or cheese, which children can eat between meals.
- Do allow children to follow their natural appetites when deciding how much to eat.
- Do encourage children to enjoy fruit and vegetables by giving them different varieties from an early age. Aim for five portions a day.
- Do invite children to help prepare food at home. With so much convenience food available, many children may never learn to enjoy cooking, and so rely on ready-made foods.
- Don't encourage a sweet tooth. If you don't add unnecessary sugar to drinks and foods, the chances are that children will never miss it.
- Don't condition children to eat extra salt by sprinkling it over food.
- Don't give skimmed or semi-skimmed milk to under-fives; they need the energy provided by the extra calories in whole milk.
- Don't give whole nuts to children under four years old in case they choke. Peanut butter and ground nuts are fine as long as the child is not allergic to them.
- Don't use lectures about the 'starving millions' to try and persuade children to eat, or force them to eat more than they want.
- Don't make children feel guilty about eating any type of food.

and supper. As long as they take regular exercise, teenagers should not have to worry about their weight.

EATING IS FUN

Eating should be one of life's pleasures. Encourage children to enjoy a family meal, and to help out with simple tasks in the kitchen such as measuring, stirring and arranging food on a plate.

Relaxed mealtimes with good food and conversation, rather than fraught occasions when children are nagged about how they eat, will encourage the building of social relationships as well as good digestion. If you eat after your children have enjoyed favourite activities such as a television programme or playing, they will be less likely to bolt their food and rush to leave the table.

THE DESIRE FOR SWEETS

Sweets have become synonymous with childhood, but there are drawbacks, as every parent knows. Sweets can spoil the appetite and cause tooth decay if eaten too frequently, and, although they provide energy, they contain no valuable nutrients. The trouble with banning sweets altogether is that children can feel deprived when their friends eat them, and may become secret sweet eaters. There is no harm in letting children have occasional sweets after meals, but do not dole them out as special treats or rewards, as this will nurture the desire for them. Ice cream and cakes are usually marginally better than sweets because there are at least some nutrients in the milk and grains.

FOODS FOR TODDLERS

After the first year, children can eat most of the dishes that are prepared for the rest of the family; though they have smaller appetites and so usually need five to six meals or snacks a day. The extra calories they consume are required for energy and growth. While a child's mother will use up around 2000 Calories a day, her two-year-old son or daughter will burn around 1200, even though he or she is only a quarter of her weight.

Children need to eat a good variety of healthy foods. Bread, cereals, fruit and vegetables should make up the major part of the diet. Protein foods can include meat, fish, soya products, pulses, and cereals. Milk is an important source of calories, and children under five should drink 600 ml (1 pint) a day. At this age there is no need to restrict fat and cholesterol as children need the extra calories; nevertheless, grilled and baked foods are always preferable to fried and fatty ones.

Many parents have a real battle on their hands when it comes to getting children to eat vegetables, but you can win children over by pandering to

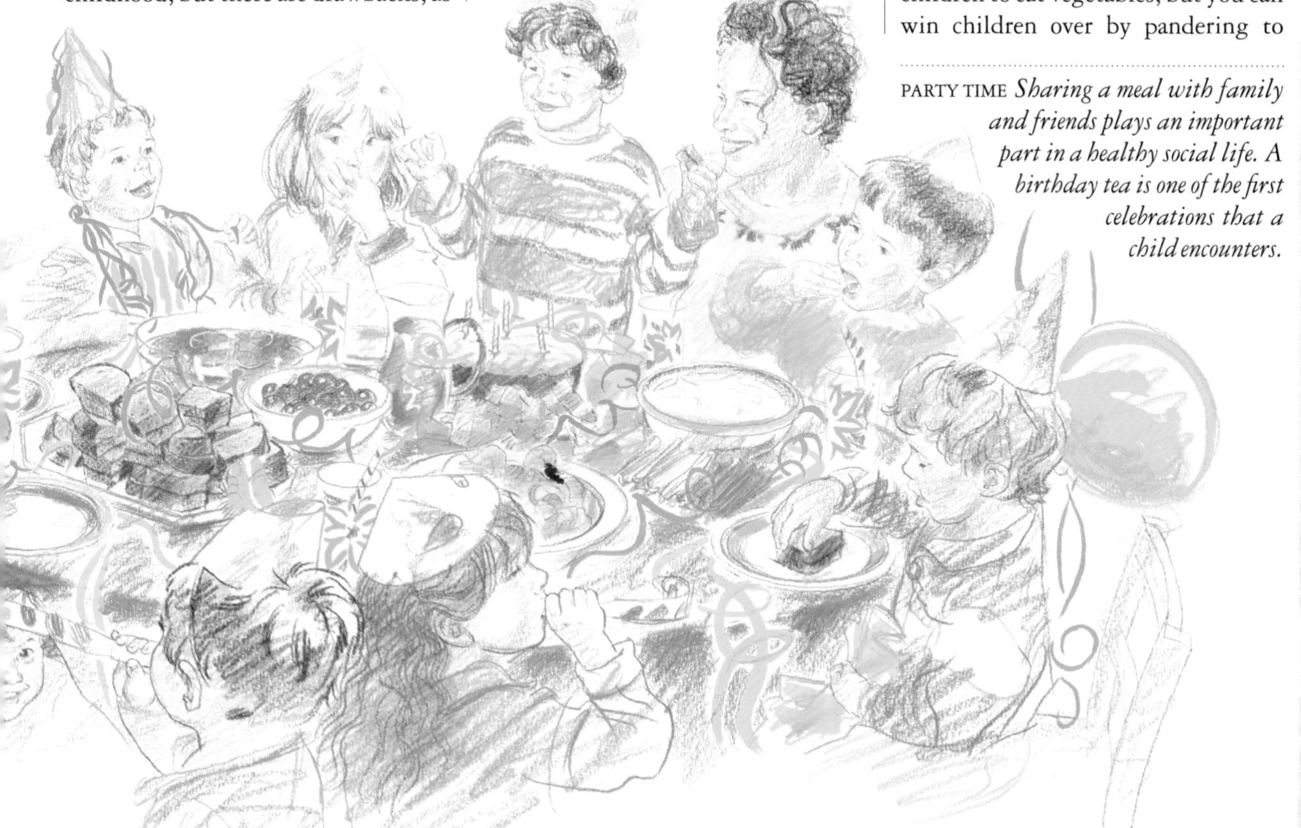

PARTY TIME *Sharing a meal with family and friends plays an important part in a healthy social life. A birthday tea is one of the first celebrations that a child encounters.*

their tastes in colour and texture. Most youngsters will screw up their faces in disgust when confronted with a plate of soggy spinach or lumpy mashed potato; they favour bright colours and smooth or crunchy textures.

When introducing new foods, try offering one at a time and give small amounts at first. It is a good idea to try out new foods at the beginning of the meal, while a child is still hungry. Stay calm if there is any resistance; children soon realise the power they have over you if you become angry and frustrated. Try again in a few days – and perhaps prepare the food in a different way, or mix it in with a favourite food. Remember that your child is bound to have some genuine dislikes.

If a child is often aggressive or tearful, and if he or she fidgets and has poor concentration, the problem may be HYPERACTIVITY. Some additives (such as a few colourings used in confectionery and certain artificial sweeteners) may cause hyperactivity. Consult a doctor if your child seems to be affected.

FOODS FOR TEENAGERS

Adolescents have an increased need for all nutrients, especially calories and protein for a strong and healthy body, and protein, calcium, phosphorus and vitamin D for proper bone formation. Because teenagers tend to start eating away from home more, they have the luxury of making their own choices for the first time, and are notorious for snacking and missing out on important meals such as breakfast. Some will use food as a way of trying to establish their identity, perhaps by becoming VEGETARIAN or going on a crash diet. Iron deficiency anaemia and ANOREXIA are relatively common problems in adolescent girls, who can become self-conscious about their bodies even before they reach their teenage years.

Food for growing up

As children grow their needs change, not only in terms of the number of calories they require, but also the amount of each food type they need to fuel growing bones and muscle. As well as changes with age there are also differences between the sexes. The chart below outlines the basic trends and recommends some good sources of calcium and iron.

AGE	CALORIES per day		PROTEIN g/day		CALCIUM mg/day	IRON mg/day	
	MALE	FEMALE	MALE	FEMALE	MALE FEMALE	MALE	FEMALE
10-12 MONTHS	920	865	14.9	14.9	525	7.8	7.8
1-3 YEARS	1230	1165	14.5	14.5	350	6.9	6.9
4-6 YEARS	1715	1545	19.7	19.7	450	6.1	6.1
7-10 YEARS	1970	1740	28.3	28.3	550	8.7	8.7
11-14 YEARS	2220	1845	42.1	41.2	1000	11.3	14.8
15-18 YEARS	2755	2110	55.2	45.0	1000	11.3	14.8
19-50 YEARS	2550	1940	55.5	45.0	700	8.7	14.8

CALCIUM – DIETARY SOURCES	IRON – DIETARY SOURCES
Milk Yoghurt Cheese Fromage frais Custard Macaroni cheese Hazelnuts Sardines Almonds White bread Dried figs Brazil nuts Porridge made with milk Tofu Prawns Spinach Parsley Anchovies Tahini paste Watercress	Dried apricot purée Lamb chops Minced beef Fortified breakfast cereals Mixed nuts and raisins Wholemeal bread Dried figs Eggs Sardines Lentils Offal Spinach Bean salad Sesame seeds Mussels Peas

SNACKS AND FAST FOODS

Instead of keeping crisps, chocolate and biscuits in the house, stock up on healthy snacks that hungry youngsters and teenagers can nibble on throughout the day.

- Bread, rolls and crackers with fillings such as peanut butter, low-fat cheese, tinned tuna or sardines and lean cooked meat.
- Rice cakes and oatcakes.
- Fresh and dried fruit.
- Yoghurt.
- Sticks of carrot or celery and cherry tomatoes with dips.
- Plain popcorn.
- Breakfast cereals.
- Baked beans on toast.
- Pasta or potato salad.
- Water, milk and fruit juice.
- Homemade soup.
- Colourful vegetable salads.

Obesity can be a problem for both sexes, and overweight youngsters should be encouraged to increase physical activity rather than to go on a diet.

Nutritional needs are particularly high during the rapid growth period of puberty. Because girls begin to grow earlier than boys they have their peak requirement for nutrients, on average, about two years earlier to coincide with this spurt of growth.

A good calcium intake is especially important at this time. All teenagers need at least three 200ml (7 fl oz) glasses of milk a day and either 45g (1½oz) of cheese or 125ml (4½fl oz) of yoghurt to meet their daily requirements. Calcium is also found in fish (especially sardines and pilchards when the bones are eaten); fortified breakfast cereals; and green leafy vegetables. Both calcium and exercise are important for the formation of strong healthy bones and the prevention of OSTEOPOROSIS in later life.

Teenagers often devour fatty and sugary foods such as crisps, chocolate, hamburgers and fizzy drinks. While hamburgers and chips may provide protein, some vitamins and minerals, they are generally low in vitamin A and fibre and do not contain much vitamin C or calcium. Most fast foods are also high in sodium and calories. It is important to provide a variety of healthy foods at home, especially fruit, vegetables, fish, whole grains, and pulses such as beans, peas and lentils.

Many teenagers skip breakfast. This can make them feel lethargic and lack concentration. A light breakfast of low-fat yoghurt and fresh fruit, or cereal and fruit juice is much better than no food at all. Alternatively, send your teenagers off in the morning with some fruit to eat on their way to school or college.

BECOMING A VEGETARIAN

Many teenagers become vegetarian out of genuine concern for animal welfare or because they do not like the taste or texture of meat. There is no reason why they should not thrive on a well-balanced vegetarian diet based around wholemeal bread, pasta, potatoes and rice eaten with a wide variety of vegetables, fruits, nuts and seeds. However, do not let your children substitute large quantities of dairy products for meat and fish, or their diet will be too high in saturated fats. Children who become vegan and cut out dairy products will need to take supplements of vitamin B_{12}, or eat fortified breakfast cereals served with soya milk or fruit juice.

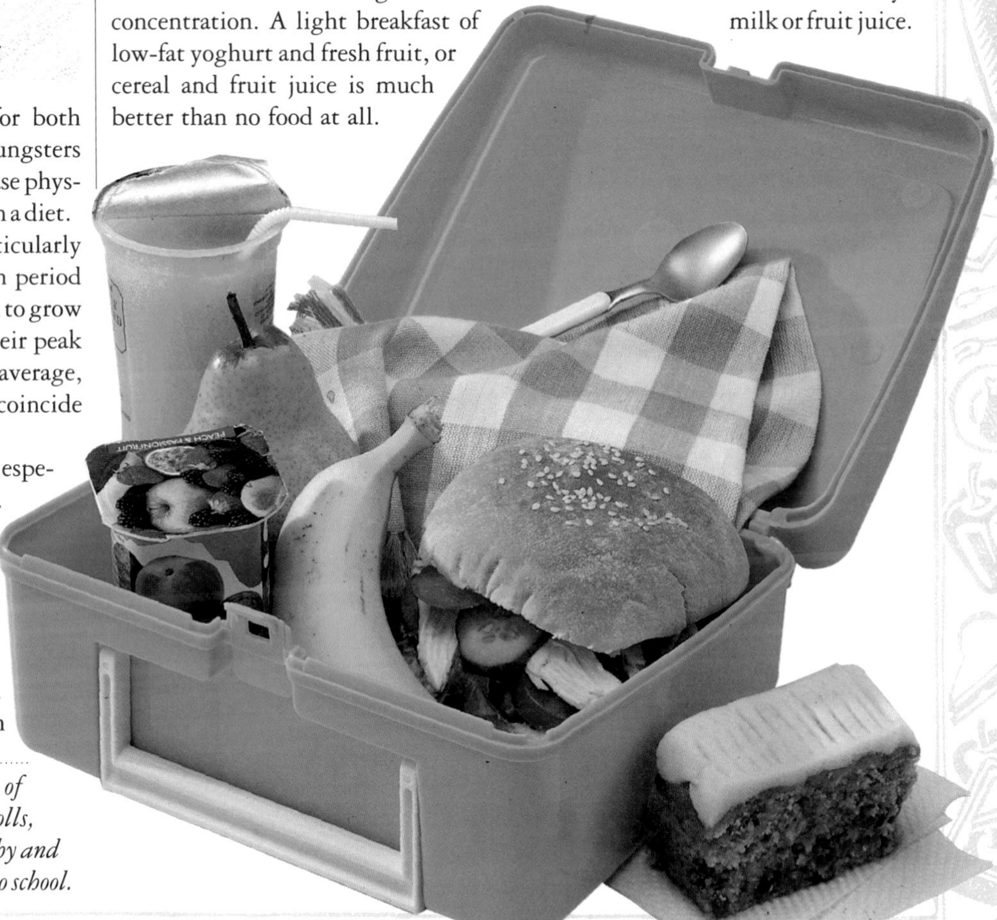

HEALTHY LUNCHBOX *A variety of foods, including sandwiches or rolls, fruit and yoghurt makes a healthy and appetising packed lunch to take to school.*

CHESTNUTS

BENEFITS
- *Low in fat*
- *Useful source of fibre*
- *High in carbohydrates*

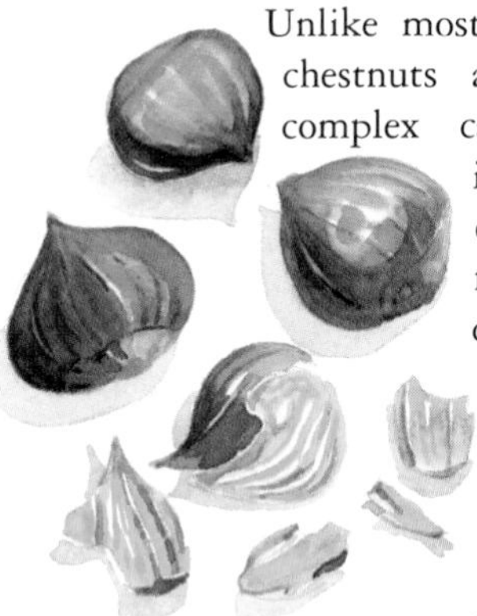

Unlike most other nuts, chestnuts are high in complex carbohydrates, in the form of starch and fibre, and also contain very little protein or fat. Brazil nuts, hazelnuts and walnuts all have more than 20 times as much fat as chestnuts. Weight for weight, chestnuts also have less than half the calories of most other nuts and a much higher water content. A 100g (3½oz) portion of chestnuts supplies about a third of the recommended daily intake of vitamin E and a quarter of the intake for vitamin B_6.

Cooking will reduce the bitterness of raw chestnuts, which is caused by the tannins they contain.

CHICKENPOX

TAKE PLENTY OF
- *Liver for vitamin A*
- *Green leafy vegetables and carrots for beta carotene*
- *Citrus fruit juices*
- *Fresh fruit and vegetables to supply vitamin C*
- *Dried fruit, nuts and seeds for energy*

Because vitamin A plays an important role in keeping mucous membranes healthy, as well as in healing the skin, people with chickenpox should be encouraged to eat a diet that is rich in this vitamin. Liver is an excellent source (but not for pregnant women), while beta carotene, which the body converts into vitamin A, is found in green leafy vegetables as well as orange fruit and vegetables. As with any fever, drink plenty of fluids. Citrus fruit juices are especially good because they supply vitamin C which is also needed for healthy skin and for helping to prevent infection. To boost energy levels, eat dried fruit, seeds and nuts.

Although following the above dietary advice will not cure chickenpox it will give the sufferer the best possible chance of recovering quickly from the illness.

AN ITCHY ILLNESS

The illness, usually caught by children, spreads through coughs, sneezes and the watery liquid contained in the blistery spots, which burst to form crusty scabs. Symptoms, which normally appear within 10 to 21 days of infection, include a fever, an intensely itchy rash, tiredness and a headache. Chickenpox is more serious in adults because they are more likely to develop pneumonia and other complications.

Chickenpox is infectious before the spots appear and for seven days after the last spots have appeared. Avoid scratching the spots or you could be left with permanent scars. For this reason young children's fingernails should be cut short for the duration of the illness. Lotions and regular warm baths may help to soothe the itching.

Once children have had the disease, they are immune for life. However, the virus lies dormant in the nervous system and causes SHINGLES if reactivated at a later date. You cannot catch shingles from someone with chickenpox, but you could catch chickenpox from someone with shingles.

A chickenpox vaccine is currently under review by the US Food and Drug Administration and may be available in the not too distant future.

CHILDREN AND DIET

See page 90

CHILLIES

BENEFITS
- *May help to relieve congestion*
- *Excellent source of vitamin C*

DRAWBACKS
- *May irritate the digestive system*
- *Require cautious handling during preparation as they can irritate the eyes and burn the skin*

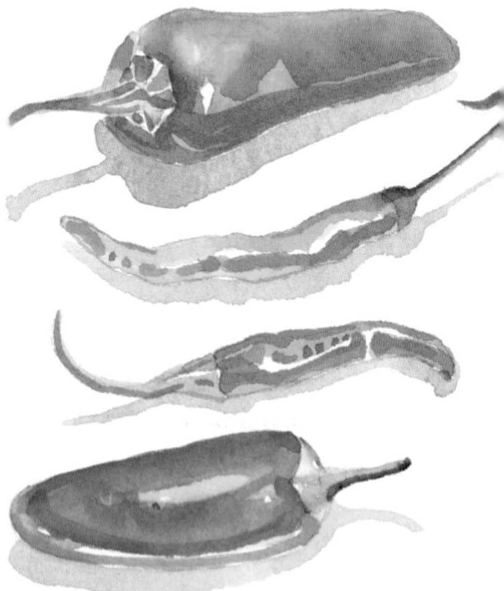

The heat in chilli peppers comes from capsaicin, a potent compound concentrated mainly in the white ribs and seeds, but also distributed unevenly throughout the flesh, to which it gives a distinctive tongue-tingling flavour.

When eaten in spicy dishes, capsaicin produces a burning sensation in the mouth, making the eyes water and the nose run. In some cases this may help to clear blocked airways by thinning down the mucus in the sinuses.

Chillies are richer in vitamin C than citrus fruits, but are unlikely to contribute much to the daily intake as

Chilli charm

What is the attraction of fiery foods such as chillies? One US psychologist has suggested that, in response to their burning taste, the brain releases endorphins – painkilling chemical compounds that, at high levels, give a sensation of pleasure. This would also account for the apparent success of crushed chillies when used to cure toothache a century ago.

they are usually eaten only in small amounts. However, some milder varieties can be eaten in larger quantities.

Some researchers have claimed that eating chillies may cause the stomach to secrete a mucus which protects its lining against irritants such as acid, aspirin or alcohol. However, the chillies themselves can sometimes irritate the digestive system and cause extensive itching in the anal area. Chillies can also act as anticoagulants and may help to lower blood pressure and blood cholesterol levels.

When chopping chillies, handle with care as the capsaicin can irritate sensitive skins and is also very painful if it comes into contact with the eyes.

CHOCOLATE AND SWEETS

See page 100

CHOLESTEROL

Despite several decades in the spotlight of medical and media concern, cholesterol remains one of the most contentious aspects of the factors that influence our health. Medical experts disagree about its relationship to heart disease, and the public is uncertain as to what cholesterol actually is. People often tend to confuse the two types of cholesterol – dietary cholesterol and blood or 'plasma' cholesterol. The first is contained in food, the other is essential for the body's metabolism.

WHAT IS CHOLESTEROL?

Each day the liver manufactures up to 1g of blood cholesterol, the fat-like, waxy material that is a component of all cells. Blood cholesterol is also involved in the creation of some hormones, and helps to make vitamin D and bile acids, which aid digestion.

The major risks of heart disease caused by high levels of blood cholesterol are rooted in genetic make-up, though diet and obesity are also important factors. While there is nothing that can be done about heredity, you can change your diet.

HOW DIET CAN HELP

Reducing saturated fats has the greatest effect of all dietary measures on blood cholesterol levels, lowering them by as much as 14 per cent. Recent US studies suggest that eating foods that contain soluble FIBRE – such as oatmeal, baked beans, pectin-rich fruits such as grapefruit, and dried fruit – can lower cholesterol levels still further. Compounds in GARLIC also suppress cholesterol production in the liver.

The amount of cholesterol in the diet is not reflected by the amount in the blood – this is mostly determined by the amount of saturated fat in the diet. Foods rich in cholesterol are now not thought to dramatically increase the risk of heart disease for healthy people. However, most experts agree that those with heart problems, a family history of heart disease, or high blood cholesterol levels, should limit dietary cholesterol.

High amounts of cholesterol are found in egg yolks, offal (particularly liver and brains) and in shrimps and prawns. But controversy colours the extent to which these sources – particularly eggs, which are low in saturated fats but high in cholesterol – influence cholesterol levels. While the World Health Organisation argues that up to ten eggs a week will not hurt you, the British Heart Foundation believes

Case study

Albert was 50 years old when his doctor discovered that his cholesterol levels were abnormally high. Albert smoked 20 cigarettes a day, and his father had died of a heart attack at 53. He was urged to stop smoking, which he has done. His doctor also advised him to reduce his saturated fat intake, which has meant sacrificing cooked breakfasts and cutting down on full-fat dairy foods. A year later, Albert's cholesterol level is back to normal and he has certainly reduced his risk of coronary heart disease.

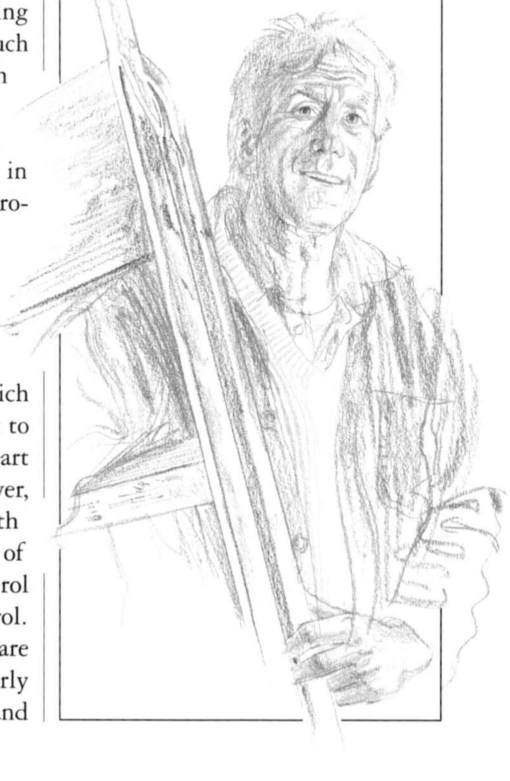

that three to four eggs a week is the safe maximum – while its transatlantic counterpart, the American Heart Association, sets the level at three.

In fact, the average daily cholesterol intake of British males is about 390 mg daily and that of women about 290 mg – enough to raise blood cholesterol levels by about 5 per cent.

Fortunately, the body can normally iron out rises in dietary cholesterol. With most people the liver automatically manufactures less cholesterol when levels from foods in the diet become too high. Even where there is a substantial intake of fats, the average healthy person is not at risk.

Because blood is mainly composed of water – which does not blend with fat – cholesterol is transported around the body attached to specific proteins called lipoproteins. There are two types of lipoproteins; low density lipoproteins (LDL) and high density lipoproteins (HDL). LDL carry about three-quarters of the cholesterol in blood, and high LDL levels usually reflect high cholesterol levels and imply a higher risk of heart disease. High levels of HDL – which carry much less fat – signal a lower than average risk of heart disease.

THOSE MOST AT RISK

High levels of LDL tend to stem from a defect (often hereditary) in a receptor in the liver which should remove them from the blood. When this receptor does not function properly a chronic furring of the arteries called ATHEROSCLEROSIS occurs. Hormonal disorders, which may affect those with diabetes or thyroid problems, can also 'switch off' the receptors.

Because the female hormone oestrogen increases both the number and effectiveness of LDL receptors, therefore helping to keep blood cholesterol levels low, women are less prone to heart disease before the menopause.

Eating to keep cholesterol in check

Until recently, many heart problems, such as angina, thrombosis and coronary heart disease, were claimed to be caused by excess cholesterol, a term which embraced both dietary and blood cholesterol. While the former can affect health, it is the latter type – where high levels are often hereditary – which is now seen as the main threat to a healthy heart. Recent research has shown that saturated and trans fatty acids can sometimes raise the blood cholesterol to unhealthy levels. A healthy diet will go a long way to protect against excessive levels of blood cholesterol, as well as lowering those that are already too high.

FOODS THAT MAY RAISE CHOLESTEROL

Hard margarine and solid cooking fats which are high in saturated fatty acids and trans fatty acids.

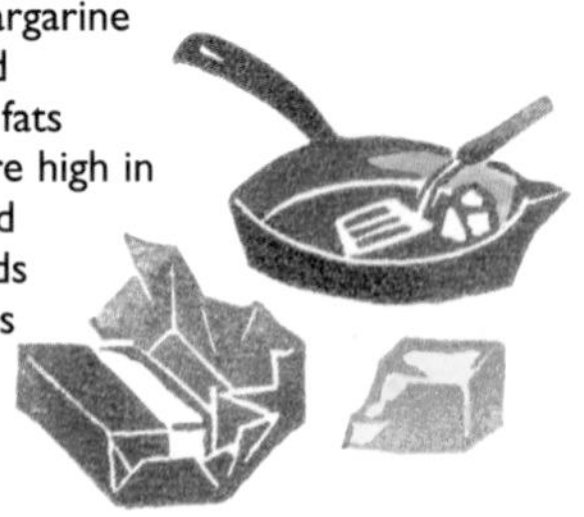

Fatty meat and meat products, such as lamb chops, mince, hamburgers, bacon, frankfurters, salamis, pâtés, pies.

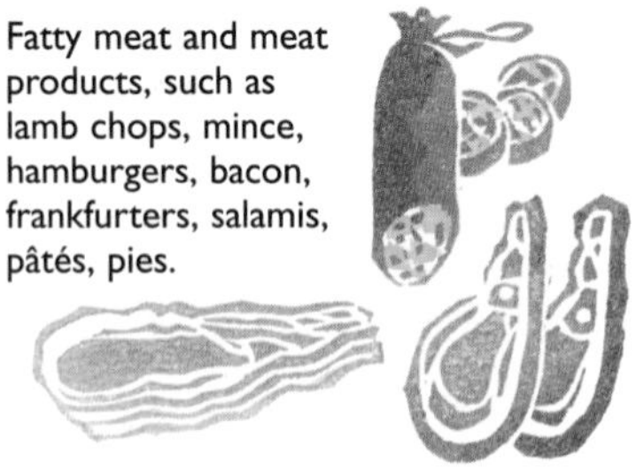

Biscuits, cakes, chocolates and pastries.

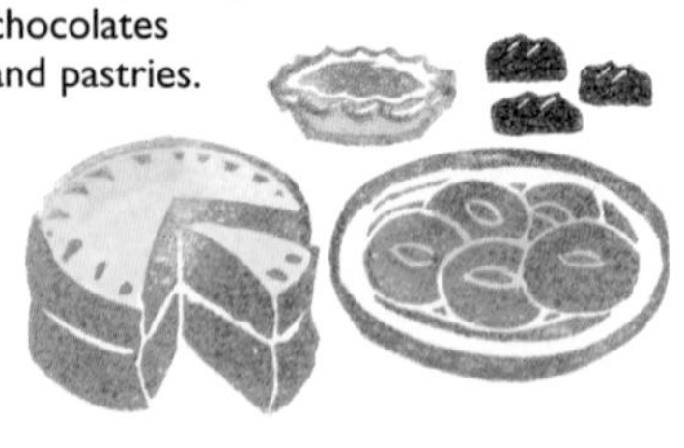

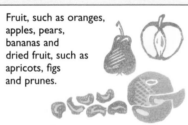

Full-fat dairy products, such as hard cheese, cream and butter.

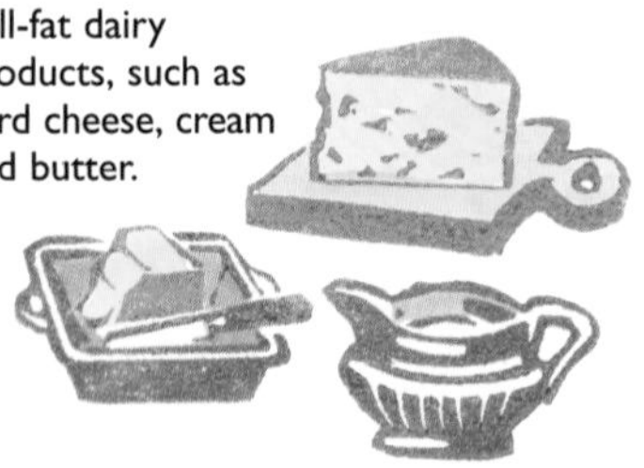

FOODS THAT MAY LOWER CHOLESTEROL

Wholemeal bread and rolls, rye crispbread and granary bread.

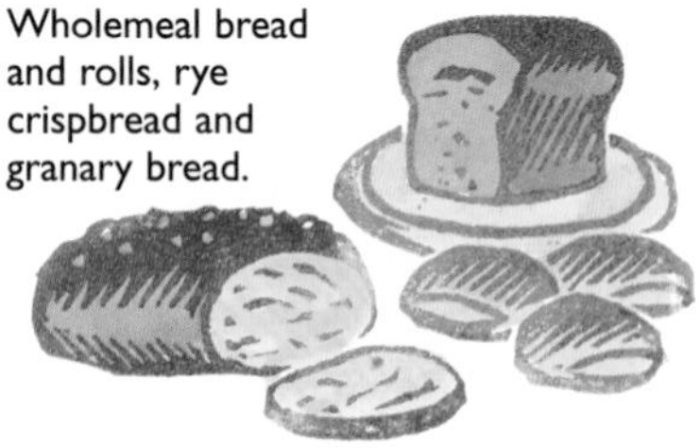

Fruit, such as oranges, apples, pears, bananas and dried fruit, such as apricots, figs and prunes.

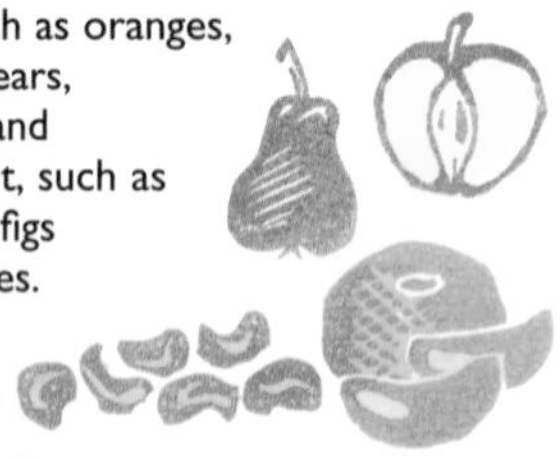

Porridge oats and breakfast cereals which contain cooked bran.

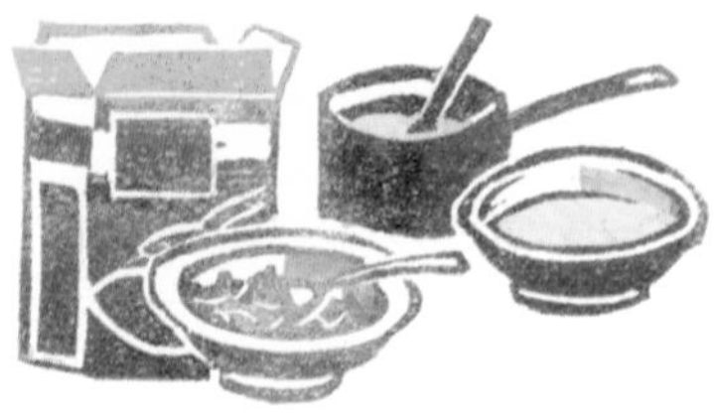

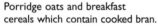

Vegetables, such as sweetcorn, mangetout, onions, garlic, broad beans, red kidney beans and haricot beans.

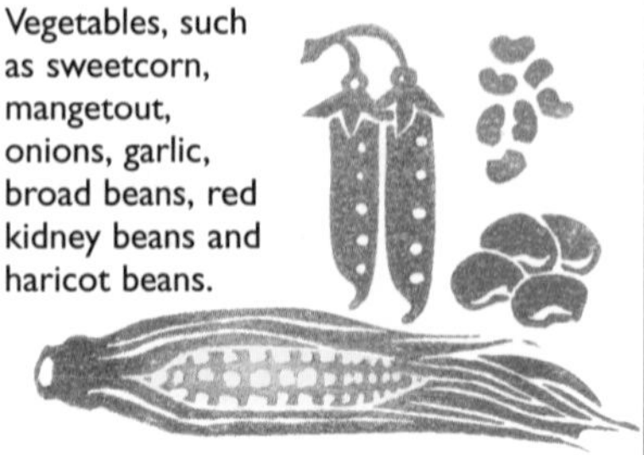

Women also tend to have higher levels of HDL, which further reduce the risks of atherosclerosis and heart disease.

Exercise often helps to lower LDL levels and raise HDL. Moderate alcohol consumption – three glasses of beer a day, or two of wine – may also increase the HDL levels in people who are not overweight. However, obesity reduces HDL levels.

Drugs used to alter the levels of the two lipoproteins tend to benefit those with high, rather than moderately raised cholesterol levels. Even when these drugs are successful, they should be accompanied by an improved diet.

How cholesterol levels are measured

Lay testing of cholesterol levels in the blood is an increasingly popular practice, but to be certain of reliable results, testing is best done under medical supervision.

Levels of blood cholesterol are measured in millimoles/litre, or (mmol/l), against which the risks of heart disease are calculated.

Cholesterol	Risk factor
Less than 5.2mmol/l	Low
5.2-6.5mmol/l	Average
6.5-7.8mmol/l	Moderate
Greater than 7.8mmol/l	High

However, when assessing the risk other factors also need to be considered. Account should be taken of any family history of heart disease as well as an individual's lifestyle. For example, a cholesterol level of 6.4 might be acceptable in a fit man with no other risk factors but worryingly high for a man who had angina, or whose family had a long history of the illness.

CIRCULATION PROBLEMS

EAT PLENTY OF

- *Oily fish*
- *Wholegrain cereals, bread and pasta*
- *Fresh fruit and vegetables*
- *Garlic and onions*
- *Low-fat dairy produce*

CUT DOWN ON

- *Fatty meat and poultry skin*
- *Processed fatty meats*
- *High-fat dairy produce*
- *Alcohol and brewed coffee*
- *Salt*

AVOID

- *Smoking*

The three major factors that cause circulation problems – including HEART DISEASE – are smoking, high BLOOD PRESSURE and high blood cholesterol levels. Obesity can lead to the last two and drinking ALCOHOL to excess is also a major cause of high blood pressure. However, as they get older, many people who are not overweight and do not smoke or drink heavily still develop high blood pressure and high blood CHOLESTEROL levels. Fortunately, a healthy diet can significantly reduce the risk of circulation problems.

Many studies have now linked excessive consumption of FATS to subsequent heart disease and other circulatory problems. There are two forms of fat: unsaturated (found in seed oils and fish oils) and saturated (mostly from animal sources). The British Government's most recent guidelines suggest that saturated fats should be limited to 10 per cent of your total calorie intake and that fats in general should form no more than 35 per cent.

Foods high in saturated fats include butter, cheese and fatty meats; less obvious sources include sausages, pork pies, biscuits, potato crisps, ice cream and chocolate. Although an excessive consumption of alcohol and sugar encourages weight gain, eating too much fat is the prime cause of obesity.

In the right quantities no fats are unhealthy, and some can actually help to prevent circulation problems. Fats from oily fish such as sardines, mackerel, herring, tuna, trout and salmon may help to prevent arterial blood clots. And replacing saturated fats in the diet with monounsaturated or polyunsaturated fats can help to counteract cholesterol build-up.

There is some evidence that garlic and onions, and also hot foods such as chillies, can act as anticoagulants and may help to lower blood pressure and cholesterol levels. A diet high in whole grains, fruit and vegetables also helps to lower cholesterol – their soluble fibre binds with cholesterol in the gut and helps the body to expel it as waste.

Drinking too much percolated or brewed COFFEE can raise blood cholesterol levels. Salt – high levels of which can be found in stock cubes, tinned soups, smoked foods and some snack foods – should be limited because excess salt in the diet has also been linked with high blood pressure, hardening of the arteries and heart disease. Nicotine also impairs the circulation.

BLOOD'S LONG JOURNEY

The circulation system carries blood to and from all parts of the body through arteries, veins and tiny blood vessels that would stretch for about 160000 km (100000 miles) if they were laid out end to end. The heart is the four-chambered pump that powers the entire system. The body's extremities, which are farthest from it, are particularly prone to circulatory problems.

The most common serious disorder associated with poor circulation is ATHEROSCLEROSIS, in which the walls of the arteries develop fatty deposits, thicken, become less supple and so impede the blood flow. This increases the risk of heart attacks, strokes and a variety of other disorders depending on which arteries are affected.

RELATED PROBLEMS

Chest pain – perhaps at times of stress, excitement or strenuous exercise – may be due to ANGINA, which occurs, in late-middle and old age, when the coronary arteries become partially obstructed as their walls thicken. Cramping calf pains during a brisk uphill walk may be caused by hardening of the leg arteries, while a stroke or dementia may be the result of a blocked artery in the brain. People suffering from DIABETES are particularly prone to circulatory disorders as thickening of the walls of the arteries is a known complication of the disease.

A condition known as RESTLESS LEGS may also be due to a circulatory disorder and is characterised by pain and an involuntary twitching in the legs which occurs particularly after going to bed. Vitamin E helps the peripheral circulatory system, so including plenty of seed oils, avocados and wheatgerm in the diet may help.

Two other circulation problems which affect the extremities include RAYNAUD'S DISEASE and chilblains. In Raynaud's disease, the fingers or toes become white and numb when cold and, when warmed, tingle painfully as the blood returns.

Chilblains usually result from exposure to cold, but they can be a problem at normal temperatures when people have poor circulation. They usually occur in fingers and toes, but they can also affect ears, cheeks and the nose. A severe itching and burning sensation results from insufficient blood reaching the affected areas which become inflamed. With chilblains and Raynaud's disease it is important to keep the extremities as warm as possible.

CIRRHOSIS

EAT PLENTY OF
- *Complex carbohydrates such as potatoes, brown rice and wholegrain bread and pasta*
- *Fresh fruit and vegetables*

CUT DOWN ON
- *Fatty foods*
- *Salt*

AVOID
- *Alcohol*
- *Highly spiced foods and pickles*
- *Barbequed foods*

Damage caused by cirrhosis – a life-threatening condition in which the cells of the liver die – cannot be repaired. However, a sensible high-carbohydrate diet can at least help to prevent further deterioration.

The first step to recovery is total abstention from alcohol, which, in the case of alcoholic cirrhosis, will already have affected the body's ability to absorb and store life-sustaining vitamins and minerals.

To replace these lost nutrients and also to regain the weight that will have been lost, sufferers should eat plenty of complex carbohydrates, such as rice, potatoes, wholegrain bread and pasta, as well as vegetables, fresh fruit, and some fish, eggs and low-fat dairy produce in order to obtain the full complement of vitamins.

The damaged livers of people with cirrhosis are often unable to cope with large amounts of fat. This is because the damaged liver has difficulty in making bile, which is needed for fat digestion. Small amounts of poultry, oily fish, lean red meat and soya products will provide low-fat protein. Fatty meats and full-fat dairy produce, such as most hard cheeses, should be avoided. The capacity to break down drugs as well as many other chemicals – particularly those found in rich and spicy foods – can also be impaired when the liver is damaged. It is therefore helpful to avoid dishes which contain a lot of spices. Avoid barbecued foods, too, as they can contain toxins.

Patients with advanced cirrhosis may suffer from oedema – popularly known as dropsy – where excessive fluid retention causes local or general

Case study

When Martin visited his local surgery with a cut hand, the doctor noticed that his liver was enlarged. Asked about his alcohol intake, Martin explained that the stress of work was such that he always drank two or three gin-and-tonics in the evening, followed by wine with his evening meal. When blood tests showed that his liver was irreversibly damaged, Martin vowed that he would never drink again – he was determined to stop his condition from deteriorating any further.

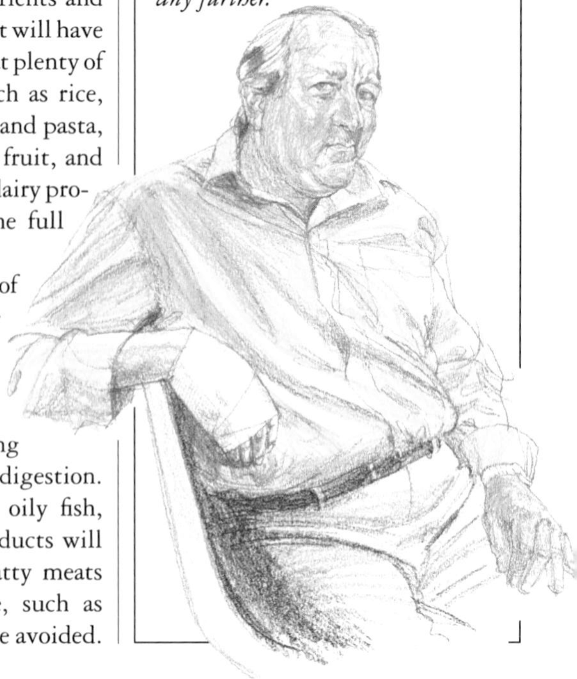

swelling of the body tissues. If this condition arises you should cut down on your salt and sodium intake.

Causes and symptoms

The most common cause of cirrhosis is persistent alcohol abuse. Other causes include viral hepatitis, malnutrition, and chronic inflammation or blockage of ducts in the liver.

As the disease develops, the normally soft liver tissue is infiltrated with fibrous scar tissue and is less able to remove toxins from the blood. The patient feels unwell and often suffers from bloating in the upper abdomen, constipation or diarrhoea, vomiting, loss of appetite and weight loss. Sometimes jaundice may also develop.

Later symptoms may include oedema and anaemia. Bleeding problems may also occur because the disease can slow down the blood-clotting mechanism.

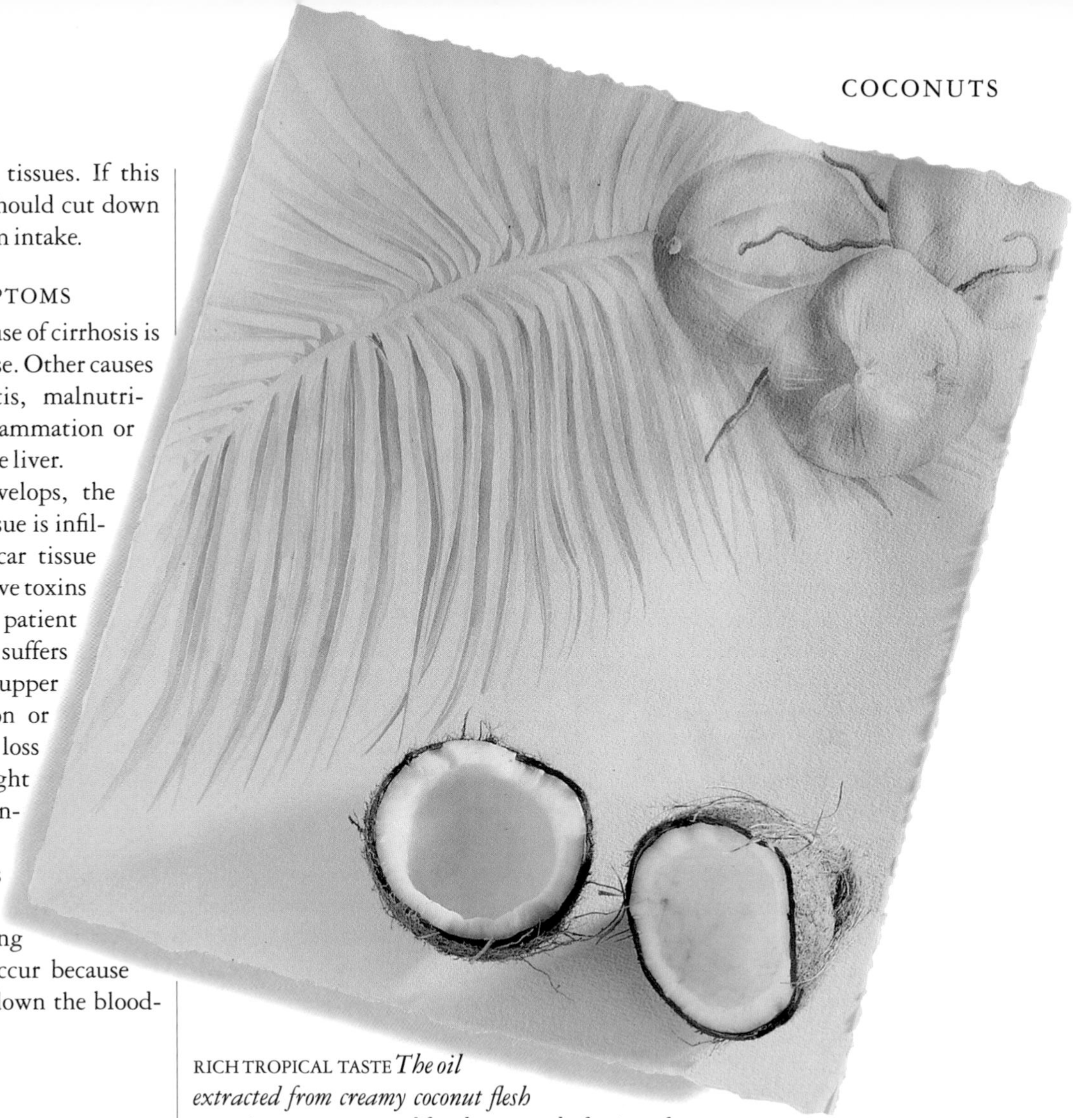

RICH TROPICAL TASTE *The oil extracted from creamy coconut flesh contains more saturated fat than even the fattiest of meats.*

Coconuts

BENEFIT
- *Useful source of fibre*

DRAWBACKS
- *High in saturated fat*
- *High in calories*

Coconut oil, used in confectionery and margarine, is one of only two plant oils in common use that are high in saturated fat (the other is palm oil). Although the oil does not contain cholesterol, the consumption of coconut oil still raises cholesterol levels in the blood which in turn increases the risk of a heart attack. Coconut oil also lacks most of the nutrients that other nut and vegetable oils contain. The coconut's flesh contains 351 Calories per 100g (3½oz), more than three-quarters of which come from saturated fat. The flesh contains plenty of dietary fibre, but is a relatively poor source of vitamin E and the minerals which most other nuts provide. Even though it is high in saturated fat, it is easily digestible, and it can be useful for people suffering from digestive disorders who have difficulty absorbing most other dietary fats.

Coconut can be eaten fresh, or it can be shredded and dried for use in desserts, ice creams and processed foods. It is best known in the British kitchen in its desiccated form, which has a slightly lower saturated fat content. Coconut milk, the sweet-tasting white fluid contained in the heart of the coconut, can be served as a drink, or used as a marinade. A cup of coconut milk contains only about 57 Calories and about 12g of carbohydrate. The protein content of fresh coconut milk is a low 0.7g per cup and there is less than 0.5g of saturated fat. The coconut milk sold in supermarkets is seldom the fresh form. It is usually produced by squeezing liquid from a mixture of grated coconut flesh and water. Its calorific and nutritional value is lower than fresh coconut milk.

Coconut cream – a rich, fatty mixture made from coconut flesh and milk – is often used in oriental curries.

CHOCOLATE AND SWEETS

While chocolate and sweets can give a boost to flagging energy levels, they should not become a habitual part of your diet. Keep them for special occasions and you will enjoy them all the more.

The feel-good factor provided by chocolate and sweets means that many people use confectionery as an instant lift when their energy levels are low. The problem is that by relying on chocolate and sweets to get that immediate blood-sugar fix, these foods can all too easily become a regular part of the diet. More often than not, sweets are merely a source of empty calories and can suppress the appetite for more nutritious food at mealtimes. Chocolate does have some nutritional value but it is high in fat and so can contribute to weight gain if eaten in excessive amounts. This is not to say that confectionery poses a health risk, merely that it should be eaten as a treat, in moderation, and not as a substitute for more nutritious food.

DID YOU KNOW?

- There is no conclusive evidence that eating chocolate causes acne or makes it worse, although acne sufferers are usually advised to cut down on chocolate.
- A small 125g (4oz) bar of dark chocolate contains more caffeine than a cup of instant coffee.
- Chocolate does less harm to the teeth than other forms of sugar confectionery.
- The cocoa tree's scientific name is *Theobroma cacao*: 'theobroma' means 'the food of the gods'.
- Sweets are a major cause of dental caries especially if consumed frequently between meals.
- The sugar in sweets does not cause hyperactivity in children, but the caffeine in chocolate can keep some people awake at night.

CHOCOLATE

According to one of the major confectionery manufacturers, people in the United Kingdom ate over £3 billion worth of chocolate in 1993 – which amounts to a hefty 8.72kg (19.2lb) per head. Chocolate enthusiasts in Britain even have their own society, which searches out good quality chocolate for its members to try. These connoisseurs are offered chocolate containing at least 50 per cent cocoa solids; some top-quality brands contain more than 70 per cent.

Nutritionally, chocolate contains some protein, variable amounts of sugar, and certain minerals. Plain chocolate is a useful source of iron and magnesium, for example, and all chocolate contains potassium. Chocolate also contains compounds which act as mild stimulants, which may also be responsible for causing MIGRAINE in susceptible people.

Because chocolate is high in fat – about 30 per cent by weight – it is also high in calories, containing around 500 Calories per 100g (3½oz).

THE FEEL-GOOD FACTOR

Chocolate is believed to boost serotonin and endorphin levels in the brain, which have an uplifting effect. The so-called 'chocolate high' is due in part to the substance phenylethylamine (PEA), which occurs naturally in the brain and is allegedly released at times of emotional arousal. Hence the traditional lover's gift of a box of chocolates, and the craving for chocolate that some people report when a relationship ends. Chocolate also contains the stimulants theobromine and CAFFEINE, which increase alertness. In addition, there are some people who find eating chocolate soothing because they associate it with comfort or reward from their childhood.

SURVIVAL RATIONS

Anyone contemplating a lake-land hike, a mountaineering expedition, or a day's fishing should consider putting a bar or two of chocolate in their lunchbox. In 1993, four Britons survived six days in the snowy wilderness of the Russian Caucasus on just three Mars bars. Expert Scottish mountaineers advise people on one-day climbs to take something hot to drink and some high-energy food – such as Kendal mint cake or bars of chocolate. Chocolate is included in the US army's daily K-rations in the field, and is even eaten by astronauts in space.

HOW IS CHOCOLATE MADE?

Chocolate is made from the fruit of the cacao tree, which is indigenous to South America. Indeed, cocoa beans – the seeds of the tree – were used as a form of money by the Aztec civilisation of Mexico some 3000 years ago. The cacao tree also thrives in west Africa and South-east Asia.

Cocoa beans undergo a considerable amount of processing before chocolate is produced. First, they are fermented

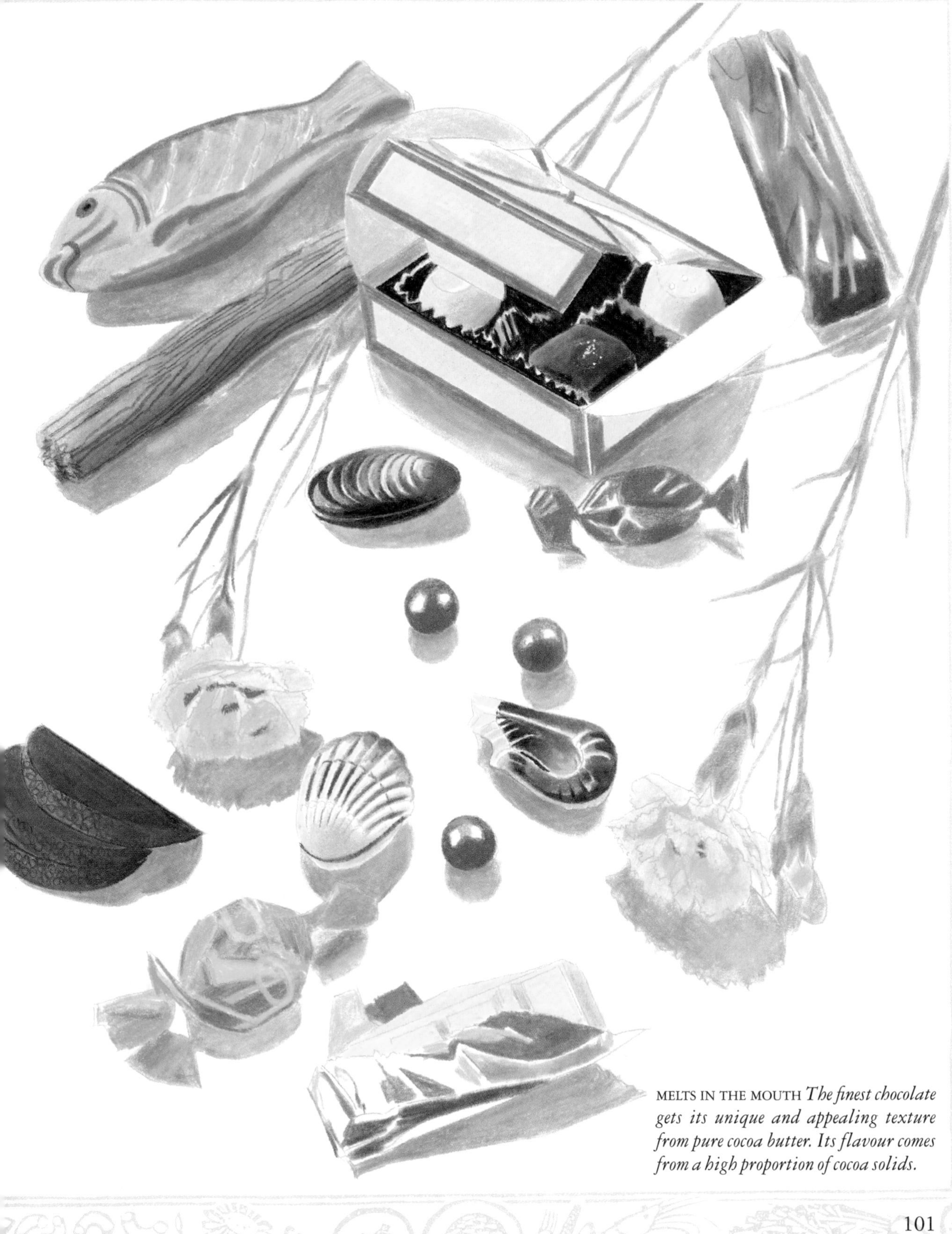

MELTS IN THE MOUTH *The finest chocolate gets its unique and appealing texture from pure cocoa butter. Its flavour comes from a high proportion of cocoa solids.*

Case study

Philip, a 46-year-old estate agent, had a very unpleasant experience with an old-fashioned dental anaesthetic as a child, and had been terrified of dentists ever since. For years, he had preferred to rely on his toothbrush, and the breath-freshening properties of peppermints – which he sucked throughout the day, assuming they were good for his teeth because they tasted similar to toothpaste. Recently, however, he had suffered from repeated toothache, and worse still, one of his teeth had broken off at gum level. Philip finally had to pluck up courage and visit a dentist, who told him that he had not seen such extensive dental caries for years. He explained that the cause was primarily Philip's mint-sucking habit, which had coated his teeth in sugar for long periods each day. With the aid of effective modern dental anaesthetics, Philip's teeth were painlessly filled and he had a crown fitted. The experience has restored Philip's faith in dentists, and he no longer relies on peppermints for fresh breath.

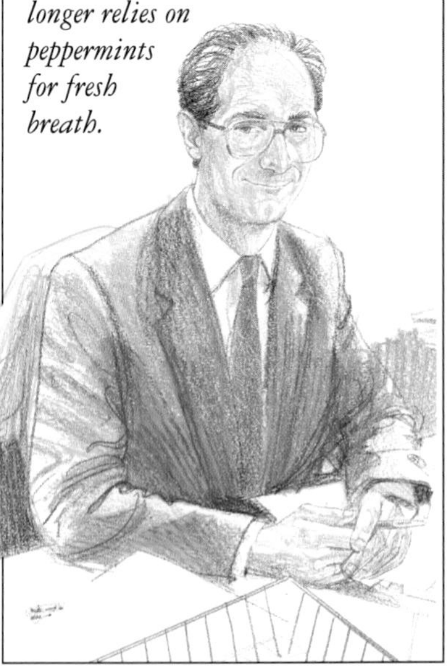

and sun-dried before being bagged for export. Chocolate manufacturers sort and clean the beans and roast them to develop their flavour. The roasted beans are then shelled and ground.

The heat of the grinding process melts the fat in the cocoa beans, resulting in a fatty material with a bitter taste called chocolate liquor. Much of the yellow fat, or cocoa butter, is separated from the liquor in a press, leaving behind a solid cake of cocoa. This is then ground and sifted to manufacture cocoa powder.

Chocolate confectionery is made by adding sugar, additional fat and milk – in the case of milk chocolate – to chocolate liquor. Traditionally, the fat added to chocolate is cocoa butter, which gives the characteristic melt-in-the-mouth texture. In the United States, cocoa butter is the only fat permitted in chocolate; in the European Union, however, some member states, including the United Kingdom, are allowed to produce chocolate containing five per cent vegetable fat, although connoisseurs generally agree that these fats produce an inferior chocolate.

SWEETS

The principal ingredient of sweets, sugar, has a rather mysterious history. No one knows when or where it originated, although it is thought that the cane may have come from Polynesia.

Almost all sweets are high in simple sugars – sucrose, glucose and fructose. They supply about 375 Calories per 100g (3½oz).

Many people regard sweets as fattening because of their high sugar content. However, this is not necessarily so, because sugar has a suppressant effect on the appetite – as many parents will testify: children who eat just a few sweets before meals often have little appetite for their food. This is worrying if it means that children satisfy their hunger with empty calories and so miss out on the vital nourishment contained in a proper meal.

CAROB – A HEALTHY SUBSTITUTE FOR CHOCOLATE?

Many health-food shops sell carob-flavoured confectionery as the healthy alternative to chocolate, largely because – unlike chocolate – it contains no stimulants. The powdered carob pod is similar in colour and fragrance to cocoa but, because its flavour is much milder, it needs to be used in larger quantities than cocoa powder. Carob flour is lower in fat and higher in carbohydrate and calcium, whereas cocoa is higher in niacin, vitamin E, iron, zinc and phosphorus.

Although carob chocolate starts out as a low-fat powder, it is far from being a low-fat food. It is usually made with coconut oil or hydrogenated vegetable oil, and the end result is often just as high in fat as chocolate.

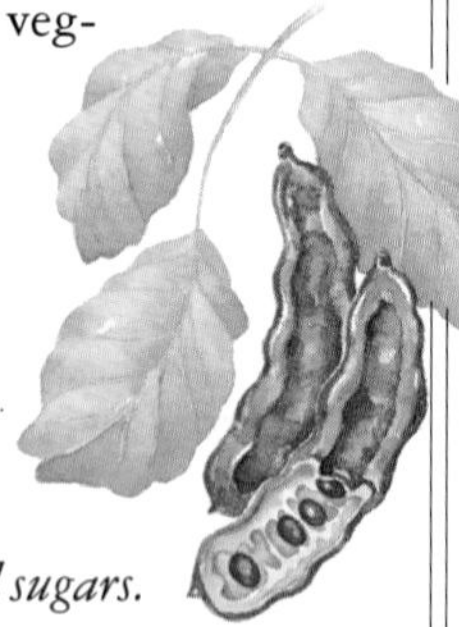

SWEET PODS
Carob pods are rich in natural sugars.

BRIGHT COLOURS AND ALLERGIES

Children love bright colours, so confectionery manufacturers produce their most colourful sweets for children. Although all permitted food colourings are rigorously tested and considered safe for people to eat, there are some which are associated with adverse reactions. The most well-known of these is tartrazine which can cause wheeziness in some asthmatics and exacerbate migraine in susceptible people. The orange colouring (E102) can also trigger nettle rash, runny nose and eyes and blurred vision. Along with other artificial colours used in sweets – including sunset yellow (E110), cochineal red (E120) and indigo carmine blue (E132) – tartrazine is on the list of ADDITIVES which the Hyperactive Children's Support Group says should be avoided.

DO CHOCOLATES AND SWEETS CAUSE TOOTH DECAY?

There is no doubt that regular consumption of sugary foods and sweet drinks leads to tooth decay. Sugar and other refined carbohydrates are fermented by bacteria in dental plaque to produce acids which dissolve tooth enamel. The harmful effects of sugar can be reduced if teeth are brushed regularly to prevent the build-up of plaque. Lollipops and sweets which linger in the mouth for any length of time cause more damage than those which are swallowed quickly.

Chocolate confectionery is less likely than other sweets to lead to dental decay. This is partly because chocolate tends to be chewed and swallowed quickly, but it could also be due either to the fat content of chocolate or to the naturally occurring tannins in cocoa, which inhibit the growth of dental plaque.

Nutritional content for various sweets

ITEM	WEIGHT	CALORIES	FAT (g)	PROTEIN (g)
After-dinner mints	40g (1½oz)	160	5	0
Chewing gum	3g or 1 stick	10	0	0
Bar of plain chocolate	40g (1½oz)	200	11	1
Bar of milk chocolate	40g (1½oz)	210	13	3
Toffees	40g or 6 pieces	180	1.5	0
Jelly beans	40g or 6 pieces	160	0	0

TOOTH-FRIENDLY SWEETS

Sweets which do not cause dental caries – and which may even actively prevent them – have now been developed. Some chewing gums are 'tooth-friendly' because, instead of being sweetened with sugar, which encourages tooth decay, they are sweetened with xylitol, made from substances extracted from birchwood, corn cobs or almond shells. These gums help in two ways: first, chewing stimulates the salivary glands, and saliva keeps the mouth clean; secondly, xylitol actually changes the composition and stickiness of dental plaque, thereby helping to reduce the incidence of dental caries. Sugar-free confectionery, in which at least half of the sweetener is xylitol, can promote dental health if eaten after meals, according to studies sponsored by the World Health Organisation (WHO). Your dentist can supply you with the addresses of mail-order suppliers.

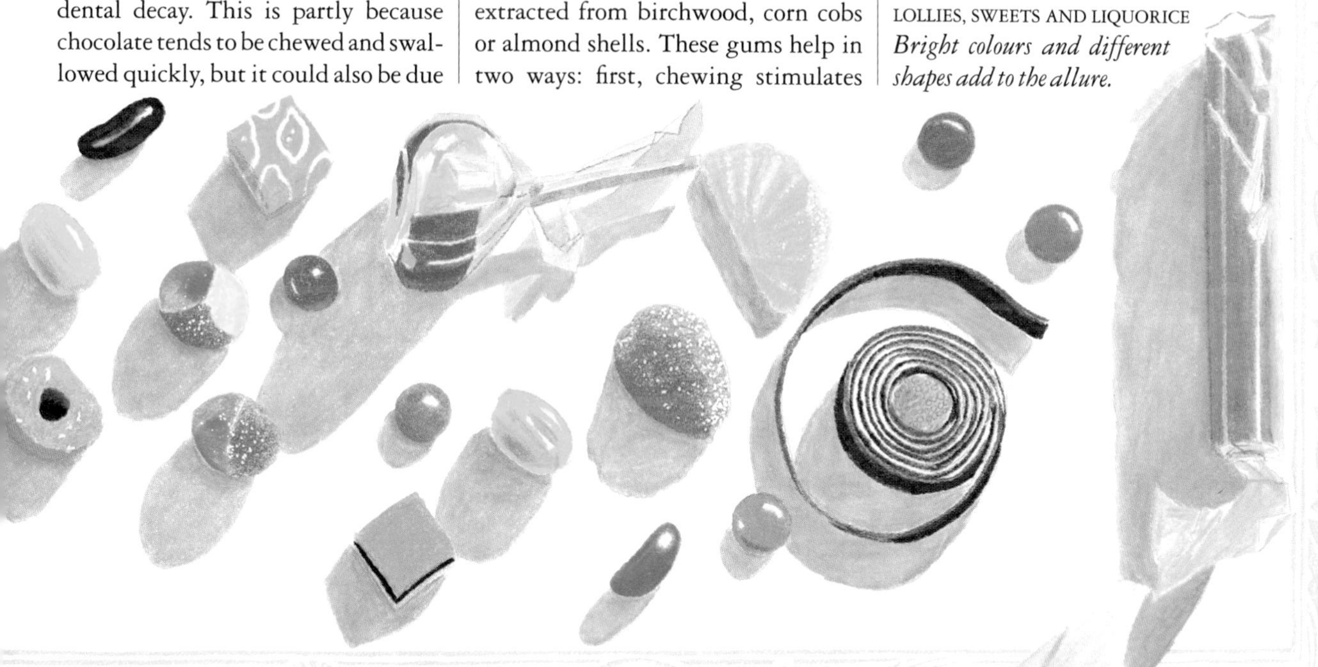

LOLLIES, SWEETS AND LIQUORICE
Bright colours and different shapes add to the allure.

Coeliac disease

EAT PLENTY OF

- *Vegetables, salads and fruit*
- *Lentils, peas, beans and nuts*
- *Cheese, milk, eggs, lean meat, poultry and fish*
- *Rice, potatoes and corn (maize)*

AVOID

- *Cereals, wheat flours, bread, pasta, cakes, batter, biscuits and oats*
- *Tinned and refined foods using wheat flour as a thickening agent*
- *Sausages and other processed meats*
- *Drinks made from barley such as beer and malted milk drinks*

A dietary disorder of the intestines, coeliac disease affects approximately one in 1500 people in the United Kingdom. The condition is caused by a sensitivity to the protein gluten, which is found in cereals such as wheat, rye, barley and oats. It occurs in adults and children, and tends to run in families. In children it may arise within a few months of taking solids such as cereals or rusks that contain gluten, but it can manifest itself at any age. Adults who develop it may have had a mild or symptomless form of the disease in childhood.

In susceptible people, gluten damages the villi – minute hair-like projections lining the small intestine – and this can inhibit the absorption of nutrients. The first signs in children are usually repeated stomach upsets and a failure to thrive. Other symptoms normally include bloating, diarrhoea, anaemia and weight loss. Adults may also experience fatigue, depression, a general loss of well-being, mouth ulcers, dermatitis or infertility. A correct diagnosis can be made only by having a biopsy, when a sample of the small intestine is removed and examined. The patient will then be put on a strict gluten-free diet. The biopsy may then have to be repeated in order to establish whether or not cutting out gluten has allowed the lining of the gut to recover. If the intestinal villi have recovered, the diagnosis is confirmed.

Case study

George, a 68-year-old retired schoolmaster, noticed that his stomach was swollen, that he was short of breath and that he looked pale. He visited his doctor who carried out a blood test which showed him to be suffering from anaemia. George underwent several investigative tests to establish the cause of his anaemia. However, no abnormalities were detected, until he underwent a biopsy of the small bowel. To everyone's surprise, the results showed that George had coeliac disease. He was put on a strict gluten-free diet. Six months later, George was feeling much better; his haemoglobin had recovered to normal levels, and a further biopsy was normal. He is still on a gluten-free regime, and remains fit and well.

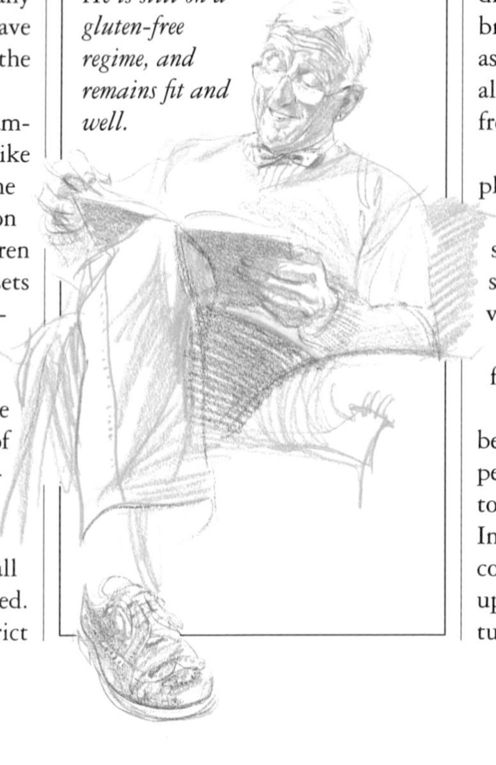

Once the disease has been identified, patients are advised never again to eat anything that contains gluten. Some people may be advised by their doctor to take extra vitamins and minerals for the first few months until they are accustomed to planning a gluten-free diet that provides all the nutrients they need. A marked improvement in health should become apparent within just a few weeks.

Avoiding gluten

Hundreds of everyday foods contain gluten: breads, cakes, biscuits and pasta, sausages bound with breadcrumbs, foods covered with batter, as well as sauces and soups thickened with wheat flour, all contain the protein. Most breakfast cereals should also be avoided.

If your baby has developed coeliac disease you will need to check the ingredients on baby foods, although most first-stage foods are gluten-free.

Always read labels of commercially prepared foods, and beware of ingredients such as flour-based binders and fillers and modified starch. Avoid drinks such as lemon barley water, and brewed drinks made with barley such as beer and stout. Communion wafers also contain gluten (although gluten-free ones are now available).

To replace any prohibited foods, eat plenty of potatoes, pulses, rice, corn and nuts. Use cornflour, rice flour, soya flour or chestnut flour to thicken sauces. Balance the diet with fresh vegetables and fruit, eggs, milk and cheese, as well as meat, poultry and fish; the fish can be fresh or canned.

Avoiding gluten is difficult, so it is best to seek the advice of an experienced dietician who can help you to maintain a balanced, healthy diet. In Britain and many other countries, coeliac societies regularly produce updated lists of gluten-free manufactured foods, as well as recipe ideas.

COFFEE

BENEFITS
- *Mild laxative and diuretic*
- *Stimulates alertness*
- *Can keep you awake when needed*

DRAWBACKS
- *A high intake of brewed or percolated coffee is linked to an increased risk of heart disease*
- *Coffee that has been brewed may raise blood cholesterol levels*
- *Can cause migraine in susceptible individuals*
- *In women, an excessive intake may increase the risk of osteoporosis in later life.*

As well as being a rich source of CAFFEINE, coffee also contains at least 300 other active ingredients, though only one of these – niacin – has any nutritional value. Niacin is produced during the bean-roasting process and one cup of coffee provides about 1mg of the vitamin. But you would need to drink about 15 cups to obtain the adult daily requirement of niacin from this source. Any other nutritional value in the drink is derived from added milk and sugar.

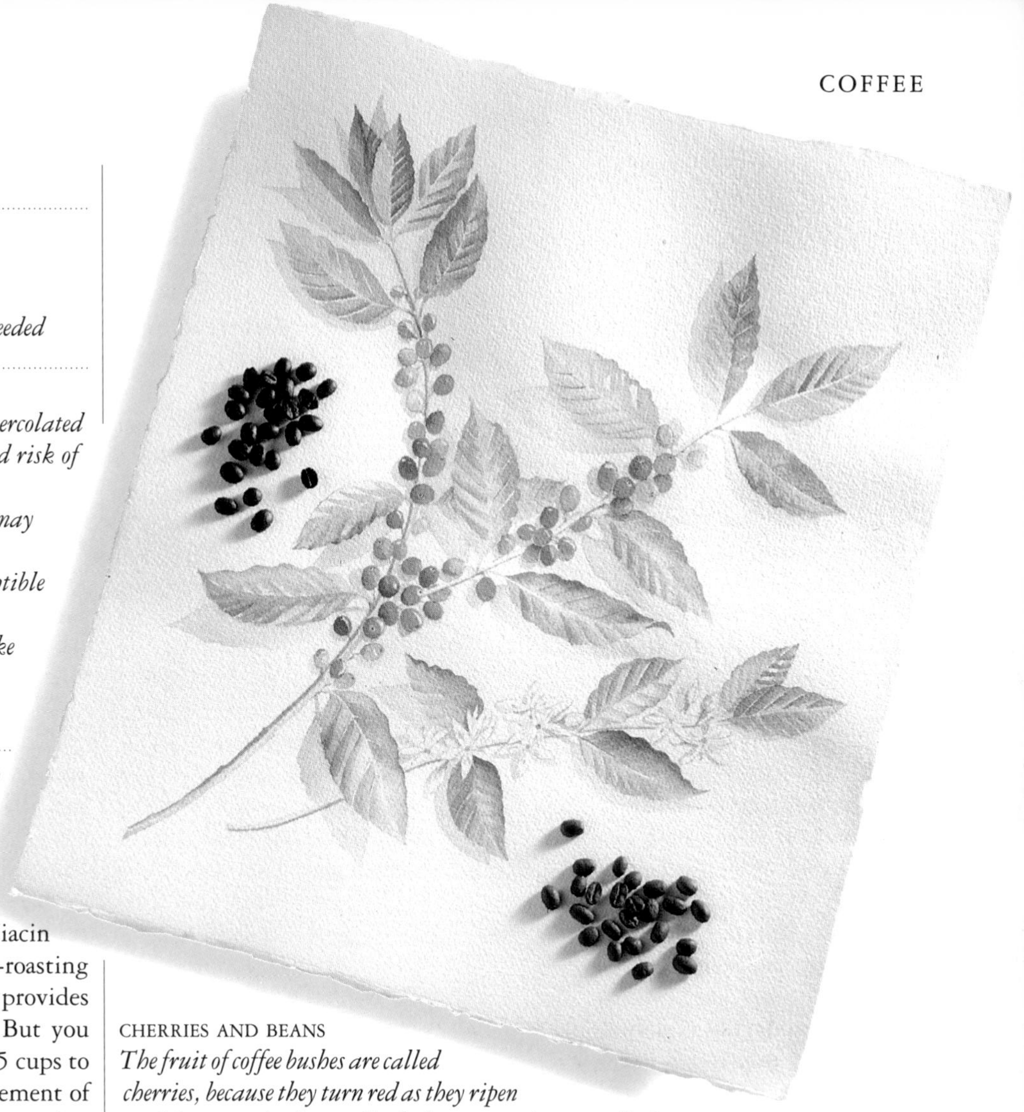

CHERRIES AND BEANS
The fruit of coffee bushes are called cherries, because they turn red as they ripen and they grow in clusters. Each cherry contains two coffee beans.

COFFEE AND CHOLESTEROL

Some studies have found that heavy coffee drinkers, who drink more than six cups of coffee a day, face an increased risk of HEART DISEASE. However, this risk is associated more with the method of preparing coffee than with its caffeine content.

When coffee is prepared in a cafetière, a percolator, by the espresso method, or by adding hot water to coffee grounds and bringing to the boil (which is a popular method in Scandinavian countries), two chemicals are released which raise blood cholesterol levels and increase the risk of heart disease. The chemicals, called cafestol and kahweol, are naturally present in the coffee bean. However, they are removed when coffee is filtered through a paper, and also during the manufacture of instant coffee.

COFFEE AND HEART DISEASE

When you drink a cup of coffee your heart rate increases and your BLOOD PRESSURE rises slightly. But, moderate coffee drinking does not cause high blood pressure; even people with existing high blood pressure do not need to stop drinking coffee altogether. Until recently it was widely held that those who had suffered a heart attack should avoid drinking any coffee, or drink only the decaffeinated varieties. It was argued that coffee, or caffeine, triggered abnormal heart rhythms, and increased the chances of having another heart attack. However, recent research carried out in Britain and the United States has indicated that drinking filtered coffee does not lead to abnormal heart rhythms among heart attack victims; so there is no need to avoid coffee if you have suffered a heart attack.

COFFEE AS A LAXATIVE

Caffeine itself is not a laxative. In fact, decaffeinated coffee is a stronger laxative than ordinary coffee and scientists are still trying to discover exactly

Real coffee: who drinks the most?

Scandinavians consume more real coffee than people living anywhere else in the world; each year they drink about 612 cups per person, made from 9kg (20lb) of coffee beans. Britons, who are better known for their tea drinking, get through 500g (just over 1lb) of coffee beans per head each year, equivalent to a mere 34 cups.

which of the other 300 organic substances in coffee beans is responsible for stimulating bowel movements. However, caffeine is a natural diuretic.

POSSIBLE HAZARDS

Suggestions that the risk of pancreatic or other types of cancer are increased by drinking coffee have been discounted, and recent studies suggest it may, in fact, decrease the risk of cancer in the large bowel.

However, women should be careful not to drink too much coffee: several recent studies indicate that women who regularly drink more than three or four cups a day face a greater risk of brittle bones (osteoporosis) after the menopause and in old age.

Coffee is among the most commonly cited MIGRAINE triggers, and many people find that it causes sleeplessness if drunk too late at night.

DECAFFEINATION METHODS

People who drink decaffeinated coffee to avoid the stimulating effect of caffeine may be exposing themselves to other chemicals. Tests on organic solvents commonly used to extract caffeine have shown at least two to be animal carcinogens; one of these is no longer employed. An older, more natural but less efficient method is a water process as caffeine is soluble in water.

COLDS

TAKE PLENTY OF

- *Fruit for vitamin C*
- *Eggs, red meat and oysters for zinc*
- *Garlic and onions which may act as natural decongestants*
- *Fluids to help prevent dehydration*

The food you eat is one of the best lines of defence against catching a cold. A balanced diet that includes plenty of fresh fruit and vegetables (see BALANCING YOUR DIET) will strengthen your immune system and help you to stay free of colds.

Once caught, there is still no effective cure for the misery of the common cold. The old adage that 'a cold lasts for seven days if you treat it, and a week if you leave it alone' may still be true. However, in its 40-year search for a cure, the British Common Cold Research Unit discovered that zinc may help to shorten the duration of a cold. Zinc is now included in some over-the-counter remedies, but not all forms of the mineral seem to work. Several trials of zinc supplements have been ineffective. Good dietary sources of available zinc include liver (not to be eaten in pregnancy), red meat, eggs and, best of all, oysters.

The Research Unit also pinpointed stress as another factor involved in people's susceptibility to colds.

COLDS AND VITAMIN C

In 1970, US biochemist and Nobel prize winner Linus Pauling wrote a revolutionary book called *Vitamin C and the Common Cold*, in which he claimed that large doses of this vitamin could decrease the severity and symptoms of a cold. While there is no clinical evidence to support Pauling's claim, many people tried the vitamin remedy and found it to be effective. It can certainly do no harm to take moderate doses of a vitamin C supplement

Natural cold remedies

- Doctors recommend that you drink plenty of fluids when you have a cold – at least six to eight drinks a day – in order to combat dehydration and keep mucus on the move. Include plenty of water, and hot drinks made with the juice of a lemon and a teaspoon of honey in a glass of hot water. The lemon juice is rich in vitamin C and the honey helps to soothe a sore throat.
- A traditional hot toddy, made with lemon or orange juice, honey, a single measure of alcohol (such as whisky) and boiling water is a time-honoured cold remedy. It may not be borne out by scientific research, but it is comforting and soothing and may help you to sleep.
- Inhale steam to relieve a stuffed-up nose. Half-fill a bowl with hot water, put a towel over your head to trap the steam and inhale for a few minutes at a time. Add some eucalyptus oil to the water for an effective decongestant.
- Aromatherapy oils can be used to keep the nasal passages clear. Mix five drops of eucalyptus with grapeseed or wheatgerm oil and rub it on your chest, or add five drops to some water in a vaporiser.
- Allow your body to rest and recover when suffering from a bout of cold or flu. If you insist on carrying on as normal, you will hinder the body's cold-fighting efforts and spread the infection to other people. Taking time off at the onset of a cold will help to shorten its duration.
- When you feel well enough, take a gentle walk and get some fresh air.

over a short period if you want to try this 'cure'. At the first sign of a cold, take two to three grams of vitamin C, or the equivalent as tablets, each day, for up to seven days. However, it is important to note that very large doses of vitamin C (more than four grams per day) should not be taken over longer periods because of the likelihood of causing kidney stones. Other side effects could include headaches, sleep disturbances and stomach upsets. Furthermore, pregnant women should not take megadoses of vitamin C or indeed any other vitamin because of potential harm to the unborn child.

How you catch a cold

Colds and flu are caused by viral infections (more than 200 of them) and are highly contagious. Coughing and sneezing in a confined space can easily spread an infection, since the mucus in the nose and throat of cold sufferers is full of viruses. These viruses can survive for several hours on objects such as doorknobs and telephones, so it is a good idea to wash your hands frequently if people around you have got colds. The chances of infection are heightened by STRESS, exhaustion, chronic sickness or DEPRESSION – all of which lower resistance. Getting wet or sitting in a draught may give you a chill but cannot give you a cold.

Garlic, herbs and spices

Garlic and onions are used as nasal decongestants for CATARRH in herbal medicine, and may help to relieve cold symptoms. Garlic also has antiviral and antibacterial properties, useful in fighting illness. You can try eating plenty of both, either raw in salads or added to cooking. Other herbs and spices that may be helpful in alleviating cold symptoms include chillies, which bring on a sweat; basil, reputed to relieve the headaches associated with colds; and cloves and ginger, claimed by some naturopaths to have an expectorant action.

Feed a cold?

Doctors recommend that you let your appetite be your guide when it comes to the old wives' tale of feeding a cold. If you feel hungry, eat plenty of citrus fruits and foods that are rich in zinc.

The traditional Jewish standby of chicken soup is also worth trying. It is a good source of protein, calories and minerals and is easily digested.

When to visit a doctor

Complications are rare, but a cold may make the body more susceptible to secondary bacterial infections, such as bronchitis, earache or sinusitis. You may need treatment if you have any of the following symptoms:

- A cough that becomes painful.
- You experience facial pain.
- One or both ears become painful.
- You have problems swallowing.
- You have breathing difficulties.
- There are traces of blood in your phlegm.
- You have a high temperature that lasts for more than 48 hours.

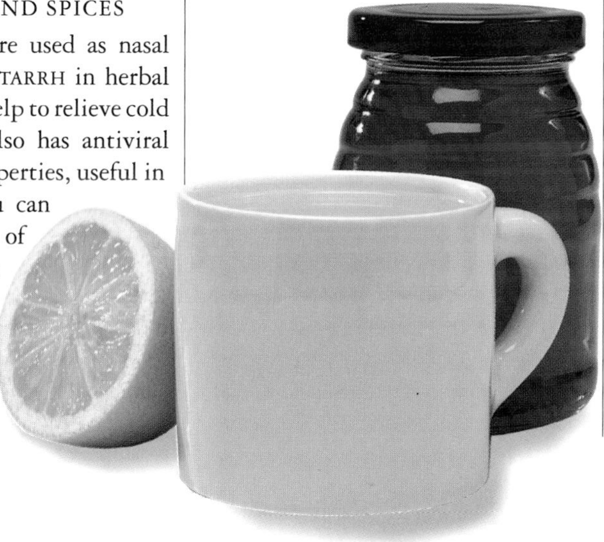

HOT TODDY *Add a measure of warming whisky to a hot honey and lemon drink.*

Colic

Babies aged between a few days and a few months often suffer from colic. It usually begins soon after birth and settles down when the baby is about three months old. Colic symptoms include sudden, severe spasms of apparent pain, which usually occur in the evening, with the baby crying loudly and continuously, frequently drawing the legs up towards the chest; the stomach is distended and tense. It may take several hours for the symptoms to abate – often after the baby passes wind or stools.

Different authorities have suggested various contributory factors, such as abdominal pain, swallowed air, underfeeding, overfeeding, intestinal allergy and even parental stress.

Colic and nutrition may be linked in some cases, according to the National Childbirth Trust (NCT) who say that some colicky babies also suffer from food intolerance. The NCT claims that, very occasionally, dairy products – especially cow's milk and cheese – eaten by a breastfeeding mother, produce colic in her baby. Other experts have blamed alcohol, caffeine and cola drinks, various fruits or spicy foods in the mother's diet, but the list is not consistent and there is no firm evidence to back these claims.

Treatment

One traditional remedy has been gripe water (a dill or fennel infusion). However, many health professionals now discourage its use; it seems that the way a baby eats may be more important. The accumulation of swallowed air in a baby's stomach is released more easily through burping if the infant feeds in a fairly upright position rather than lying down. After feeding and winding, it is suggested that the baby be laid down on the right side rather than the left so that any air still trapped in the stomach is not forced into the intestine where it may cause discomfort.

Holding a baby upright during an attack or laying the infant across your knee, or over a warm hot water bottle, while gently patting or rubbing the back, may also have a soothing effect.

COLITIS

EAT PLENTY OF

- *Fruit and cooked green leafy vegetables for soluble fibre*
- *Oily fish such as salmon, sardines and mackerel for vitamin D*
- *Foods rich in beta carotene*
- *Liver for vitamin A, unless pregnant*

AVOID

- *Bran, nuts, seeds and sweetcorn*

Although diet cannot cure colitis – more correctly known as ulcerative colitis – adjustments to the diet may help to reduce some of the symptoms to a more tolerable level. For example, a diet rich in soluble FIBRE, is recommended for people who have colitis, although foods high in insoluble fibre, such as bran, nuts, seeds and sweetcorn, are probably best avoided. This fibre may further irritate the colon, stimulate bowel contractions and so increase the likelihood of diarrhoea.

Colitis is an inflammatory disease of the colon or rectum. It affects about four to six people in 100000, and is slightly more common in women than in men. The onset of ulcerative colitis peaks between the ages of 20 and 25 years. The prognosis for sufferers depends on the severity and duration of the active disease: when the disease is active, it produces swelling, bleeding and ulceration of the lining of the colon and causes pain and urgent diarrhoea. Although some 60 per cent of sufferers have only a mild form of the disease, at least 30 per cent will require surgical removal of part or all of the colon within the first three years. And as many as 97 per cent of people who develop ulcerative colitis will have at least one relapse over a ten-year period.

Adequate nutrition is very important in colitis, especially if you are recovering from a flare-up or are reducing your intake of food in order to lessen diarrhoea. Care should therefore be taken to include adequate protein, calories, vitamins A, C, D, B_{12} and folate, calcium, iron and zinc. This means eating as wide a variety of foods as possible without exacerbating the inflammation. Eat liver once a week for extra vitamin A (except when pregnant) and orange-fleshed fruits and vegetables for beta carotene, which the body converts to vitamin A. Fresh or canned salmon, sardines and mackerel provide vitamin D. Liver, fish, pork and eggs are all good sources of B_{12}; dark green leafy vegetables supply folate and, like fruit, contain soluble

Case study

Five years ago, Jim was diagnosed as having ulcerative colitis. He had been able to keep his condition under control and stay active by eating a high-protein diet, which also supplied plenty of soluble fibre. Recently, however, he had an attack of vomiting, with abdominal pain, a high fever and severe bloody diarrhoea. Jim was taken to hospital where the doctors suspected that his deterioration could have been due to a lapse in his usual strict diet control. It turned out that they were correct: Jim, believing that he could relax because he had been free of trouble for years, had been indulging in his favourite 'fast foods' such as milk shakes, crisps, fizzy drinks and burgers, forsaking his previously prescribed diet. Unfortunately, his most recent fast-food binge proved to be the last straw. On arrival at the hospital he was pale and weak, suffering from anaemia due to blood loss through his colon – which had become inflamed. In the intensive care unit he was given high-calorie fluids and protein via a drip to correct his dehydration and two units of blood to help his anaemia. Fortunately, he responded to the treatment. When Jim left hospital, he was again put on a diet high in protein and soluble fibre, and also prescribed supplements of folic acid, vitamin B_{12} and iron. He now attends the hospital for regular check-ups to ensure that his diet provides him with all the nutrients he needs. After such a scare, Jim has vowed never to revert to his bad old eating habits that could put him back into hospital.

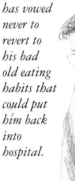

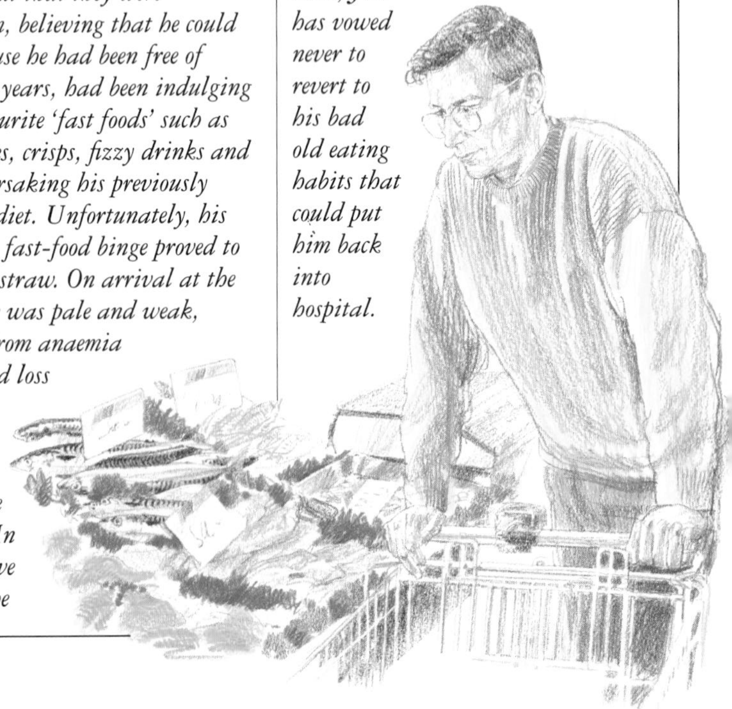

fibre; cheese and yoghurt are good sources of calcium; and zinc is found in seafood, especially oysters.

ANAEMIA is a fairly common problem with ulcerative colitis, as there is often bleeding from the area of inflammation. It is important, therefore, to eat plenty of dietary iron. The most available form of iron is in red meat, especially liver. To help the body to absorb iron from vegetables, meals should contain a good source of vitamin C such as fresh orange juice.

CONSTIPATION

TAKE PLENTY OF

- *Unpeeled fruit, green leafy vegetables, wholegrain cereals and wholemeal bread, for insoluble fibre*
- *Water – at least 1.7 litres (3 pints) a day*

CUT DOWN ON

- *Refined carbohydrates*

A diet that is low in fruit, vegetables and whole grains, coupled with a lack of physical activity, has made constipation a common problem in the West. Constipation can have serious long-term implications; regular bowel movements indicate a healthy bowel and reduce the risk of large-bowel disease, particularly cancer of the colon.

Although regular bowel movements are essential to health, many people wrongly assume that a daily bowel action is necessary and that anything less is constipation. In fact, perfectly normal bowels may empty anything from three times a day to once every three days.

There are two types of constipation. Atonic constipation is due to a lack of muscle tone. It occurs when the diet is low in fluid and FIBRE, or as the result of insufficient physical exercise. Spastic constipation is characterised by irregular bowel movements. It may be due to nervous disorders, excessive smoking, irritating foods or obstruction of the large bowel.

A diet high in refined foods and low in complex carbohydrates (such as wholemeal bread and pasta), fruit and vegetables will be deficient in fibre.

Fibre and some forms of starch are fermented in the large bowel and provide the bulk that helps to stimulate the muscles of the colon so that digested food can be pushed through the gut. Compounds in certain foods such as coffee, rhubarb and prunes also have the same effect.

If a low-fibre diet is combined with a low fluid intake – you should aim to drink at least 1.7 litres (3 pints) a day – the dense mass of digested food in the colon becomes further dehydrated, making it dry and hard and therefore more difficult to move through the system. This causes a rise in pressure in the bowel and discomfort. The longer the digested food residue remains in the bowel, the more water is reabsorbed from it, the harder it gets and the more difficult it becomes to pass.

Regular physical activity helps to stimulate bowel movements, whereas sitting still for long periods can cause constipation. Constipation may also be caused by bad toilet habits, such as not defecating when the need arises. Excessive long-term use of laxatives can also interfere with the proper function of the colon, which comes to depend on them; they should be used as infrequently as possible.

RECIPE FOR RELIEF

The average daily consumption of fibre in the United Kingdom is around 12g, while the Government advises 18g. There are two types of fibre: soluble, which helps to regulate blood sugar and blood cholesterol levels, and insoluble, which helps to prevent constipation as it works as a bulking agent

The 'bran revolution' in perspective

In 1972, a British doctor, Dr Dennis Burkitt, began to publicise his theory that constipation, caused by lack of fibre in the diet, went on to be a factor in diverticulitis – a form of colonic inflammation – and even led to cancer of the bowel. Around the same time, Commander T.L. Cleave, a surgeon, suggested that the low-fibre diet served up to seamen caused constipation – the biggest health problem in the Royal Navy – and that this could be a precursor of varicose veins and haemorrhoids.

As a result of all the publicity, bran became increasingly popular, and by the 1980s it had become almost an obsession with some people. Unfortunately, excessive consumption of bran can cause problems, such as abdominal bloating and flatulence. And bran contains a substance called phytic acid which inhibits the body's absorption of certain minerals, especially iron, to the extent that large intakes of bran can contribute to anaemia.

Women at risk of osteoporosis should also be wary of eating too much bran, as it may impede the uptake of dietary calcium. Finally, researchers in Manchester found that more than half of patients with irritable bowel syndrome actually felt worse after eating bran.

Wheat bran is insoluble fibre, colloquially known as roughage. This type of fibre is also found in fruit and vegetable peels. But oat bran, like fruit and vegetable pectin, is a soluble fibre – a type of fibre that lowers blood cholesterol levels.

in the gut. It is best to eat foods that are naturally high in fibre rather than processed foods that have an artificially high fibre content. Avoid the side effects of a sudden increase in dietary fibre by gradually adding it to your diet. Begin by increasing your fluid consumption; aim for at least 1.7 litres (3 pints) a day – more in hot weather. If you are used to eating only white bread, start by taking half your bread as wholemeal, and eat porridge or muesli in the morning.

Add two teaspoons of BRAN to a small tub of live yoghurt or to your cereal each day for a week, increasing it to three teaspoons in the second week, by which time you can replace the rest of your white bread intake with wholemeal. There may be some discomfort in the form of wind and bloating at first, particularly once you add 100g (3½oz) of dried fruit to your daily diet and extra fresh fruit, cooked green leafy vegetables and salads.

The optimum amount of fibre varies from one individual to another, and you should try to determine just how much your body seems to be happiest with. In any event, do not rely solely on bran to provide all the fibre you need. It can have a harsh effect over prolonged periods. Consult a doctor if constipation is prolonged or if there is abdominal pain.

TOO MUCH OF A GOOD THING

In 1990, the *Journal of the American Medical Association* reported on a man who, on his doctor's advice, ate a bowl of bran every morning to relieve his constipation. Ten days later he had to undergo major surgery for the removal of a clump of bran that had completely blocked his gut. The man had been taking diuretics, and not drinking enough fluids. This unusual episode highlights the dangers of eating too much bran, and the importance of having an adequate fluid intake.

CONVALESCING DIET

A proper period of convalescence – a quiet time to recover after illness – was once considered an essential part of medical treatment. The pressures of modern life often conflict with the body's natural need to recuperate, but resuming a normal routine too soon after surgery or a bout of flu can delay full recovery for several weeks.

Use your common sense when deciding on the amount of rest you need. Be kind to yourself but do not be overly cautious; a positive attitude can do wonders for speeding up the recovery process. Modern research suggests that patients should get up and walk about as soon as possible. Prolonged bed rest causes calcium to be lost from the skeleton and can also increase the risk of thrombosis.

STOCK UP ON GOODNESS

In general, a convalescing diet should always be nutrient-rich, appetising, easy to eat and readily digestible. Essential nutritional elements are plenty of vitamin C and zinc to help any wounds to heal and iron to ensure a healthy level of oxygen-carrying haemoglobin in the bloodstream.

Choose a diet that includes plenty of fruit, vegetables and starchy carbohydrate foods, with fish, poultry and dairy produce to provide easily digestible protein. And try to eat foods that will give your immune system the best chance of making a quick recovery and fighting off any secondary infections. The precise diet required depends upon the type of illness from which you are recovering. For example, if you have undergone major abdominal surgery it is best to avoid high-fibre foods as these can cause bloating and can irritate scar tissue. Many people suffer loss of appetite during or after illness, so attractive presentation of food in appropriate sized servings is especially important in helping a convalescent back to full health. There is nothing more off-putting than being presented with a mountain of food when you only feel like eating a mouthful or two.

EATING FOR FITNESS

Malnutrition regularly causes complications in hip fracture cases, and can almost double the number of days in hospital. Post-operative recovery is delayed by pressure sores and poor wound healing due to an inadequate intake of vitamin C. Even fit elderly people can recover from infections more quickly through modest levels of vitamin and mineral supplements.

People who have been ill or who have undergone surgery tend to have different requirements to those who are well. Because feeling ill often suppresses the appetite, it may be sensible to eat numerous small meals rather than trying to adopt a more conventional eating pattern. The body needs concentrated nutrients to fuel its recovery, so the conventional wisdom of eating a high-fibre, low-fat diet that applies to healthy people is inappropriate for many convalescents, and

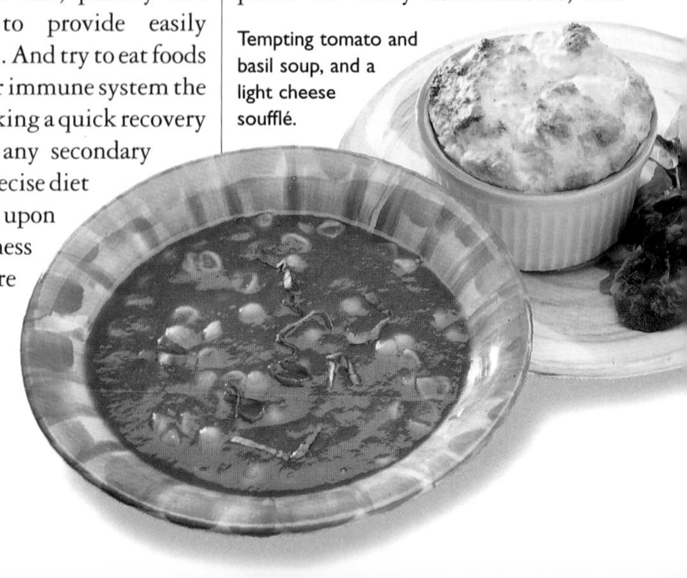

Tempting tomato and basil soup, and a light cheese soufflé.

may even delay recovery. For example, a diet high in fibre and carbohydrates may be so filling that the convalescent is not able to eat enough to supply all the necessary nutrients. Generally, if patients feel like eating something, it is usually sensible to give it to them.

WHAT TO CHOOSE

A week of convalescent meals might include the following:

- Breakfasts – porridge made with whole milk; full-fat yoghurt served with honey or soaked dried fruits; croissants; poached eggs on toast.
- Lunches – fish in a white sauce, or meat with gravy; cheese dishes such as soufflé or macaroni cheese; chicken with herbs. Eat plenty of vegetables, and also include a starchy food such as pasta, rice, bread or potatoes. Alternatively, choose a hearty soup for your main course. Desserts such as yoghurts and baked custards are light yet nourishing.
- Suppers – choose lighter meals in the evenings: salads, soups made with root vegetables, fruit salads, and warm milky drinks to help you sleep.
- Snacks – fresh fruit; dried fruit; fresh nuts and seeds; half a sandwich and a glass of milk.

ROAD TO RECOVERY *Meals for convalescents should both look and taste appealing, without being dauntingly large.*

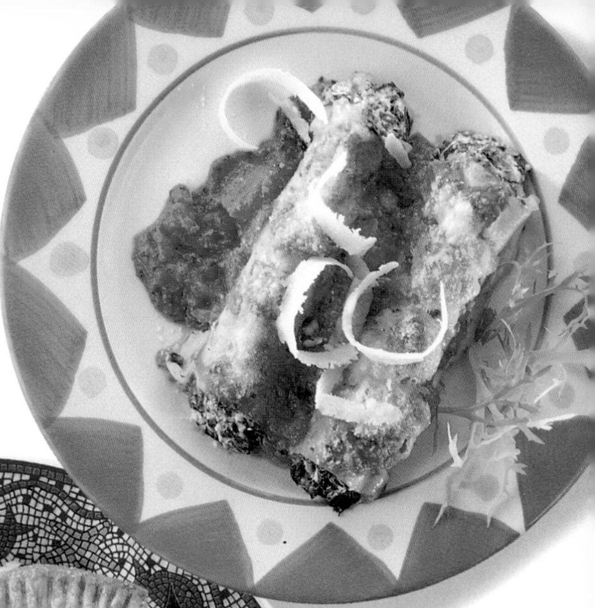

Cannelloni with a delicate spinach and ricotta filling and fresh tomato sauce provides a nutritious vegetarian meal.

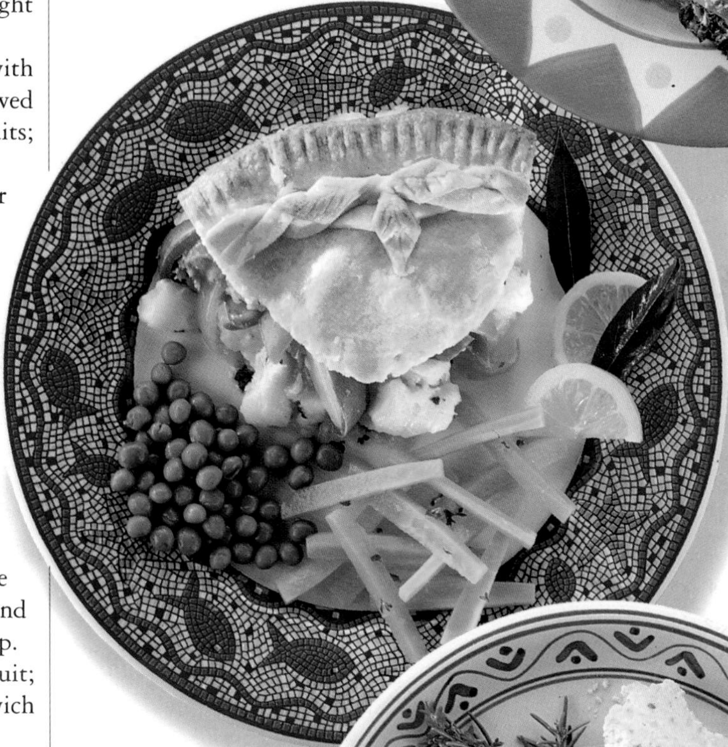

Chunky fish pie topped with light shortcrust pastry and served with fresh vegetables is a tempting meal to help speed recovery.

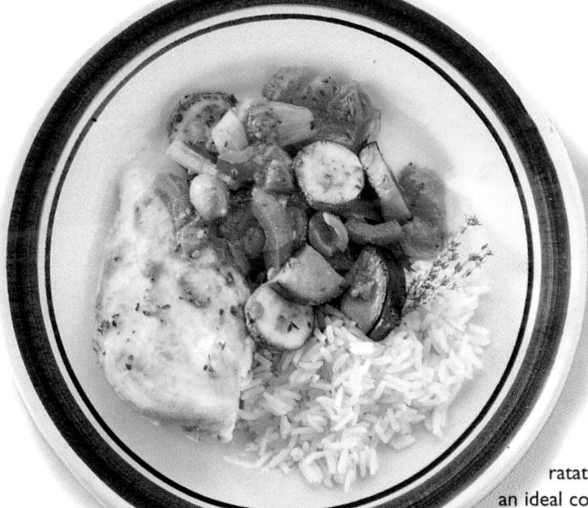

Fragrant chicken provençal with ratatouille and rice is an ideal convalescent meal.

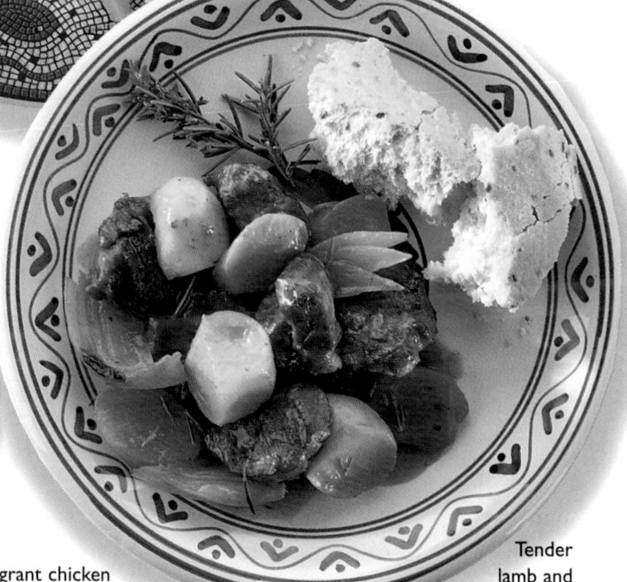

Tender lamb and warming winter vegetable casserole is served with nutritious granary bread.

CONVENIENCE AND FAST FOODS

A diet consisting solely of convenience and fast foods is unlikely to be healthy. But with a little care you can enjoy regular takeaways and still achieve a healthy balance of nutrients.

Technological advances have dramatically increased the quality and range of convenience meals that are now available. Vacuum packed or frozen precooked meals ready for the microwave, packets of soup, cake, dessert and sauce mix, instant mashed potato and frozen fish fingers are just a few of the time-saving foods that many people now rely on.

Although pre-prepared meals save time, they do not always measure up nutritionally to fresh HOME COOKING. This is because each time they are heated they lose some of their vitamins, and many 'heat-and-eat' meals have already been cooked before they are reheated – resulting in further nutrient losses. Convenience foods also tend to contain more sugar, salt and fat than most other foods.

However, there are increasing numbers of 'healthy' or calorie-counted meals, usually identified with healthy eating symbols, the word 'lite', or the manufacturer's own brand name for their low-calorie products. Some labels claim 'reduced' or 'controlled' sodium, but these may still contain considerable amounts of salt.

'JUNK' FOOD?

'Junk' food is a blanket term used to describe a vast range of convenience foods, from instant desserts and sweets to burgers and chips, fizzy drinks and instant noodles. Public opinion is mixed. At one extreme, there are people who believe these foods are almost poisonous and, at the other, there are those who live on them. Junk foods are undeniably unhealthy if they are eaten to the exclusion of all else. Diets that are based on convenience and fast foods can be deficient in vitamin C, iron, folate and riboflavin; low in fibre; and high in calories, fat and sodium.

So whether you enjoy frozen pizza or ready-made lasagne, try to redress the balance by adding some vegetables, salad or fruit.

THE PRICE OF CONVENIENCE

A meal in a packet is a useful standby, especially in families who like to eat different things at different times, and for people who work late. It is often cheaper than a takeaway and a convenient alternative to cooking from scratch – and it saves on washing up. International dishes are now widely available, with Italian and Indian meals topping the popularity list.

The 'healthy' versions of most dishes – whether lasagne, curry, or cauliflower cheese – are more expensive than their standard equivalents, but may be worth choosing if they are lower in fat, particularly saturated fat, and lower in calories. However, the levels of fibre and sodium in the standard and 'lite' varieties of most ready meals are usually similar, and in some cases they may even be higher in the 'lite' versions. Unfortunately, there is often a price tag for convenience: ready meals can cost significantly more than the homemade alternative. Although some ready-made foods are sold as 'complete' meals, they are rarely a good source of vegetables or starchy foods. It is a good idea, therefore, to add extra vegetables or a salad along with a starchy food, such as brown rice or a wholemeal roll.

SAFETY FIRST

Although food manufacturers and retailers have improved hygiene and food safety at many stages of the food chain, precooked foods found in chill cabinets may still be a source of FOOD POISONING, caused mainly by listeria and salmonella. Consumers need to store and cook these foods carefully, to prevent proliferation of bacteria. This means bringing food home as soon as possible after purchase, not letting it get too warm, and storing it in a refrigerator or freezer; checking and adhering to use-by dates; following microwaving guidelines carefully – being sure to observe standing times; and making sure that food is piping hot throughout before eating.

MEALS FOR CHILDREN

Many convenience foods are specifically aimed at children. Typical 'economy' fish fingers are usually made with minced fish pieces, shaped and coated in breadcrumbs then dyed with natural colours such as annatto and turmeric. Although highly processed, these are a nutritious and safe way of feeding fish to children.

Instant pudding mixes are often regarded as a good way to get children to take milk, because the majority come in powdered form and are reconstituted with milk. But a typical list of ingredients in a packet of instant

How to balance convenience or fast foods with other meals

The trouble with many fast foods is that they tend to be high in fat, salt or sugar, or all three, and often do not provide a balanced meal. The pros and cons of some popular meals are discussed in this table, and the 'healthy balance' column suggests a suitable second meal for that day which will compensate for any nutritional deficiencies or excesses.

ADVANTAGES	DISADVANTAGES	HEALTHY BALANCE
FISH AND CHIPS		
This meal is a good source of vitamins B_6 and B_{12}; high in protein and carbohydrate; contains some calcium, phosphorus, manganese, iron, thiamin and potassium. 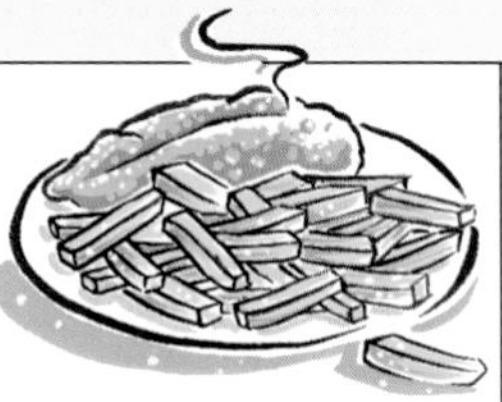	High in fat but low in fibre; low in vitamins A, C, D, folate and beta carotene. Depending on the portion size, the meal contains between a third and a half of the recommended daily amount of fat.	Salad made with lettuce, tomatoes, onion, feta cheese, olive oil and lemon juice: this is low in calories but contains vitamins C, E, folate and beta carotene.
SANDWICH AND AN APPLE		
This depends on the type of bread, the filling, and the amount of filling used. Tuna and lettuce on wholemeal bread, and an apple with its skin, offers a balanced meal, with some useful fibre. 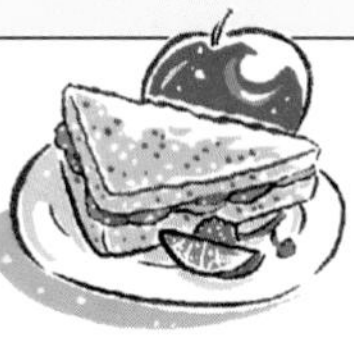	Again, this depends on the filling; a prawn and mayonnaise sandwich on buttered bread has double the calories and three times the fat of the tuna salad version.	Beef stew with mashed potatoes and carrots: high in protein and beta carotene. The beef is also a good source of B vitamins, iron, potassium and zinc.
PIZZA		
Depends on the topping. High in carbohydrate; a wholemeal base increases fibre. A cheese and tomato topping provides protein, vitamin E, calcium and phosphorus. 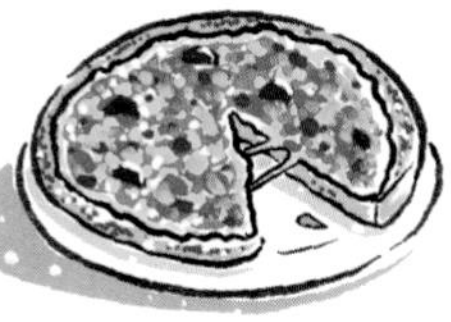	Often high in fat and low in protein; sometimes high in sodium; if topped with blue cheese, salami, pepperoni or ham, the fat level is increased and the salt can be as much as doubled.	Chicken and vegetable casserole: high protein from chicken, beta carotene from carrots; fibre and vitamin C from vegetables.
DONER KEBAB IN PITTA		
Good protein, iron and zinc; a balanced meal containing folate, vitamin C and beta carotene if plenty of salad is incorporated in pitta. 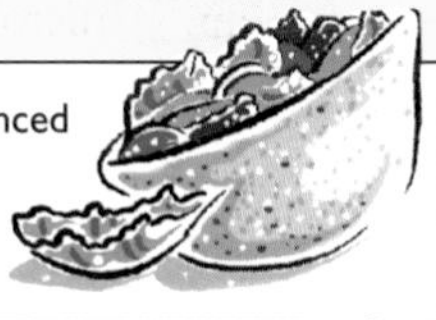	Often fatty, as outlets may use cheap cuts of high-fat lamb; low in fibre, vitamin A, D, E and folate. A possible food-poisoning risk.	Kedgeree made with brown rice, and a green salad: this is a low-fat meal providing moderate protein, good fibre and vitamins B and C.
BEEFBURGER, CHIPS AND MILK SHAKE		
High in protein, carbohydrates and calcium; contains vitamin A, phosphorus, vitamin B_{12} and riboflavin. 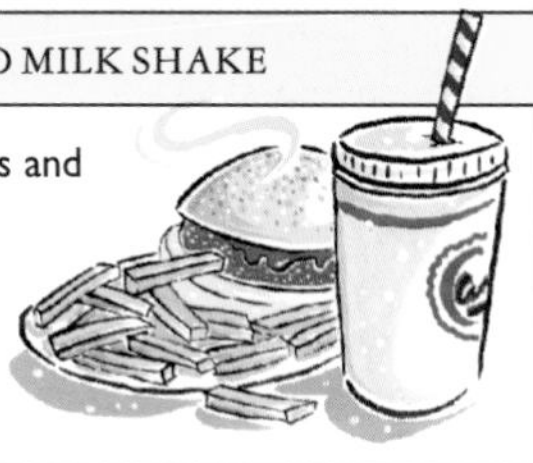	High in fat, especially saturated fat; high in cholesterol, sodium and possibly artificial colours and flavourings; low in fibre and vitamin C.	Wholemeal pasta salad with a selection of raw or lightly steamed fresh vegetables: pasta provides fibre; vegetables supply vitamin C and beta carotene; broccoli is a source of iron.
HEAT-AND-EAT CHICKEN CURRY AND RICE		
High in protein, high in carbohydrates; source of B vitamins, phosphorus and zinc. 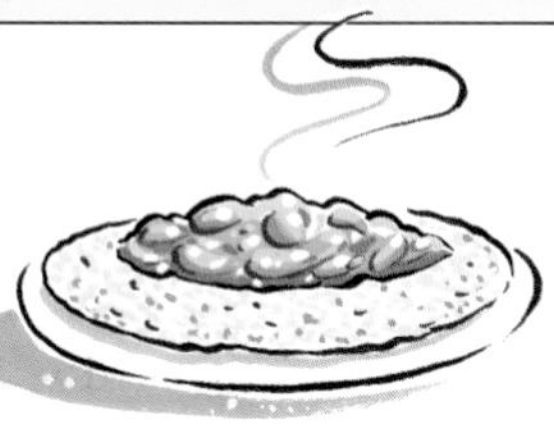	High in calories and probably fat; low in vitamin C due to lack of vegetables; low in dietary fibre; high in sodium.	Herb omelette with wholemeal bread and tomato and watercress salad: this meal is low in calories and a moderate source of fibre; it provides protein, beta carotene, vitamins A, C, and D, as well as B vitamins.

dessert includes sugar, modified starch, hydrogenated vegetable oil, emulsifiers (propylene glycol monostearate, lecithin), gelling agents (disodium monophosphate, sodium pyrophosphate), lactose, flavourings, whey powder, caseinate and colours (carmine, annatto). These puddings also tend to be high in saturated fat: yoghurt and fresh fruit would be a nutritious and convenient alternative.

THE ADDITIVE FACTOR

Instant packet soup is very different from homemade soup because it is made of a blend of dry constituents. It may contain some of the labelled flavour (beef, chicken or tomato, for example), but most of the ingredients – which include maltodextrin, hydrogenated vegetable oil, monosodium glutamate (MSG), sugar, emulsifiers, stabilisers, flavourings and colour – would rarely, if ever, be added to a homemade broth.

Although ADDITIVES are often viewed with suspicion, they have their plus points too: their presence is often vital if food is not to spoil, and many enhance its taste, texture or colour. All additives undergo rigorous safety checks, and allergic reactions are very rare – only about one person in 2000 is known to have an adverse reaction to additives. Adverse reactions to everyday foods such as eggs, milk, wheat, nuts and shellfish are much more common. Indeed, many experts place food additives quite far down the list of potential food hazards.

FAST FOODS

Fast food may be defined as any food you take away, which is ready to eat, whether a hot meal, such as a beefburger and chips, or a ready-made chicken salad sandwich and a doughnut. Fast food is more varied and of a higher quality than it was ten years ago. Nevertheless, a typical fast-food meal of cheeseburger and chips with apple pie and a large cola contains between 1100 and 1200 Calories. This amounts to 60 per cent of the recommended daily calorie intake for the average seven to ten-year-old, with many of these calories coming from saturated fats and sugar. The cola alone, apart from its caffeine and colouring, contains more than eight teaspoons of sugar. Although such a meal is rich in many nutrients, it tends to be low in others. A diet based on fast foods is not a recipe for good health – it will probably not supply enough vitamin A, C, D or E, or sufficient amounts of trace minerals and fibre.

One of the problems with fast foods is that they 'crowd out' fresh fruits and vegetables. They tend to be high in fats (mainly saturated fats), sodium or sugar, and low in fibre. Consequently, eating fast food to the exclusion of nutritious alternatives that would balance the diet increases the risk of OBESITY and related disorders such as heart disease and cancer.

Some takeaway meals may be cooked well in advance of their sale and kept warm for many hours. This increases the risk of bacterial proliferation and consequent food poisoning.

A GROWING MARKET

The fast-food industry is growing rapidly: McDonald's, the world's largest hamburger chain, serves at least 13000 customers a minute, or more than 98 million every week. This is not surprising, since fast foods are usually so affordable and convenient. They appeal to all ages, and most chains offer menus created specifically for children. A survey has found that more than 40 per cent of 16 to 18-year-olds buy takeaway food at least once a week, with hamburger and chips being the most popular order.

For most people, fast-food outlets still supply only a small percentage of their weekly food intake. And there is no need to worry about eating fast food from time to time.

GOOD AND BAD NEWS ON FAST FOODS

Unlike packaged foods with their comprehensive labels, fast-food outlets do not have to list the ingredients used or their quantities, although

HOMEMADE FAST FOOD *There are many dishes that can be prepared at home in the same time that it takes to heat a 'convenience' meal, or to go to a Chinese or Indian takeaway, for example, and pick up a ready-to-eat meal.*

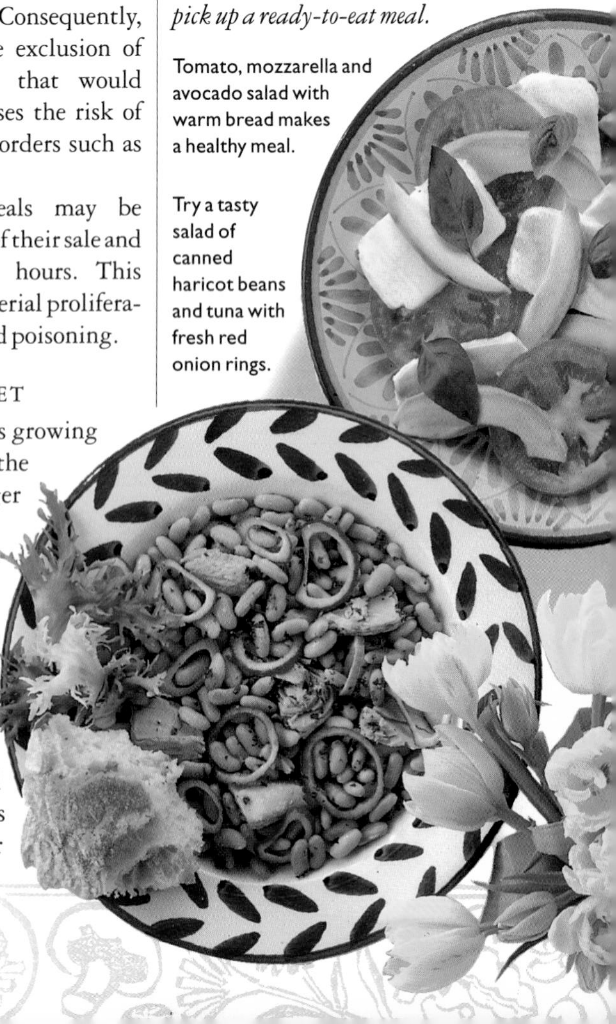

Tomato, mozzarella and avocado salad with warm bread makes a healthy meal.

Try a tasty salad of canned haricot beans and tuna with fresh red onion rings.

some chains will now give you comprehensive information sheets if you ask for them. The quality of fast foods has improved greatly over the past decade. Many outlets have responded to criticism and decreased the calorie, fat and sodium content of their foods, and several now fry in vegetable oil rather than animal fats.

In any case, chips are not inherently unhealthy: they are a good source of potassium and contain some vitamin C. What should be avoided, if possible, are chips cooked in animal fats or hydrogenated fats. Thick-cut chips are healthier than thin or crinkle-cut ones, because they contain less fat: when thick chips are cooked, they have a smaller surface area, relative to their weight, through which to absorb fat. Fresh fried fish from fish-and-chip shops is an excellent source of protein; if the oil is really hot, the batter absorbs little fat – but weight-watchers can always discard the batter.

The same goes for fried chicken, when the high fat content can be substantially reduced by discarding any skin or breadcrumb coating. In the USA, many fast-food outlets offer skinless versions and 'non-fried' chicken; however, this is roasted, and is often still high in fat.

Pizza may be comparatively higher in carbohydrate and lower in fat than traditional fried fast food – but it still contains high fat levels. Pitta bread stuffed with salad and felafel (small deep-fried chickpea balls) is a healthy alternative. And a baked potato with tuna and salad filling makes a balanced meal.

WHAT TO CHOOSE IN THE BURGER BAR

By choosing foods carefully from fast-food menus, you can select a reasonably well-balanced meal, while limiting your intake of some of the more harmful ingredients.

- Choose small plain burgers as opposed to giant burgers with all the trimmings.
- Skip the mayonnaise and melted cheese. By leaving them out, you can save nearly 200 Calories on a king-sized burger and reduce your fat intake.
- Order milk instead of a milk shake, or a low-calorie soft drink instead of a conventional one.
- Choose a smaller portion of french fries and have a side salad.
- Don't be persuaded to eat larger helpings than you really need.

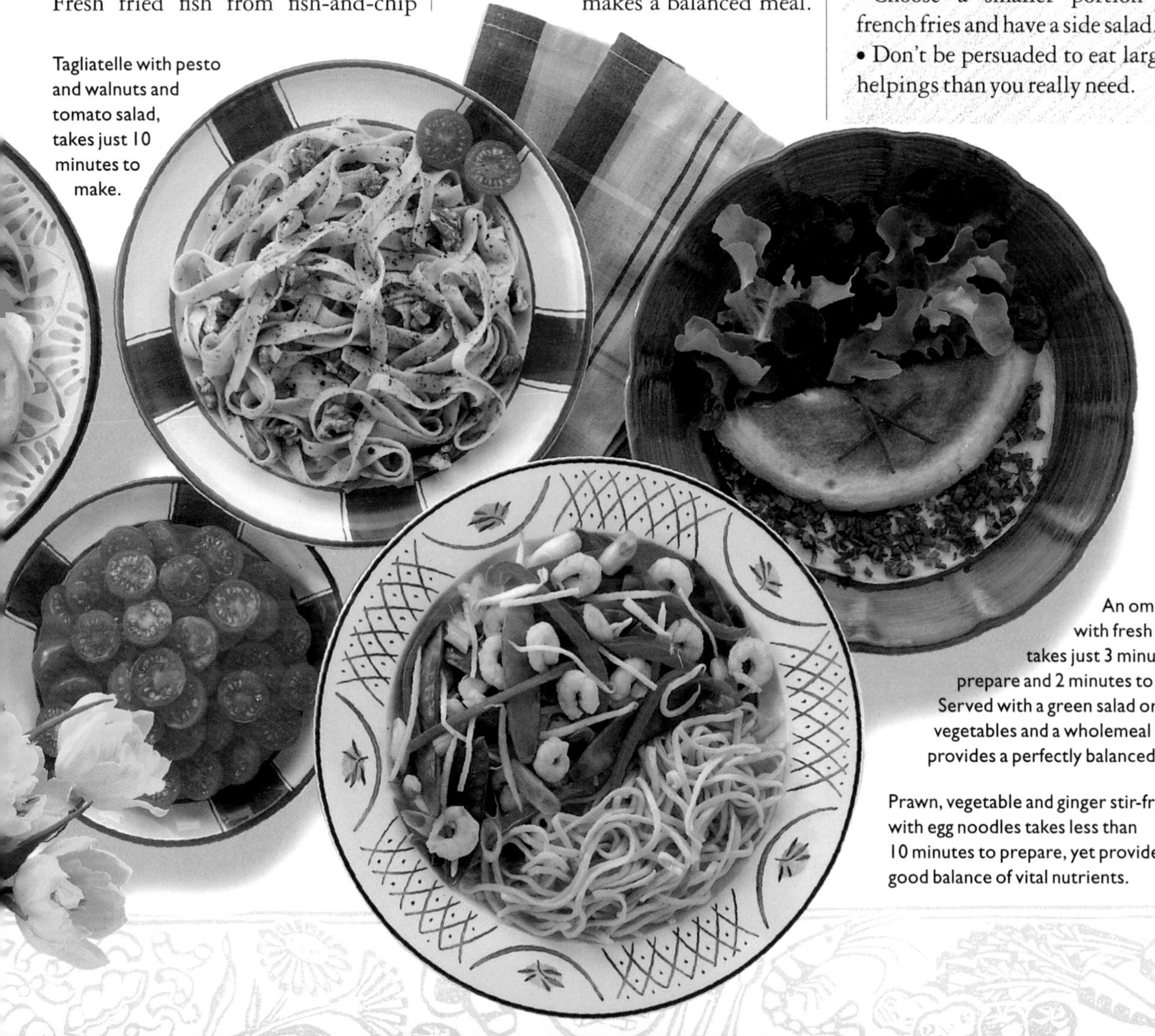

Tagliatelle with pesto and walnuts and tomato salad, takes just 10 minutes to make.

An omelette with fresh herbs takes just 3 minutes to prepare and 2 minutes to cook. Served with a green salad or fresh vegetables and a wholemeal roll, it provides a perfectly balanced meal.

Prawn, vegetable and ginger stir-fry with egg noodles takes less than 10 minutes to prepare, yet provides a good balance of vital nutrients.

COT DEATH

Cot death, also known as Sudden Infant Death Syndrome, has been the subject of intense research in recent years. No definitive cause has been identified. There are almost twice as many cot deaths in winter than in summer and it is the most common cause of death in babies between one week and one year old.

Diet is among the many factors being examined in a bid to find out what makes some babies susceptible, although smoking by mothers appears to pose the main threat.

VITAMIN C AND SMOKING

Infants who are deficient in vitamin C may be more susceptible to respiratory infections; such infections are also more prevalent in winter when the body's vitamin C levels may be lower. It is known that women smokers have lower blood levels of vitamin C than non-smokers and the same may be true of babies who inhale their parents' cigarette smoke. However, a more direct link with smoking has been established. Several studies have shown that the babies of mothers who smoke during pregnancy run a higher risk of cot death.

Other studies have suggested that marginal deficiencies of selenium and biotin may be involved in cot death.

Non-dietary factors linked with cot deaths include the baby's sleeping position. Parents are now advised to lay babies on their backs rather than on their stomachs. The incidence of cot death has fallen markedly since this advice was given. It is also suggested that babies' bedrooms are kept warm rather than hot – between 16°C and 20°C (61°F and 68°F) and that to prevent infants from wriggling down under the covers and getting overheated, their feet should be almost touching the end of the cot.

COUNTRYSIDE FOODS

See page 118

COURGETTES (ZUCCHINI)

BENEFITS

- *Low in calories*
- *Good source of beta carotene*
- *Useful source of vitamin C and folate*

Courgettes, a type of small young marrow, have tender edible skins and this is where most of the nutrients are found. A 100g (3½oz) portion of lightly boiled courgettes provides over a quarter of the vitamin C and a sixth of the folate an adult needs each day, while containing only 19 Calories. (The same amount, shallow-fried, provides around 63 Calories.) Courgettes also supply beta carotene which the body converts to vitamin A.

Orangey-yellow courgette flowers can be served raw, in salads, or hot – stuffed with finely chopped vegetables.

CRAMP

TAKE PLENTY OF

- *Water before, during and after exercise to prevent dehydration*
- *Foods rich in calcium, such as dairy products and sardines*
- *Nuts and seeds for magnesium*
- *Sources of riboflavin (vitamin B_2) such as fortified breakfast cereals and yoghurt*
- *Avocados and vegetable oils for vitamin E and fish or eggs for vitamin B_{12} if the problem is night cramps*

A prolonged, painful and involuntary contraction of a muscle is known as cramp. Any muscle can be affected, but these spasms commonly occur in the calf or the foot. The best way to alleviate the problem is with massage and stretching; however, nutrition is possibly the most effective way to prevent cramp occurring.

CRAMPING YOUR STYLE

When cramp occurs during or immediately after exercise, it is likely to be the result of a gradual build-up of lactic acid, which is a by-product of muscle activity. If the exercise has been fairly vigorous and the weather very hot or humid, the cramp may be due to dehydration caused by excessive sweating. An isotonic drink will help to replace lost fluids and salts as quickly as possible.

To prevent dehydration, drink plenty of water before, during and after exercise – about 1 litre (1¾ pints) per hour of activity. Salt tablets are unnecessary, except in the tropics. Vitamin B_2, found in fortified breakfast cereals, yoghurt and lean meat, may be useful for cramps in athletes, as well as for cramp associated with pregnancy and diabetes.

Leg cramps may signal a lack of calcium, needed for muscle contraction. Foods high in calcium are dairy products, sesame seeds and sardines eaten with their bones. Magnesium, too, may be helpful – seeds and nuts are excellent sources. Calf pains experienced during a brisk walk may be due to narrowing of the arteries.

NIGHT CRAMPS

Eating foods high in vitamin E may help to improve the poor circulation that can cause night cramps. Night cramps in the elderly may also be helped by vitamin B_{12}, found in foods such as fish, eggs, cheese and pork.

A DIFFERENCE OF COLOUR *Weight for weight, yellow and green courgettes both provide similar amounts of nutrients.*

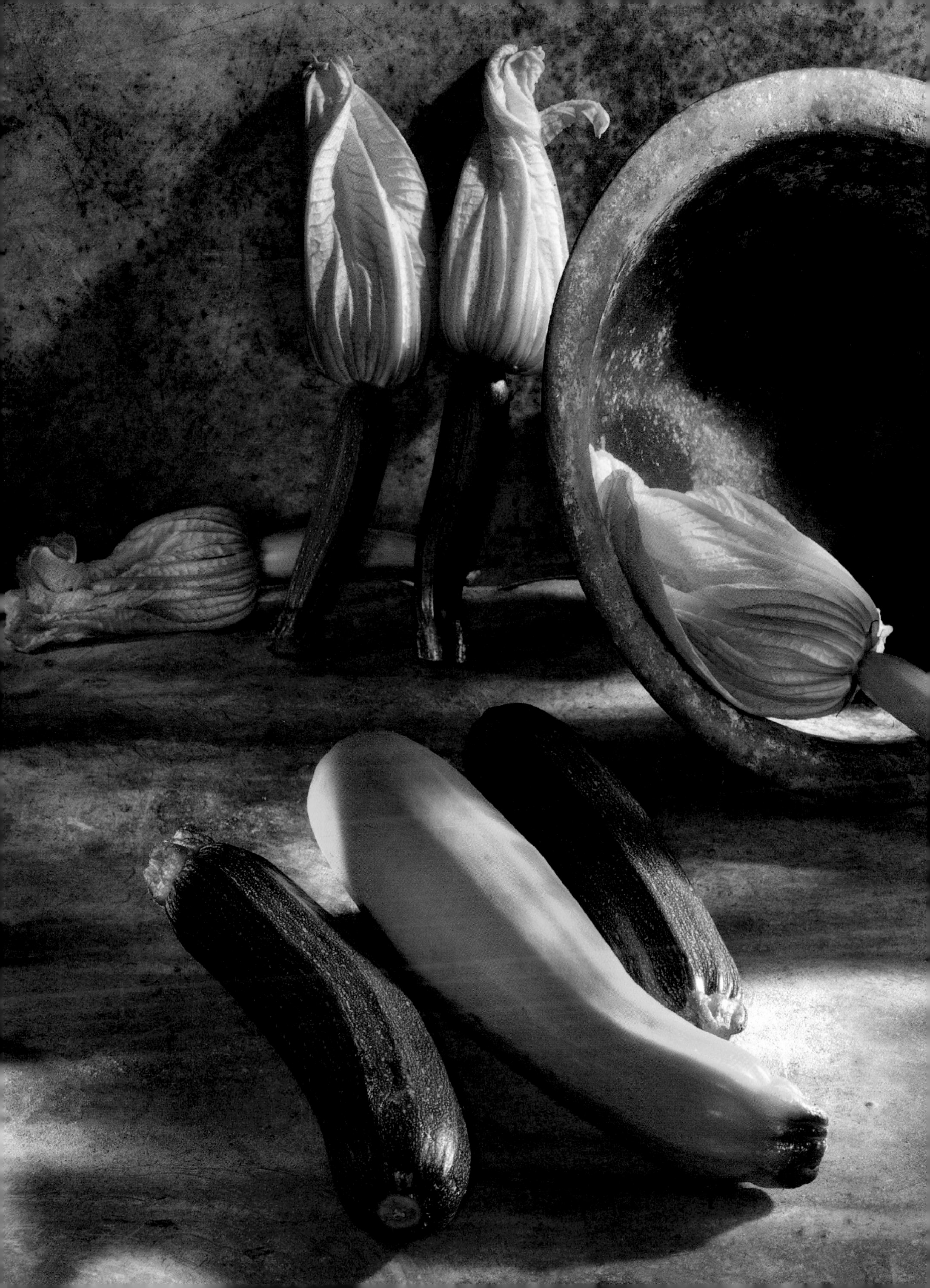

FOODS FROM THE COUNTRYSIDE

For centuries, people have gathered foods from the wild, both for nourishment and to use as natural medication – to treat ailments from rheumatism to influenza, and eczema to cystitis.

The British countryside offers a wealth of delicious – and free – foods. From moors and meadows to hedgerows, woodland or seaside, each habitat has its own unique larder.

HEDGEROW

Hedgerows are a rich hunting ground for wild berries, fungi and salad leaves.

Blackberries ripen from late August until early October. Avoid fruits growing beside busy roads and, wherever you pick from, wash the fruit before eating it. Blackberries supply useful quantities of dietary fibre, vitamin C and manganese, while in herbal medicine blackberry leaf tea is used as a tonic for dysentery and diarrhoea, and as a gargle for sore throats.

Dandelions, found throughout the countryside, are available almost all year round. The fresh young leaves have a slightly bitter flavour and are an enlivening addition to any salad. They contain beta carotene, calcium, potassium and one-and-a-half times as much iron as the same quantity of spinach. Dandelion is a natural diuretic, hence the colloquial name wet-the-bed in parts of England and *pissenlit* in France. However, unlike many diuretics, dandelion does not cause potassium depletion, because its own high potassium content is enough to replace any excreted in urine. In natural medicine, dandelion is prescribed to cleanse the blood and to treat skin disorders such as eczema.

Giant puffballs look like enormous white eggs, and can grow as large as footballs. The whole fungus is edible as long as the flesh is pure white throughout, which indicates freshness. Slice the puffball into large 'steaks' and fry in butter; smaller ones may be toasted like marshmallows.

Goose grass (or cleavers) is eaten young as an alternative to spinach in soups. In herbal medicine, it is used as an anti-inflammatory and as a diuretic. An infusion, made by pouring boiling water onto the leaves and straining after 10 minutes, can be used as a tonic for tonsillitis and adenoid problems.

Hazelnuts are ready for picking in late September. Keep them in their

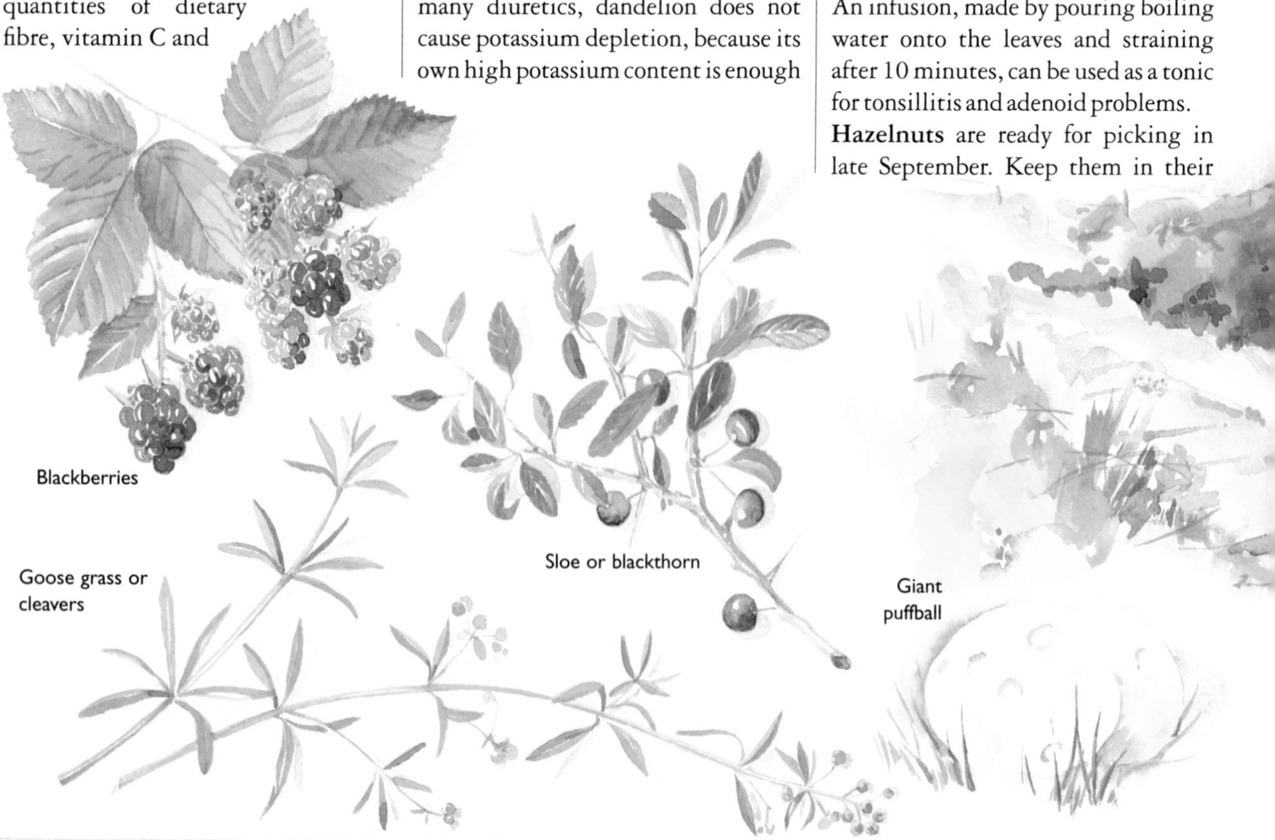

shells until you are ready to eat them, so as to prevent them from drying out.

Sloe (or blackthorn) berries are dark blue, with a dusty bloom. They are small and bitter and grow on the spiny blackthorn bush. Pick sloe berries in late autumn and use them to make a clear jelly to accompany meat, or add them to gin to make sloe gin.

Stinging nettles lose their sting when they are cooked. They contain beta carotene, vitamin C, calcium, iron and potassium. Nettles, like dandelions, are a natural diuretic. In herbal medicine, the juice of the leaves is mixed with honey and used to treat asthmatic complaints. A soup or tea made with nettle leaves is believed to help eczema sufferers, and nettle leaves are also used to treat rheumatic and arthritic conditions. In summer, a fresh bunch of nettles hung in a larder will help to keep it free of flies. Pick young, pale green nettle tops in spring, because by June they become coarse and bitter. To avoid being stung, wear gloves when picking and preparing the nettles. Do not pick from roadside verges where the soil may be polluted or the plants themselves might have been sprayed with herbicides. Rinse the nettles and discard any tough stalks before steaming or boiling; they have a slightly acidic flavour, and are traditionally used as an alternative to spinach in soups or quiches.

Wild rose (or dog rose) blooms adorn the hedgerows in early summer. The small orange-red rosehips usually appear between late August and October. Weight for weight, rosehips contain eight times as much vitamin C as oranges, with 100 g (3½ oz) supplying seven times an adult's daily requirement. In the form of rosehip syrup, they became an important source of vitamin C for British children during the Second World War when citrus fruit were often impossible to find. Rosehips contain tiny seeds covered in spiky hairs which can irritate the digestive tract, so the stewed fruit should be sieved before it is used in cooking.

Poisonous berries

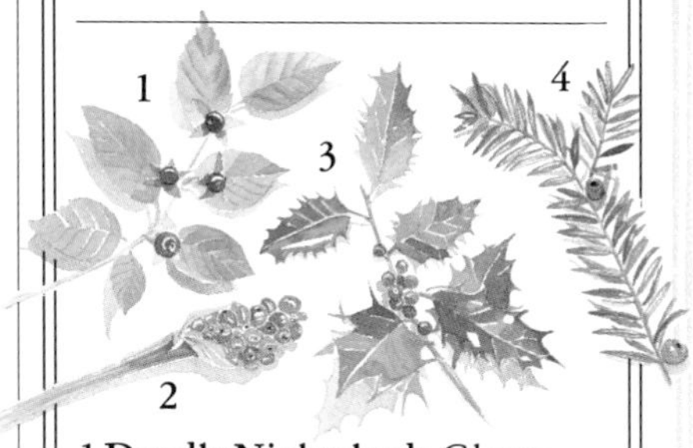

1 Deadly Nightshade Glossy black berries in August. Just two or three are enough to kill a child.

2 Cuckoo Pint (Lords and Ladies) In spring, the clusters of highly poisonous orange-red berries appear on a 30 cm (12 in) stalk.

3 Holly Bright red poisonous berries appear in late autumn and remain on the tree until February.

4 Yew All parts of the yew tree are poisonous, especially the seed, hidden inside the slimy red berry.

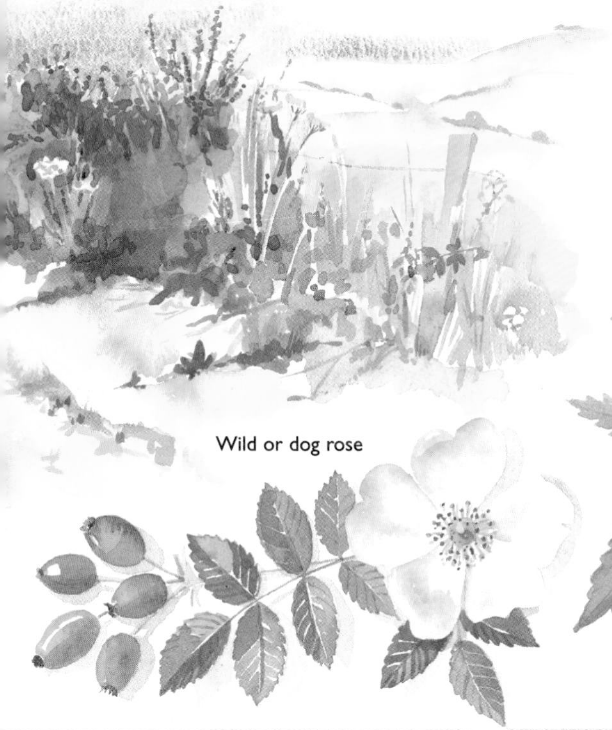

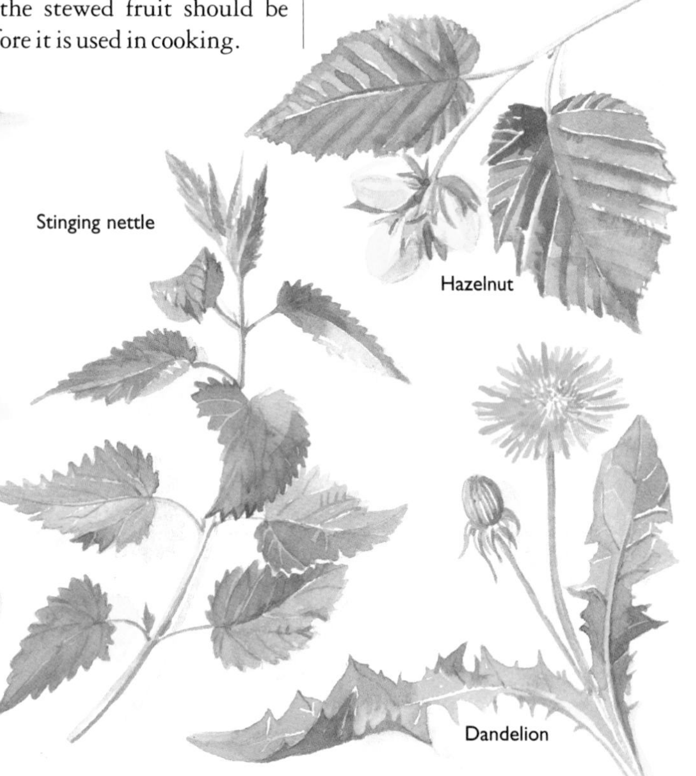

WOODLAND

Deciduous woods, especially beech, provide a good environment for summer leaves and autumn fungi.

Chickweed is easily identified by its tiny, white, star-shaped flowers. The bright green stems and oval leaves can be cooked as a vegetable. Herbalists prescribe chickweed tea to treat rheumatism, while in traditional medicine, a poultice of chickweed was applied to soothe wounds and help to heal skin disorders such as eczema.

Crab apples are sour yellow-green (sometimes turning red) fruits, about the size of gooseberries, which may be picked from August to November. They contain potassium and vitamin C and make one of the best jellies of all wild fruits.

Elder flowers and berries have long been used in folk medicine as remedies for colds, flu and other respiratory ailments; they are also mildly laxative. The cream-coloured flowers are picked in May to make cordials and wine. In autumn, the tiny black-purple berries – rich in beta carotene and vitamin C – can be made into jelly or boiled with sugar and strained to make a soothing linctus for sore throats and coughs.

Horseradish is a large white tap root supporting large dark green crinkly leaves. It is peeled and grated to make horseradish sauce, but be sure to peel the root under a running tap and grate it in the open air, or the pungent fumes will burn your eyes. In herbal medicine, horseradish is used to stimulate the circulation and help the digestion. It contains a very antiseptic volatile oil which is partially excreted through the urinary tract, so it may also help to treat infections such as cystitis.

Rowan (or mountain ash) trees grow in dry woodlands and upland areas. The clusters of brilliant orange-red berries, which appear in autumn, make a sharp-tasting jelly. In herbal medicine, the fruit forms the basis of an astringent gargle for sore throats, and in the 19th century, rowan berries were used to treat scurvy, the disease of vitamin C deficiency.

Sweet chestnuts ripen and fall in late October. They are low in protein and fat, and high in carbohydrates and fibre. CHESTNUTS can be eaten raw but taste sweeter when roasted.

Walnut trees can sometimes be found in old woodland and parks. The nuts are best in early November when they are fairly ripe and dry. Pick walnuts green and 'wet' in July for pickling – they should be soft enough to pass a skewer through. Do not eat them raw as they contain cyanide, which is destroyed by pickling. Pickled walnuts are an excellent source of vitamin C. Gargling with the pickling vinegar is said to soothe sore throats.

Wild garlic is found in damp woodland and hedgerows. It has clusters of star-shaped white flowers, and its leaves, which look like those of lily-of-the-valley, can be eaten as a vegetable. In herbal medicine, wild garlic is prescribed to reduce blood pressure and high blood cholesterol levels, as well as for colds, flu and bronchitis.

Rowan or mountain ash

Sweet chestnut

Wild garlic

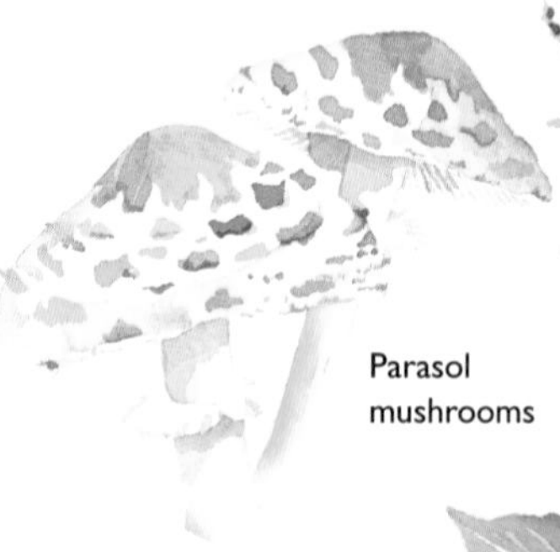

Parasol mushrooms

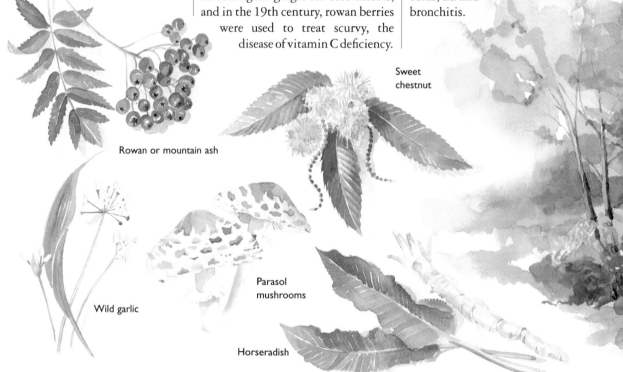

Horseradish

Fungi can be found growing wild in many parts of Britain, and there are well over a hundred edible varieties. Most of them contain B vitamins, copper, protein and fibre. Hunt in beech woods in late summer and early autumn, before the first frost, for easily identified varieties such as chanterelles – brilliant yellow trumpets – and horns of plenty, which are dark brown and cornet-shaped. Two varieties which favour woodland clearings are scaly parasol mushrooms – which grow up to 18 cm (7 in) across and are shaped like old-fashioned beehives – and meaty-flavoured ceps, which are dome-shaped and have porous sponge-like undersides; avoid ceps tinged with red or purple as these may be poisonous. The easiest fungi to recognise are field mushrooms, which grow on open pastures. The gills are pink but turn brown with age. Fungi are not renowned for their medicinal properties and in Britain, they are seldom, if ever, used as folk remedies.

Learn to recognise poisonous as well as the edible varieties, so you know which to avoid.

Poisonous fungi: some can kill

1 Yellow Stainer White cap yellowing with age, yellow staining at base of white stalk. Easily mistaken for field or horse mushroom, it can be recognised by cutting swollen base of stalk which goes a deep yellow. Vomiting and coma.

2 Panther Cap Smoky brown cap with flaky white scales; white stalk which has a series of rings around the base. Possibly deadly.

3 Destroying Angel Pure white cap, gills and stem – which is shaggy with a ragged ring. Deadly.

4 Fly Agaric Bright red cap with white scales; white gills and white scaly stem. It is especially tempting to children. Rarely fatal, but causes hallucinations and violent stomach upset.

5 Red-staining Inocybe Light brown conical cap with a pinkish flush or, occasionally, red veins. Distinguished by its gills which turn red when bruised. Deadly.

6 Death Cap Greenish or pale yellow tinged with green; white stalk and white gills; the cut flesh has a sweet, slightly sickly smell. It grows hidden in undergrowth and is the deadliest known fungus. Its poisons take effect in 6-24 hours, and there is no known antidote.

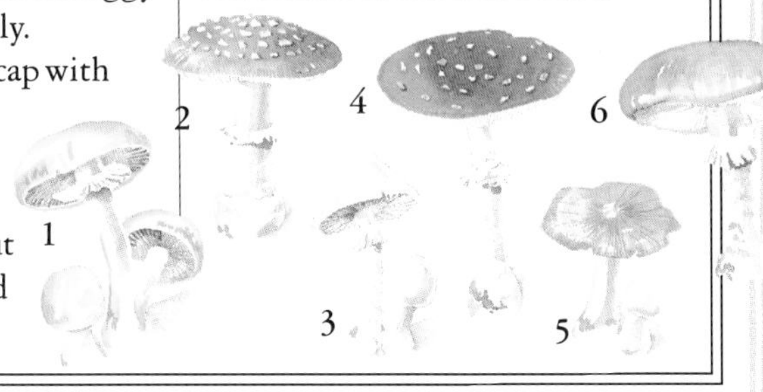

Collect fungi in an open basket so that the spores can drop (to perpetuate the species), and to prevent them from deteriorating or becoming slimy due to lack of air. Keep the stalks intact for accurate identification, and double-check each specimen with an illustrated reference book once you get home.

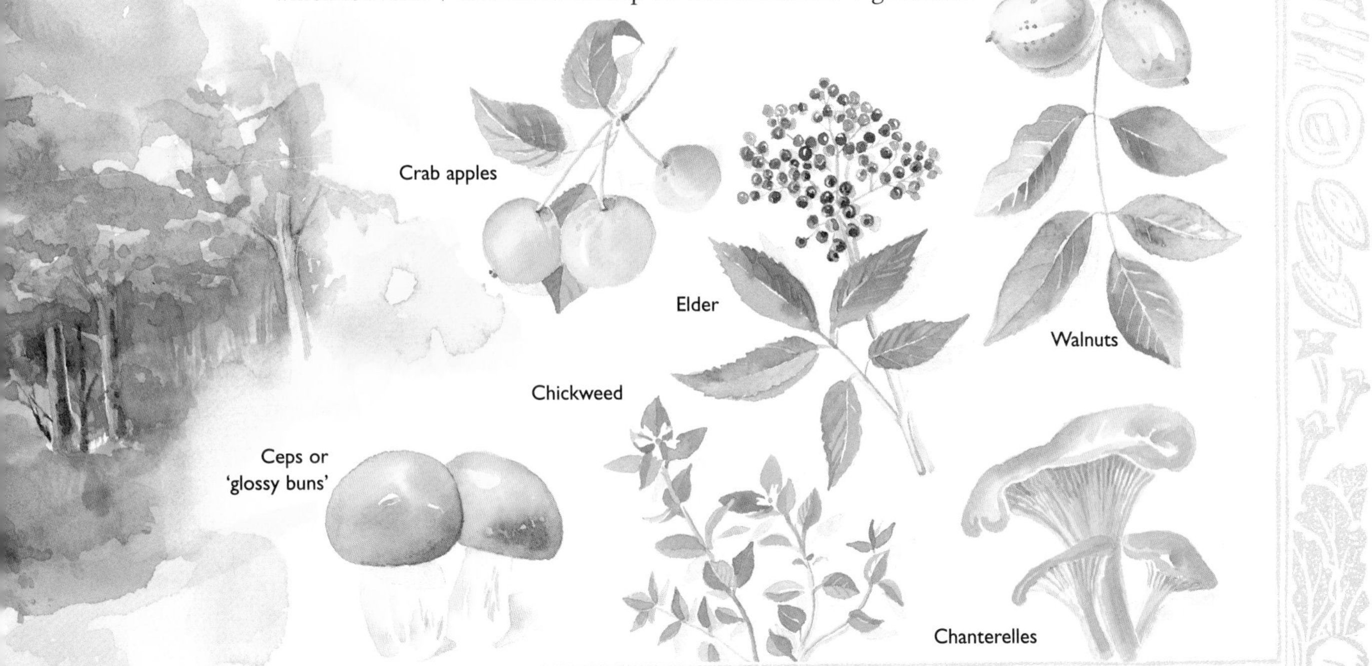

MOORLAND AND MEADOW

Wherever you hunt for free foods, remember not to strip one plant of all its leaves or berries, but take small amounts from several so as not to affect their appearance or health.

Bilberries are small, juicy bluish-black fruits with a 'tart' taste that grow on low shrubs. Their pigment is a powerful antioxidant, and they are a good source of vitamin C. They are antibacterial, and may be useful in fighting urinary-tract infections, diarrhoea and some eye disorders.

Field mushrooms are the most easily identifiable of all edible fungi, as they look like the cultivated variety. They are a good source of copper.

Good King Henry is one of the goosefoot family, named for the shape of the leaves. It grows to about 60 cm (2 ft) and is eaten in the same way as spinach; rich in iron, calcium and vitamin C and thiamin, it is more nutritious than either spinach or chard.

Sorrel has arrow-shaped leaves with a sharp, lemony flavour. It is best eaten raw in salads when it is an excellent source of beta carotene and vitamin C. Sorrel is high in oxalic acid which may inhibit absorption of iron and calcium and predispose susceptible people to kidney stone formation.

Wild celery, similar to garden celery, is eaten in soups and stews. It has diuretic properties and is reputed to help treat arthritis, rheumatism and gout. It is also mildly sedative.

Wild chicory, related to cultivated endive, is a tall plant with pale blue flowers. Its ragged, slightly bitter leaves can be added to salads and are an excellent source of beta carotene, vitamin C and potassium. It is used in herbal medicine to stimulate the appetite. Its roasted and ground root may be added to coffee, giving it a slightly bitter taste, and it can also be used as a coffee substitute.

Dos and don'ts

When gathering wild produce, it is important that you follow a few safety rules and precautions:

- Do study the subject carefully by reading clearly illustrated books before foraging for foods.
- Do be sure which mushrooms are toxic and which are safe.
- Do follow the country code.
- Do obey 'No Trespassing' signs.
- Do adopt the golden rule, 'if in doubt, leave alone'.
- Don't collect wild foods near cultivated crops as these may have been sprayed with pesticide.
- Don't pick near busy roads where hedges and verges may be contaminated by exhaust fumes.
- Don't encourage children to forage for 'free' foods unless they are accompanied by an adult.

Wild strawberries are an excellent source of vitamin C. In folk medicine, strawberries are believed to cleanse the digestive system, to eliminate kidney stones and to relieve joint pain.

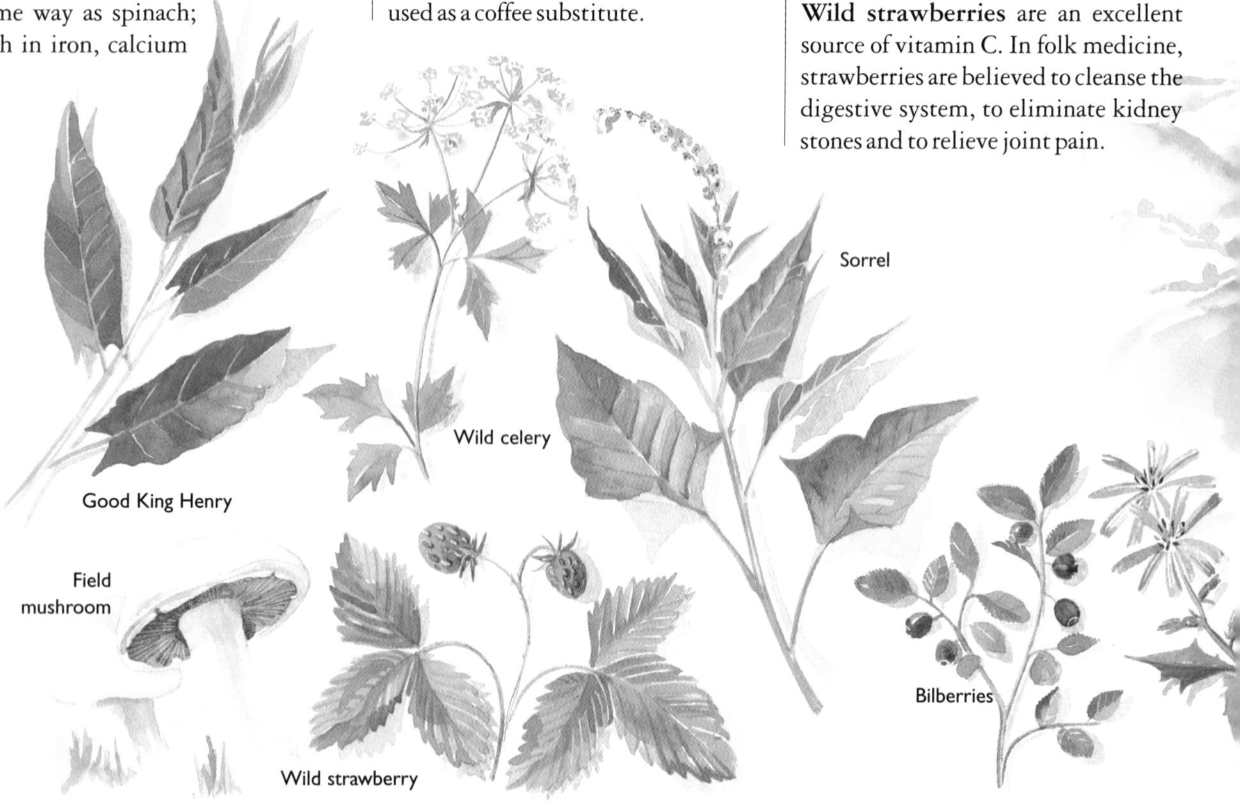

SEASIDE

May and June are the best months to gather most seaweeds. Before cooking seaweed, be sure to wash it thoroughly in plenty of fresh water to remove sand, shells and other debris. Seaweeds are rich in iodine, a mineral not widely found in other foods. This iodine content has made seaweed important in many parts of the world to treat goitre, an enlargement of the thyroid gland. Seaweeds also contain other useful minerals, especially potassium and calcium.

Laver is an easily recognised seaweed, common on rocks and stones all round the British coast. It is a translucent, thin, wavy-edged frond attached to the rock by a small disc-shaped holdfast. Laver should be well washed and simmered until it becomes a purée resembling well-cooked spinach. In South Wales this purée, known as laverbread, is coated in oatmeal, then fried and served with bacon and eggs.

Marsh samphire (or glasswort) is abundant on muddy salt marshes. The plump, shiny stems grow like tall, bushy desert cacti. In June or July the young shoots make a crisp salad; in late summer the older plants are served like asparagus. Eat boiled by using the teeth to strip the fleshy part of the plant from its tough central spine.

Sea beet (or sea spinach), which grows just like cultivated spinach, can be picked from June to October from coastal paths and sea walls. Sea beet is an excellent source of beta carotene, and also supplies iron, magnesium, potassium and calcium. It is used in the same way as garden spinach.

Cockles and mussels

The seashore is a good hunting ground for SHELLFISH, such as mussels or cockles. However, because these molluscs feed by filtering sea water, they may become contaminated with sewage particles. Select areas away from sewage or refuse outlets and do not collect molluscs during the warm months when bacteria can multiply rapidly, causing food poisoning. Clean them carefully and eat on the day they are collected. Make sure that all shellfish are alive immediately before cooking, as dead shellfish decompose very quickly and are all too likely to cause food poisoning.

Emergency action

If a poisonous plant, fungus or berry – red berries are particularly attractive to small children – is eaten, go straight to the nearest hospital, taking a sample of the substance eaten with you. Do not drink anything as this may speed up absorption of the poison. Inducing immediate vomiting may help to prevent the poison from entering the bloodstream.

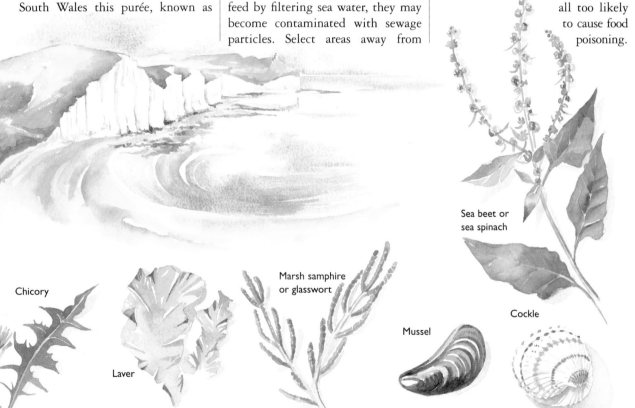

CRANBERRIES

BENEFIT
- *Juice helps to fight bladder, kidney and urinary-tract infections*

The juice of these scarlet berries has long been used as a home remedy for cystitis and other bladder, kidney and urinary-tract infections, especially in their native North America.

Initially, the scientific explanation for this was based on the high acidity content of the cranberries. It was thought that they raised the acid levels of the urine, thereby killing the bacteria responsible for the infection. However, scientific research undertaken in Ohio, USA, suggests that cranberries contain a substance that stops the infectious bacteria from clinging to the cells that line the urinary tract and bladder, preventing them from multiplying. Further research undertaken by Israeli scientists comparing a variety of juices indicates that the only other fruit to have a similar effect is the blueberry, a member of the same botanical family.

Many urologists recommend drinking a couple of glasses of cranberry juice daily as a preventive measure and to help to control mild infections. If symptoms persist, seek medical advice as medication may be necessary.

Commercially produced cranberry juice is high in added sugar, which may not be evident from its tart taste. Consequently, it may not be suitable for certain people such as diabetics.

BOUNCING BERRIES

Cranberries are known as bouncing berries because good ones do, literally, bounce. People used to tip them down steps to test them – the bad ones remained where they fell and the good ones kept on bouncing.

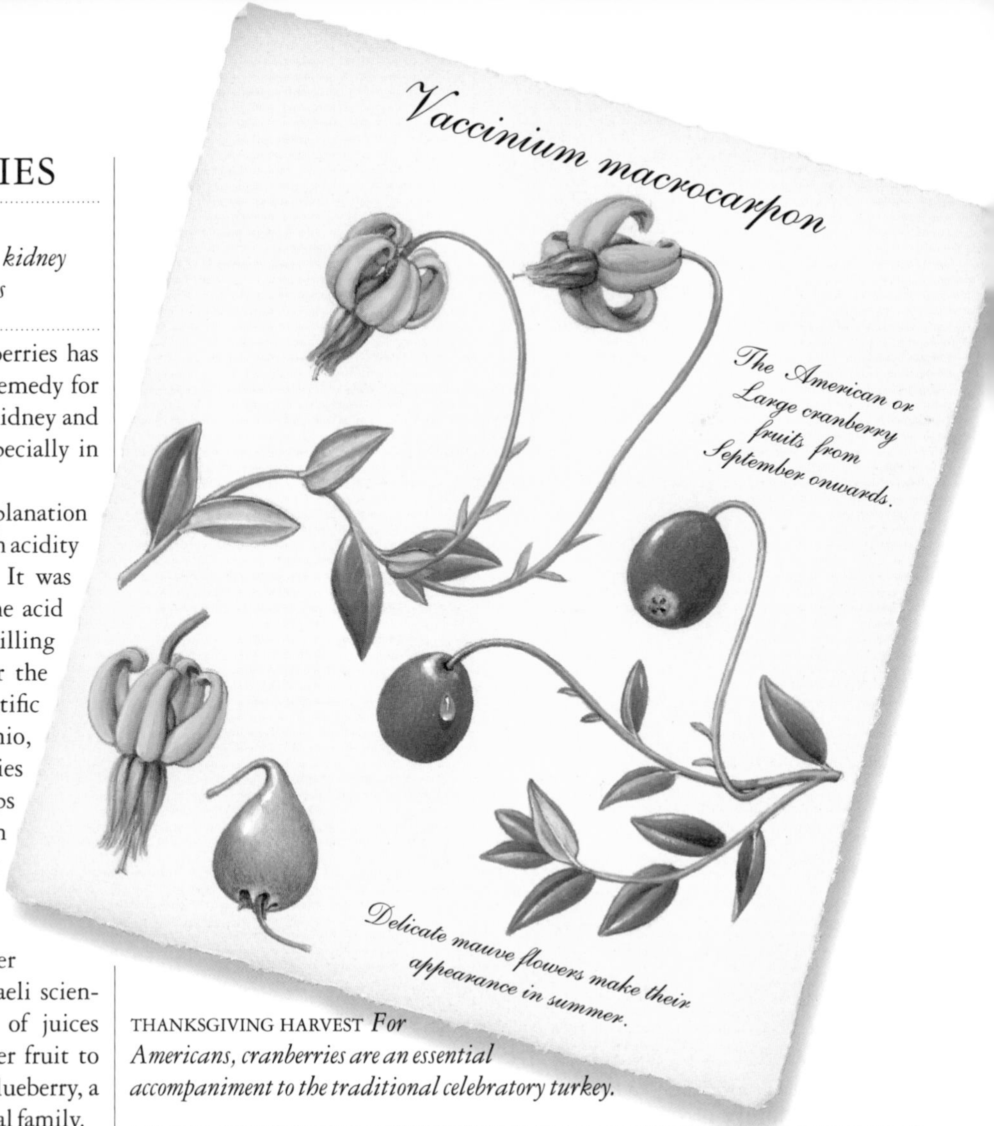
Vaccinium macrocarpon
The American or Large cranberry fruits from September onwards.
Delicate mauve flowers make their appearance in summer.

THANKSGIVING HARVEST *For Americans, cranberries are an essential accompaniment to the traditional celebratory turkey.*

CROHN'S DISEASE

EAT PLENTY OF
- *All nutritious foods, according to your personal tolerance*

People diagnosed as suffering from Crohn's disease often have a tendency to malnourishment either as a result of the effects of the inflammation in their intestine, or from changes they have made to their diet. It is therefore essential for anyone with the condition to plan their diet carefully.

Crohn's disease is an inflammatory bowel disease that can affect any part of the gastrointestinal tract. It is most often diagnosed in people between the ages of 15 and 35. Symptoms of the disease usually fluctuate in severity, and may include internal pain, fever, diarrhoea and weight loss.

The causes of Crohn's disease are not fully understood. It may be an auto-immune response in which the body attacks its own intestinal tissue, as the result of an infection or a reaction to stress or other environmental factors. It has been suggested that the high incidence of the disease among people who eat a highly processed Western-style diet may be significant, while a nine-year study in Uppsala, Sweden, reported by *The Lancet* in 1994 found a link between Crohn's disease and measles. More newborn babies in central Sweden went on to develop Crohn's disease than expected during the research period, in which there were five epidemics of measles.

Crohn's disease remains something of a mystery to the medical profession and as yet there is no cure, but effective medical treatment usually involves anti-inflammatory drugs. Many sufferers will need surgery to the most affected areas of the intestine at some time. Poor nutrition may be a result of the inflammation, which can cause the wall of the intestine to become scarred and thickened, obstructing the passage of food. Patients can also suffer from a loss of appetite.

Eating often becomes more difficult when the disease flares up. If the small intestine is inflamed, or if there is a narrowing of the bowel, eating may cause painful cramps. In this case, avoiding foods high in fibre may be helpful. Vitamin and mineral supplements may be given to those so severely affected they have difficulty absorbing any nutrients from food.

Food intolerance (see ALLERGIES AND FOOD INTOLERANCE) is now thought by most experts to be an important factor in Crohn's disease. Many sufferers have reported that their symptoms seem to be made worse by particular foods. The foods most often cited are grains (wheat, oats, barley, rye and maize), yeast, dairy products, nuts, raw fruit, shellfish and pickles.

Evidence suggests that medically supervised exclusion diets have benefited more than 50 per cent of people affected by Crohn's disease. Patients can try eliminating particular foods, one at a time, from their diet for a few weeks to see if this brings an improvement, but care must be taken not to eliminate too many essential foods.

Possible vitamin and mineral deficiencies depend on the location of the inflammation as well as the drugs prescribed, but they often include folate, found in liver, leafy green vegetables and pulses. Sufferers may also have low reserves of other B vitamins, including thiamin (B_1), which is present in potatoes, pork, offal, seeds and cereals; riboflavin (B_2), which is obtained mainly from eggs, meat, poultry, fish and dairy products, as well as from yeast extract and fortified breakfast cereals; and vitamin B_6, which is found in wholewheat bread, nuts and soya beans. Vitamin B_{12} may also need boosting by eating lean meat, fish, milk or fortified breakfast cereals.

Other possible vitamin deficiencies include vitamin C, which is found in fresh fruit and vegetables – particularly blackcurrants and citrus fruits; vitamin D, found in fish such as herring, salmon and sardines; and vitamin K, provided by green vegetables, liver and tomatoes.

Levels of essential minerals may also become too low. Dairy foods, sardines and green leafy vegetables are valuable sources of calcium. Iron levels can be boosted by eating offal, oily fish and dark green leafy vegetables. And people with Crohn's disease often need more magnesium, which can be obtained by eating fish and shellfish. Liver, fish and wholegrain cereals can help to compensate for the reduced absorption of selenium. Zinc levels can be increased by eating seafood, beef, pork, dairy products and chicken.

There is some evidence that vitamin E – found in seed oils, wheatgerm, green leafy vegetables and eggs, for example – may help to reduce bowel inflammation. However, this has yet to be proved by scientific studies.

There are no specific foods that are known to cause Crohn's disease and none that are known to cure it. However, by eating a balanced nutritious diet, avoiding only the foods that you are sure make your symptoms worse, you will minimise at least some of the disease's unpleasant effects.

Case study

Peter is a 34-year-old aircraft engineer for whom shift work is a way of life. When, over a six-month period, he suffered from repeated episodes of diarrhoea and stomach-bloating, he simply put it down to the new shift pattern he had started at work. His family and friends, on the other hand, had noticed that he seemed to be losing weight and kept on telling him how ill he looked. Peter refused to listen, and it was only when he started to feel unwell that he realised there might be cause for concern. Medical investigation revealed that he was suffering from Crohn's disease.

Peter's doctor prescribed low-dose steroid drugs to be taken in conjunction with a high-fibre, high-protein diet and vitamin supplements. After six weeks, Peter no longer experienced abdominal pains or diarrhoea, and he slowly began to feel better and put on weight.

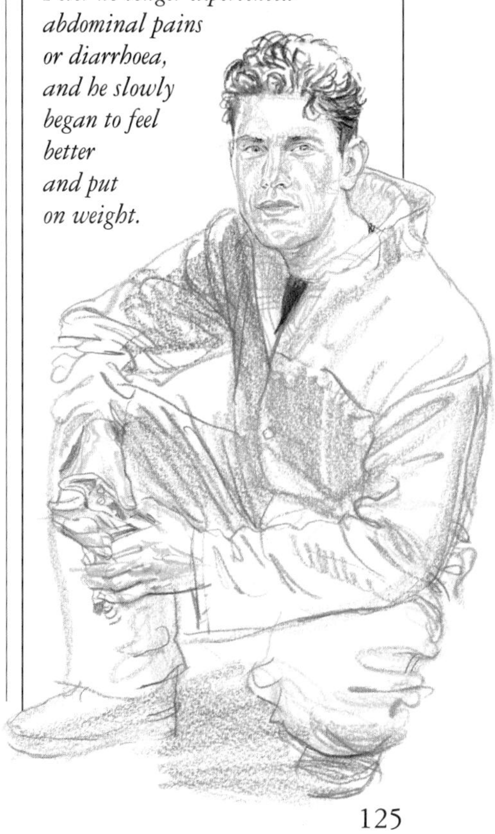

CUCUMBER

BENEFIT

- *Low in calories*

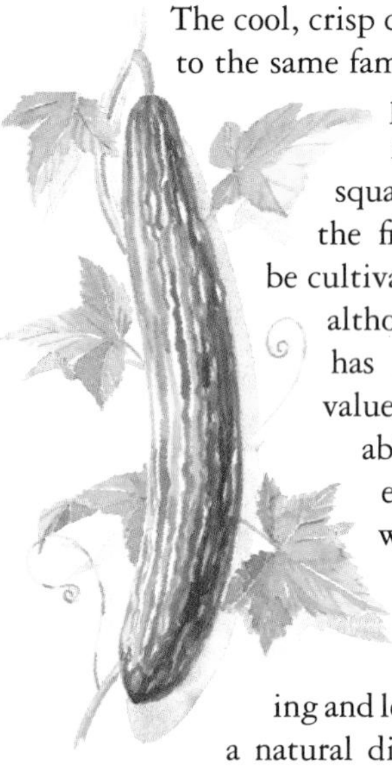

The cool, crisp cucumber belongs to the same family as courgettes, pumpkins, watermelons and other squashes. It was one of the first vegetables to be cultivated in the world, although it actually has little nutritional value. Its most remarkable quality is an exceptionally high water content – 96.4 per cent – which makes it both refreshing and low in calories. It is a natural diuretic, but not a particularly powerful one.

Although cucumbers have long been valued as an ingredient in skin-care preparations, there is no scientific proof that their extract is beneficial to the skin or that slices placed over the eyes will have a reviving effect.

CYSTIC FIBROSIS

EAT PLENTY OF

- *Protein-rich foods, such as meat, poultry, fish and eggs*
- *Fats, including dairy produce, oils and fatty fish*
- *Simple carbohydrates such as sugary foods and sweets, and complex carbohydrates such as bread, potatoes and pasta*

AVOID

- *Low-calorie or fat-reduced products*

A combination of a high-energy, high-protein diet, medication, physiotherapy and exercise can enable people suffering from cystic fibrosis to have a better quality of life. There is no cure for the disease, but the correct diet is vital in helping sufferers to stay well enough to fight off further infections and other disorders associated with it.

This hereditary, life-threatening condition is caused by a defect in the gene that controls the passage of salt and water across cell membranes. About 1 in 25 people in Britain carry the defective gene, but a child will develop the disease only if both parents carry the genetic fault. If this is the case, there is a one in four chance of producing a baby with cystic fibrosis (inheriting a defective gene from each parent); a one in two chance of having a baby that is completely healthy but a carrier (inheriting a faulty gene from one parent and a normal gene from the other); and a one in four chance of producing a normal baby (inheriting normal genes from both parents). Most people with the disease are diagnosed before the age of two.

Cystic fibrosis makes huge energy demands on the body, and infants and children with the condition have ravenous appetites because they have difficulty eating and absorbing nutrients. The illness causes a failure of the glands that produce mucus in the lungs and pancreas, with the result that instead of the thin mucus normally produced to keep the airways moist, a thick, sticky mucus builds up in the lungs. This can cause vomiting, respiratory infections and, in the long term, a severe reduction in lung efficiency – all of which increase the need for nutrients to be provided in the diet.

Mucus also builds up in the pancreas, blocking the ducts that allow enzymes to travel from the pancreas to the intestine where they are needed to digest food. As a result, food, especially fat and protein, is not properly digested or absorbed, causing diarrhoea and deficiencies in the essential fat-soluble vitamins A, D, E and K. About 85 per cent of people with cystic fibrosis suffer from what is termed pancreatic insufficiency, so they need to take pancreatic enzymes in capsule form to help them digest their food – together with vitamin and mineral supplements.

A diet that provides lots of calories, fat, simple and complex carbohydrates, protein, salt and water (needed because of the diarrhoea and vomiting) is also vitally important. A high-fibre, low-fat diet – which is normally accepted as 'healthy' – is totally unsuitable because it gives a feeling of being full long before the increased nutritional demands have been met. In adults suffering from cystic fibrosis, this type of diet can result in weight loss. In children, it can lead to insufficient weight gain and poor growth.

Energy and protein are the most important factors in the normal, everyday diet for people with cystic

High energy, high protein

All the foods people are normally told to eat in moderation are included in the 'recommended' list for people with cystic fibrosis:

- Meat, fish, cheese, pulses or nuts at each meal, including breakfast.
- Butter, margarine, oils, crisps, fatty meats, fried foods.
- Sugar, honey, jam, chocolate, cakes, sweets, fizzy drinks.
- Up to 1 litre (1¾ pints) of whole milk per day. It can be fortified by adding dried milk powder.
- Breakfast cereals, rice, potatoes, pasta and bread. Add milk or butter to increase calorie intake.
- Fruit and vegetables provide vital vitamins, but should not be eaten at the expense of higher energy foods. Add sugar, cream and butter to increase calories.

fibrosis, but especially if they have frequent chest infections or lose a lot of fat in their stools. No one can say precisely how much greater the energy needs are for people with cystic fibrosis because they vary from one individual to another. One person may need only 5 per cent more than the normal adult requirement, whereas another may need as much as 100 per cent more. However, the Cystic Fibrosis Trust recommends a dietary intake guideline of between 20 and 50 per cent more calories than the national recommendation for age and sex, and twice as much protein.

Getting enough fat and protein in the form of dairy produce, oils and meat is more important than any worries about blood cholesterol. Fatty fish such as salmon, mackerel and sardines are good sources of protein, fat and essential fatty acids. Other suitable fatty foods include sausages, ice cream, pastry, cream, nuts, chocolate and crisps. Butter or margarine should be added to vegetables to boost the calorie count, and foods should be fried for the extra fat content.

If DIABETES is not a complication (it can occur as the disease develops because of damage to the pancreas), sugary foods, sweets and sweet drinks should all be part of the diet because they are easily absorbed and provide plenty of energy. Meals should be supplemented with calorie-rich snacks throughout the day; they too should preferably contain protein.

Salt is also an essential part of the diet. Cystic fibrosis affects the sweat and parotid glands, causing them to excrete abnormal amounts of salt in perspiration, tears and saliva, especially during hot weather and when exercising for extended periods. However, there is usually no need to add excessive amounts of salt to food.

It is possible for people with cystic fibrosis to become vegetarian or even vegan, but it can be difficult to achieve the right balance of protein and calorie intake. You should always see a dietician or doctor before making any changes to your diet.

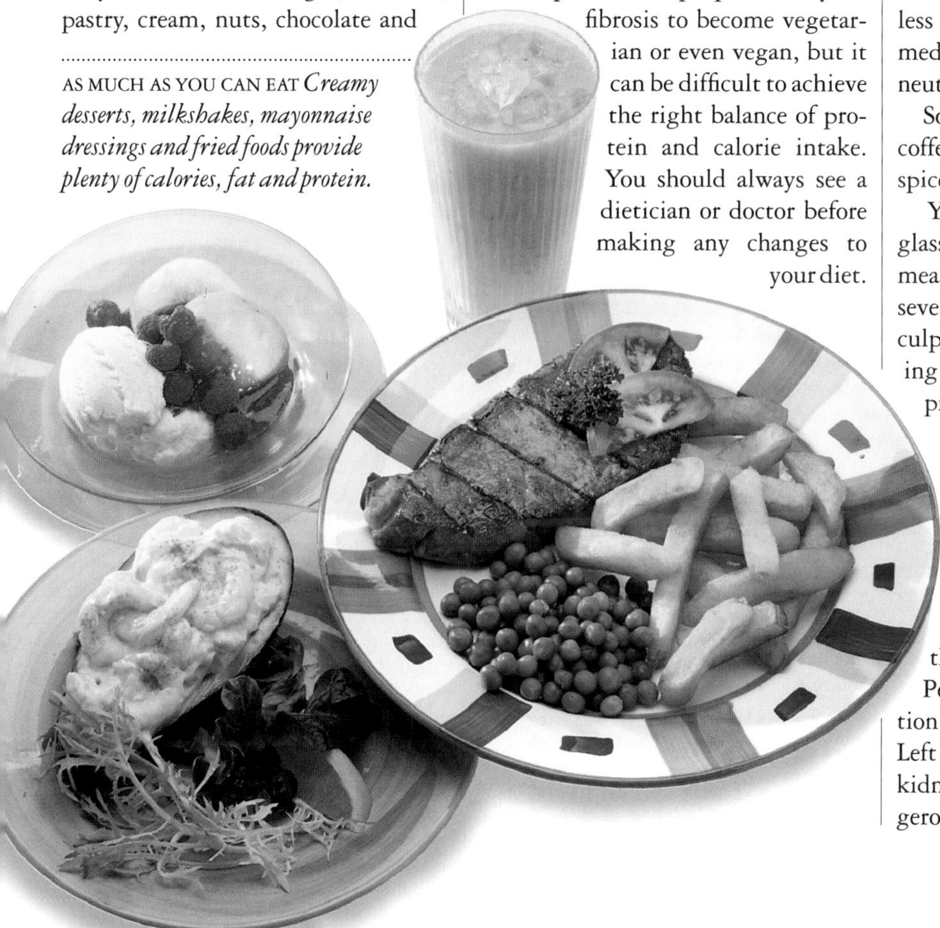

AS MUCH AS YOU CAN EAT *Creamy desserts, milkshakes, mayonnaise dressings and fried foods provide plenty of calories, fat and protein.*

Cystitis

TAKE PLENTY OF

- *Water or other fluids – at least 2-3 litres (3½-5¼ pints) a day*
- *Cranberry juice*

CUT DOWN ON

- *Hot, spicy foods*
- *Tea, coffee and fizzy drinks*

Thousands of women – and some men as well – suffer from cystitis. This painful bladder infection makes people want to pass water frequently but, when they try, they can normally only pass a small amount of urine – and the act of urination causes a painful burning sensation.

The most important dietary rule for cystitis sufferers is to drink plenty of fluids – at least 2-3 litres (3½-5¼ pints) a day – to dilute the urine. This makes it less acidic, so passing water is less painful. Taking the prescribed medication, potassium citrate, also neutralises the urine.

Some cystitis sufferers find that tea, coffee, fizzy drinks, chilli peppers and spices make their symptoms worse.

You may like to try drinking a daily glass of cranberry juice as a preventive measure. Cranberry juice, according to several studies, appears to prevent the culprit bacterium, *E. coli*, from sticking to the walls of the urinary tract, protecting against the infection. In the USA, the Harvard Medical School conducted a six-month study among 153 elderly women, which found that those drinking a daily glass of cranberry juice were much less likely to show signs of cystitis than those who were not.

People with any urinary tract infection should always consult a doctor. Left untreated, it may turn into a kidney infection, which can be dangerous and difficult to cure.

Dates

BENEFITS
- *Useful source of vitamin C*
- *Rich in potassium (when dried)*
- *Gentle laxative*

DRAWBACKS
- *May trigger migraines*
- *Dried dates are high in sugar, which can cause tooth decay and gum disease*

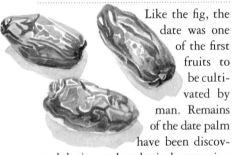

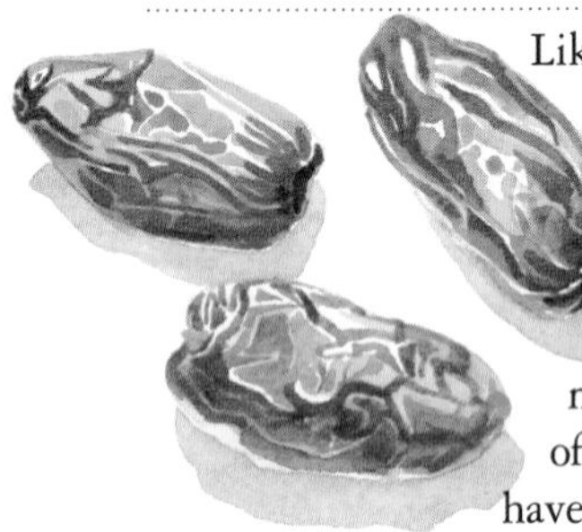

Like the fig, the date was one of the first fruits to be cultivated by man. Remains of the date palm have been discovered during archaeological excavation of several Stone Age sites.

Both fresh and dried dates are a nourishing food. A 100g (3½oz) portion of the fresh fruit contains 107 Calories. The same weight of dried dates supplies 227 Calories.

Fresh dates are the better source of vitamin C – 100g (3½oz) provides almost a third of the recommended daily intake. They are also a useful source of soluble fibre, making them a gentle laxative which does not irritate the bowel or stomach.

Dried dates are richer in potassium than the fresh fruit and a more concentrated source of nutrients such as niacin, copper, iron and magnesium. A 100g (3½oz) portion contributes around one-eighth of the recommended daily intake of each.

Dates, however, also contain tyramine (an organic compound found in foods such as certain dairy and yeast products), which is known to trigger migraines in susceptible people.

Anyone eating dried fruit as a healthy alternative to sweets should be aware that dates are high in sugar. Eating dried dates too often can lead to dental caries and gum disease because the sugar content is readily fermented in the mouth to form dental plaque.

Depression

EAT PLENTY OF
- *Whole grains, peas, lentils and other types of pulse*
- *Fresh fruit and vegetables*
- *Lean meat, poultry and offal*
- *Fish and shellfish*

CUT DOWN ON
- *Alcohol*
- *Caffeine, in tea, coffee or colas*

If you are taking certain antidepressants:
AVOID
- *Canned and processed meats*
- *Calves' or chicken liver*
- *Beer, red wine and liqueurs*
- *Processed or ripe cheese*

Just when a balanced, wholesome diet is needed most, people who are suffering from severe depression neglect their body's needs. The illness is quite distinct from a normal, reactive response to disappointment and often leaves some people with no appetite at all, while others go on binges or develop cravings for carbohydrates.

As a result, victims of depression may often suffer from nutritional deficiencies or imbalances – particularly a lack of B vitamins and vitamin C, and of the minerals calcium, copper, iron, magnesium and potassium. The precise relationship between different nutrients and the brain's chemistry is still unclear but malnourishment or weight problems clearly contribute to morale spiralling downwards.

This is particularly true of people suffering from ANOREXIA, when an abnormal diet and low self-esteem are both common causes of depression. The MENOPAUSE – when hormonal changes may be a contributory factor – and premenstrual tension are also associated with the condition. In this case the vitamin B_6, which is sometimes prescribed for premenstrual tension, may also help to fight depression.

Nutritional guidelines from the Department of Health offer pointers on nutrition for sufferers of depression. Plenty of whole grains and pulses, and regular amounts of lean meat, offal, oily fish, shellfish and eggs, will supply B vitamins, iron, potassium, magnesium, copper and zinc. A high intake of fresh fruit and vegetables (such as asparagus, broccoli, cabbage, melon, oranges and berries) will supply ample vitamin C. Dark green leafy vegetables will improve levels of calcium, magnesium and iron; dried fruit will provide potassium and iron, while dairy produce (preferably low-fat) will boost reserves of calcium.

Too much caffeine (more than four cups of coffee or six cups of tea a day) can exacerbate depression. Since caffeine also contributes to sleeplessness, and insomnia is one of the symptoms of depression, sufferers should avoid drinking tea or coffee before going to bed. People should be aware that the headaches and lethargy, which are symptoms of sudden caffeine withdrawal, can last from one to three days before real improvements are felt.

People suffering from depression should cut down on their alcohol intake – not only because more than one or two drinks can have an adverse effect on mood, but also because it can sabotage healthy nutrition by suppressing the appetite.

In susceptible people, certain foods can also cause depression. If you suspect that there is a link between a food sensitivity and your state of mind, try eliminating the culprit foods from your diet to see if this brings relief.

THE DRUG DIMENSION

People taking antidepressants that contain monoamine oxidase (see MEDICINES AND DRUGS) should avoid any food or drink that contains high levels of tyramine. These include various types of alcohol such as beers, liqueurs, red wine, sherry and vermouth, as well as processed or ripe cheese, calves' or chicken liver, salamis, tinned meats, soya sauce, yeast extracts, herring and kippers. Other foods that should be limited and contain lower levels of tyramine include bananas, avocados, figs, chocolate, products containing vanilla, and drinks such as hot chocolate, cola and coffee; you should not consume more than three cups a day.

A reaction between tyramine and chemicals in some antidepressants and tranquillisers can affect the nervous system, causing symptoms which include palpitations, nosebleeds and headaches. Very rarely, blood pressure can rise so high that it can lead to intra-cranial bleeding and even death.

Women whose depression stems from taking an oral contraceptive may benefit from increasing their intake of vitamin B_6 – found in lean meats, whole grains, pulses, wheatgerm and dark green vegetables – but this has not been scientifically proven.

Another form of depression, which is prevalent in northern climates, is SEASONAL AFFECTIVE DISORDER (SAD), caused by the effects of light deprivation. It can usually be treated with full-spectrum light therapy.

DIABETES

Glucose, a form of sugar carried in the bloodstream, is a vital source of energy. For the body to function efficiently, however, levels must be kept within narrow limits. Too much glucose in the blood indicates development of the ailment known as diabetes mellitus. Its symptoms are thirst, frequent urination due to excess glucose, weight loss, tiredness, recurrent infections, problems with vision, and, in severe cases, coma. Too little glucose, resulting in low blood sugar, or HYPOGLYCAEMIA, can also result in a coma.

Carbohydrates – sugary or starchy foods such as chocolates, cakes, biscuits, bread and potatoes, or fruit and jam – send up the levels of sugars in the blood. Under normal circumstances, a proper balance is soon restored through the action of insulin – a hormone produced by the pancreas.

If the body's output of insulin is too low, or the insulin produced is ineffective, the blood glucose remains high. This is how hyperglycaemia (high blood sugar) is caused.

Excess glucose in the blood is excreted. Consequently, one test for diabetes is to measure the level of glucose in the urine. Treatment always involves a carefully controlled and healthily balanced diet that restricts the patient's intake of simple carbohydrates and reduces concentrated sugar and sugary drinks.

Diabetes takes two main forms. Insulin-dependent diabetes mellitus (IDDM, formerly referred to as juvenile onset diabetes) usually develops in childhood, but it can develop at any age and often occurs where there is a family history of any form of diabetes. Non-insulin dependent diabetes mellitus (NIDDM), as its former description – late onset diabetes – implies, tends to be much more common among older people. IDDM stems

Case study

When Amy, a normally energetic 14-year-old, began to suffer from headaches, aching joints, a dry mouth and general listlessness, she thought at first that it was flu. However, when her parents took her to the doctor, blood and urine tests revealed diabetes mellitus.
Amy was given fluids, glucose and insulin via an intravenous drip and she soon recovered. She was able to return to school after two weeks, injecting herself with insulin twice a day and monitoring her blood sugar levels. She already ate high-fibre, low-fat meals without any added sugar, the only change to her diet is that now she has a small snack before her energetic games of netball. Amy is successfully controlling her condition and leads an active life.

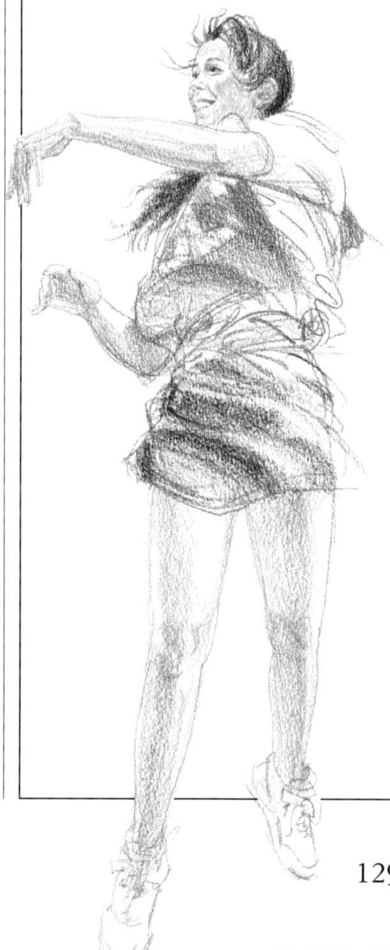

from an inability of the pancreas to produce insulin because of damaged or destroyed cells. This form of diabetes must be treated regularly with insulin injections. Diet plays no part in causing IDDM, although breastfeeding may offer some protection against it developing. In susceptible individuals it can be sparked by viral infections such as a previous attack of mumps or German measles.

NIDDM, which affects some 15 per cent of the population over the age of 50, apparently results from impaired secretion of insulin or a resistance to the hormone by the body's tissues. It can often be treated by diet alone, although some sufferers need medication. People need insulin injections if other methods fail to control their condition. Weight reduction is very important for diabetic people who are overweight because obesity increases their resistance to insulin.

It is essential for both groups of diabetics to eat regularly to prevent low blood sugar levels. Some insulin-treated diabetics need to eat every 2 or 3 hours and may also require snacks between meals. If hypoglycaemia occurs, glucose is needed as soon as possible. The British Diabetic Association advises that 15g (½oz) of glucose or sucrose should be given – as tablets or, preferably, in solution. If hypoglycaemia occurs before meals are due, their timing needs to be advanced and enough carbohydrate should be consumed immediately to prevent any recurrence.

All diabetics should carry a card describing their treatment and stating the measures to be taken in an emergency. Since it is possible to have a mild form of diabetes without any of the obvious symptoms, it pays to have regular check-ups after the age of 50.

Who is at risk?

One person in every 50 in Britain and one in every 20 in the United States suffers from diabetes, but fewer than half of these cases are diagnosed. In Britain, diabetes is most common among the elderly, particularly people who are overweight, and those of Asian origin. Diabetes is not caused by eating too much sugar or the wrong kind of food, nor can it be 'caught'.

Dietary guidelines

There are general dietary guidelines that diabetes sufferers can follow to help keep their blood sugar levels under control:

- Avoid being overweight. Make sure you eat a balanced, healthy diet based on suitable foods. If you do need to lose weight, see your doctor or nutritionist to formulate a diet tailored to your needs.
- Eat regular meals; exactly how many and how often can usually be decided by what is convenient.
- Eat more starchy, high-fibre foods such as wholemeal bread, beans, peas and lentils. All of these foods cause only a gradual rise in blood sugar because the fibre content slows down the release of glucose.
- Cut down on sugary sweetened soft drinks, cakes, confectionery and chocolate. The sugar is absorbed quickly and therefore causes blood glucose levels to rise more rapidly.
- Eat lots of fresh fruit and vegetables for soluble fibre and vitamins. Fruit makes an ideal snack or pudding, but beware of eating very sweet fruits such as grapes or mangoes in large amounts because of their effect on your blood sugar level. If you do eat tinned fruit, choose those canned in natural juice rather than syrup. Dried fruits such as dates are a concentrated form of sugar and so should only be consumed in small quantities.
- Ensure that you have portions of meat, eggs or cheese as part of at least two of your meals each day. Keep the portions small if you are worried about gaining excess weight, and remember that fish and pulses are alternative sources of protein.
- Cut down on fats, which aggravate the diabetic's increased risk of coronary heart disease.
- Limit salt and salty foods, because of the diabetic's increased susceptibility to high blood pressure. Be aware of hidden salt in many tinned, smoked and processed foods.
- Keep alcohol consumption at moderate levels, remembering that low-sugar diet beers and lagers tend to have a high alcohol content.
- Although artificial sweeteners may be useful, special diabetic products are usually unnecessary.
- Drink water, or sugar-free drinks.

DIET AND DIABETES

Anyone with diabetes needs a carefully planned diet prepared with expert help. Although the dietician's general advice will be similar for most diabetics, individual needs will differ slightly – depending on the type of diabetes and other factors such as body weight and how physically active the person is. As well as following a general nutritional regime, the pattern of eating must also take into account the timing and type of any insulin injections and of the diabetic's sensitivity to insulin and other drugs.

The consumption of special, commercially produced diabetic foods is discouraged by the British Diabetic Association, who feel that the very

KEEPING CONTROL *Diabetes does not usually demand specially prepared meals, just a well-balanced and healthy diet.*

A thickly cut wholemeal sandwich with poached salmon is a nutritious snack.

Balance pasta with vegetables and a low-fat sauce for a tasty main course.

Risotto with a little chicken makes a satisfying main meal.

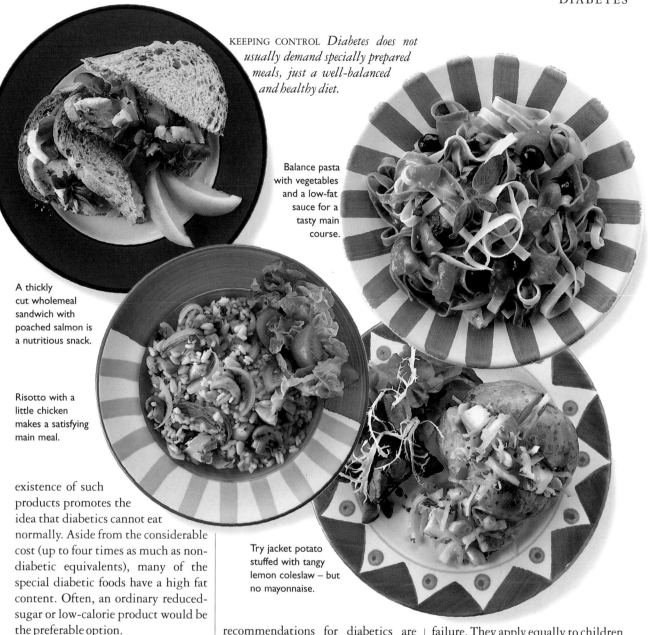

Try jacket potato stuffed with tangy lemon coleslaw – but no mayonnaise.

existence of such products promotes the idea that diabetics cannot eat normally. Aside from the considerable cost (up to four times as much as non-diabetic equivalents), many of the special diabetic foods have a high fat content. Often, an ordinary reduced-sugar or low-calorie product would be the preferable option.

Until the 1970s, diabetics were advised to follow a high-fat and low-carbohydrate diet. However, since then, increasing evidence has linked high-fat diets with heart disease – to which diabetics are particularly prone – and emphasised the benefits offered by carbohydrates in reducing coronary risk. The ability to control blood glucose levels in diabetes by eating foods that are rich in carbohydrates has also been recognised. Today, recommendations for diabetics are based on a diet that is high in complex carbohydrates, high in fibre and low in sugar and fat.

The aims of such a diet are to stop immediate symptoms (often through diet and exercise alone in cases of NIDDM) and reduce the risk of hypoglycaemia, which mainly affects those with IDDM. These diets are also designed to avoid the long-term complications associated with diabetes – heart disease, eye problems and kidney failure. They apply equally to children and teenagers with diabetes, although a doctor and specialist paediatric dietician will usually be involved on a regular basis to take account of changing needs because of physical growth.

Women should be aware that it is possible to develop 'gestational' diabetes during pregnancy. This usually disappears six weeks after the birth, but there is a 40 per cent chance that the woman will go on to develop NIDDM over the next 20 years.

DIETS AND SLIMMING

Forget about regimes of self-denial, nobody can keep them up for long. You need a diet that you can follow for life, and the new ground rules for losing weight are as easy as they are effective.

The Western world is obsessed with dieting. Fatty foods and sedentary lifestyles are often to blame for obesity, while glamorised images of reed-thin models and 'muscle men' encourage people to aspire towards an unrealistic body shape. Whether the reasons for dieting are cosmetic or health-related, slimming need not involve fad diets or peculiar eating patterns. A sensible balanced diet based on moderate quantities of foods that are low in fat will help most people to lose weight safely.

The successful slimmer loses weight slowly and surely, and establishes a healthy eating and exercise pattern that will last a lifetime, so that weight loss is permanent. Energy is measured in calories, and the aims of a slimming diet are to bring about weight loss by reducing your calorie intake from food and drink, and increasing your calorie output with exercise, so that the body uses up more energy than it takes in. In this way, the body's stores of fat tissue are gradually reduced.

NO MORE CALORIE COUNTING!

You may be relieved to learn that obsessive calorie-counting is now viewed as a rather old-fashioned and impractical way to lose weight. If you concentrate on cutting your fat intake, it is not necessary to count calories, and the diet remains satisfying as fairly generous amounts of starchy foods, grains and vegetables can be eaten. Just make sure you have a good understanding of which foods are calorie-laden, and avoid them. You obviously have to use your common sense and refrain from eating vast amounts of low-calorie foods because any surplus will still be stored as fat. Moderation is the key. Eat only when you are truly hungry, and stop when you feel satisfied and full.

FADS AND FALLACIES

Calorie intake can be reduced in a variety of ways, but not all slimming plans are scientifically based, and some of them can actually be quite dangerous. Faddy regimes neither encourage healthy eating habits nor establish safe and permanent weight loss.

Food combining diets, based on the HAY DIET, do help you to lose weight – but only because of the increased intake of fruit and vegetables at the expense of more calorific foods – and because the food combinations are so limited. Dieting 'magic potions' that claim to help you lose weight while you continue to eat normal meals cannot work; weight can be lost only by reducing calorie intake or increasing the amount your body uses up by taking more exercise.

Crash diets which include low-calorie meal replacement drinks, soups and snack bars cannot provide the same balance of nutrients as ordinary healthy food. The success of any crash diet is short-lived because water and protein are lost from the body, rather than excess body fat. Once normal eating is resumed, body fluids are quickly replaced and there is an immediate weight gain. Slimming then becomes even more difficult the next time around – a phenomenon known as the 'yo-yo' effect. Slimmers who get into a cycle of yo-yo dieting have a tendency to put on more weight every time they eat 'normally'. It is now thought that this is probably due to a repeated cycle of deprivation and bingeing, rather than any fall in the dieter's metabolic rate.

Fasting, when a person stops eating but drinks plenty of water, can be a dangerous practice; it may lead to lowered blood pressure and heart failure. Even when fasting is conducted under medical supervision, it is very rare for weight loss to be sustained once normal eating is resumed.

A HEALTHY SLIMMING DIET?

A slimming diet must provide all of the nutrients that the body needs. As these nutrients have to come from a lower calorie intake, it is important to cut right down on confectionery, cakes, biscuits, and sugary and alcoholic drinks, which are relatively high in calories but low in nutrients. The diet should be based on lower-calorie, nutritious foods such as vegetables, fruit, lean meat, poultry, fish, low-fat dairy products, bread and cereals.

Of all the major components of food, fat is the most concentrated source of energy. At nine Calories per gram, fat provides more than twice as many calories as protein and carbohydrate at four Calories per gram. Reducing the amount of fat in the diet is therefore the most effective way to reduce calorie intake. Pure alcohol has seven Calories per gram, so cutting down on alcohol is also an effective way to help weight loss.

There is a misconception that starchy staple foods such as bread, rice potatoes and pasta are fattening. In fact, these are medium-calorie foods. Provided they are not eaten with a lot of fat, these staples can be eaten in fairly large amounts on a slimming diet. Starchy foods help to satisfy the appetite because they are filling rather than fattening. Wholegrain foods such as wholemeal bread and brown rice are preferable to refined foods, as they provide significantly more vitamins, minerals and fibre.

A healthy slimming diet should also include plenty of salads, vegetables and pulses (beans, peas and lentils). Fresh fruit makes a good choice for a low-calorie dessert.

Fat-fighting tips

In order to help reduce your fat intake, choose lean cuts of meat and trim all visible fat before cooking. Avoid high-fat meats such as sausages, bacon and minced beef. Poultry should be eaten without the skin, and fish should be steamed, grilled, baked or micro-waved rather than fried. Sweet and savoury pies and pastries, biscuits, cakes, crisps and nuts are all high in fat and are best avoided on a slimming diet. Replace full-fat dairy products with low-fat alternatives.

You will probably lose 1.3kg (3lb) or more during the first week of any diet, due to an initial loss of water from the body. Thereafter, it is best to aim for a steady weight loss of 450-900g (1-2lb) a week, which will result in a reduction of body fat. Increasing your calorie expenditure through regular exercise – three times a week for a minimum of 20 minutes – will help to burn fat, and tone up the muscles for a leaner shape. (See also OBESITY and ENERGY, EXERCISE AND VITALITY.)

Balancing your slimming diet

When dieting, it is important to make sure that the foods you eat are nourishing. If you eat a wide variety from the food groups below, you should obtain optimum levels of each of the nutrients required for good health.

FOOD TYPES	TIPS
STARCHY FOODS	
Rice, bread, potatoes, cereals, pasta and other starches are the staple foods in your diet; everything else revolves around them. Contrary to popular belief, starchy foods are not fattening. Breads and cereals contain no more calories per gram than lean meat and far less than fats.	Choose speciality breads that taste good on their own without spreads. Serve pasta and rice with tomato-based vegetable sauces, avoiding any made with cheese, cream, butter or lots of oil. 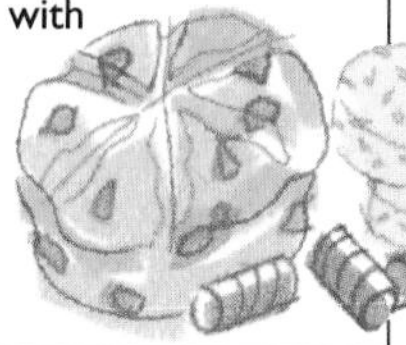
FRUIT, VEGETABLES AND SALADS	
Include a wide variety of fresh fruits, vegetables and salad leaves. 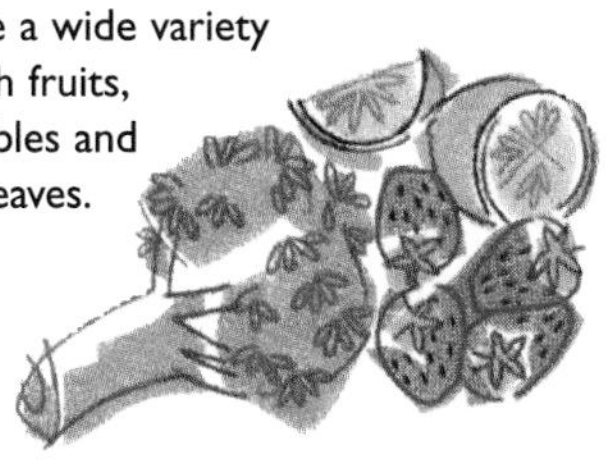	Go easy on dried fruit and avocados; dried fruit is high in sugar and avocados are high in fat. Avoid fattening salad dressings such as mayonnaise; make your own based on lemon or lime juice and low-fat yoghurt. Do not eat fried potatoes, such as chips, or potatoes baked with a cheese sauce.
MILK, CHEESE AND YOGHURT	
Eat moderate amounts of low-fat dairy products. 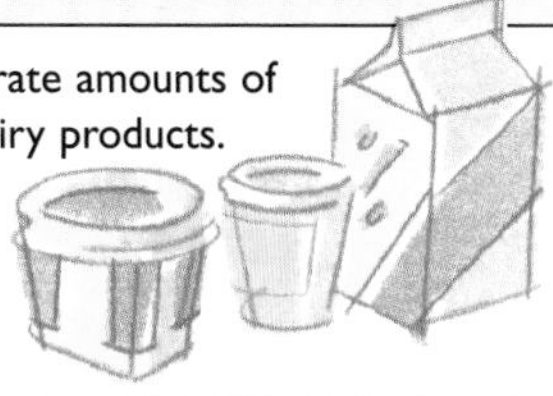	Choose skimmed or semi-skimmed milk, low-fat yoghurt and low-fat cheeses such as fromage frais, cottage cheese and ricotta. Avoid milk shakes made with whole milk.
PROTEIN	
Choose lean meat (such as game) with all visible fat trimmed off, poultry with the skin removed, fish and pulses (lentils, split peas and dried beans). 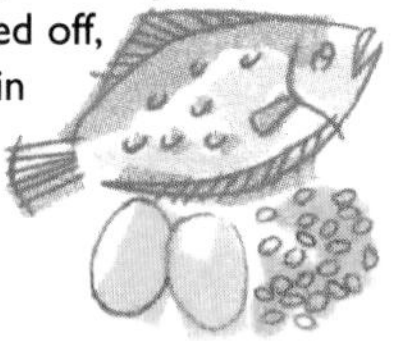	Steam, grill, bake or poach – but do not fry. Eat nuts, nut butters and seeds in moderation. Avoid high-fat meat products such as pies, pasties, sausages and beefburgers. White fish such as cod is less fattening than oily fish. Avoid fish canned in oil, or drain well.
FATTY AND SUGARY FOODS	
Use low-fat spreads. Use oil – even olive oil – sparingly. The occasional (once or twice a week) sugary treat will do no harm, as sugar is not blamed for obesity. Cutting down on fats is the best approach when you are dieting.	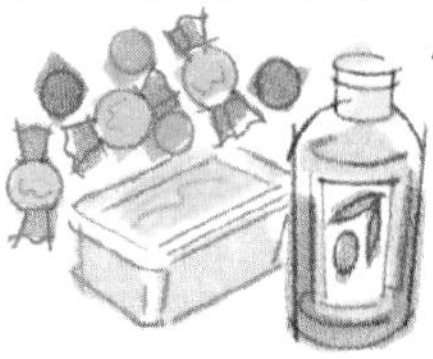 Avoid all crisps, biscuits, cakes and pies as they contain a lot of hidden fats.

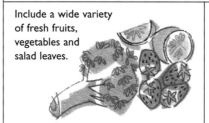

DIARRHOEA

TAKE PLENTY OF

- *Water to replace lost fluid*
- *Bananas for potassium*
- *Boiled white rice and dry white toast for low-fibre carbohydrate*
- *Apples, which naturopaths believe help to cleanse the digestive system*

AVOID

- *All other food for the first 48 hours*
- *Alcohol and caffeine for at least 48 hours after the symptoms have gone*

If you have an attack of diarrhoea – where you pass loose, watery stools frequently – it is important to replace the body's lost fluids and salts. Rehydration preparations are available from chemists, but you can make your own by adding one teaspoon of salt and eight teaspoons of sugar to 1 litre (1¾ pints) of boiled water. When symptoms begin, drink about a litre (1¾ pints) of this mixture every 2 hours: roughly 150ml (¼ pint) every 15 minutes. This simple solution replaces bodily fluid reserves faster than ordinary water can. In fact, it has saved millions of lives since it was discovered in 1974 when it was hailed by *The Lancet* as 'one of the greatest medical breakthroughs of the 20th century'. The solution is also useful during endurance exercise such as marathon running or distance cycling.

As soon as you feel like eating – but preferably not within the first 24 hours – follow a diet of bananas, boiled rice, apples and white toast (known as the 'brat' diet). The bananas provide potassium, which is vital for controlling the body's fluid balance; and boiled white rice and white toast provide low-fibre carbohydrate that will not irritate the bowel. Naturopaths believe that apples have a cleansing action on the digestive system.

Eat small amounts of these foods at regular intervals and after 48 hours introduce boiled potatoes, cooked vegetables and eggs. If the symptoms begin to subside, you can gradually go back to a normal diet, leaving milk and other dairy products until last.

Herbal teas can help to replace lost fluids, and some have a soothing effect on the digestive tract. Try two cups a day of raspberry-leaf tea (except in early pregnancy) or up to three cups a day of ginger tea, sipped slowly. Avoid caffeine and alcohol for at least 48 hours after an attack of diarrhoea; both can have a dehydrating effect as they stimulate the kidneys to increase the output of urine.

Diarrhoea can be either acute – short-lived – or chronic and recurrent. Chronic diarrhoea may be a sign of a serious illness and a doctor should be consulted. Acute diarrhoea may be caused by overindulgence in laxative foods such

Travellers' diarrhoea

Diarrhoea is one of several factors that can affect TRAVELLERS' HEALTH in many parts of the developing world, such as most of Asia, Africa, Central and South America. Southern Europe, the Caribbean, Russia and Japan are moderate risk areas; western Europe, North America and Australia carry the least risk.

If hygiene is doubtful, avoid raw fruit and salads. Drink bottled or boiled water, and do not put ice in drinks unless you are sure of its source. Avoid cold buffets as these are a haven for bacteria and germ-carrying flies. Never eat undercooked meat or poultry, and beware of raw fish and shellfish.

Case study

After two weeks of persistent, mild diarrhoea, Don, a merchant banker, decided to visit his doctor. He felt bloated and had noticed that his symptoms were worse when he drank milk or food containing it. Careful questioning showed that the diarrhoea had started after Don had returned from a business trip to St Petersburg. With this in mind the laboratory searched for and found cysts of the parasite Giardia lamblia. *The doctor explained that other cases of giardiasis had been reported among visitors to St Petersburg and that* Giardia lamblia *was presumed to be in the water supply. Don was treated with antibiotics and his diarrhoea quickly cleared up. Don was told that when the gut has become inflamed it can be intolerant of lactose (a sugar found in milk and milk products), and he was warned that if his symptoms recurred he should follow a low-lactose diet, avoid spicy food and cut down on alcohol. He was also advised in future to drink boiled or bottled water when visiting a foreign country.*

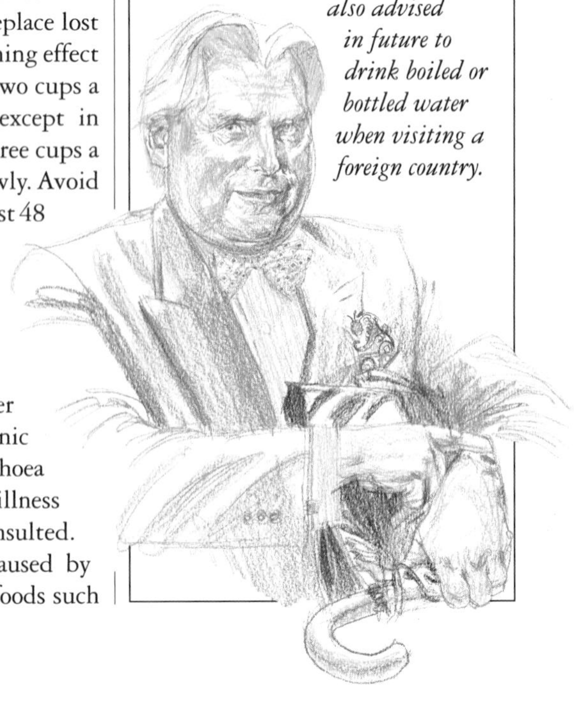

as figs, bran, prunes or dried fruits, but it is far more commonly the result of a food-borne infection. When it is caused by FOOD POISONING, diarrhoea may last anything from 6 hours to three days. Diarrhoea can be life-threatening to very young children and also to the elderly as a result of the dehydration it causes. In these instances, medical advice should be sought as soon as possible.

DIETS AND SLIMMING

See page 132

DIGESTION AND DIGESTIVE PROBLEMS

See page 136

DIURETICS

EAT PLENTY OF
- *Fruit, especially bananas, and vegetables, for their potassium*

CUT DOWN ON
- *Salt*

AVOID
- *Salted and pickled foods*

Drugs that encourage the elimination of water and salt from the body are called diuretics. Natural diuretics include caffeine, parsley, asparagus, celery and dandelion leaves – nicknamed as 'wet-the-bed' in parts of England and *pissenlit* in France.

Diuretics are prescribed specifically to lower BLOOD PRESSURE and to treat heart failure and other severe conditions. They reduce fluid and salt in the body and alleviate the symptoms of oedema – fluid retention, usually in the feet and ankles. The effects can be dramatic, with swollen feet and hands visibly regaining their normal shape.

Unfortunately, many diuretics also stimulate calcium excretion and may promote mineral loss from the bones. They may also cause excessive amounts of potassium to be lost in the urine. Low levels of potassium in the blood can produce unpleasant side effects, including appetite loss, constipation, weak muscles, memory loss and confusion. More seriously, potassium deficiency can interfere with the normal functioning of the heart.

If you are taking diuretics, it is important to eat plenty of food sources of potassium, unless your doctor advises you against doing so. Bananas and potatoes are both good sources of the mineral. Dandelion leaves, eaten in salads or used like spinach, offer the double bonus of being diuretic and a source of potassium.

Because one of the functions of a diuretic is to eliminate salt, eating salty foods is counterproductive. Use less salt in cooking and at the table, and avoid smoked foods such as bacon, tinned or dried soups, stock cubes and other foods with high levels of additives based on SALT AND SODIUM.

DIVERTICULITIS

TAKE PLENTY OF
- *Fresh fruit and vegetables*
- *Wholemeal bread, porridge and brown rice*
- *Water*

CUT DOWN ON
- *Refined carbohydrates, such as biscuits, cakes and sweets*

The inadequate amount of fibre eaten in the West has meant that increasing numbers of people are suffering from disorders such as CONSTIPATION, HAEMORRHOIDS and diverticular disease. The latter is extremely common among people in late middle-age and the elderly; women are particularly susceptible. Acute episodes of diverticulitis can be treated in hospital with antibiotics and intravenous fluids.

The condition arises as a result of a build-up of pressure in the large bowel which causes weakened areas of the bowel wall to balloon outwards, forming sac-like diverticula. If these sacs become infected and inflamed, the condition is called diverticulitis.

Soothing herbs

People with diverticulitis may find some relief from their symptoms by drinking a cup of peppermint or camomile tea after meals to soothe local irritation or inflammation. Both have traditionally been used by herbalists to treat digestive problems, but peppermint in particular is believed to relax intestinal muscles, thereby relieving any pain.

A HIGH-FIBRE DIET

A diet high in vegetables and wholegrain cereals may help to prevent diverticular disease. In fact, the incidence of the disorder is about 30 per cent lower in vegetarians than in meat eaters. Cut down on refined foods and instead eat wholemeal bread, muesli or porridge daily, along with plenty of other fibre-rich foods, such as pulses, vegetables, fresh and dried fruit. Some studies have suggested that bran may exacerbate diverticular disease once it is established, so it is best to obtain your fibre from wholefoods.

With a high-fibre diet, drink plenty of water – at least 1.7 litres (3 pints) a day – to help the digested food pass easily through the system.

DIGESTION AND DIGESTIVE PROBLEMS

Most people experience indigestion occasionally, but others suffer from it day after day. Yet with a little attention to diet, most of the uncomfortable symptoms can be eased or eradicated altogether.

Even before you have taken the first taste of any food, its aroma triggers the digestive system. Then, with the additional spur of flavour, saliva moistens drier food and makes chewing easier while providing enzymes which begin to break down starch; food should always be chewed thoroughly. Once chewed, the food is carried through the oesophagus to the stomach, where acids and enzymes start to work on the protein content.

When the food has been reduced to a porridge-like consistency it moves through the small intestine, where digestive juices from the pancreas and gall bladder break down the protein further, as well as fats and carbohydrates. Absorption of nutrients occurs mainly in the small intestine, leaving waste matter to travel through the large intestine and out of the body. FIBRE and resistant starch are fermented in the large bowel and provide the bulk that helps to stimulate the muscles of the colon so that digested foods can be pushed through the gut. A daily fluid intake of at least 1.7 litres (3 pints) will help to prevent the dense mass of digested food in the colon from becoming dehydrated and difficult to move through the system.

An efficient digestive system is vital for good health. Without it, vitamins, minerals, trace elements, fats, proteins and carbohydrates cannot be absorbed by the body and used to build and maintain its cells.

The intestine has a remarkable ability to heal itself. It replaces its lining every 72 hours and reacts swiftly to expel harmful substances. However, a diet high in refined and nutritionally deficient foods, as found in a typical Western diet, can lead to problems. Common complaints range from FLATULENCE and INDIGESTION, to DIVERTICULITIS and PEPTIC ULCERS.

Indigestion is often the result of eating large meals quickly or late at night. If you suffer from indigestion at night, try spreading your eating more evenly through the day. Cut down on fatty foods which stimulate the output of acid in the gut. Too much alcohol also increases stomach acidity.

CONSTIPATION, flatulence and bad breath, often caused by fermented fibre, can also result from poor eating habits. Repeated attacks of severe pain, especially following heavy, fatty meals, may be a sign of gallstones. A bloated abdomen (due to distension of the intestine) or pain, especially in the lower left side of the abdomen, accompanied by wind and alternating diarrhoea and constipation, may be a sign of IRRITABLE BOWEL SYNDROME. Long-term alcohol abuse can result in GASTRITIS and ulcers.

COLITIS, particularly in the form of CROHN'S DISEASE, reduces the amount of nutrients absorbed during digestion. Colitis sufferers are advised to eat a diet rich in soluble fibre. Foods such as bran that contain a lot of insoluble fibre are not fully digested in the small intestine and are best avoided.

Ulcers, heartburn and indigestion can often be eased by taking antacid remedies which act to neutralise the acid in the stomach. However, antacids often include aluminium hydroxide and their prolonged use can inhibit the absorption of phosphorus.

EAT PLENTY OF
- *Fresh fruit*
- *Vegetables and vegetable juices*
- *Herbs and certain spices*

DRINK
- *At least 1.7 litres (3 pints) of water daily*

CUT DOWN ON
- *Refined carbohydrates*
- *Deep-fried foods and other foods with a high fat content*
- *Alcohol*

HEALING HERBS

Herbs and some spices may help a troubled gut by easing flatulence and colic. Most of the HERBS AND SPICES that are traditionally used in cooking aid digestion, so use plenty of mint, dill, caraway, horseradish, bay, chervil, fennel tarragon, marjoram, cumin, cinnamon, ginger and cardamom. Camomile tea may also help.

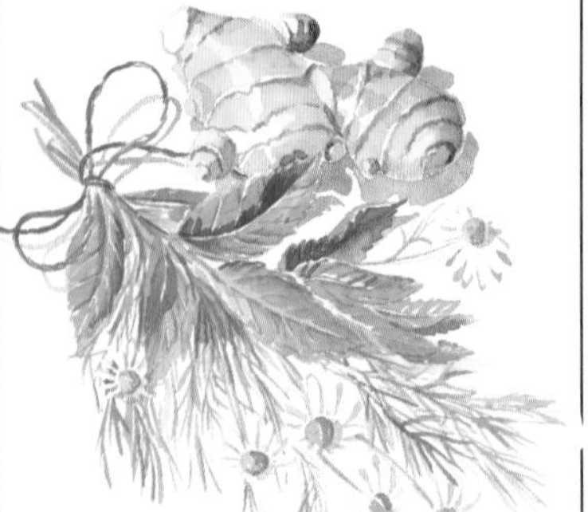

If you often suffer from indigestion or if you suspect that you have an ulcer, you should consult your doctor.

Some people have specific food intolerances and allergies. The most common intolerance, which affects 5 per cent of adults in western Europe, is an inability to digest the sugar lactose found in milk and dairy products. COELIAC DISEASE – an intolerance of gluten, which is found in wheat and some cereals – is also on the increase.

Case study

Margot enjoyed the dinners she attended with her Rotarian husband. Unfortunately, she often felt bloated after the meals, and would develop embarrassing wind and burning pains that travelled from her stomach to her chest. She attributed this to her hiatus hernia. Margot's doctor advised her to lose weight, eat smaller meals and avoid fatty food and alcohol. This she did and the bouts of indigestion became less frequent. Margot soon began to enjoy after-dinner socialising at the Rotary dinners as well as the food.

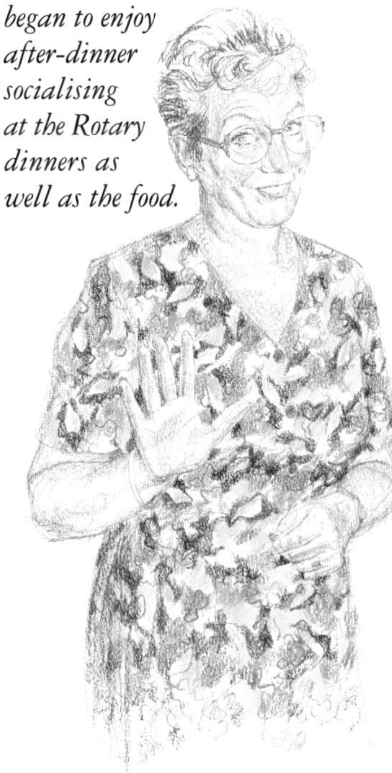

Calming a troublesome gut

In the vast majority of cases, digestive problems can be eased simply by watching what you eat. However, if the disorder is severe or does not respond to the changed diet after more than a few days, consult your doctor.

FOODS TO AVOID	FOODS TO EAT
COELIAC DISEASE	
Wheat and cereals which contain gluten, flour products, tinned foods that flour may have been used to thicken, and beer.	Fresh fruit and vegetables, pulses, nuts, poultry, cheese, rice and potatoes. 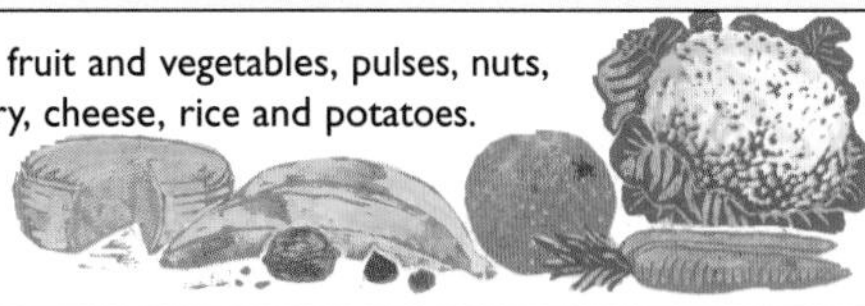
COLITIS (INCLUDING CROHN'S DISEASE)	
Wheat bran, nuts, seeds, sweetcorn and all foods known to contain substances to which you are susceptible.	Porridge, apples, dried fruit, oily fish, liver, parsley, lentils and watercress. People with Crohn's disease often require extra zinc, calcium, magnesium, B vitamins and vitamins C and K. 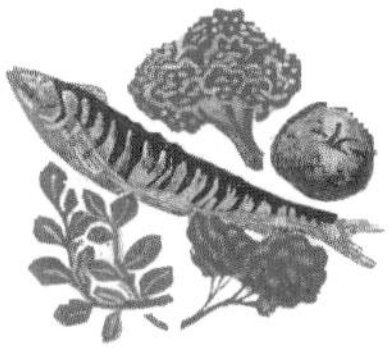
DIVERTICULAR DISEASE	
Refined carbohydrates: replace them with wholegrain types.	 Plenty of cooked green leafy vegetables, porridge and apples, wholemeal bread, brown rice and other wholegrain cereals.
FLATULENCE	
Gradually cut down on pulses – such as peas, beans and lentils – Brussels sprouts and cabbage.	Plenty of live yoghurt, peppermint and fennel teas, herbs such as thyme, sage, caraway and fennel seeds, which help digestion. 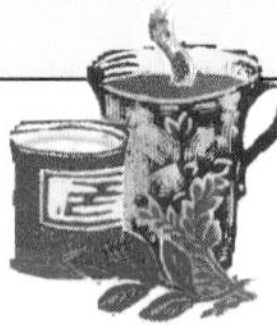
GASTROENTERITIS	
For the first 48 hours of the illness, avoid foods not listed opposite.	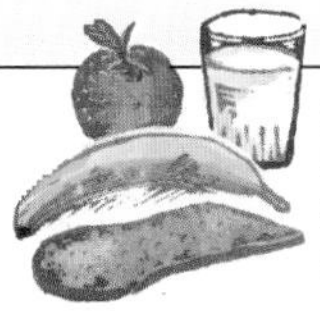 Bananas, apples, boiled white rice and dry white toast. Plenty of water to replace lost fluids. Camomile tea may also help.
INDIGESTION	
All acid foods (particularly those made with vinegar), raw onions, chillies, fatty or fried foods, coffee and alcohol.	Fibre-rich foods such as wholemeal bread, brown rice and vegetables. Angostura bitters, or beer made from hops, half an hour before a meal stimulate digestive juices. 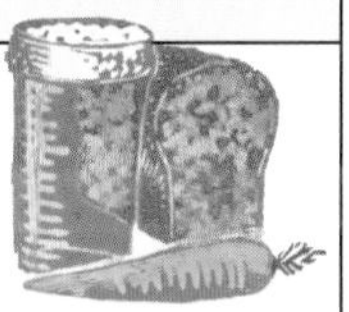
IRRITABLE BOWEL SYNDROME	
Wheat bran, pulses and any foods to which you have an allergy or intolerance.	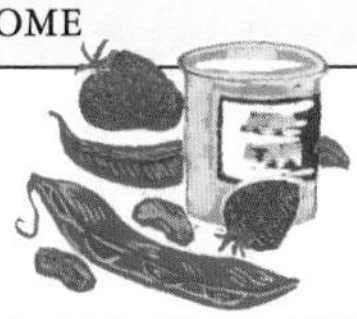 Plenty of fruit and vegetables for their soluble fibre, and live natural yoghurt for the beneficial bacteria it contains.

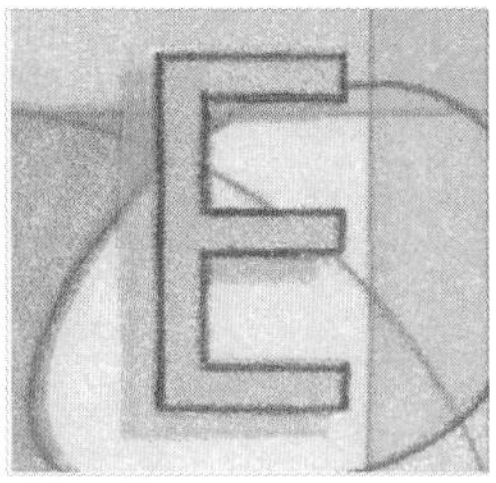

EAR DISORDERS AND HEARING PROBLEMS

EAT PLENTY OF

- *Garlic, onions and chilli peppers when mucus is a problem*

CUT DOWN ON

- *Foods high in saturated fats, which may contribute to deafness*

The ears are responsible for your hearing and sense of balance – they prevent you from falling over. These sensitive organs are a triumph of miniaturisation: the inner ear, although no bigger than a hazelnut, contains as many circuits as the telephone system of an average city. But the ears are easily damaged and if they become infected a great deal of pain in the ear or face can result. Ear problems should never be ignored. Whether you experience dizziness, impaired hearing or pain, consult your doctor promptly.

EARACHE

Usually, earache is due to an infection triggered by CATARRH. Glue ear is the result of a build-up of sticky mucus behind the eardrum, and it mainly affects young children. Now, a possible link has been discovered with bottle-feeding. When a child is breastfed, the action of sucking on the breast exercises a muscle that helps to open the Eustachian tube, which connects the middle ear to the back of the throat and drains away any fluid. In bottle-feeding the teat does not reach as far into the mouth, and the muscle is not exercised in the same way.

DEAFNESS

There are two main kinds of deafness: conductive deafness is usually curable and is due to something hindering the transmission of sounds to the inner ear; nerve deafness occurs when the auditory nerve is damaged.

One form of nerve deafness may be triggered by an excessive intake of saturated fats in the diet, which tends to promote ATHEROSCLEROSIS in the tiny blood vessels of the ear, causing a blockage. Several studies have suggested that low-fat diets are associated with better hearing, and that many patients with hearing problems have either raised blood cholesterol levels, or are obese – or both. Consequently it makes sense to maintain a healthy weight and to avoid foods that are high in saturated fats – such as butter, fried foods and fatty red meats – which raise blood cholesterol levels.

Naturopaths believe that diet can affect the functioning of the ears and may recommend foods rich in vitamin A and thiamin, thought to help repair damaged cell tissue in the ear and to strengthen the auditory nerve. Vitamin A is found in liver and as beta carotene in apricots, carrots, mangoes and spinach, while wholemeal bread contains thiamin. You may be advised to avoid dairy products and to eat garlic, onions, horseradish and chilli peppers to reduce mucus production, although there is no scientific proof that such measures will be effective.

Aeroplane ear

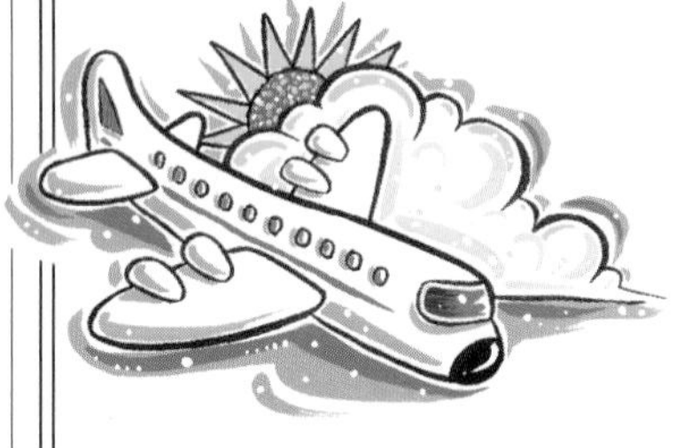

An uncomfortable sensation of tightness in the ears experienced during or after flying in an aircraft can be relieved by sucking or chewing something, particularly during take-off and landing. The sensation can be relieved by holding the nose, shutting the mouth and trying to blow until there is a popping sound and pressure is released. Temporary deafness after a flight is quite common and will usually wear off within 48 hours.

ECZEMA

AVOID

- *Any foods that exacerbate or trigger your eczema, such as milk and eggs*
- *Touching materials or foods known to cause contact dermatitis*

There is some evidence to suggest that eczema is linked to a food allergy in up to half of reported cases, or even more where the sufferers are children; the main culprits are thought to be milk and eggs. However, other potential links between this skin ailment and diet have yet to be proved.

There are two types of eczema: contact eczema, which is more commonly known as contact dermatitis, and atopic eczema. Contact eczema develops on people whose skin is sensitive to particular irritants, such as wool or nylon clothing, metal, make-up, detergents, various chemicals or sunlight; food irritants include raw fish, garlic and onions. Atopic eczema often affects people with a family history of asthma, hay fever or hives (also known as urticaria or nettle rash). Eczema in

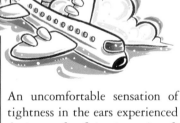

Case study

Nasreen, a pretty four-year-old girl, had been irritated for several months by an itchy rash on her wrists. When the rash spread to her face her mother became distraught with worry. She confided in her mother-in-law who was convinced that Nasreen's rash was due 'to something she eats'. When presented with the child, the doctor was sceptical but under the grandmother's insistence agreed to ask a dietician to advise the family about an exclusion diet. Initially, Nasreen was kept off milk for six weeks, with no success. When eggs were excluded from her diet, however, Nasreen's eczema improved dramatically – to the surprise of the doctor and delight of her family.

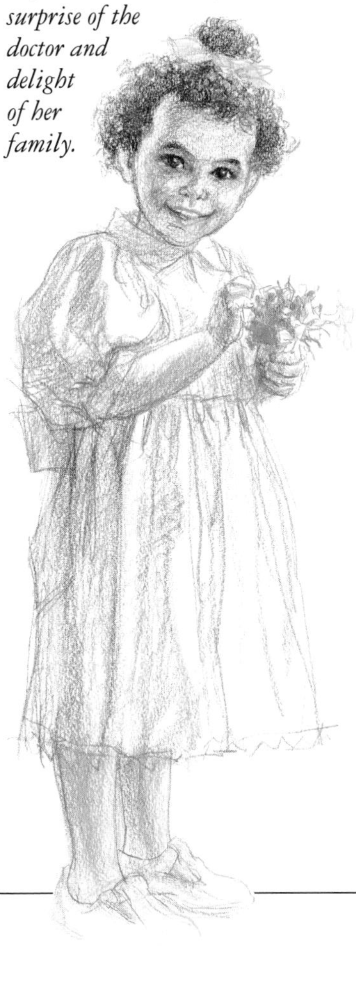

babies and small children is often atopic; fortunately, many children do eventually grow out of it.

In both types of eczema, the symptoms include redness of the skin, severe itching, pinhead-sized blisters that may weep, and dry, flaking skin. Anybody with eczema should consult a doctor, who may prescribe skin creams or ointments.

ECZEMA AND ALLERGIES

The importance of the link between eczema and allergies is still the subject of fierce debate. Apart from eggs, milk and other dairy produce, suspect foods include fish, shellfish, wheat, tomatoes, nuts, soya products, yeast and certain additives. If you eliminate such foods completely from your diet for two weeks and the condition improves, it suggests that a food might be contributing to the problem. Reintroduce the 'banned' foods slowly, one by one, and if the eczema returns, there is a good chance that you have found the food which contains the allergen triggering your dermatitis.

Some babies develop eczema when their mother stops breastfeeding and starts to give formula milk, which may indicate an intolerance to cow's milk. If, however, a baby who is being breastfed develops eczema, the mother should consider consulting a dietician about her own diet since babies rarely react to the mother's milk itself.

SUPPLEMENTS MAY HELP

Evening primrose oil has been shown to help in some cases of eczema, according to studies quoted in *The Lancet*, but some experts still dispute this. Other studies have shown that fish-oil supplements give relief to atopic eczema. However, this does not mean that eating fish will have the same effect, since fish is also a relatively common trigger for allergic reactions. The possible link between eczema and zinc deficiency has also been examined but anecdotal evidence of eczema sufferers being successfully treated with zinc supplements has not been backed up by scientific studies.

CABBAGE POULTICE

Although there is no scientific evidence to support the claim, traditional medicine has long held that fresh green cabbage leaves (especially Savoy cabbage) can help to relieve eczema. Wash, pound and warm the leaves, then use a bandage to hold several layers of them in place on the affected areas every morning and night.

Chinese herbs

Medicinal plants from China have, in recent years, gained a reputation for successfully treating atopic eczema. In particular, people with severe, widespread, very dry atopic eczema often find Chinese herbs succeed where orthodox medicine has failed.

The National Eczema Society advises that patients have liver function tests and a full blood count before beginning treatment, and thereafter at regular intervals. The 'tea' is made by boiling Chinese herbs in water for half an hour or more to make a decoction. This is taken for several months, during which time the patient's progress is monitored by the practitioner, who will make any necessary alterations to the formula. One drawback is that the tea has a very pungent and bitter flavour.

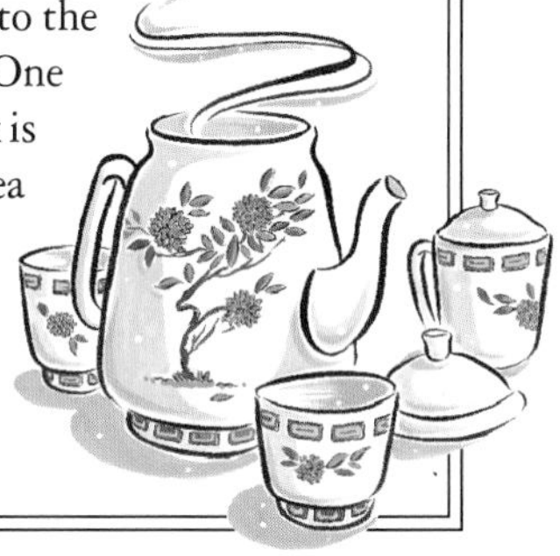

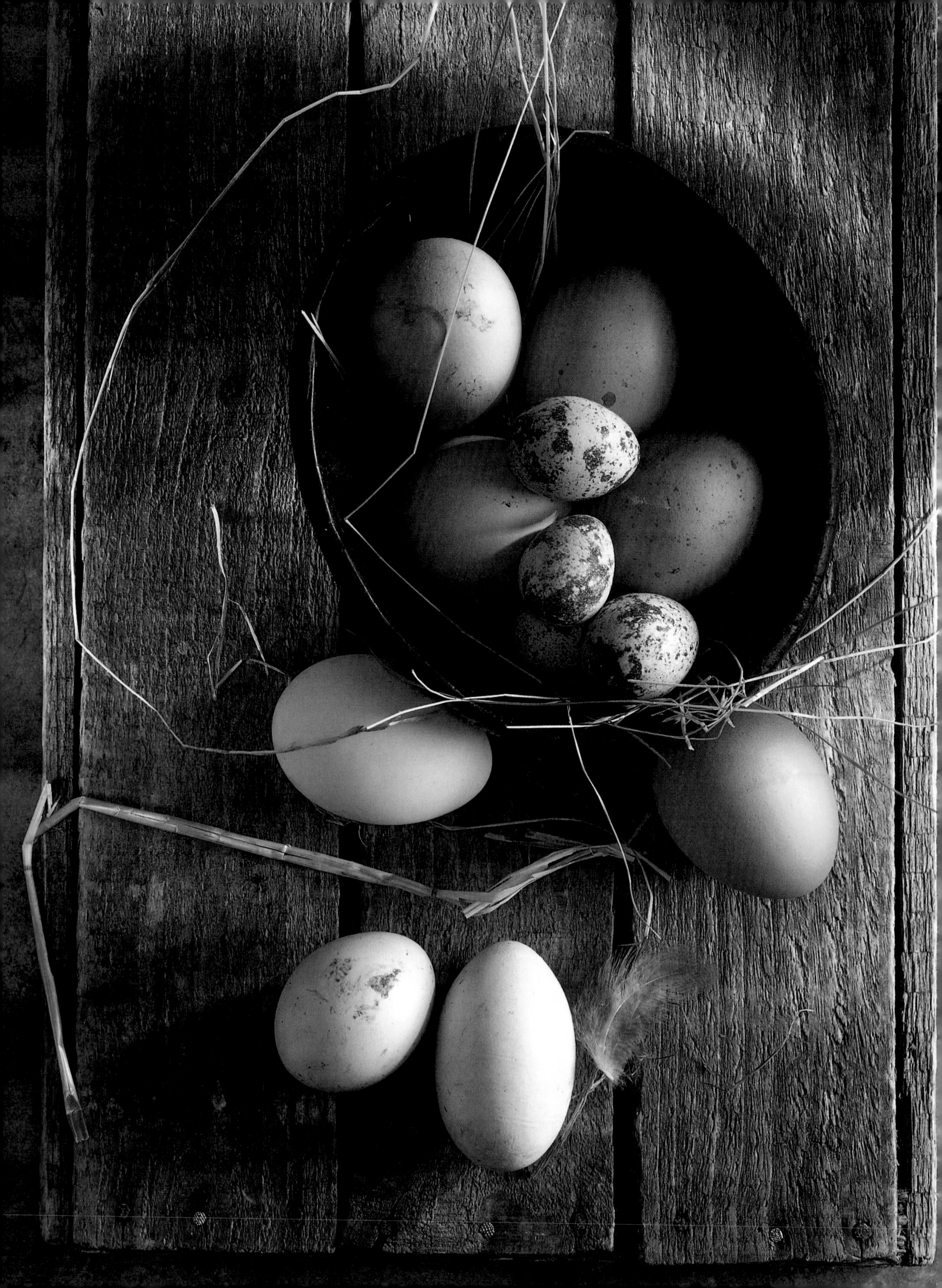

EGGS

BENEFITS

- *Excellent source of vitamin B_{12}*
- *Convenient source of protein*
- *Rich in vitamins and minerals*

DRAWBACKS

- *High cholesterol content*
- *A common cause of food allergy*
- *Risk of salmonella poisoning if not thoroughly cooked*

An egg is designed by nature to provide protein, vitamins and minerals for the developing chick. Despite widely publicised concern over cholesterol and salmonella, eggs remain a popular and inexpensive source of nourishment. Cooking does not alter their nutrient content significantly.

Eggs supply a multiplicity of vitamins and minerals. In particular, they are an excellent source of vitamin B_{12}, which is vital for the nervous system, and are an important source of this vitamin for vegetarians.

The lecithin in egg yolks is also rich in choline, which is involved in the transport of cholesterol in the bloodstream and in fat metabolism. It is also an essential component of cell membranes and nervous tissue. Even though the body is able to make enough choline for its normal needs, it has been reported that additional amounts provided by the diet may be helpful in treating the accumulation of fat in the liver, as well as certain types of neurological damage.

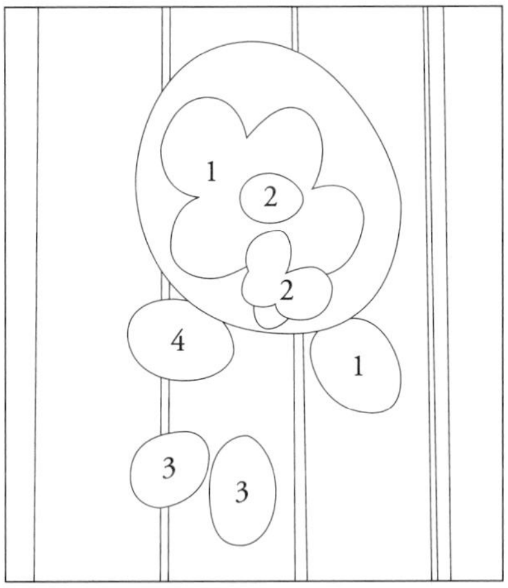

NUTRIENTS IN A SHELL *Eggs are a source of nourishment throughout the world. Those that are most readily available in Britain include eggs from hens (1), quails (2), bantams (3) and ducks (4).*

CHOLESTEROL CONCERN

How many eggs is it safe to eat before the CHOLESTEROL contained in their yolks becomes a problem? The British Heart Foundation recommends eating no more than four eggs a week; the World Health Organisation, however, suggests an upper limit of ten eggs per week from all sources, such as mayonnaise, biscuits, cakes and mousses.

A large egg contains 6-8g of protein and 5-7g of fat, of which less than 2g is saturated. A single egg yolk provides about 448mg of cholesterol. In Britain, the average daily cholesterol intake is 390mg for men, and 290mg for women. In fact, the greater health concern is not dietary cholesterol but excessive blood cholesterol manufactured by the liver from saturated fats. Consequently, the relatively high cholesterol content of eggs is only of concern to people who already have raised blood cholesterol levels.

CONFUSING EGG LABELS

Labels such as 'farm' or 'country fresh' can conjure up misleading images; the hens that laid them may well have been raised in batteries. The term 'free range' may suggest chickens pecking freely in a farmyard, but by law it can be applied to the eggs of any battery hens with daytime access to open runs.

The tags 'barn' or 'perchery' eggs can be similarly misleading. These are often laid by hens held in coops slightly less cramped than batteries, but without access to open-air runs. Whatever the labelling, always reject any eggs that have cracked or blemished shells. It is a myth that brown eggs are better for you than white – both are equally nutritious.

Eggs should be stored in the main part of the refrigerator rather than in the fridge door. Keep them in a bowl so that air can circulate freely, or, if they have not been date-stamped, in their original box so that you know how old they are. Store them with the pointed end down, so that the yolk remains centred in the egg away from the air pocket at the large end of the egg. They will keep for up to three weeks.

The salmonella scare

Only one egg in every 7000 harbours salmonella bacteria (which are passed on by the hen and are not due to unhygienic living conditions). Nevertheless, Britain's Department of Health recommends that you avoid eating raw eggs in any form, and also warns of the risk of salmonella poisoning posed by partly cooked eggs; the elderly, the sick, young children, pregnant women, people with AIDS and others whose immunity has been compromised by illness, are particularly vulnerable.

Caesar salads, fresh mayonnaise, egg-based sauces and mousses can all contain raw eggs. Eggs must be cooked properly to destroy bacteria. To be absolutely certain, you should boil eggs for at least 7 minutes, poach them for 5 minutes, and fry eggs for 3 minutes on each side. Both the yolk and the white should be firm. Omelettes and scrambled eggs should be cooked until dry. Duck eggs must be cooked for at least 5 minutes, and should be used in baking rather than eaten boiled or poached.

Emphysema

EAT PLENTY OF

- *Foods that provide vitamin C, such as citrus fruits and blackcurrants*
- *Sources of beta carotene, such as carrots, apricots and spinach*
- *Foods that supply vitamin E, such as wholegrain cereals and sunflower oil*

AVOID

- *Smoking*

Heavy smokers and people living or working in polluted atmospheres are at risk from this progressive and incurable disease of the lungs.

For smokers, the best way to prevent emphysema is to give up immediately, but if you cannot, make sure that your diet is rich in the ANTIOXIDANT nutrients. These include vitamin C (found in fresh fruit, especially citrus fruits and blackcurrants); vitamin E (found in wholegrain cereals, wheatgerm, nuts and seeds) and beta carotene (found in carrots, apricots, mangoes, spinach and broccoli).

Antioxidant vitamins neutralise FREE RADICALS, which can damage living cells and cause degenerative diseases. Although free radicals are always present in the body, their numbers are increased by air pollution and the smoke from cigarettes.

Emphysema occurs when tiny air sacs in the lungs become inflamed, and the walls between them rupture, forming large, scarred sacs. This causes lung stiffness, and a reduction in the area of the lungs through which oxygen can be absorbed. More effort is then needed for the lungs to expand, which puts a strain on the heart pumping blood into the lungs. Even the slightest exertion – such as walking across a room – increases the work rate of the heart to deliver enough oxygen. In the majority of cases, the added strain eventually leads to heart failure.

Energy, Exercise and Vitality

See page 144

Epilepsy

TAKE PLENTY OF

- *Pulses and meat to supply vitamin B_6, zinc and magnesium*
- *Calcium-rich dairy produce, especially milk that has been fortified with vitamin D*
- *Rice, wholemeal bread, pineapple, blackberries and figs, for manganese*

AVOID

- *Excessive amounts of alcohol*
- *Evening primrose oil*

One in every two hundred Britons has epilepsy, a disorder triggered by imbalances in the brain's electrical impulses. Epilepsy may be caused by brain damage resulting from injury before, during or after birth, by a tumour, a childhood fever, or by an infection. It is sometimes hereditary, but occasionally no cause can be found. A lack of vitamins appears to spark some epileptic attacks, which has prompted doctors to look more closely at the possibility of treating the ailment through diet.

Epileptic seizures vary in intensity and their frequency ranges from brief spells of memory and concentration loss known as absences (previously called *petit mal*) to convulsions that may occur several times a day. Stress, tiredness, too much alcohol, a bout of fever, and menstruation are all potential triggers of an attack.

Drugs are used to treat all forms of epilepsy. In fact, medication keeps 80 per cent of people with epilepsy free from seizures. However, because some of the drugs can have harmful side effects, there is growing support among doctors for drug therapy to be used in conjunction with dietary methods in the control of epilepsy.

Some studies show that in rare cases a lack of vitamins B_6 and D can prompt epileptic attacks. Vitamin B_6 is supplied by meat, whole grains and pulses. Vitamin D is found in most oily fish and some animal products, particularly in cheese and fortified milk. Anyone suffering from epilepsy should take vitamin supplements only under medical supervision.

Certain minerals also appear to help some individuals. Magnesium (abundant in wholemeal flour, millet, figs, meat, fish, nuts and pulses); zinc (in meat and offal, wheatgerm, nuts, crab, oysters and lentils); and calcium (mainly found in milk and milk products) have all been found to help to prevent convulsions in some people.

While it is still highly controversial, preliminary evidence suggests that there may be a link between congenital seizures and a deficiency of the trace mineral manganese in the mother's diet. Good sources of manganese include rice, wholemeal bread, wheatgerm, buckwheat, lima beans, nuts, cockles, sardines, blackberries, figs and pineapple.

In a small number of cases, nutritional deficiencies and low blood sugar have been implicated in epileptic seizures. People with epilepsy should therefore maintain their blood sugar levels by eating normal, well-balanced meals at regular intervals.

Mixed salads and raw fruit are said by some alternative practitioners to be particularly effective in reducing the number and intensity of attacks.

Excess alcohol consumption may precipitate an attack in some susceptible people with epilepsy. Evening primrose oil has also been found to trigger attacks in some individuals, and for this reason is best avoided.

EYE DISORDERS

EAT PLENTY OF

- *Carrots, sweet potatoes and dark green vegetables, for beta carotene*
- *Fruit and vegetables for vitamin C*
- *Seafood and wheatgerm for zinc*
- *Lean meat, poultry, fish, nuts, whole grains, seeds and green vegetables for their B vitamins*
- *Seed oils and avocados for vitamin E*

A healthy, balanced diet has a role to play in maintaining good eyesight, with vitamin A holding the key to many eye disorders. Beta carotene, which the body converts to vitamin A, is found in yellow and orange-coloured fruit and vegetables (apricots, mangoes, carrots, sweet potatoes and squashes) and in dark green, leafy vegetables such as spinach and kale.

In the developing world, vitamin A deficiency is the most common cause of blindness in people under the age of 21. The first sign of this deficiency is usually night blindness – an inability to adapt to low light intensity.

MACULAR DEGENERATION

Caused by the deterioration of part of the retina, macular degeneration is a major cause of blindness in the elderly. One of the major risk factors is prolonged exposure to bright light, and this has led to the view that damage to the retina is caused by FREE RADICALS.

As vitamin E and beta carotene are believed to protect against free radical damage, research has focused on diet and foods rich in these two nutrients.

A study at Harvard Medical School found that the degree of degeneration was correspondingly less in those who had a higher consumption of dark green vegetables which contain beta carotene. Scientists speculate that lutein and zeaxanthin, two 'relatives' of beta carotene, build up in the retina. There, they filter out the rays at either end of the light spectrum that cause damage over many years, thereby making the eye less vulnerable.

Certain vitamins and minerals have been claimed to help to retard macular degeneration: eat plenty of fresh fruit and vegetables for vitamin C; wheatgerm, seafood and pulses for zinc; lean meat, poultry, fish, nuts, whole grains and green vegetables for B vitamins; and include cold-pressed seed oils and avocados for vitamin E. Bioflavonoids, which are found in the pith of citrus fruits, may also help.

CONJUNCTIVITIS

The delicate membrane covering the front of the eye can become inflamed as the result of an infection or an allergy, producing the condition known as conjunctivitis or 'pink eye'.

If the redness forms a ring around the front of the eye, it may be due to a deficiency of riboflavin. Soreness and a reddening and cracking at the outer corners of the eyes may also signal a lack of this B vitamin, which is found in milk, whole grains and offal.

GLAUCOMA

A build-up of fluid pressure in the eye is known as glaucoma. It is most common among people aged 40 or over and tends to run in families. Symptoms include blurred vision, a halo effect around lights and difficulty seeing in the dark. Glaucoma has been linked with a deficiency of thiamin, found in meat, fish, poultry, whole grains, pulses and nuts, and of vitamin A, abundant in liver and eggs, and also derived from orange-coloured plant foods that contain beta carotene. Seek medical attention immediately if any of the above symptoms appear.

CATARACTS

This painless clouding of the lens of the eye is most common among the elderly, but can occur in younger people because of a rare metabolic defect. It is believed that cataracts are the result of oxidation occurring in the lens of the eye, and vitamin C may help to protect against this type of damage. Other studies indicate that riboflavin, found in milk, wholegrain cereals and yeast extract, may also offer some protection. The ability of the eye to metabolise a sugar called galactose appears to decrease as we grow older. This, combined with a high level of galactose in the blood, which occurs in the inherited condition known as galactosaemia, may also trigger the formation of cataracts.

OTHER EYE PROBLEMS

Diabetics are prone to a condition in which the capillaries in the retina leak fluid or break. This is a major cause of blindness. Supplements of vitamin C have been found to have some protective effect upon the blood vessels of diabetics, so it is possible that a high intake of vitamin C, from fresh fruit and vegetables, may be helpful. Good overall control of diabetes appears to result in fewer eye complications.

Styes – small red boils on the glands that lubricate the eyelashes – are caused by bacteria and usually come to a head and heal in a few days. Recurring styes may be a sign of poor nutrition, stress or of being run-down.

Night sight

Were you told as a child to eat your carrots, because they would make you see better in the dark? This is more than merely an old wives' tale. Night blindness, or poor vision in the dark, is usually a sign of a deficiency of vitamin A, which carrots can help to replace. This is because carrots are an excellent source of beta carotene, which the body converts into vitamin A.

Energy, Exercise and Vitality

Plenty of rest, the right foods, fresh air and regular exercise can add years to your life, lift the spirits and help to protect against illness and the pressures of modern life.

All the energy people need comes from food; it is burned by the body, and is measured in calories. Vitality is a feeling of well-being that enables you to sail through a busy day and yet have energy to spare at the end of it. To achieve this good-to-be-alive feeling, you need to insure that you eat high-energy, low-fat foods, take regular exercise and allow yourself time to unwind and recharge your batteries.

Starch for stamina

Carbohydrates – the starches and sugars which are abundant in plant foods such as fruit, vegetables, pulses and cereals – are excellent foods for physical energy.

Although fat and, to a lesser extent, protein also supply fuel for the body, most energy needs are met by carbohydrates because many of them break down easily into glucose – the most accessible source of energy for the body. In Britain, the Department of Health believes that the right mixture of nutrients for energy is at least 50 per cent from carbohydrates (most of which should be starch, not added sugars), less than 35 per cent fat and 10 to 15 per cent protein.

When sugars are eaten in the form of foods such as fruit, they provide energy along with valuable vitamins, minerals and fibre. Table sugar, however, provides energy but no nutrients, which is why it is said to contain 'empty calories'. It is healthier to obtain your sugar from fruit and fruit juice. Starchy foods, for example pasta, rice, potatoes and bread, are well known energy boosters. Many athletes eat a lot of complex carbohydrates, such as pasta, while training and in the run-up to a competition in order to build up their body's energy stores.

However, the body absorbs different carbohydrates at different rates, depending upon how quickly they release sugar into the bloodstream. For a quick spurt of energy, eat bananas, dates, raisins, dried apricots, bread, rice, cornflakes, wheat-based cereals or muesli made with flaked wheat. For a steadier stream of energy, try eating plenty of baked beans, lentils, porridge oats, oatmeal biscuits, muesli made with oats or cracked wheat, peas, pasta, potatoes and apples which are all digested more slowly.

Eating little and often

Some nutritionists believe that 'grazing' on small snacks throughout the day can help to keep energy flowing. If you do not have time for three meals a day, it is better to eat little and often: breakfast followed by a mid-morning snack, a light lunch, a mid-afternoon snack and then a light supper. Do not starve yourself for most of the day and then eat a large meal late at night as this may encourage weight gain.

EAT PLENTY OF
- *Quick-boost snacks such as bananas, dates, raisins and dried apricots*
- *Starchy foods such as pasta, brown rice, potatoes and wholemeal bread, for a steady stream of energy*
- *Fruit and vegetables*

CUT DOWN ON
- *Sugary foods that contain hardly any nutrients*
- *Alcohol and caffeine drinks*

Feeling alert

Because food affects the chemistry of the brain, eating the right foods at the right time of day can make a difference to your mental alertness. While a meal that is rich in starch can improve your physical endurance, it can also have a calming, sedative effect on the brain, which is why you often feel sleepy after a lunch based on pasta or potatoes. It is a good idea to eat carbohydrate food in the evening to help you to relax and promote a good night's sleep.

Recent research in the USA has focused on the controversial theory that protein foods stimulate brain activity by encouraging the brain to produce its own form of chemical stimulant. A group of nutrition scientists has measured the brain's reactions to different types of food and now claims that people who eat a high-carbohydrate lunch are less alert following the meal than people who eat a small, high-protein lunch. However, research into the subject is continuing.

Stimulants

Caffeine is a stimulant found in coffee, tea and cola drinks. Coffee has excited much controversy, but one cup can improve alertness without doing any harm. However, if you need an hourly drink of coffee simply to keep going, you risk fatigue, anxiety, insomnia and shaking. Try to cut down on caffeine gradually, by spacing out your cups of coffee for longer and longer intervals; do not suddenly give it up entirely as withdrawal symptoms can include headaches, nausea, irritability and marked mood swings.

Slim, trim and fit

If you eat more food than your body uses up in energy, the surplus calories are stored as fat. The only sensible and effective way to lose weight is to combine a healthy low-fat diet with regular aerobic exercise such as walking, cycling or jogging. Aerobic exercise speeds up the breathing, raises the heart rate and helps to burn body fat. So if you are overweight, review your eating habits and try to take more

How to build your own exercise programme

The reason why exercise makes you feel wonderfully alive is because it triggers the release of endorphins – chemicals in the brain that make you feel generally happier, calmer and more clear-headed. The following tips will help you to build regular exercise into your life.

- Choose something that you will enjoy doing regularly for half an hour at least three times a week. It is much better to do a little exercise regularly than to make a big effort just once in a while.
- Whatever exercise you decide to do, always start gently and build up slowly and surely.
- Try to choose your activity so that it matches your particular fitness need. For example, try yoga for improving flexibility, weight training for strength, or brisk walking or swimming for endurance.
- Find physical activities that free the mind. Long-distance walking, cycling or swimming allow your mind to roam freely, while the ancient Chinese art of Tai chi is a form of moving meditation.
- If you are not sufficiently motivated to exercise alone, try training with a friend, taking part in a team game, or joining a group such as a ramblers' association.
- Try to choose more than one type of exercise. Variety will help to keep your exercise programme interesting and enable you to work on different parts of your body.

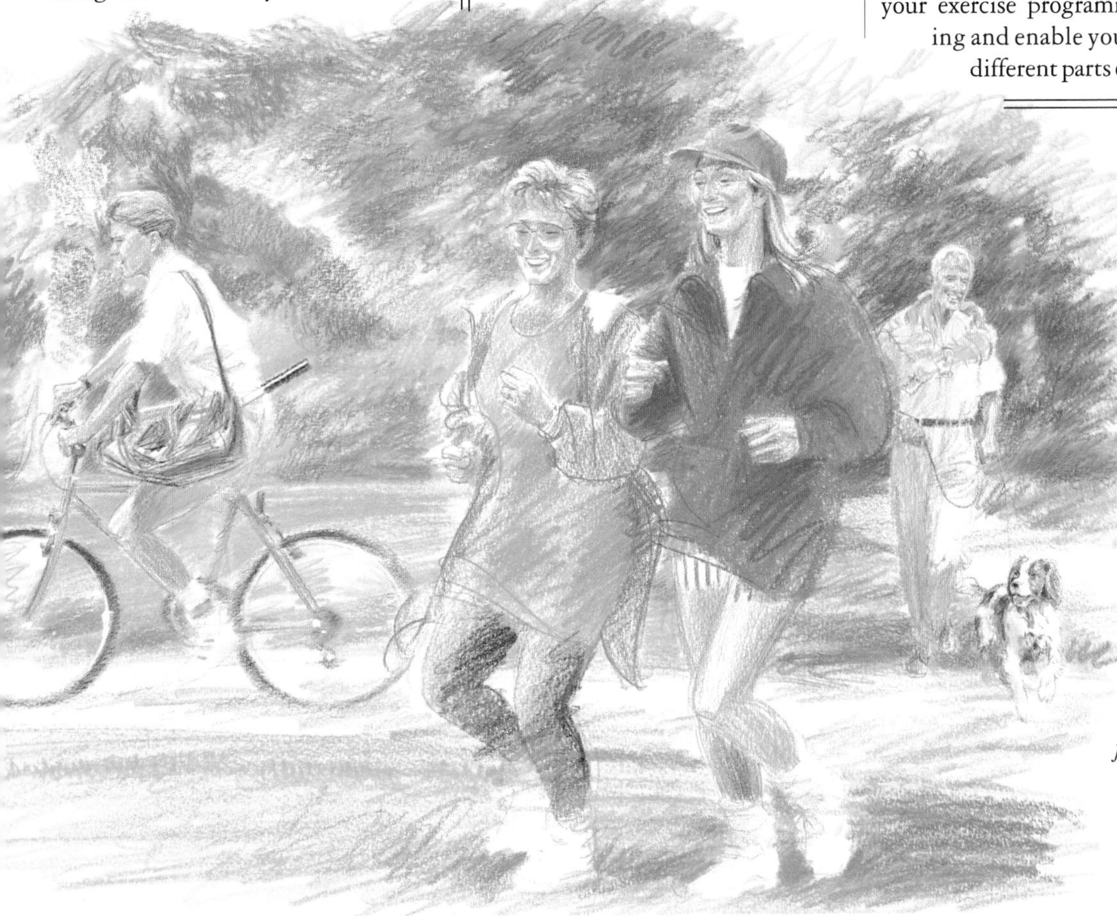

FIT FOR LIFE
No matter how fit you are now, exercise will help to boost energy levels and your sense of well-being.

Keeping energy levels high

Long hours spent working, a poor diet and not enough rest deplete the body's store of nutrients and cause fatigue. Knowing what will reinforce the benefits of your exercise programme – and what will undermine it – will help you to stay fit.

VITALITY ROBBERS

- **Alcohol** In excess, alcohol can interfere with the quality of your sleep. Stick to safe limits and have one or two alcohol-free days a week.
- **Smoking** Nicotine stimulates the brain initially, but then acts as a depressant. Smoking also increases the rate at which the liver uses up micronutrients, especially the B vitamins and vitamin C. It also makes extra work for the antioxidants that help to detoxify the body.
- **Anxiety and stress** Make a habit of doing something every day that takes your mind off your problems, whether it is exercise, meditation, listening to music or gardening. Do it until you feel relaxed.
- **Allergies** Fatigue can be the only symptom of an intolerance or allergy to particular foods, which may be worth considering as the cause of unexplained lethargy.

VITALITY BOOSTERS

- **Sleep** A good night's sleep, or a cat nap during the day will rest your mind and boost energy levels.
- **Breakfast** You will feel lethargic if you force your body to keep going all morning without any fuel. Eat a sustaining breakfast such as wholemeal toast, wholegrain cereal, porridge, or fresh fruit and yoghurt.
- **Fresh air** A bracing walk can do wonders when you are feeling tired.
- **Deep breathing** Bringing oxygen into your body is a good way to release tension and increase energy levels. Relax and breathe in through your nose and count to four. Breathe out through your mouth (keeping your jaw relaxed) and count to eight. Repeat until you are refreshed.

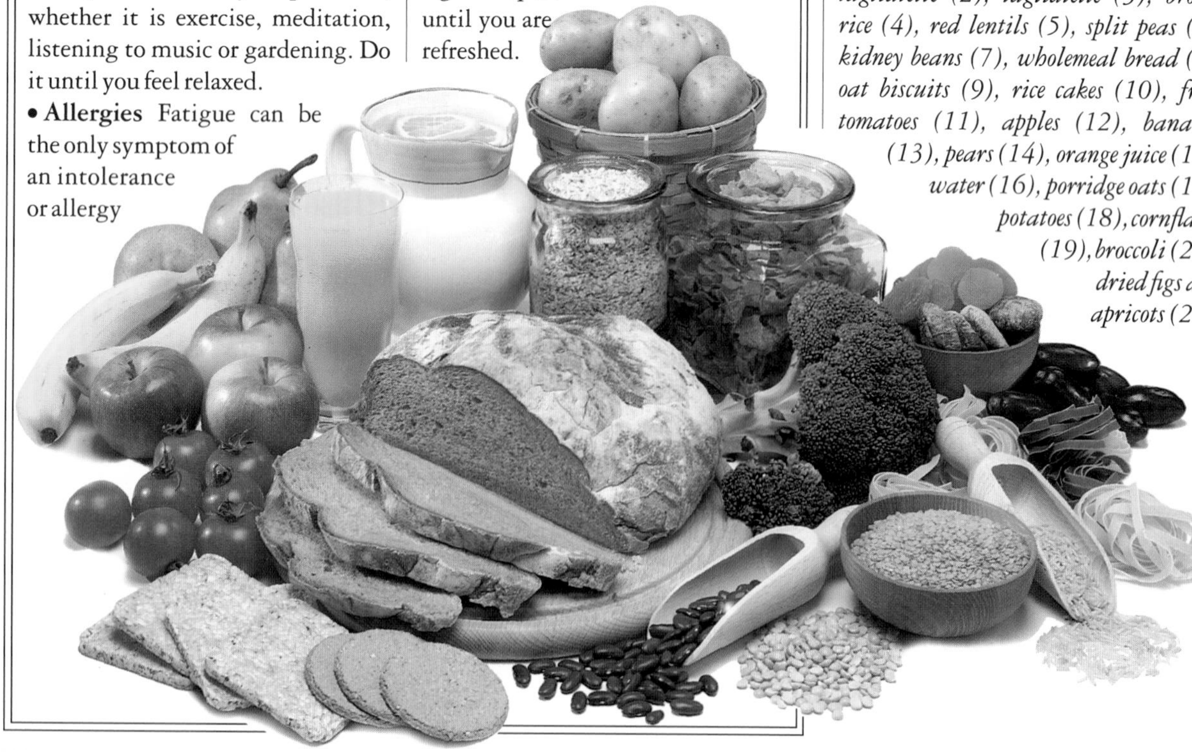

exercise. It is sensible to consult your doctor before starting a weight-loss diet or a new exercise programme.

Clearing out toxins to restore vitality

Many naturopaths believe in spring-cleaning your body once or twice a year with a detoxification diet. It is thought to help cleanse the digestive system and rid the body of waste products, improving digestion, energy and the condition of the skin. A typical detoxification programme will recommend

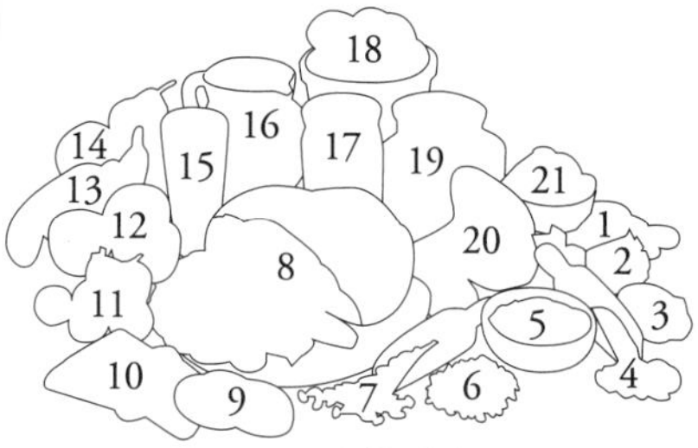

FOOD FOR ENERGY *All of these nutritious foods are particularly useful for avoiding low energy levels: dates (1), spinach tagliatelle (2), tagliatelle (3), brown rice (4), red lentils (5), split peas (6), kidney beans (7), wholemeal bread (8), oat biscuits (9), rice cakes (10), fresh tomatoes (11), apples (12), bananas (13), pears (14), orange juice (15), water (16), porridge oats (17), potatoes (18), cornflakes (19), broccoli (20), dried figs and apricots (21).*

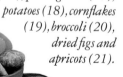

that you consume only fruit juice, fruit, salads and plenty of water for the first two days, and then spend five or more days eating healthy meals consisting of fresh fruit, raw and steamed vegetables, homemade soup, nuts, seeds, whole grains, fish, and poultry without the skin. No dairy products, wheat, red meat, coffee or alcohol are allowed. However, a little weak tea or herb tea is usually permitted.

There is limited scientific evidence that detoxifying diets can cleanse and rejuvenate the body, and most doctors argue that the body is quite capable of eliminating toxins without special diets. But naturopaths argue that a little extra help is necessary to counter the effects of pollution as well as the additives and impurities in some foods. Many people claim that it leaves them revitalised. Check with your doctor before starting a detoxification diet and limit the regime to two weeks.

How to bring exercise into your life

You do not have to invest in expensive equipment or join a gym to make exercise a part of your life. There are plenty of different forms of activity that can easily be built into your routine. Some forms of exercise – dancing, for example – are as sociable and as fun as they are energy-boosting; others, such as walking, may already be part of your lifestyle.

EXERCISE	ADVANTAGES	ACTION PLAN	TIPS/RISKS
Walking	Gentle and easy to fit into your lifestyle. Stimulates the heart, lungs, muscles and mind. Studies show that even very gentle walking may prolong your life by keeping you mobile and burning calories.	Aim for 10 or 15 minutes a day to start with and build up to at least 30 minutes. Swing your arms and walk fast enough to work up a slight sweat; you should be slightly out of breath.	Always wear comfortable, sturdy shoes. Try to use the entire foot by placing it down on the back of the heel and then moving through the length of the shoe to the toes.
Jogging	Helps to prevent heart disease and high cholesterol levels, high blood pressure and a wide variety of other health problems. Jogging also triggers the release of endorphins – chemicals in the brain that elevate your mood and reduce anxiety.	Start with some brisk walking and jogging about twice a week for two weeks, being careful not to overdo it. Gradually build up your speed, distance and the number of times a week that you can go jogging.	The greater risks are to knees, ankles and feet. Well-cushioned shoes help to protect your knees and hips. If you are overweight, consult your doctor before taking up jogging.
Swimming	Works most of the major muscle groups and gives an excellent aerobic workout. Improves strength, stamina and suppleness with little risk of any damage to the joints. Suitable for pregnant women, as well as people who are unfit or overweight.	If you get bored swimming up and down lanes, or if you cannot swim at all, consider trying some pool exercises and join an aqua-aerobics class. Swimming and water exercise are good complementary activities.	Shower thoroughly and disinfect any cuts after swimming. Never swim until at least 1 hour after eating. Do not struggle to keep your head out of the water – it puts a considerable strain on your neck and back.
Cycling	Medical experts maintain that cycling is one of the best types of exercise, suitable for people of most ages and levels of fitness. It builds muscular endurance and tones leg muscles.	Consider investing in an exercise bike; the aerobic benefits are the same as with a real bike and you can cycle in any weather. Use a real bike for leisurely weekend rides.	Choose a bicycle that suits the kind of cycling you will be doing and one that is the right size. Wear fluorescent or reflective clothing on the road.
Aerobics classes	Energetic type of exercise performed to music with a clear, simple beat. Aerobics improves the efficiency of your heart and lungs and as a result can help to reduce the risk of heart disease and circulation problems.	Aerobic exercise can be either low or high impact (the force with which the feet hit the ground). Start with low impact, when one foot always stays on the ground, and progress gradually to high impact if you wish.	Doctors usually advise people who have heart disease, are overweight, or who have problems with their lower back, knees, ankles or hips to avoid any kind of high-impact class.
Dancing	Good for all levels of fitness. Ballroom for general mobility; barn dancing for aerobic exercise; Latin American for strength and flexibility; tap or Irish step-dance for lower body strength.	Watch or take part in classes in your area until you find a dance style that appeals to you, and enjoy yourself. All forms are sociable and fun.	Some forms of dance, such as ballet, jazz and contemporary, are physically demanding and may not suit people who have joint problems.

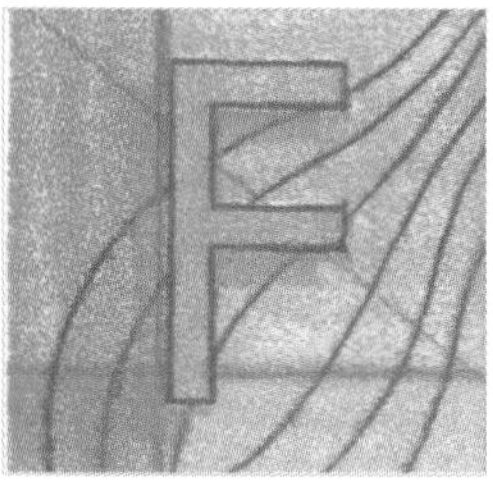

FAINTING

There are a number of possible causes for a temporary loss of consciousness. Even healthy people can faint from shock, dehydration, from standing too long in one position, or anything else that causes a sudden drop in blood pressure and therefore a brief interruption in the flow of blood from the heart to the brain.

It is not unusual for recurrent fainting to be a symptom of an underlying condition that requires treatment. ANAEMIA, HEART DISEASE and CIRCULATION DISORDERS can all be a cause. Medical treatment and an appropriate diet that helps to control the underlying problem are essential. See a doctor if you suffer from recurrent fainting.

FATIGUE

EAT PLENTY OF

- *Iron-rich foods such as lean red meat*
- *Zinc-rich foods such as shellfish*
- *Dark green vegetables for folate*
- *Complex carbohydrates such as pasta*
- *Meat, fish and eggs for vitamin B_{12}*

CUT DOWN ON

- *Sugar, cakes, biscuits and sweets*
- *Caffeine in tea, coffee and colas*
- *Alcohol*

Fatigue or tiredness is a common symptom that has many causes. It can result from illness, stress or lack of sleep. One of the most common causes of fatigue is ANAEMIA, which results from a reduced capacity to deliver oxygen to the tissues. It often occurs as a result of chronic illness, but it can also be due to a faulty diet.

The most common form of anaemia to affect women is caused by iron deficiency, as a result of poor diet, blood loss or illness. The main source of iron in the diet is meat, especially liver; non-meat sources for vegetarians and vegans include beans, lentils, dark green leafy vegetables, nuts, wheatgerm and sunflower seeds. However, some people with anaemia – mainly women – often need iron supplements and not just food sources of iron.

Two other nutrients, vitamin B_{12} and folate, are also needed for blood formation. Folate is found in wholegrain cereals, liver, dark green leafy vegetables and nuts. Vitamin B_{12} is found in meat, fish, eggs and dairy foods, so may be lacking in vegetarian and vegan diets. Some studies have found that vitamin B_{12}, when given by injection, can decrease tiredness.

Diets that are high in refined carbohydrates or low in calories, iron or zinc can also cause fatigue.

Refined sugar and readily digested starches (which are found in confectionery, biscuits, cakes and pastries) give you a sudden surge of energy because they reach the bloodstream quickly. In susceptible people, blood sugar (glucose) levels then tumble about half an hour later with a resulting feeling of tiredness. Long gaps between meals can also cause low blood sugar levels, so try to eat regular healthy snacks such as fresh fruit or a packet of nuts and raisins.

You can help to keep blood sugar levels on an even keel by cutting down on refined sugar, and getting into the habit of eating little and often – four to six small meals a day. Complex carbohydrates such as bread made from wholemeal flour, oat-based products and cooked pulses provide a much slower, steadier release of energy.

Nutrients for fatigue

- Starchy carbohydrate foods such as pasta to improve stamina.
- Folate for the formation of red blood cells, found in liver, meat, green vegetables and nuts.
- B_{12} for a healthy nervous system and formation of red blood cells.
- Iron to help prevent anaemia, taken with vitamin C, which helps the body to absorb it.
- Zinc, for energy metabolism.

People who are crash-dieting will not be taking in enough calories to sustain their body's normal functions, and will tend to lack energy. Crash diets are ill advised; it is better to lose weight slowly and surely – about 0.5-1kg (1-2lb) a week – by cutting down on fat. A gram of fat contains twice as many calories as a gram of protein or carbohydrate. To lose weight without fatigue, replace fatty foods with carbohydrates such as fruits, bread, pasta and oat-based foods.

Zinc is essential to many of the body's enzymes, so is vital for energy metabolism. Good sources are red meat and seafood – especially oysters.

While alcohol may seem like a good pick-me-up after a hard day, it causes fatigue and so makes you feel worse rather than better.

STIMULANTS

Caffeine in tea, coffee and colas brings short-term relief from fatigue, but an excessive amount (more than six cups a day) may well leave you feeling tired.

OTHER CAUSES

The underlying causes of prolonged fatigue can range from physical illnesses such as GLANDULAR FEVER and

MYALGIC ENCEPHALOMYELITIS (ME) to psychological conditions such as STRESS and DEPRESSION. A lack of stress or stimulation can also cause fatigue.

Lack of exercise can be another cause of fatigue. This is because taking regular exercise will increase the oxygen storage capacity of the muscles and stimulate the immune system. It may be the last thing you feel like doing when you are tired, but exercise should leave you feeling invigorated. (See also ENERGY, EXERCISE AND VITALITY.)

FATS

See page 150

FENNEL

BENEFITS

- *Seeds are good for digestion and may help to prevent colic in infants*
- *Low in calories*

DRAWBACK

- *High in nitrates*

There are two types of fennel: Florence fennel and garden fennel. Almost every part of both varieties can be used for culinary purposes, but it is the seeds which are renowned for their medicinal properties.

Florence fennel has a hard, bulbous, fleshy base with a crunchy texture, and a delicate but distinctive liquorice flavour. It is eaten raw in salads but can also be boiled or braised. Garden fennel has dark green spindly stems and feathery leaves. Their refreshing, delicate aniseed flavour complements fish and seafood. Fennel contains beta carotene – which the body converts into vitamin A – and folate, which is needed for blood formation. At only 12 Calories per 100g (3½oz), it makes a low-calorie addition to a healthy salad. Like CELERY, however, fennel can be high in nitrates.

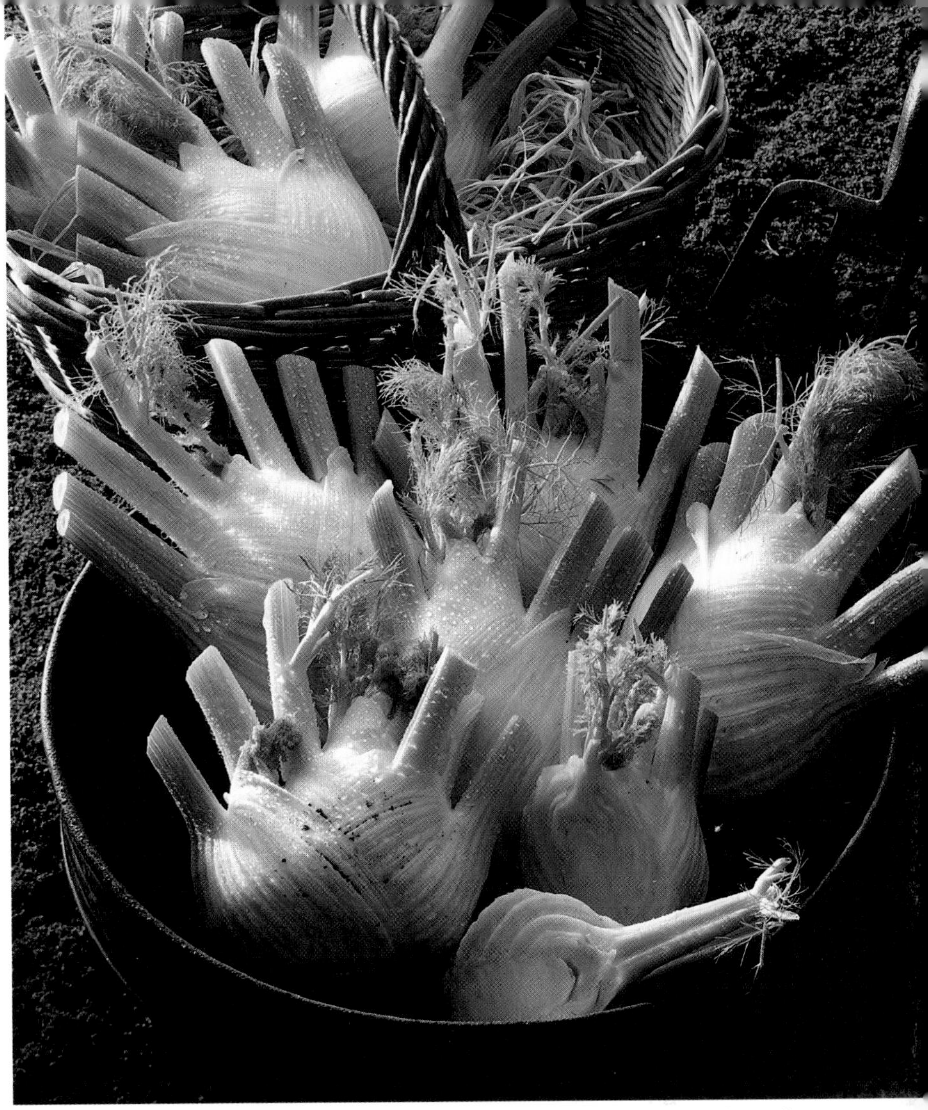

FOOD AND PHARMACY *Florence fennel is a versatile vegetable; every part can be used in cooking. The seeds have been popular since ancient times as both a spice and a medicine.*

An ancient remedy

In India, toasted fennel seeds are chewed after eating to prevent bad breath and to help digestion. In classical Greece and Rome, the seeds were eaten to prevent obesity. Both the Ancient Greek physician Hippocrates and, 2000 years later, the English herbalist Nicholas Culpeper, recommended fennel tea (one cup per day) to stimulate milk production in nursing mothers. A teaspoon of cooled, weak fennel tea can be used as gripe-water for infants.

FENNEL SEEDS

Aromatic fennel seeds are one of the world's oldest spices. In traditional medicine across the world they have long been used to make a tea to help a range of digestive problems from hiccups to colic. Fennel tea has a refreshing taste and can help to ease FLATULENCE and bloating. However, fennel seeds are thought to encourage menstruation and should therefore be avoided during pregnancy.

FATS: HOW TO ACHIEVE A HEALTHY BALANCE

The role of fats in the diet has excited much controversy and debate in recent years. Eating too much of certain types is harmful but others are vital for the body and can help to prevent disease.

Dietary fats are the most concentrated source of calories. Weight for weight, they contain more than twice as many calories as carbohydrate or protein; 25g (1oz) of fat has 225 calories. However, glucose and alcohol are more easily converted into immediate ENERGY and fuel.

Fats make food tasty; they give it a smooth creamy texture and carry compounds that impart flavour and smell. Certain fats are essential for childhood growth, healthy development and regulating the body's metabolism. The Department of Health in Britain has suggested that fats should provide around 35 per cent of total calories; in the United States, however, the recommended level is 30 per cent.

Surveys have shown that the typical Western diet has a fat content of 40 per cent or more. This is divided almost equally into visible oils, spreads and meat fat and the invisible fats which are present in foods such as cheese, milk, meat products, biscuits and nuts. A high-fat diet is likely to lead to obesity because fatty foods are so rich in calories. Obesity and high intakes of certain types of fat can contribute to ailments such as ATHEROSCLEROSIS, HEART DISEASE and forms of CANCER.

BENEFITS
- *Rich source of calories for energy*
- *Provide fat-soluble vitamins A, D, E and K*
- *Supply essential fatty acids for healthy skin and regulating body functions*
- *Make food tasty and palatable*

DRAWBACKS
- *High intakes of saturated fats can increase the risk of heart disease*
- *High-fat diets may lead to obesity and may increase the risk of cancer of the breast, bowel and pancreas*

DIFFERENT TYPES OF FAT AND WHY THE BODY NEEDS THEM

Eating too many fats and oils of any kind may prove harmful, but excluding them from the diet deprives the body of important nutrients. Dietary fats from oily fish, fish oils, vegetable oils and full-fat dairy products, between them, supply the fat-soluble vitamins A, D, E and K and are also required to absorb them.

The body needs at least 25g (1oz) of fat a day to absorb these fat-soluble vitamins and also beta carotene (found in leafy green and also orange vegetables, and orange and yellow fruits), which the body can convert into vitamin A.

When fats are removed from dairy products, the foods lose much of their vitamin A content. Low-fat yoghurts, skimmed milk and cottage cheese are poor sources of vitamin A; the vitamin is added to margarines to make them more nutritious.

While fat intake can often be sensibly reduced in adults, the diets of children under five should not be similarly restricted. From weaning onwards, children's likes and dislikes are developing and change quite frequently. They need a wide choice of foods to make sure they obtain enough calories and vitamins, as well as all the essential fatty acids; these are vital for healthy growth and development.

THE ESSENTIAL FATTY ACIDS

Fats are made up of fatty acids. There are two main types – saturated and unsaturated. Fats rich in saturated fatty acids, such as butter and lard, tend to be solid at room temperature; fats rich in unsaturated fatty acids, such as vegetable oils, tend to be liquid. The unsaturated fatty acids can be subdivided into monounsaturated and polyunsaturated.

Saturated and monounsaturated fatty acids are not strictly required in the diet because the body can make its own from carbohydrates, alcohol or proteins. However, it cannot make certain polyunsaturated fatty acids (essential fatty acids) which must be supplied by foods that contain them.

There are two families of these essential polyunsaturates: the omega-6 family derived from linoleic acid and found in vegetable oils such as olive and sunflower oil, and the omega-3 family derived from linolenic acid and found in some vegetable oils such as soya bean and rapeseed oil, in walnuts and in oily fish such as sardines, herring, mackerel and salmon.

Omega-6 fatty acids are needed as part of the make-up of all cells in the body and to produce hormone-like substances called eicosanoids which help to control a wide range of functions including inflammation and blood flow. Deficiency in omega-6 fatty acids (sometimes found in babies fed on skimmed milk and patients

The family tree of fats

Fats and oils contain many different fatty acids which affect the body in varying ways. Most simply, they are classified as saturated and unsaturated. Unsaturates are further subdivided into monounsaturates and polyunsaturates. Trans fatty acids are created in food processing and also occur naturally in beef, mutton and dairy products.

THE FATS IN EVERYDAY FOODS

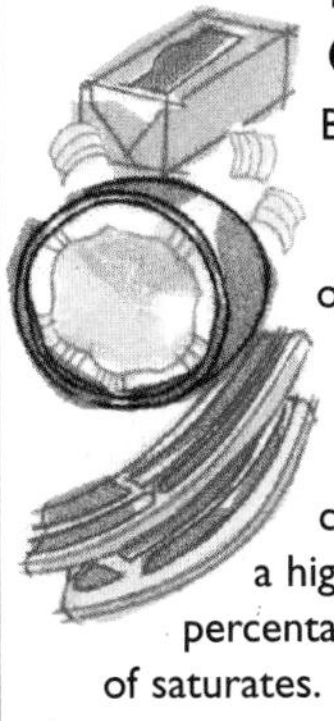

Saturated (fatty acids)
Butter, hard cheese, palm and coconut oil, and also fatty meat products contain a high percentage of saturates.

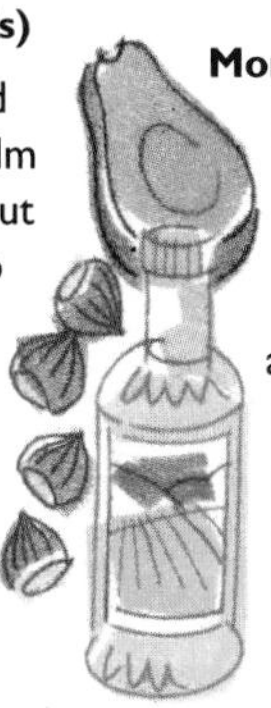

Monounsaturated (fatty acids)
The principal sources are olive oil, rapeseed oil and foods such as avocados, nuts and seeds (olive oil, rapeseed oil and some nuts also contain important polyunsaturates).

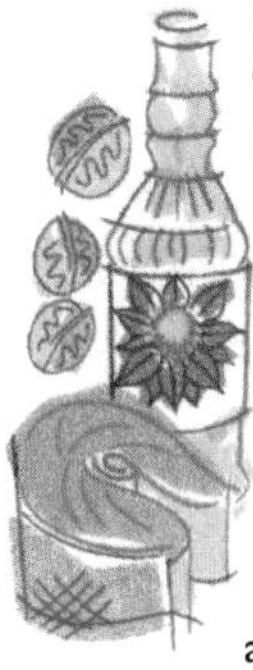

Polyunsaturated (fatty acids)
Foods high in polyunsaturates include most vegetables oils, fish oils and oily fish. These also contain the essential fatty acids which are grouped in two families.

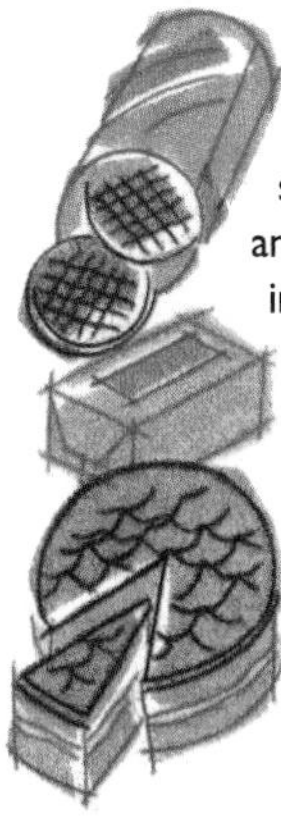

Trans (fatty acids)
Hydrogenated oils such as margarine and fats which are industrially hardened to avoid rancidity, and processed foods such as biscuits, pies, cakes and crisps are the major sources of trans fatty acids in the diet.

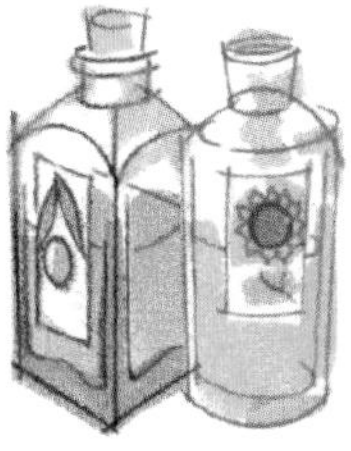

Omega-6 (derived from linoleic acid)
Good sources include olive oil and sunflower oil.

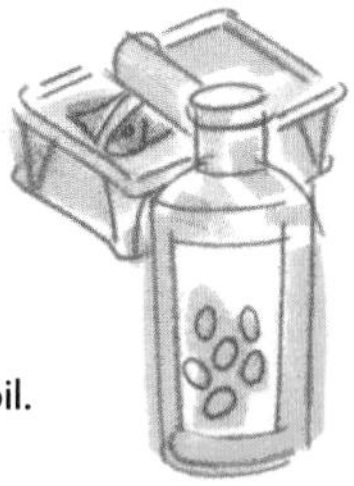

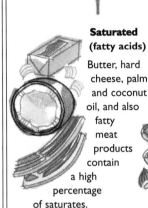

Omega-3 (derived from linolenic acid)
Good sources include soya bean and rapeseed oil, walnuts, and oily fish such as sardines, mackerel and salmon.

FAT CHEMISTRY *Fatty acids are made up of carbon, hydrogen and oxygen in varying proportions. A fat is saturated when its molecules hold the maximum amount of hydrogen; monounsaturates have a little less while polyunsaturates have the least. Trans fatty acids can be created by the hydrogenation process.*

unable to absorb fats) can lead to poor growth, skin problems, blood clots, and an impaired immune system.

An adult requires about 4g (⅛oz) omega-6 fatty acids a day (equivalent to two teaspoons of sunflower oil or a handful of almonds or walnuts); more may offer some protection from heart disease. An upper daily limit of 25g (1oz) is suggested as very high intakes may be harmful because they increase the production of FREE RADICALS. Linoleic acid has also been shown to promote tumour growth in animals.

Omega-3 fatty acids are needed in smaller amounts (about 1-2g) per day which can be obtained from a 100g (3½oz) portion of herring, one to two teaspoons of rapeseed oil or a handful of walnuts. They are required as structural components of the brain and the retina of the eye during early development. They reduce inflammation and the tendency of blood to clot, and have also been shown to be helpful in the treatment of heart disease, psoriasis and ARTHRITIS.

WHY SOME TYPES OF FAT SHOULD BE RESTRICTED

Medical research and population studies have fuelled the theory that high intakes of saturated fats which occur naturally in meat and dairy foods increase blood CHOLESTEROL levels and the risk of coronary heart disease. The industrial hardening of oils to make them solid at room temperature (such as hydrogenated hard margarines) converts unsaturated fats into saturated fats. Partial hydrogenation (used in making softer margarines and other processed foods) can change unsaturated fatty acids into trans fatty acids. Unlike the natural 'trans fats' found in some foods of animal origin, trans fats produced by hydrogenation have also been linked to heart disease.

The latest recommendations from the British Department of Health are that saturated fats should make up about 10 per cent of the calories in our daily diet, that trans fats should account for 2 per cent, and that unsaturated fats should make up the balance.

Replacing both trans and saturated fats with naturally occurring monounsaturate-rich fats (such as olive oil) or polyunsaturate-rich fats (such as sunflower oil) lowers blood cholesterol levels. These unsaturated fats are also the major dietary source of vitamin E which may protect against heart disease and atherosclerosis.

A low intake of animal fats and a high intake of olive oil is thought to contribute to the low rate of heart disease in Mediterranean countries such as Greece, Italy and Spain. The Inuit people of Greenland also have a low incidence of heart disease; medical experts believe that this is because the fish and marine animals which they eat in large quantities are low in saturated fat and high in omega-3 fatty acids.

High intakes of fish oil may also protect against cancer of the breast, bowel and pancreas which are associated with obesity and excessive total fat intake. The omega-3 polyunsaturated fatty acids that fish oils contain have been shown to inhibit tumour growth in animals. In several human studies, fish oils appear to protect against cancer of the colon.

Changing your fat intake

It is advisable to spread butter more thinly or to replace it with a low-fat spread or soft margarine that is high in polyunsaturates and low in trans fats. Semi-skimmed or skimmed milk should be used in place of full-cream milk (but not in infants' diets).

Some days, eat nuts and oily fish for protein rather than foods which contain animal fats. When eating meat, choose lean cuts and trim off the excess fat. The cooking method is also significant; it is much healthier to stew or grill rather than fry in extra fat.

Use liquid vegetable oils (rapeseed, sunflower, safflower or olive oils) for cooking rather than hard fats.

Carefully inspect food labels. Some manufacturers already specify polyunsaturated, monounsaturated and saturated fat contents of prepared foods. The hydrogenated fat content will also have to be declared under forthcoming European legislation.

The different sources of fat in the British diet

A trip to any UK supermarket or grocery store reveals the great British weakness – fatty foods, from meat products to a multitude of delicious and tempting sweet and savoury snacks. Little wonder that fat consumption in Britain is among the highest in the world. The chart below shows the various sources of fat in the British diet. It appears that red meats, dairy products and sweets far outweigh the sources of healthier fats such as fish.

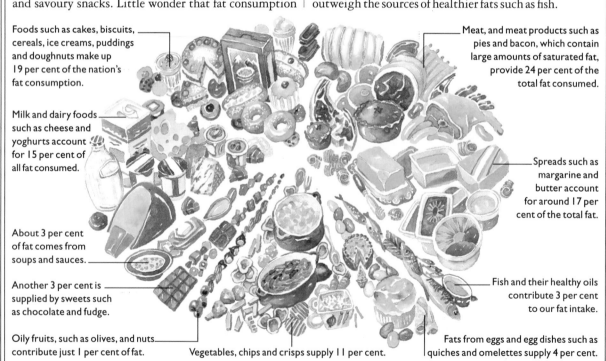

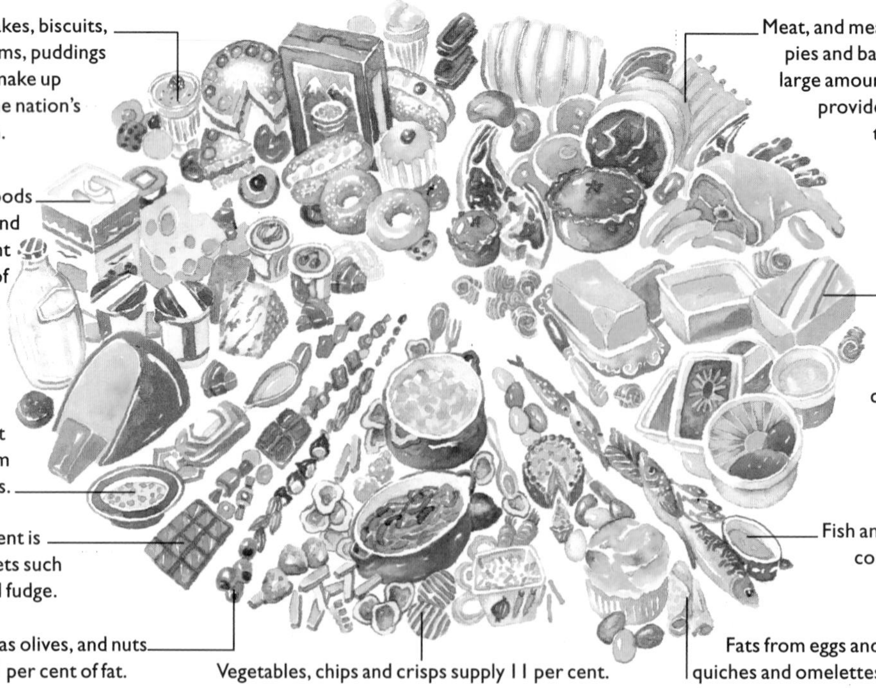

Foods such as cakes, biscuits, cereals, ice creams, puddings and doughnuts make up 19 per cent of the nation's fat consumption.
Milk and dairy foods such as cheese and yoghurts account for 15 per cent of all fat consumed.
About 3 per cent of fat comes from soups and sauces.
Another 3 per cent is supplied by sweets such as chocolate and fudge.
Oily fruits, such as olives, and nuts contribute just 1 per cent of fat.
Vegetables, chips and crisps supply 11 per cent.
Fats from eggs and egg dishes such as quiches and omelettes supply 4 per cent.
Fish and their healthy oils contribute 3 per cent to our fat intake.
Spreads such as margarine and butter account for around 17 per cent of the total fat.
Meat, and meat products such as pies and bacon, which contain large amounts of saturated fat, provide 24 per cent of the total fat consumed.

National diets and how they affect the risk of heart disease

In a bid to pinpoint a cause for the many coronary disorders prevalent in the West, researchers are increasingly looking at evidence from other cultures whose diets are quite different from our own.

What the Japanese eat

It is no coincidence that the Japanese whose diet contains just over 30 per cent fat (mostly polyunsaturated), compared with 40 per cent in Britain and 55 per cent in Denmark, should also enjoy one of the lowest rates of heart disease in the world.

Their cuisine is strongly associated with fish in forms such as sushi, sashimi and tempura; on average the Japanese eat 100g (3½oz) a day. However, the staple food is rice. A basic meal includes steamed rice, a soup such as miso (made with soya bean paste) and small side dishes which may contain meat, vegetables

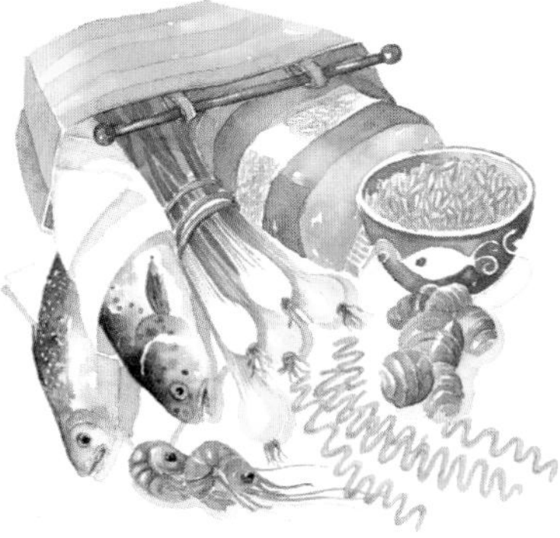

(including seaweed), seafood, fish, eggs, chicken and noodles, in different sauces and combinations.

As in the West, the Japanese eat three meals a day. Traditionally, breakfast consists of rice and a miso soup made with ingredients such as seaweed, tofu or leek and a side dish such as grilled fish. A typical lunch might contain chicken and vegetables cooked in soup stock blended with eggs and served on rice. Dinner, the most important meal of the day when the family gathers together, may include a little grilled fish as well as a meat dish such as stewed beef and potatoes, served with boiled greens, miso soup and rice.

The Mediterranean diet

Although people living in France, Greece, Spain and Italy eat slightly more fat than the British, most is

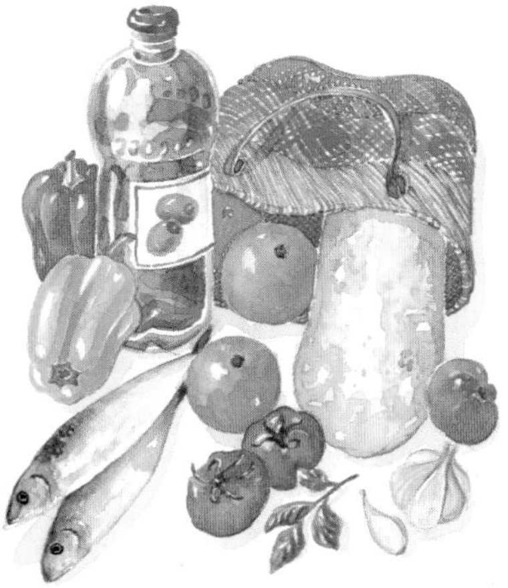

unsaturated and their risk of fatal heart disease is between a quarter and half the rate in the UK.

Staple foods of the Mediterranean countries are rice, bread, potatoes, pasta or cereals such as couscous, accompanied by plenty of vegetables.

Olive oil is widely used in cooking; other sources of fat include nuts, seeds and oily fish such as sardines. Butter consumption in Spain, Portugal, Italy and Greece, but not in France, is far lower than in the UK.

Mediterranean breakfast is light – frequently made up of rolls, coffee, and fruit juice, or fruit. Lunch may include bread or pasta to accompany a protein dish of meat, fish or poultry, sometimes with a vegetable. At both lunch and dinner, salad is served, often as a course on its own. Dinner is typically an extended meal of several courses, accompanied by wine.

People living in southern Europe, eat more pulses, nuts and vegetables than the British; on average the Mediterranean diet includes five servings of fruit and vegetables a day compared with only two in Britain.

British meals

The UK diet is traditionally high in saturated fats from animal sources.

Typically, British people eat one portion of fish, two portions of beef and lamb, three portions of pork and poultry and seven portions of other meat or meat products every week. They drink 2 litres (3½ pints) of milk a week – equivalent to a glass of semi-skimmed and a glass of whole milk a day; other dairy foods such as cheese and yoghurt, make up 15 per cent of the total fat consumed.

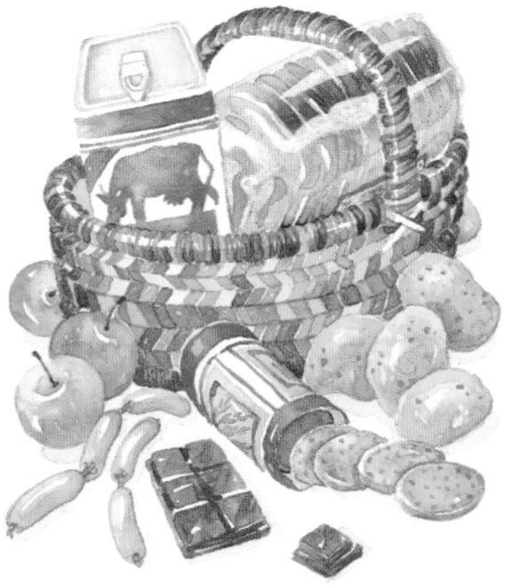

Fat spreads account for 16 per cent; however, margarines are now more popular than butter.

In Britain, vegetables make up 11 per cent of the fat intake, but half of this comes from roast and fried potatoes, including chips.

FEVER

TAKE PLENTY OF
- *Fluids, especially fruit juices*
- *Frequent small, light meals*

The normal human body temperature averages 37°C (98.6°F); it is lowest in the morning and rises in the evening. A few people have a 'normal' temperature as much as 0.6°C (1°F) above or below the average. Someone is said to be feverish if his or her temperature rises above its own norm. Fever is a symptom of an underlying problem, usually a sign that the body is fighting infection. It is often accompanied by other symptoms, such as sweating, shivering, thirst, flushed skin, nausea, aching and diarrhoea.

Sweating, the body's response to a raised temperature, results in the loss of fluid. So it is important to drink at least 1.7 litres (3pints) of fluid a day to prevent dehydration. If a feverish person does not feel thirsty, it may be easier for him or her to take a small volume regularly: a 200ml (7fl oz) glass of fruit juice diluted with an equal volume of water at hourly intervals is a good way to replace lost fluids.

As well as losing fluids, the body burns energy rapidly during a fever. However, people with fever often lose their appetite, so it may be difficult to persuade them to eat; furthermore, when people have diarrhoea, or are vomiting, it is better that they do not eat at all, in order to give the gut a chance to recover.

Children's temperatures can rise rapidly, but a high temperature (over 38.9°C, 102°F) does not necessarily reflect the severity of an illness. Doctors treat illnesses, not raised temperatures, and parents concerned that their child is ill should, of course, seek medical advice. You can cool a feverish child with paracetamol, and by sponging his or her limbs with tepid water. In adults, if a fever persists for more than three days or is accompanied by other symptoms such as severe pain, neck stiffness, dislike of light or a purplish rash, consult the doctor.

Feed a fever – not a cold

A bout of fever can leave the body exhausted and depleted of vitamins and other nutrients. Thus there is no medical basis for the saying, 'Feed a cold and starve a fever'. If anything, you need more calories than normal if you have a raised temperature. In fact, your metabolic rate rises by about 7 per cent for every 1°C your body temperature rises above normal.

The trouble is, fever usually contributes to a poor appetite, so a patient with a fever should drink plenty of liquids such as diluted fruit juices and, if not suffering from diarrhoea or vomiting, be encouraged to eat light, nourishing meals. They may be tempted by nutritious snacks such as home-made soups, custards or bananas.

FIBRE

BENEFITS
- *Helps to prevent constipation*
- *May protect against large bowel disease, including cancer*
- *Helps to lower blood cholesterol*

DRAWBACKS
- *Too much fibre can lead to flatulence and other digestive problems*
- *A high-fibre diet can restrict calorie intake*
- *Can reduce calcium absorption*

All plant foods and their products contain some fibre – such as cellulose, pectins and gums that make up their cell walls – which is not digested but nevertheless plays a number of important roles in the body's food cycle. The effects of fibre appear to have been known since Biblical times but only in recent years has its importance in preventing disease and maintaining health begun to be fully understood.

Some researchers suggest that a deficiency of fibre in Western diets may contribute to such widespread illnesses as diabetes mellitus, coronary heart disease and digestive problems.

Our main sources of fibre are cereals, vegetables, fruits, pulses, nuts and seeds. Most cereal fibre is found in the outer layers of grains, which are removed in the refining process. This is why wholegrain products such as brown rice, wholewheat pasta and wholemeal bread offer the best sources of fibre, though white bread still contains useful amounts.

DIETARY SOURCES

There are two main types of dietary fibre – soluble and insoluble. Though most plant foods provide both types, oat bran and pulses are particularly good sources of soluble fibre, and wheat, maize and rice of insoluble fibre. Because of their ability to retain water, acting like a sponge in the stomach and the gut, both types of fibre increase stool bulk while making stools softer and easier to expel.

The Department of Health argues that the amount of fibre in the average British diet should increase by almost 40 per cent – or by at least 5g a day, from the current average of 13g to 18g. They advise people to eat more complex carbohydrate foods such as wholemeal bread, potatoes, rice and pasta, and more fruit and vegetables.

Fibre can help to prevent CONSTIPATION by increasing stool bulk; it speeds up the passage of food residues through the large intestine, keeps the intestines in good order and reduces the risk of bowel disorders. Eating one extra slice of wholemeal bread a day will provide an extra 5 g of fibre

Although fibre is not digested, it nourishes bacteria in the large bowel and the subsequent fermentation produces volatile (light and easily absorbed) fatty acids, which are used as a source of energy by the gut wall. It may also help to prevent the build-up of carcinogens. Soluble fibre helps to reduce blood cholesterol levels because it can bind to cholesterol in bile – the yellowish liquid secreted by the liver which helps to break down fats in the small intestine. Some cholesterol may then be removed with the fibre as waste rather than being reabsorbed.

In the small intestine, soluble fibre also slows the absorption of glucose into the bloodstream preventing a sudden rise in blood sugar level which is particularly beneficial for diabetics.

The level of minerals such as calcium and iron absorbed by the body may be reduced when they combine with some forms of insoluble and unprocessed fibre – especially wheat BRAN and brown rice, which contain phytic acid. Too much fibre in the diet may prevent children from obtaining sufficient calcium, and women may fail to absorb sufficient iron. However, unless fibre intake is much higher than the recommended 18g a day, it is unlikely to interfere with the body's mineral supply. Digestive disorders are a more common result of eating too much fibre from one food source, such as bran. Eating fibre from a variety of different foods will help to prevent any potential adverse effects.

Fibre in everyday foods

While fibre has little or no nutritional value, it forms an essential link in the body's digestive chain. Soluble and insoluble fibre are both important. Some plant foods provide both sorts – apple peel, for instance, is insoluble cellulose, while the flesh is an excellent source of the soluble fibre, pectin.

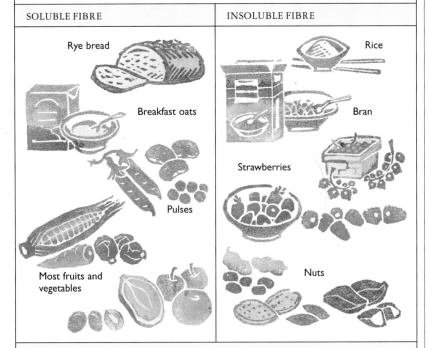

SOLUBLE FIBRE

INSOLUBLE FIBRE

SOLUBLE AND INSOLUBLE FIBRE

Wheat bran and whole grains are our main sources of combined fibre types. Dried fruits are particularly good sources of both forms.

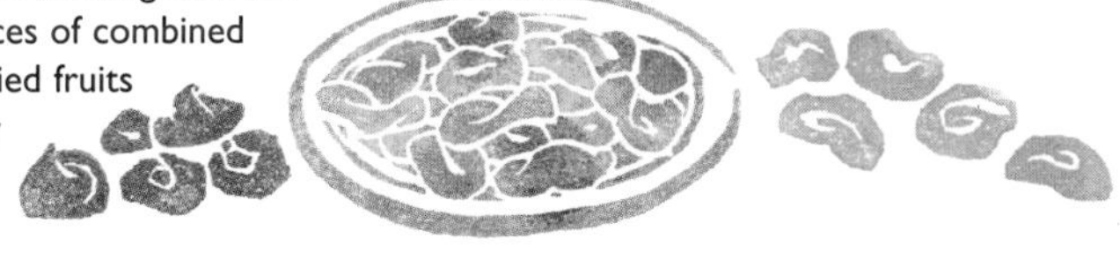

Brown bread versus white – 2000 years of debate

Medical historians argue that the Bible provides the first written record of the apparent benefits of a high-fibre diet, citing the fact that after ten days of eating vegetables and drinking only water, Daniel and his companions were healthier than the other young men who ate rich food and drank wine at the king's table.

The discussion surrounding the comparative merits of brown and white bread seems to have gone on for more than 2000 years. In early civilisations such as ancient Greece, breads baked from white flour were widely regarded as a symbol of riches and status. However, Hippocrates – known as the Father of Medicine – advised his wealthy patrons and patients to follow the practice of their servants and eat wholemeal bread 'for its salutary effect upon the bowel', while nearly 1000 years ago, the Persian physician Hakim urged his patients to eat only wholewheat chapattis, the local unleavened bread.

FIGS

BENEFITS
- *Dried figs are high in fibre, which helps to prevent constipation*
- *Dried figs are rich in potassium*

DRAWBACKS
- *Dried figs are high in sugar and can contribute to tooth decay*
- *Dried figs may be contaminated with toxins from mould*

Since fresh figs bruise easily and do not travel well, around 90 per cent are dried for export from the southern European countries where they grow. Nevertheless, fresh figs – both the black and green varieties – are increasingly available in UK supermarkets. Weight for weight dried figs provide roughly six times as many calories as fresh figs. Drying also concentrates the nutrients to make them a rich source of potassium and a useful source of calcium, iron and magnesium.

Dried figs contain pectin – a form of soluble FIBRE which can help to reduce blood cholesterol levels – and also insoluble fibre, which helps the movement of food through the gut, so preventing constipation and other bowel disorders. A handful of dried figs will usually have a laxative effect while syrup of figs is a traditional remedy for constipation.

However, dried figs are also high in sugar, and if eaten too frequently can cause tooth decay. They are also prone to mould contamination and may contain mould toxins such as aflatoxins, which are potentially carcinogenic.

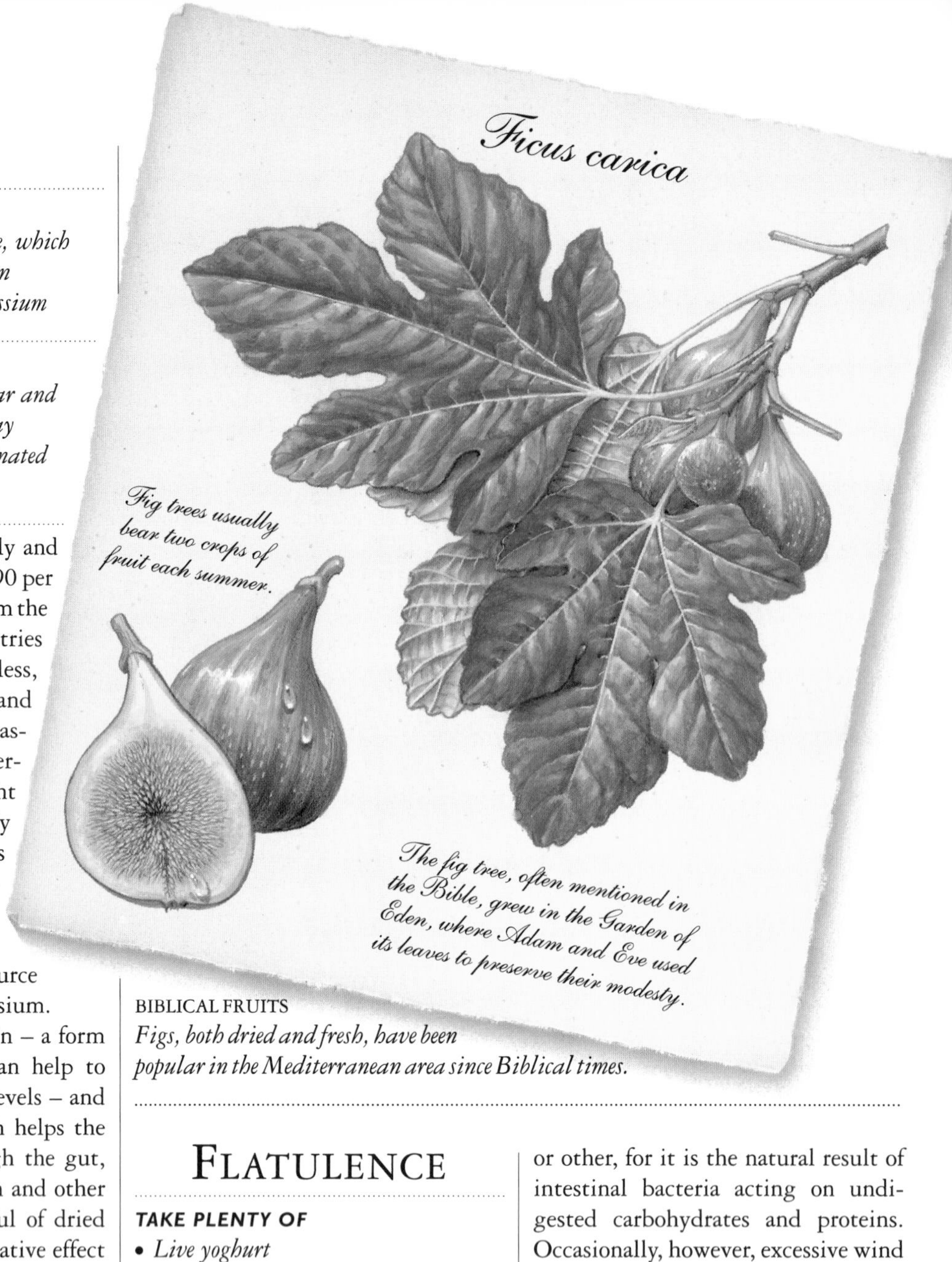
Ficus carica
Fig trees usually bear two crops of fruit each summer.
The fig tree, often mentioned in the Bible, grew in the Garden of Eden, where Adam and Eve used its leaves to preserve their modesty.

BIBLICAL FRUITS
Figs, both dried and fresh, have been popular in the Mediterranean area since Biblical times.

FISH

See page 158

FLATULENCE

TAKE PLENTY OF
- *Live yoghurt*
- *Herbs known to aid digestion*
- *Peppermint and fennel teas*

CUT DOWN ON
- *Pulses, such as peas, beans and lentils*
- *Brussels sprouts, cabbage and artichokes*

Excessive wind, or flatulence, causes uncomfortable bloating that can be relieved only by bringing up the wind or by expelling it through the anus. We all suffer from wind to some degree or other, for it is the natural result of intestinal bacteria acting on undigested carbohydrates and proteins. Occasionally, however, excessive wind may be a symptom of another condition, such as chronic constipation, a stomach ulcer or Crohn's disease. Swallowing too much air while eating can also cause flatulence.

Some people are more susceptible to wind than others. Avoiding heavy meals, eating slowly and not gulping liquids, especially fizzy drinks, will all help to minimise flatulence. Another helpful measure is to add herbs or spices which aid the digestion to foods such as Brussels sprouts, pulses and cabbage that commonly cause wind. Lemon balm, rosemary, sage, thyme, summer savory, caraway and fennel seeds are all helpful.

Except for lentils and split peas, which do not need to be presoaked, soaking dried PULSES in water for several hours or overnight before cooking them in plenty of fresh water helps to reduce the indigestible sugars responsible for causing wind.

The use of high-fibre foods such as BRAN to treat constipation and other digestive problems often causes a dramatic increase in wind. It is therefore a good idea to increase fibre intake by gradually introducing high-fibre foods. As the digestive system adapts to the higher intake, this uncomfortable side effect should subside.

A carton of live yoghurt each day can help to maintain levels of the bacteria vital to digestion. Even people with lactose intolerance, in whom milk and milk products normally cause flatulence, may be able to digest live yoghurt. Mint or fennel tea after a meal has long been used as a digestive aid while peppermint tea relaxes the muscles of the colon helping to relieve the discomfort of excessive wind.

FOOD CRAVINGS

EAT PLENTY OF

- *Low-fat, complex carbohydrates and bulky foods, such as rice, potatoes, wholegrain bread and pasta, at regular intervals*

EAT IN MODERATION

- *The foods you fancy*

AVOID

- *Being hungry*

When the appetite for certain foods is very strong and runs out of control it is described as a craving. Merely having marked preferences for particular foods does not constitute a craving; nor does buying snacks on an impulse. A craving is much more than this – it is an insistent desire that you will go to some lengths to satisfy.

Cravings for high-calorie sweet foods or any foods with a high fat content can cause enormous problems for people trying to watch their weight. To cope with a craving, certain preventive measures should be taken. Never go hungry – it can make you sluggish and depressed and can lead to binge eating. Fill up with low-calorie, high-fibre fresh fruit, vegetables and grains. Do not forbid yourself the food you crave but eat only a little of it.

A NUTRITIONAL NEED?

In the past, it was thought that food cravings indicated specific nutritional shortfalls, and that we craved certain foods because, like animals, we knew instinctively that they would make up for deficiencies in our diet. Some experts still feel that this 'wisdom' of the body plays a part in cravings.

However, as the foods we crave tend not to be the healthiest or the most nutritious, it is now widely believed that the mind plays a more important role than the body. Food can be an emotional crutch; many people know that they crave certain foods when they are under stress or depressed. For other people, the trigger is suggestion; a spontaneous craving can be sparked by the sight or smell of a particular food.

The cravings which are most often reported include chocolate, sweets and other high-sugar, high-calorie foods, although cravings for healthy foods such as fruit or vegetables could well pass unnoticed because they would not be perceived as a problem.

Women report food cravings more often than men, and people who are on diets also seem to be susceptible. Some women report their strongest cravings during the week before the onset of menstruation or during pregnancy, which suggests that some physiological component, such as a change in hormone balance, may be partly responsible. Before menstruation, the appetite increases and the metabolic rate decreases. The cravings – often for sweet fatty foods – experienced at this time are thought to be the result of wide fluctuations in blood sugar levels caused by hormonal changes.

People over 65 have fewer cravings than younger people, possibly because as the sense of smell and taste weakens with age, the appetite also diminishes.

For dieters, cravings are probably psychological. It seems that the very process of self-denial results in powerful, and even obsessive, yearnings.

If you are driven to the kind of binge eating that causes OBESITY or are caught in the bingeing and purging cycle of BULIMIA, you need to seek professional help.

Pica – a bizarre phenomenon

There are numerous cases, worldwide, of people craving non-foods such as clay, earth, chalk, laundry starch or coal. This phenomenon is known as pica – the word comes from the Latin for magpie, because of the bird's omnivorous nature. It can affect both sexes, but is most likely to occur in children.

Pica should always be vigorously discouraged as filling up with non-foods can cause malnutrition, poisoning and various other problems. Clay-eating, for example, causes severe constipation and impacted faeces. Pica poses a threat to pregnant women because it can cause ANAEMIA or blood poisoning and is associated with poor foetal development.

FISH: FOOD FROM RIVER AND SEA

Their nutritional benefits have long been recognised; however, researchers are still discovering how the regular consumption of fish can help to prevent life-threatening strokes and heart disease.

Fish contain so many important nutrients, including protein, that they should form a major part of our diet. In fact, in Britain, we eat far less than we used to; a decline in fish consumption has been one of the major dietary changes this century.

Just one small portion of fish (100g, 3½ oz), supplies between a third and a half of the protein required each day. Most fish are also rich in vitamin B_{12}, which is vital for a healthy nervous system, and iodine, which the thyroid gland needs to function effectively.

Fatty fish such as salmon or herring contain at least twice as many calories as white fish. Unlike saturated animal FATS however, unsaturated fish oils are highly beneficial. Studies have found that people who eat oily fish at least once a week are less likely to suffer from heart disease or stroke.

OMEGA-3

Most experts believe that it is the omega-3 fatty acids in the fish which help to protect against heart and circulation problems; they are thought to reduce the risk of thrombosis and may also improve the flow of blood through small blood vessels.

Studies have shown that the consumption of oily fish helps to relieve some symptoms of psoriasis. This may be due to the omega-3 fatty acids or to the large amounts of vitamin D in oily fish such as herring and mackerel.

Scientists have also discovered that omega-3 fatty acids are essential for the healthy development of the eyes and brain; in particular, mothers-to-be should include them in their diet.

The British Government's 1994 COMA report on cardiovascular disease suggests a daily intake of 0.2g of omega-3 fatty acids (1.5g a week); other nutritional experts believe that 0.5g-1g a day (up to 7g a week) would have a more protective effect.

Fish that are farmed, such as salmon and trout, contain similar levels of omega-3 fatty acids to the wild varieties and, because they consume a similar diet, differ little nutritionally.

POTENTIAL DRAWBACKS

Eating raw fish – used in Japanese dishes such as sushi and sashimi – carries a risk of getting worms as fish act as intermediate hosts for many parasitic worms. Fish such as cod must be cooked to ensure that all worms and their eggs are killed.

Oily fish such as herring and mackerel must be cooked and eaten fresh as they spoil rapidly and can cause stomach upsets and a skin rash; this is known as scombroid poisoning and is thought to result from bacteria growth on the fish. The term 'holy mackerel' stems from the days when markets in Cornwall were given a special licence to open on Sundays to sell the day's catch while it was still fresh.

Another hazard of eating fish is the danger of bones becoming caught in the throat, which can cause choking; all bones should be removed from fish served to children.

Steaming, baking or grilling fish is best for your health. Laboratory studies suggest that smoking and pickling fish can produce compounds which may be carcinogenic if eaten to excess.

POLLUTED WATERS

Fish are also highly vulnerable to contamination by pollution. This is not a problem in the seas around Britain, but chemical pollution has occurred in rivers, affecting freshwater stocks.

In 1994, one in ten samples of farmed salmon, that were tested in Britain by government officials, contained residues of a potentially toxic pesticide – ivermectin – which is not

CHOICE CATCH *A giant tuna – tail up – with a salmon above and a pair of gleaming mackerel beneath. Oily fish such as these are rich in many healthy nutrients.*

JAPAN'S DANGEROUS DELICACY

In Japan, the eating of *fugu* – a great delicacy prepared from the flesh of the pufferfish or blowfish – has been likened to a game of Russian roulette. The ovaries, roe and, in particular, the liver of the fish all contain a potent toxin. One wrong move with the knife during preparation can cause this poison to leak into the fish. The substance is so powerful that consuming just a drop quickly leads to paralysis, and then death. Restaurant chefs who would like to be entrusted with *fugu* preparation must undergo a seven-year apprenticeship. Despite this caution, *fugu* remains the principal cause of fatal food poisoning in Japan; according to official statistics, dozens of people die from it every year.

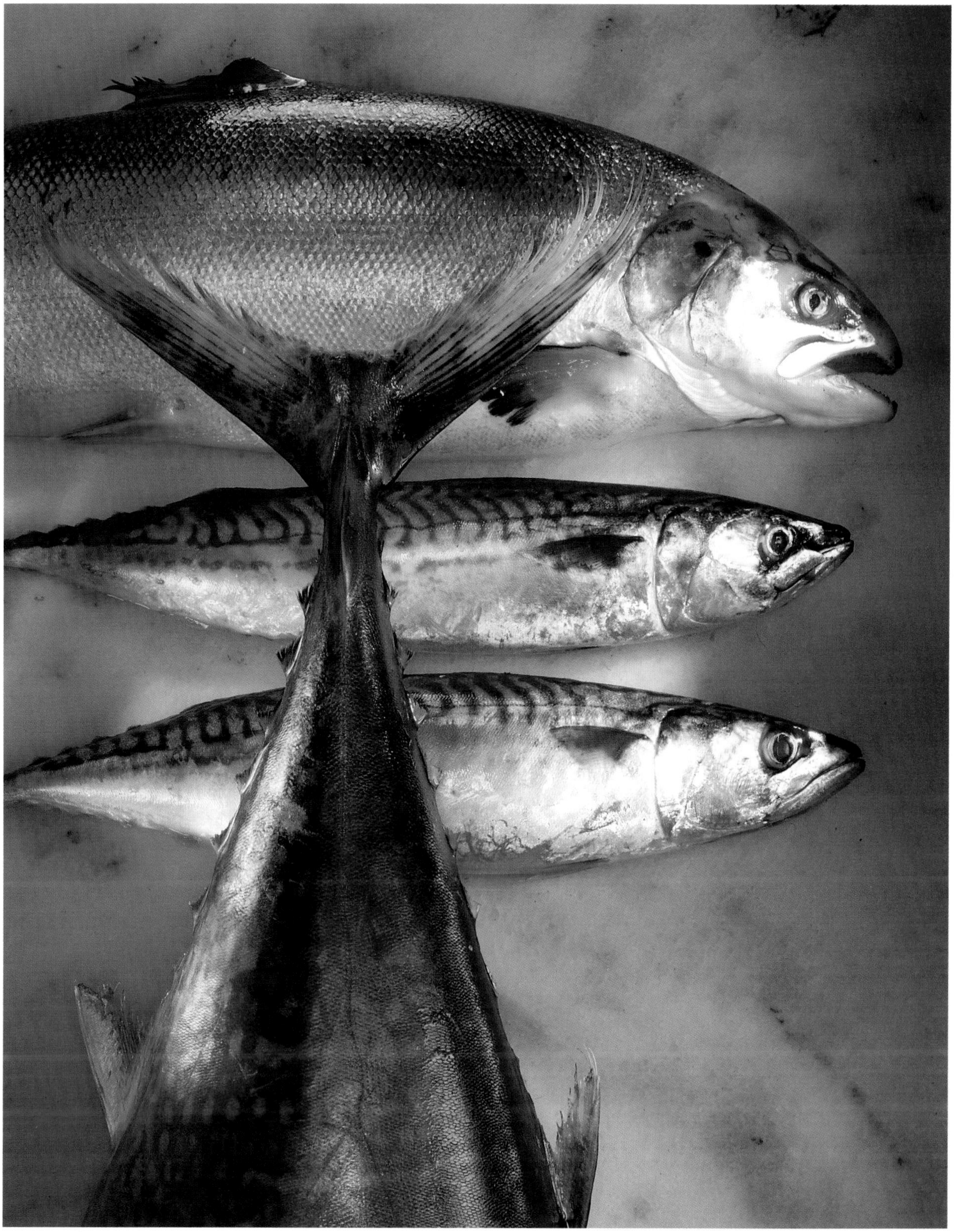

licensed for the marine environment and may have been used illegally to kill sea lice which prey on farmed fish. Elsewhere freshwater fish have suffered from accidental or illegal spillage of industrial and agricultural chemicals in rivers and streams.

In many of the Great Lakes of North America, fish are contaminated with cadmium and mercury from industrial discharges from smelting works and are not safe to eat because deposits of these heavy metals in the body can damage the human nervous system. In parts of the Indian Ocean and in the Caribbean, the fish can accumulate natural toxins from plankton in the food chain that can cause paralysis and, in the most severe cases, death.

The amount of mercury in tinned tuna is now monitored routinely as a result of past concern about the high levels present. As swordfish can also contain natural accumulations of heavy metals such as mercury, it is not advisable to eat them too frequently.

High levels of other chemical pollutants called polychlorinated biphenyls (PCBs) have been reported in fish liver oils from the Baltic Sea. Generally, levels of PCBs are low in fish from the Atlantic and Pacific Oceans. Most commercially available fish oils are monitored for these pollutants and the levels present are no cause for concern.

Why fish oils are so good for us

Available as a food supplement in capsule or liquid form, fish oils can be divided into two categories: fish liver oils (from cod, halibut and shark), and fish body oils, normally derived from anchovies, sardines, and capelins and menhaden (small fish from North Atlantic waters).

The term cod liver oil defines oils derived from cod and also from pollack, saithe and whiting. The oil extracted from the fish livers is deodorised and then vitamin E and antioxidants are added to prevent it from going rancid.

The oil is an excellent source of vitamins A and D. Two teaspoons (10ml) of cod liver oil typically provide about 1200μg of retinol (vitamin A), 20μg of vitamin D and about 2g of omega-3 fatty acids – more than enough to meet an adult's recommended daily intake and to offer some protection against various circulatory and skin disorders. Fish oil capsules are usually fortified with vitamins A and D but contain less omega-3 fatty acids. Because of its high concentrations of these vitamins, cod liver oil has long been used to prevent and treat conditions such as xerophthalmia, a progressive eye disease due to vitamin A deficiency, and rickets, a bone disease caused by lack of vitamin D.

Halibut liver oils and shark liver oils contain higher concentrations of retinol and there have been occasional cases of vitamin A poisoning in people who have taken excessive amounts. Shark liver oil also contains squalene, which the body synthesises to produce cholesterol and which may raise blood cholesterol levels. As a result, researchers are divided on the benefits of these oils. However, it has been claimed that other substances in shark liver oil called glyceryl ethers may help to protect against cervical cancer.

Fish body oils tend to contain substantially less vitamin A and vitamin D but are rich in omega-3 fatty acids. Controlled clinical trials, carried out in the United Kingdom, Scandinavia and the United States, suggest that supplements supplying 2-3g of omega-3 fatty acids can provide mild relief for symptoms of psoriasis and rheumatoid arthritis.

White fish species

Cod and haddock (which is a smaller member of the cod family) store their fat reserves in the liver – cod liver oil is rich in vitamins A and D. The flesh is low in these vitamins and contains little fat, but it is high in vitamin B_{12}.

The hard roe of cod is eaten boiled and also used in the Greek dip, taramasalata. It is rich in omega-3 fatty acids but high in cholesterol. Salted and smoked cod and haddock are high in sodium; people suffering from high blood pressure should avoid them.

Flatfish such as sole, plaice and flounder all have a similar nutritional composition. They are low in fat (1-2 per cent by weight), high in protein (16-18 per cent by weight), and are easy to grill. Frying can quadruple the calorific value of a 100g (3½oz) portion; flatfish take up slightly more oil than round fish because of their greater surface area. Unlike oily fish, they are not a useful source of vitamin D. However, they are rich in vitamin B_{12}.

Oily fish species

Tuna is rich in vitamin D, vitamin B_{12} and omega-3 fatty acids. Tinned tuna retains a high vitamin content but is a poor source of omega-3 fatty acids as most of the fish oil is removed before canning. A 100g (3½oz) portion of tuna canned in vegetable oil contains more than twice as many calories as tuna canned in brine, but similar amounts of sodium.

Because they live for 30-40 years, tuna which feed in contaminated water can accumulate high levels of metals in their flesh – particularly mercury, cadmium and lead. Levels are now monitored and fish from seas around the United States and Europe are not thought to be contaminated.

Mackerel are rich in omega-3 fatty acids, vitamin D and selenium. Their fat content varies according to season. It is lowest after spawning in the summer, when it is about 5 per cent fat by weight, and highest in December, when it is about 25 per cent fat. An average fish that weighs 200g (7oz), however, will supply about 6.5g of omega-3 fatty acids.

In New Zealand, where the soil is low in selenium, mackerel is the main dietary source; severe selenium deficiency can affect the heart.

Herring, which is equally rich in omega-3 fatty acids, is also susceptible to spoilage. This is why many methods of preserving the fish have evolved including pickling, salting and smoking. Pickled herrings are high in salt which can contribute to increased blood pressure. They also contain histamine and tyramine which can trigger migraines in susceptible people.

The healthiest way of preparing herring is to steam, grill or fry them; frying does not increase the fat content as heating cooks out their own oils.

Sardines are an inexpensive and useful source of protein, iron and zinc plus all the other nutrients associated with oily fish. Typically they contain about 10 per cent fat by weight; when canned in vegetable oil, they contain approximately 14 per cent and when canned in tomato sauce about 10 per cent. Fresh sardines are usually grilled.

Salmon and trout belong to the same fish family; they are all rich in the protein, essential fatty acids and vitamins A, B_{12} and D – common to all oily fish.

CARTILAGINOUS FISH

Dogfish, shark, skate and ray are primitive fish with uncalcified skeletons and large oily livers. The flesh is firm and generally low in fat, varying between 1 and 10 per cent by weight. They must be cooked and eaten fresh as they quickly develop an 'off' taste.

Fish facts and food values

NUTRIENTS PER 100g (3½oz)	DID YOU KNOW?
WHITE FISH SUCH AS COD, HADDOCK, PLAICE, SKATE, SOLE, WHITING	
Calories: 96-104 Protein: 19-23g Iron: 0.4-1mg Fat: 0.6-2g 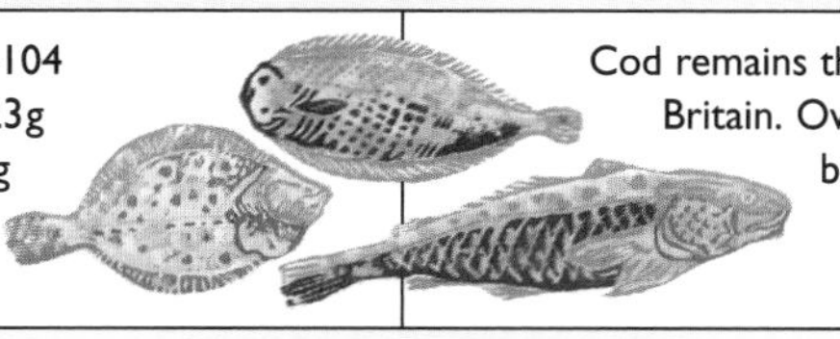	Cod remains the most popular fish in Britain. Over 15000 tonnes were bought by consumers in 1994 – more than half of it frozen.
OILY FISH SUCH AS HERRING, MACKEREL, SALMON, SARDINES, TROUT	
Calories: 135-240 Protein: 20-26g Iron: 0.4-2mg Fat: 5-17g oily fish are an excellent source of omega-3 fatty acids and also vitamin B_{12} (6-28µg) 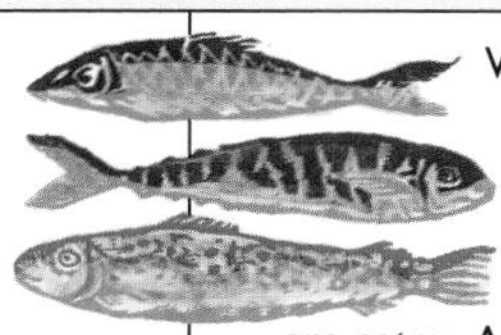	Whitebait, the young of various oily fish such as sardines, anchovies and herring, are an excellent source of calcium as both the bones and flesh are eaten. A 100g (3½oz) portion contains more than the recommended daily intake.
TINNED FISH SUCH AS ANCHOVIES, SARDINES, TUNA	
Calories: 99-280 depending on whether fish is canned in oil or brine Protein: 19-27g Iron: highest in fish paste (9mg) and sardines (3.0mg) Fat: 0.6g (tuna in brine) to 20g (anchovies in oil)	Although oily fish are an excellent source of omega-3 fatty acids, tinned tuna provides very little as most of the oil is removed before canning. Whitefish are not canned as the flesh tends to discolour. 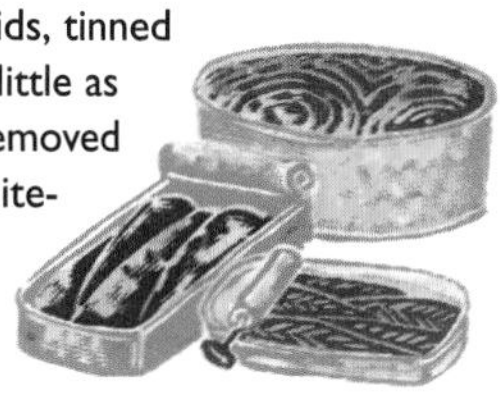
SMOKED FISH SUCH AS MACKEREL, SALMON, KIPPERS	
Calories: 142 (salmon) to 354 (mackerel) Protein: 19-25g Iron: 0.6-1.6mg Fat: 4.5g (salmon) to 3g (mackerel)	Smoking fish does not destroy their vitamin D content, nor their beneficial omega-3 fatty acids. In Britain, kippers are still the most popular type of smoked fish. 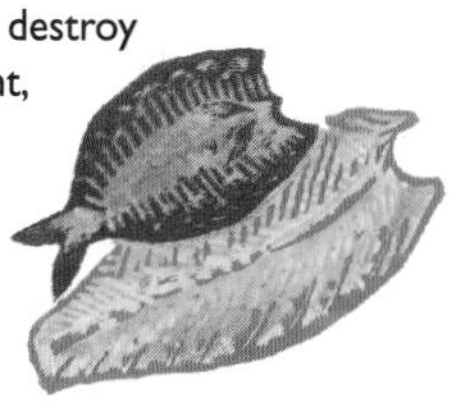
FISH FINGERS	
Calories: 200 Protein: 15g Iron: 0.8mg Fat: 9g 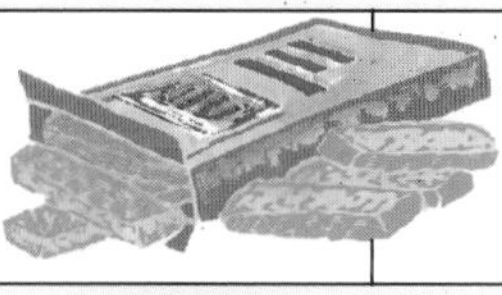	Fish fingers, introduced in Britain by Bird's Eye in 1955, remain very popular. Some 22000 tonnes are consumed each year – a quarter by adults aged over 45.
CAVIAR	
Calories: 92 Protein: 10.9g Iron: 0.5mg Fat: 5.4g 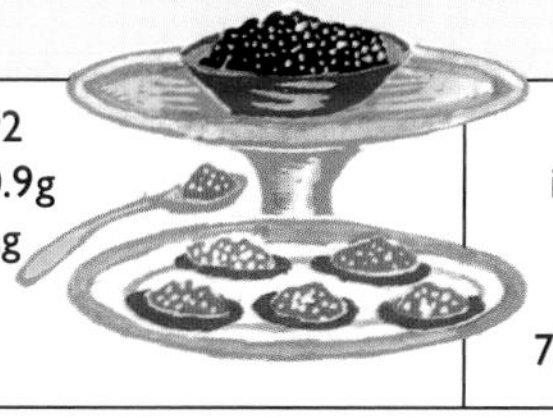	Gout sufferers may avoid caviar because it is high in purines. The real thing – sturgeon roe from the Caspian Sea – is also very expensive. Best Beluga caviar costs around 70 times as much as substitute lumpfish roe.

FOOD POISONING

Many people suffer from food poisoning at some time in their lives. The incidences of food poisoning from bacteria and viruses are on the increase: in 1994 in England and Wales alone, there were some 87 000 reported cases – up from nearly 65 000 in 1992 – and it is estimated that as many as ten times this number go unreported.

Most foods harbour bacteria, and if foods are not kept in the right conditions – which means keeping cold foods chilled and hot foods piping hot – such bacteria can breed rapidly and cause food poisoning. Contaminated foods left for more than an hour and a half at a warm temperature provide the ideal conditions for bacterial proliferation, which makes food poisoning much more common in warm weather.

Foods to be particularly careful of include undercooked poultry and meat; unpasteurised milk products; rice which has been kept warm for long periods or inadequately reheated; shellfish from dubious sources; spoilt oily fish; cooked meat products; and raw and lightly cooked eggs, or those with cracked shells.

The Department of Health advises people not to eat raw eggs, and not to serve soft-cooked eggs to pregnant women, infants, the sick or the elderly. Pregnant women should also avoid pâté, and soft-rinded cheeses such as Brie and Camembert as they are prone to contamination by *Listeria monocytogenes*, which can harm the foetus.

MINIMISING THE RISKS

Two of the most important sources of food contamination are nasal and faecal transference, so people should always wash their hands before touching any food, and avoid blowing their nose when handling food. Pets also carry bacteria and should be kept out of the kitchen and away from the dinner table when people are eating. Because food poisoning is more common in summer than in winter, it is particularly important to store food properly through the hotter months. Make sure that the temperature inside the refrigerator is between 0°-5°C (32°-41°F). If your refrigerator has no built-in temperature display, it is worth buying a special thermometer. Check the dates on goods, always use food within the recommended period and ruthlessly discard any food that looks, smells or tastes off.

Case study

To celebrate her entry into professional tennis, Jean's friends organised a party. The next day, she felt sick with a headache and assumed that she had overdone it with the wine. By lunchtime Jean had been sick a couple of times, felt hot and had stomach pains.
Within the hour she had profuse, watery diarrhoea. Jean went to her doctor who sent for tests at the local laboratory which isolated a strain of the salmonella bacteria.
She remembered that she had eaten some lightly boiled ducks' eggs at the party – they were the prime suspects. All that Jean could do was rest, take plenty of fluids and let the illness run its course. After two days she felt better and was soon ready to play tennis again.

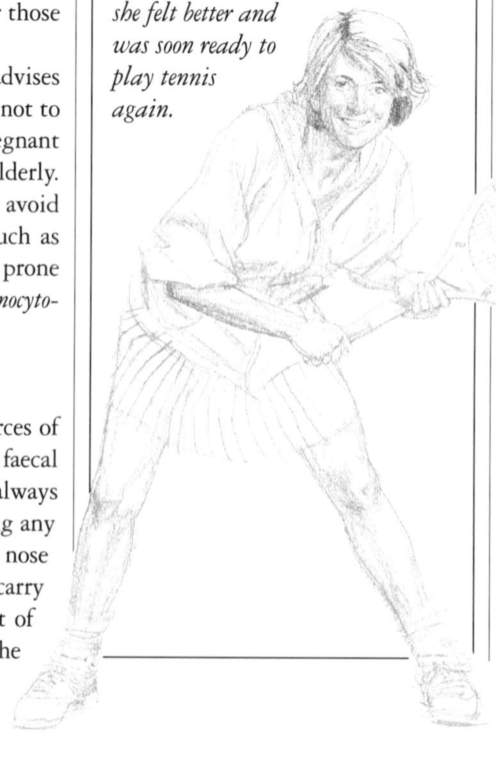

Unfortunately, many bacteria do not obligingly signal their presence in this way, so careful refrigeration, hygienic preparation and thorough cooking at an adequate temperature are also essential.

HIGH RISK FOODS

The people most at risk from food poisoning – pregnant women, the elderly, the very young, the chronically sick and those with compromised immune systems, such as anyone with cancer or AIDS – should be especially careful about eating the following foods.

Eggs are a major source of salmonella bacteria, a common cause of food poisoning, symptoms of which include abdominal cramps and vomiting. The bacteria thrive in custards, salads and other dishes incorporating raw or lightly cooked eggs, particularly when such dishes are not refrigerated. You can destroy salmonella by boiling eggs for 7 minutes, poaching them for 5, or frying them for 3 minutes on each side. Avoid foods which incorporate raw eggs, such as freshly made mousses, and sauces like mayonnaise and hollandaise.

Poultry is a source of salmonella and campylobacter bacteria, which are both common causes of headaches, nausea, vomiting and diarrhoea lasting for anything up to five days. Chicken and turkey should be thawed completely in a cool environment such as a refrigerator or larder (but not on the kitchen worktop which is generally too warm) and cooked to an internal temperature of at least 80°C (176°F). They should never be eaten if the meat appears pink or bloody: make sure the juices run clear when a skewer is inserted into the thickest part of the thigh. However careful you are about cooking, if you handle raw meat or poultry – or use your hands to make a meat loaf – and then touch an ice cube for a drink, say, or any food which will not be heated, you will spread bacteria.

Stuffing can harbour bacteria that has spread from the raw meat, since it seldom reaches a safe temperature inside the bird. Stuff poultry just before cooking and re-weigh the bird to calculate cooking time to include the weight of the stuffing or, preferably, cook stuffing in a separate roasting dish. To be extra safe, test stuffing with a meat thermometer before eating – it should have reached a temperature of at least 75°C (167°F).

Pork and beef may harbour salmonella or other bacteria. Pork, in particular, should never be eaten pink because it may also be contaminated with a parasitic worm infection called trichinosis (it should be cooked to an internal temperature of 75°C, 167°F).

Steak tartare, although considered a delicacy, poses a particularly high risk, as it is made with raw beef and raw egg yolk. It may therefore harbour salmonella, *E. coli* and other bacteria.

Soft-rinded cheese, unpasteurised milk and cream, coleslaw, salads, inadequately cooked chilled foods and pâté can all contain *Listeria monocytogenes*, which causes listeriosis. The illness may cause flu-like symptoms or, more seriously, meningitis. In pregnancy, it can cause a miscarriage or damage the unborn child.

Seafood, such as mussels, oysters, or prawns, can precipitate quite violent food-poisoning symptoms. This is usually due to sewage pollution in the water where the shellfish feed. Spoiled oily fish such as mackerel, herring or tuna (especially when served raw, as in

What's your poison?

If you have symptoms of food poisoning, try to work out when you ate a suspect meal as this can help to determine which bacteria are responsible. If fever develops or the symptoms persist for more than a couple of days, consult your doctor.

BACTERIA	SYMPTOMS
BACILLUS CEREUS	
Found in cooked rice which has been kept warm or inadequately reheated: cooked rice should be kept very hot, or cooled quickly and refrigerated.	Severe vomiting within 1 hour of eating rice, or diarrhoea later. Recovery is rapid.
CAMPYLOBACTER JEJUNI	
Usually due to cross-contamination, such as blood from raw poultry dripping onto cooked foods or salad.	Fever, abdominal pain and nausea followed by bloody diarrhoea; symptoms appear within 2-6 days and last 1-10 days.
CLOSTRIDIUM BOTULINUM (BOTULISM)	
A very rare and deadly form of poisoning found in inadequately sterilised tinned or bottled vegetables, meats or fish.	Within 18-36 hours, it causes slurred speech, difficulty in swallowing, blurred vision, paralysis and respiratory failure.
CLOSTRIDIUM PERFRINGENS	
This bacterium is associated with warm meat, gravy and stuffings; typically, a casserole or saucepan of mince sitting over a low heat, or in a warm room.	Abdominal cramps, diarrhoea and headache; occasionally vomiting and fever too. Incubation from 6-12 hours; normally a full recovery is made after 24 hours.
ESCHERICHIA COLI (E. COLI)	
A severe form of poisoning found in poorly cooked beefburgers and other minced products, associated with poor kitchen hygiene in fast-food outlets.	Vomiting and severe diarrhoea which is often bloody; symptoms occur within 12-72 hours, and last for up to 10 days; patients often require hospitalisation.
LISTERIA MONOCYTOGENES	
Lives undetected, causing no problems, in the intestines of many people and animals. Mainly found in soft cheeses, and can reproduce at refrigerator temperatures.	Sudden flu-like symptoms, anything from 4 hours to several days after ingestion. Can damage the foetus. Also very serious in babies, the elderly and the sick.
SALMONELLA	
Usual sources are raw or lightly cooked eggs, undercooked poultry and also cooked foods or salads which have been left unrefrigerated for several hours.	Nausea, abdominal pain, fever, vomiting and diarrhoea; within 8-36 hours. A common food-borne infection; major outbreaks can involve thousands of people.
STAPHYLOCOCCUS AUREUS	
Many people carry *staphylococci* bacteria, and can easily transfer them to foods. Common culprits are ham, poultry and cream or custard-filled baked goods.	Abdominal pain, nausea, vomiting and diarrhoea within a few minutes to 6 hours; occasionally chills, weakness and dizziness.

Dos and don'ts

• Do remember that bacteria are found on all the foods that people eat. Therefore it follows that any food can become contaminated with poisonous bacteria.
• Do wash your hands before you handle any food, and cover up any cuts or sores with a plaster.
• Do remove stuffing from cooked poultry before refrigerating.
• Do keep a separate chopping board for raw meat, poultry and fish. Always store cooked and raw food separately.
• Do ensure meat is well cooked.
• Do reheat cooked food thoroughly, and never reheat it more than once.
• Don't keep cooked dishes warm over a very low heat, as bacteria multiply rapidly in warmth.

ushi), can cause scombroid poisoning. Its symptoms are a sharp, peppery, burning sensation in the mouth, diarrhoea and vomiting, hot flushes, headache and a bright red rash.

If you get food poisoning

Food poisoning symptoms take effect anything from a few minutes to several days after eating the culprit food. Typical symptoms include nausea, stomach pain, vomiting, diarrhoea, and sometimes fever. In most cases such symptoms are unpleasant but they are not life-threatening; botulism, a rare form of food poisoning, is the exception, and requires immediate medical attention.

Vomiting is the natural way for the body to expel bad food, and in cases of poisoning it should be endured rather than cured. The major hazard from food poisoning, especially in the young or the sick, is dehydration and a loss of essential minerals from the body. It is crucial to replace lost fluid, salt and sugar. Sip dilute solutions of sugar, glucose or honey and, if there has been a high fluid loss, a little salt in boiled water while the symptoms persist. Camomile tea is gentle on the stomach and has soothing properties.

The last thing you want to do after a bout of sickness is to eat, but when you start to feel better, try a banana to help settle your acid stomach, and some live yoghurt to restore protective bacteria in the gut. Build up your strength with a bland diet: the Harvard Medical School advocates the 'brat' diet – bananas, rice, apples and toast – for the first 24 to 48 hours.

Fractures

EAT PLENTY OF

- *Dairy products, nuts and pulses which are good sources of calcium*
- *Oily fish for vitamin D*

AVOID

- *Bran products, unleavened bread and brown rice*

Anyone who has just sustained a fracture can facilitate the healing process by eating foods which help to build bones. In order for calcium to be deposited in the bones, the body needs an adequate supply of vitamin D as well as calcium. It is therefore important to take plenty of milk, cheese and yoghurt, nuts and pulses, for their calcium, and oily fish for its vitamin D.

Even the fittest athletes can break bones, although serious injuries are less likely when bones and joints are supported by well-developed muscle tissue. Fractures are more common in elderly people, who tend to fall more often. Even minor accidents, which one would not expect to inflict severe damage, can cause fractures in people whose bones are weak and brittle. This brittleness most commonly occurs in post-menopausal women whose bones are weakened through OSTEOPOROSIS. Anyone with OSTEOMALACIA will also be prone to fractures.

It is sensible to avoid the major dietary sources of phytic acid, such as bran and brown rice, because it inhibits calcium absorption. It may also be worth avoiding foods which contain oxalic acid, such as rhubarb and spinach, because oxalates also inhibit absorption of the mineral.

Eating calcium-rich foods – such as milk and other dairy produce, green leafy vegetables, and tinned sardines with their bones – in childhood and adolescence, can help to prevent bones becoming brittle when you get older. However, bone weakness may be the result of other underlying diseases or long-term drug treatment.

Free radicals

The unstable atoms or molecules known as free radicals are produced by the body as a consequence of its normal metabolism, and as part of its natural defence against disease. Sometimes, however, the body over-reacts, increasing its free radical production and releasing more of the unstable atoms or molecules than it needs. Factors that can spark their overproduction include cigarette smoke, smog, overexposure to ultraviolet light, illness and even intense exercise.

Free radicals contain at least one unpaired electron (or negative charge), making them highly reactive. As soon as they are produced, they search for other molecules with a positive charge with which they can react – this reaction is called oxidation. Free radicals can oxidise – and so damage – DNA and cell membranes, opening the way for cancers and diseases to develop. They are linked to the appearance of brown patches on the skin of elderly people. But although free radicals have been associated with ageing, cancer, atherosclerosis, high blood pressure, osteoarthritis and immune deficiency, the role they play in the development of these conditions is still the subject of extensive medical research.

However, it is generally believed that if free radicals reach and attack the DNA in the nucleus of a cell, the cell mutation which can result may cause cancer. It has also been observed that when blood cholesterol is oxidised by free radicals it is more damaging to the artery than 'native' cholesterol – so implicating free radicals in the development of heart disease.

The body has defence mechanisms against free radicals: ANTIOXIDANT enzymes and nutrients in the blood serve to 'mop up' free radicals and render them harmless. Protective nutrients include iron, zinc, copper, manganese and selenium (which help to make up protective antioxidant enzymes) as well as vitamins A, C and E. Certain other plant substances also provide protection against free radical damage; these include beta carotene and bioflavonoids.

FROZEN FOOD

BENEFITS

- *Most nutrients are retained well*
- *Most foods retain their natural colour, texture and flavour*

DRAWBACKS

- *Vegetables lose some vitamins during the blanching process*
- *Foods with a high water content may lose their firmness once thawed*

Supermarket freezer cabinets offer a huge range of commercially frozen produce and CONVENIENCE FOODS. The maximum recommended storage times – after which quality will begin to deteriorate – must be clearly shown on their labels. (See PREPARING, COOKING AND STORING FOOD.)

Freezing delays food spoilage by slowing down the enzyme activity which breaks down food. It also makes the water in food unavailable, and so checks the growth of bacteria, which need moisture to multiply.

Blanching – exposure of fruit or vegetables to high heat through boiling, steaming or microwaving – is used to inactivate certain enzymes and yeasts which would otherwise continue to break down cells, albeit very gradually, after freezing. Blanching causes a loss of some vitamin C and other heat-sensitive vitamins such as thiamin and folate. Despite these losses, vegetables and fruits frozen in peak condition are often more nutritious than their 'fresh' counterparts. This is because fruits and vegetables start to lose vitamin C from the moment they are picked, but commercial growers can freeze crops almost immediately after picking. Fresh soft fruit and green vegetables can lose as much as 15 per cent of their vitamin C per day if kept at room temperature.

There are virtually no nutrient losses from fish, meat or poultry, because protein as well as the vitamins A and D are unaffected by freezing.

YOUR DEEPFREEZE

Unless you have a self-defrosting freezer, you will need to defrost your freezer regularly. Once emptied, wash out the freezer with warm water and bicarbonate of soda, which cleans efficiently without leaving a smell behind. Allow the freezer temperature to drop down to -18°C (0°F) before restocking it. Pack frozen food as close together as possible in the freezer: it is both more efficient and more economical. Food which has been frozen and thawed should never be refrozen.

FRUIT

See page 166

FUNGAL INFECTIONS

Fungal infections can occur at any time without any obvious trigger. The infections can be severe if the immune system is seriously impaired, as in patients undergoing chemotherapy, for example. Try to eat a balanced diet and cut down on alcohol, which is known to impair the immune system.

Warmth, moisture, irritation and chafing of the skin all help fungi (which are naturally present on the body) to proliferate. This can give rise to diseases. The skin, nails and genitals are most commonly affected, but in rare cases, the lungs and other organs may be susceptible. Antibiotic treatment, which rids the body of the harmful organism but also destroys the 'friendly' bacteria that control fungal populations, can also leave a person open to fungal infection. Eat plenty of YOGHURT to replace bacteria in the gut destroyed by antibiotics.

TYPES OF FUNGAL DISEASE

The most common fungal infections are candidiasis (THRUSH) and tinea. Candidiasis commonly arises in the mouth and genitals. There are several types of tinea, and all cause itchy, red, scaly patches on the skin. Ringworm affects the scalp or neck (*Tinea capitis*) or the non-hairy parts of the body (*Tinea corporis*); jock (or dhobie) itch (*Tinea cruris*) affects the groin area; and athlete's foot (*Tinea pedis*) affects the spaces between the toes and the soles and sides of the feet. Badly damaged skin can suffer secondary bacterial infections. Tinea infections are highly contagious and can be spread via hairbrushes, clothes and direct contact.

FRUIT: A VITAL SOURCE OF VITAMINS

Although most fruits are sweet, they tend to be relatively low in calories. Better still, they are a good source of fibre and are packed with nutrients – especially vitamin C.

One reason why the much-vaunted Mediterranean diet is considered to be so good for the heart is because it includes plenty of fresh fruit. The World Health Organisation recommends that everyone should try to eat at least five portions of different fruit or vegetables each day.

A 'portion' of fruit counts as a single fruit, such as an apple or orange; a cup of small fruit such as grapes or raspberries; or a glass of pure fruit juice. You can include dried, tinned and frozen fruit as part of your quota, but tinned fruit is often sweetened in syrup, and contains less vitamin C. Where possible, buy fruit that has been canned in its own juice without added sugar.

Fruit is a valuable source of ANTIOXIDANTS, such as bioflavonoids and vitamin C, which may help to protect against degenerative diseases including cancer and heart disease. As fruit is low in calories, it is an excellent food for anyone trying to lose weight.

NUTRIENTS AND FIBRE

Fresh fruit and juices provide most of our daily intake of vitamin C, with citrus fruit (oranges, lemons, grapefruit and tangerines) being the most important source. Other top vitamin C providers include kiwi fruit, strawberries, raspberries, blackcurrants, mangoes and papayas.

Fruits with orange or deep yellow flesh, such as apricots, mangoes and cantaloupe melons, get their colour from a yellow-orange pigment called beta carotene, the plant form of vitamin A. Other carotene pigments such as lycopene are found in red fruits and these, along with beta carotene, are thought to protect against FREE RADICALS and possibly cancer. Fruit is rich in potassium, especially bananas and dried fruits. Potassium helps to regulate blood pressure. It works in tandem with sodium to regulate the body's fluid balance.

Another reason why fruit is so important to the diet is because it contains both soluble and insoluble fibre. The insoluble fibre helps to prevent constipation and is associated with a reduced risk of colon cancer, while the soluble fibre can help to lower blood cholesterol levels. Citrus fruit and dried fruits (such as figs, dates, apricots and raisins) are particularly good sources of fibre.

PESTICIDES

Most nutritionists agree that the benefits of eating lots of fruit far outweigh any possible risks to your health from chemical pesticides. The use of these chemicals is controlled by law and levels in foods must remain within predetermined safe limits. Pesticides are applied to crops to ensure that the produce is of a high quality and free

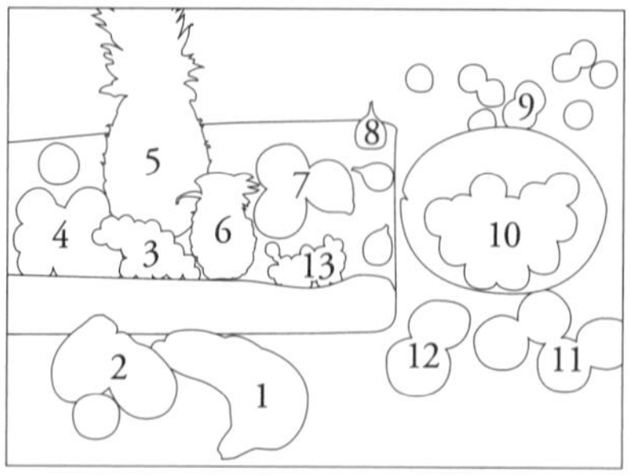

FRUIT COCKTAIL *As well as providing vitamins and minerals, fruit supplies carbohydrates. Choose from bananas (1), papaya (2), grapes (3), clementines (4), pineapples (5, 6), lemons (7), figs (8), apricots (9), plums (10), satsumas (11), guavas (12) and raspberries (13).*

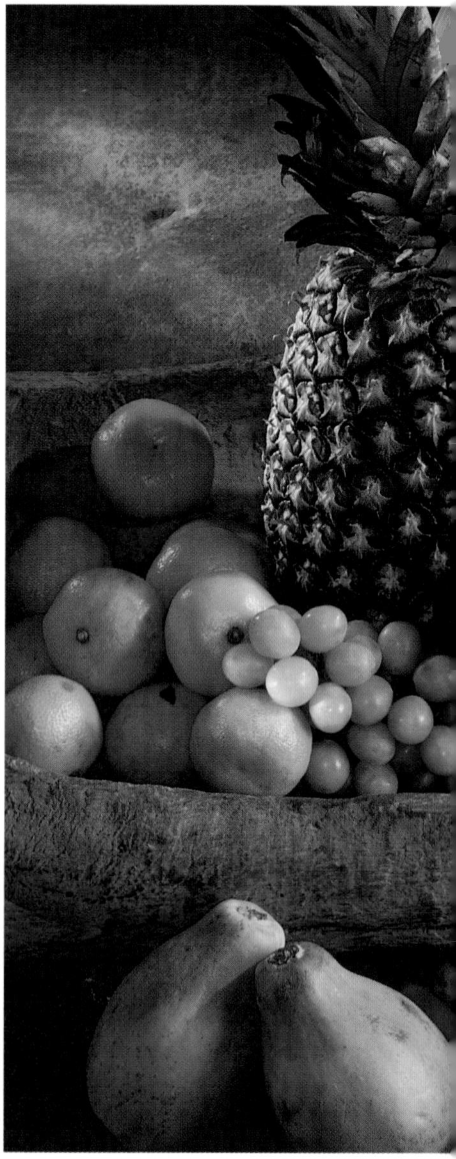

from pests and diseases, and in most fruit the levels are so low that they pose no hazard to health – even for children.

However, because it is assumed that people do not eat citrus peel, the rinds of many citrus fruits are coated in fungicides to prevent mould growth. It is therefore sensible to use untreated fruit when making marmalade or candied peel or wash the fruit thoroughly in clean running water. If you still feel sceptical about the use of chemicals, you could consider buying organic fruit which has been grown without pesticides. But beware of fruit that is mouldy or blighted with spots – it may contain natural carcinogens.

It is thought that there is relatively little difference in the nutritional value of organic and ordinary produce. Some surveys have suggested that organic fruit may have a lower water content and so be more concentrated in terms of vitamins and minerals – and possibly also flavour. However, a low water content could be nothing

BENEFITS

- *Contains antioxidants which may help to protect against cancer*
- *Rich source of potassium which helps to regulate blood pressure*
- *Provides most of our daily intake of vitamin C*

DRAWBACK

- *Fruit juice can contribute towards tooth decay*

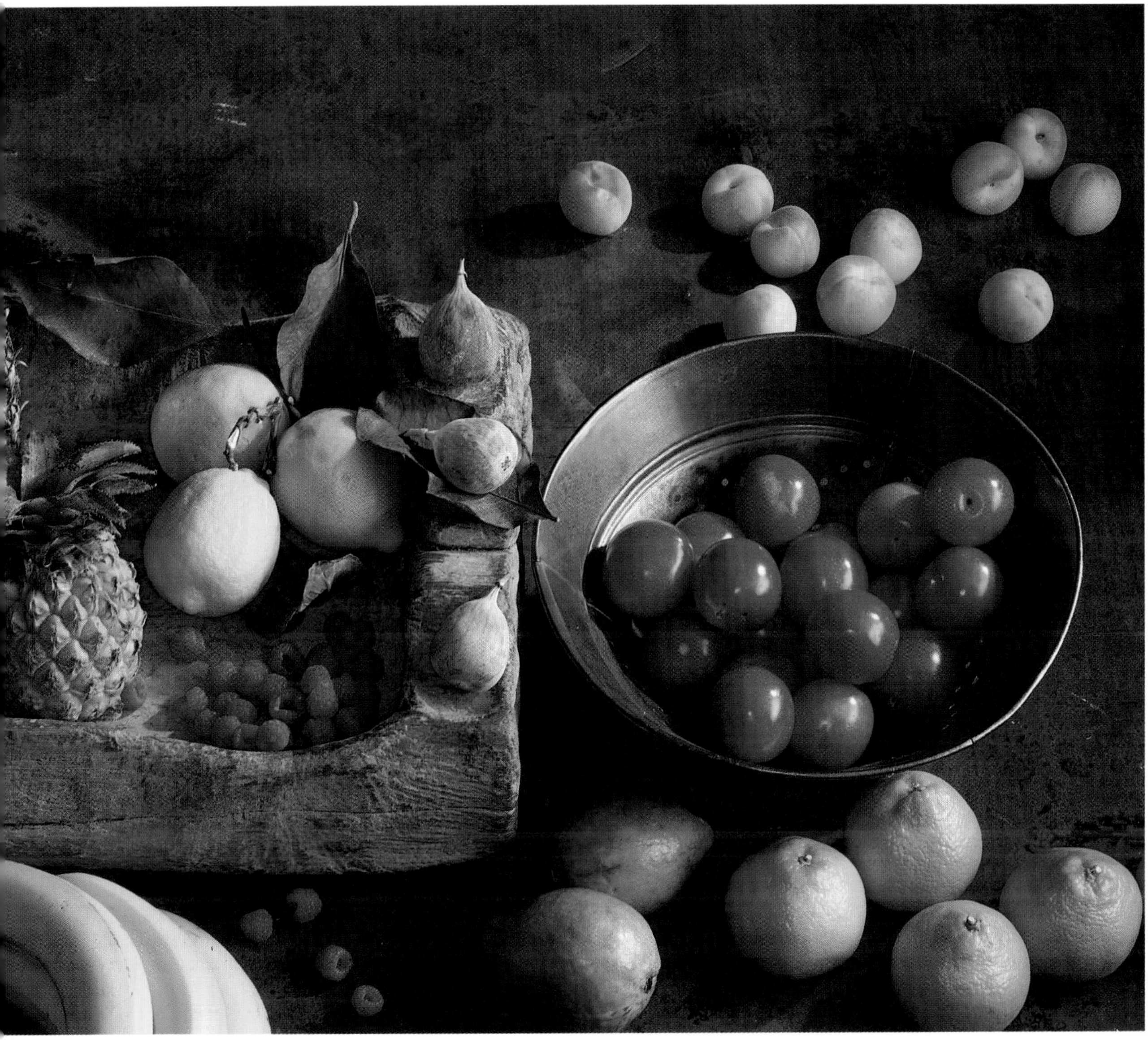

BERRIES

Berries are divided into soft types, such as strawberries and raspberries, and firm ones such as currants and cranberries. These fruits supply varying amounts of vitamin C for a strong immune system, and potassium which has a vital role in maintaining the body's mineral and fluid balance. All berries have ANTIOXIDANT properties, and so may help to prevent degenerative diseases such as cancer. Most fruit, but especially berries, contain salicylates – aspirin-like compounds that can cause reactions in susceptible people. Fresh berries are low in calories, but commercially canned berries may contain extra sugar and more calories.

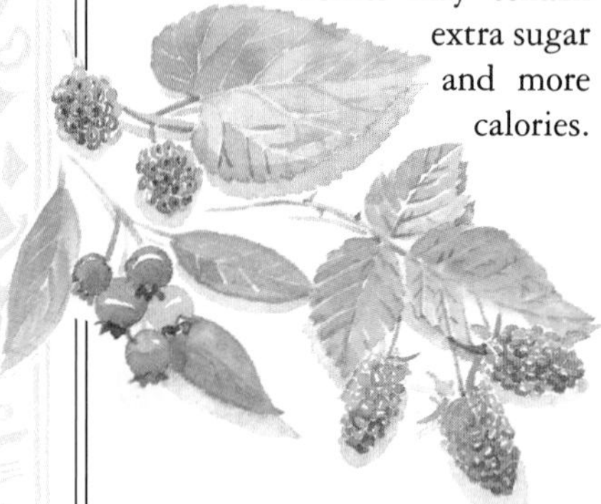

more than a sign of dehydration, resulting from the way the fruit has been stored and transported.

FRUIT JUICE

Freshly squeezed juices have been used as health cures in Europe since the 19th century, and naturopaths believe that juices can help to cleanse the body by flushing out waste products and harmful toxins. There is, however, no medical evidence for this claim.

Fruit juice is a good source of vitamin C, and the extracting process results in only a small loss of this vitamin. But it should be noted that the combination of high acidity levels and simple sugars in fruit juice can contribute to TOOTH AND GUM DISORDERS, although the risk is lessened if consumed with a meal.

There are so many different kinds of fruit juice that it can be confusing when trying to make a choice. Some of the terms that you will encounter in the shops are listed in the next column.

Freshly squeezed (grapefruit and orange juice). The only type of juice that can truly call itself 'natural' and 'pure' because it has undergone no processing except the extraction of the liquid from the fruit.

Freshly pressed (tomato and apple juice). In the case of tomatoes, the fruit is pulped shortly after picking and then pasteurised. In the case of apples, the fruit is milled, pressed, pasteurised and filtered to remove the heavier sediment, and a small amount of vitamin C (ascorbic acid) is added to prevent it going brown.

Made from concentrates The fruit is squeezed, then the juice is heated so that its water content evaporates, resulting in a thick concentrate which is pasteurised. Water is added back before packaging. Vitamin C losses are usually fairly small.

'Premium' or 'supreme' A mix of freshly squeezed fruit and juice from concentrates. The ratio of fresh fruit juice to juice from concentrates does not have to appear on the label.

Pasteurised This has twice the shelf life of fresh juice because it has been

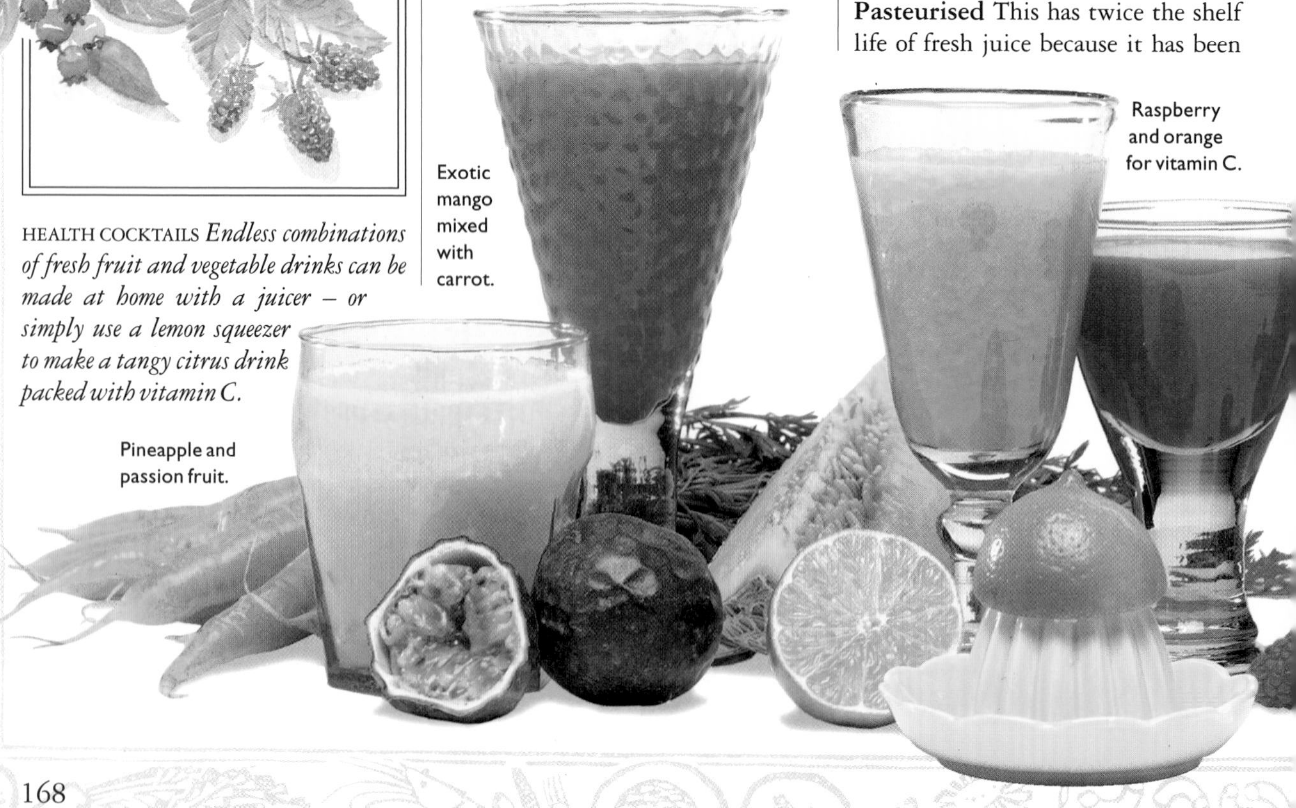

HEALTH COCKTAILS *Endless combinations of fresh fruit and vegetable drinks can be made at home with a juicer – or simply use a lemon squeezer to make a tangy citrus drink packed with vitamin C.*

Exotic mango mixed with carrot.

Raspberry and orange for vitamin C.

Pineapple and passion fruit.

heated briefly to kill off some of the bacteria. The pasteurisation process destroys little of the vitamin C content.

DRIED FRUIT

Drying is almost certainly the oldest way of preserving fruit. Although dried fruits are considered to be one of the great health foods because they are a good source of fibre, and a concentrated source of nutrients such as iron and potassium, they also contain a lot of sugar and are high in calories. Common dried fruits include raisins from several varieties of grape; currants from small seedless grapes; and prunes from plums. Dates are the fruit of the handsome date palm, and are common in the Middle East.

Dried figs are especially useful if you suffer from constipation, as they are high in fibre. If it is energy that you need, raisins and dried apricots make excellent snacks for a quick energy boost. Dried fruits can also be used as a sweetener; try chopping them into breakfast cereals and yoghurt.

A refreshing drink squeezed from pink grapefruit.

Combine the sharp taste of cranberries with apple juice.

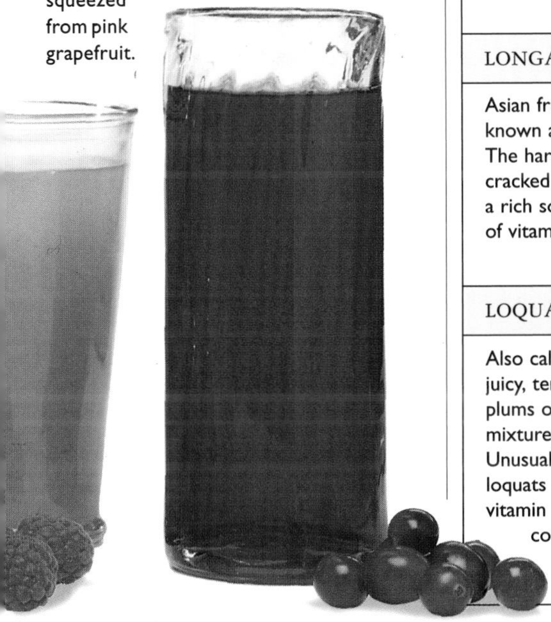

Exotic fruits

Nowadays, supermarket shelves contain a wide choice of fruits from around the world, thanks to modern techniques of transport and storage. All tropical fruits, from pomegranates to cape gooseberries, have unique flavours and textures, and most are good sources of nutrients.

CAPE GOOSEBERRIES

One of the prettiest fruits, cape gooseberries (of the *Physalis* family) are also known as Chinese lanterns. They contain useful amounts of beta carotene and vitamin C, for a strong immune system, as well as potassium, for healthy blood pressure.

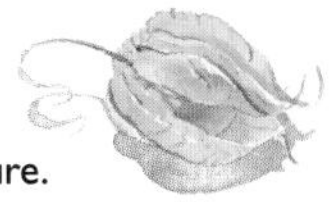

LYCHEES

Originally from China and related to longans. Most people consume tinned lychees, but fresh fruits are available from November to January, and have a sweetly perfumed aroma that is reminiscent of elder flowers. Lychees are an excellent source of vitamin C.

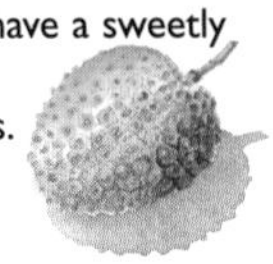

CUSTARD APPLE

Generic name given to a tropical family (*Annona*) of some 60 fruits. All are heart-shaped with scaly skins. They are a good source of potassium and vitamin C.

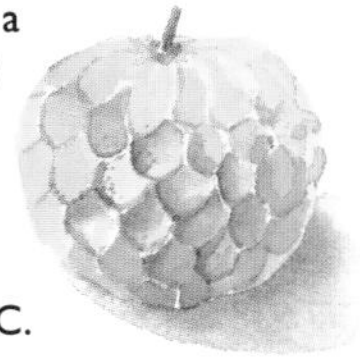

PASSION FRUIT

One of the most fragrant and distinctive tasting of all tropical fruits; native to Brazil and also known as granadilla which means 'little pomegranate'. They contain useful amounts of vitamin C.

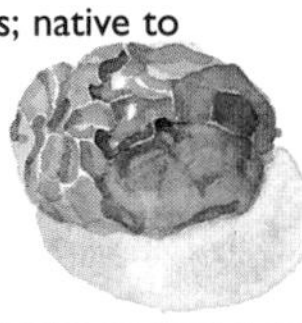

KUMQUATS

The smallest of all citrus fruits, originally from China. Unlike other citrus fruits, kumquats have a sweet edible rind. They contain useful amounts of vitamin C.

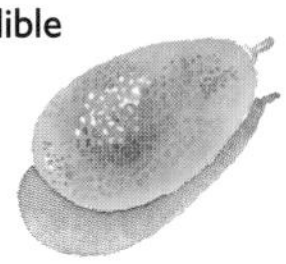

PERSIMMON

The national fruit of Japan; also known as Sharon fruit. Persimmons supply useful amounts of vitamin C, and are a good source of beta carotene and potassium.

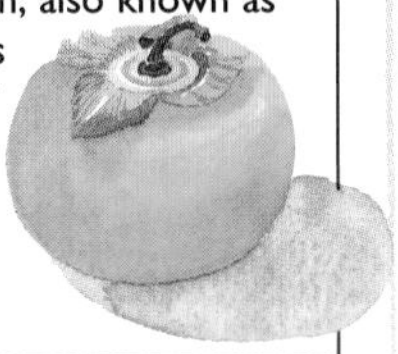

LONGANS

Asian fruits related to lychees, also known as dragon's eyes. The hard shell is easily cracked. Longans are a rich source of vitamin C.

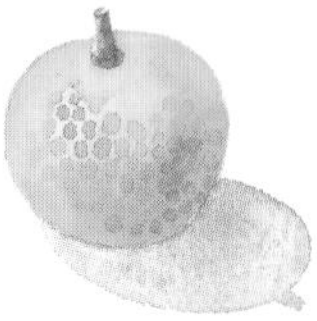

POMEGRANATE

A symbol of fertility in folklore throughout the world. This fruit is a good source of vitamin C and a useful source of fibre if you eat the seeds.

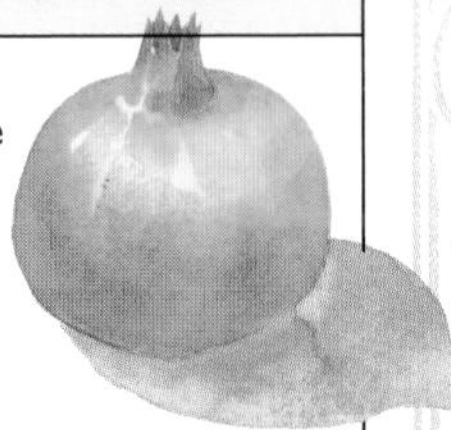

LOQUATS

Also called Japanese plums, loquats have a juicy, tender flesh that is reminiscent of plums or cherries. They taste like a mixture of apple and apricot. Unusually for a fruit, loquats contain no vitamin C. They do contain beta carotene.

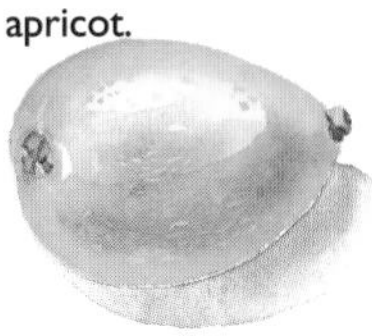

POMELO

Ancestors of the grapefruit, pomelos (or pummelos) originated in South-east Asia. Like most citrus fruits, pomelos are an excellent source of vitamin C.

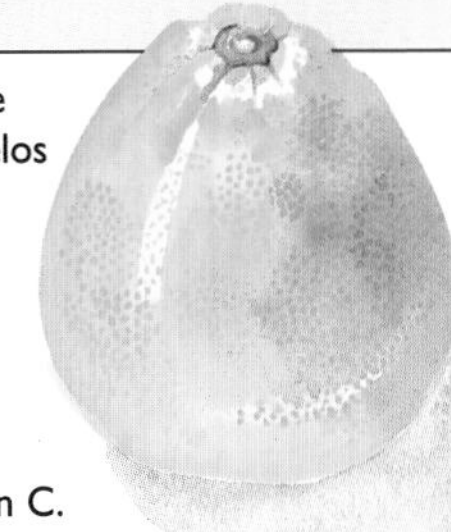

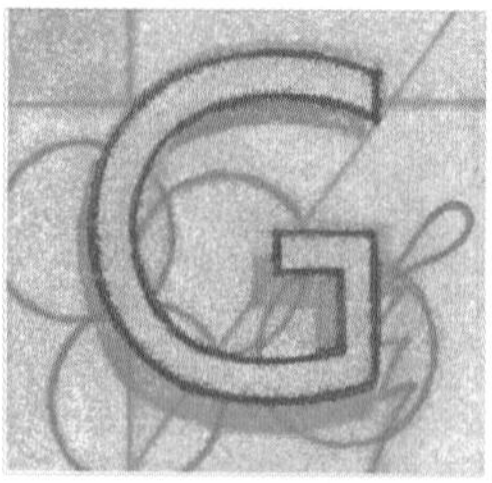

GALLSTONES

EAT PLENTY OF

- *Starchy foods, such as bread and rice*
- *Fresh fruit and vegetables*
- *Oat bran and pulses, for soluble fibre*

AVOID

- *Fried and fatty foods*
- *Obesity*

Hard lumps of cholesterol, calcium or bile pigments can form 'stones' in the gall bladder or bile duct. It is the crystallisation of these substances that causes the gallstones. The crystals latch on to a protein fragment and gradually build up layer on layer.

Gallstones often go undetected until they begin to cause pain. Symptoms range from mild upper abdominal discomfort to severe pain with vomiting, in which case surgery may be necessary to remove the stones or the whole gall bladder. However, if the symptoms settle down after the initial bout of pain, a low-fat, high-fibre diet can help to prevent stones becoming any larger and discourage the formation of new ones.

Diet cannot shrink existing stones, but small ones may be excreted into the gut. Sufferers should eat more starchy foods, such as bread and rice, as well as more fresh fruit and vegetables for fibre. They should avoid fatty meals and fasting, both of which can precipitate an attack, and cut down on refined foods, fat and red meat. A study of more than 700 women showed that meat eaters were twice as likely to have gallstones as vegetarians. It was concluded that the higher incidence of gallstones in these women was because they ate more fat and less starch and fibre than the vegetarians.

A high cholesterol level in the blood and bile can contribute to gallstone formation. A high intake of soluble fibre, which can help to reduce blood cholesterol, may therefore help to prevent the development of gallstones. Oat bran and pulses are good sources of soluble fibre. Research also suggests that cynarin, found in ARTICHOKES, may have a beneficial effect on gallstones. Curiously, a moderate intake of alcohol and caffeine has been linked to a lower incidence of gallstones.

WHO IS AT RISK?

Obesity can be a contributory factor in developing gallstones, although many slim people suffer from them too. In the UK, gallstones are twice as common in women as men; 10 per cent of women aged over 40 develop stones.

GAME AND GAME BIRDS

BENEFITS

- *Low in fat and calories, compared with untrimmed meat from farm animals*
- *Excellent sources of protein*
- *Rich in B vitamins*
- *Rich in iron*
- *Good source of phosphorous and they contain potassium*

DRAWBACK

- *Danger of biting or swallowing lead shot in wild game*

Because they live in a harsh environment, wild game can rarely afford to build up the fat reserves that are typical of many domesticated animals. Hence there is little or no fatty tissue to be trimmed from game, as is often necessary with beef, lamb and pork. But once the meat has been trimmed, lean cuts of both game and domesticated animals have a similar fat and

What is in your game pie?

Wild game is generally considered healthier than farmed meat. If you bag your own, there is the benefit of physical exertion while out hunting. The chart below gives details of game's nutritional benefits. The recommended daily allowance for phosphorus is 550mg; for potassium 3500mg; and for iron 8.7mg.

FOOD per 100g (3½oz)	FAT (g)	PROTEIN (g)	PHOSPHORUS (mg)	POTASSIUM (mg)	IRON (mg)
Roast venison	6.4	35	290	360	7.8
Stewed rabbit	7.7	27.3	200	210	1.9
Stewed hare	8.0	29.9	250	210	10.8
Roast pheasant	9.3	32.2	310	410	8.4
Roast grouse	5.3	31.3	340	470	7.6
Roast partridge	7.2	36.7	310	410	7.7
Roast wood pigeon	13.2	27.8	400	410	19.4

calorie content. Like all meat, game and game birds provide abundant amounts of protein and are rich sources of B vitamins and iron. They are also good sources of potassium, which is needed for the maintenance of all cells, and phosphorus, which is essential for healthy bones and teeth.

Rabbit, hare, venison and a wide range of game birds are now available in good butchers and larger supermarkets throughout the year. Prices are often very reasonable during the shooting season (which varies for different game species), while at other times – when only frozen game is available – it can be very expensive.

Much of the game sold in Europe is wild, but in the United States hunters are usually not allowed to sell their quarry, so most retail game has been farmed. With wild game any risk of contamination by antibiotics, artificial growth hormones or pesticides is minimal. Reared game, however, is not always clear of these chemicals.

TOUGH OLD BIRDS

As game and game birds tend to be more active than domesticated animals, their meat tends to be tougher. This is mainly due to the collagen of their muscles being more resistant to breakdown during cooking than the collagen found in meats from domesticated animals. It is important, therefore, that game meats are prepared and cooked in the correct way.

Hanging game helps to tenderise it and improve its flavour. If you are unsure how long you should hang game, ask your local butcher for guidelines. The age of the animal and the temperature of the room can make quite a big difference. In cold conditions pheasants may need to be hung for as long as two to three weeks, but if it is warm, a day or two may be enough. Game birds that have been frozen should not be hung after they have been thawed. Roasting is the best way of cooking all young game birds. A hot oven gives a brown, crispy skin – but game should never be overcooked. Rabbit is best cooked in a traditional stew and venison usually needs long, slow cooking for tender and flavoursome meat.

Although lead is an accumulative poison and you should try to avoid ingesting any pellets, swallowing one by mistake will not normally cause any ill effects. Remove the lead shot from wild game as you prepare it for cooking, and warn any diners that there may still be some in the meat because lead shot can damage teeth.

GARLIC

BENEFITS

- *Daily doses may help to lower blood pressure and blood cholesterol*
- *Acts as a nasal decongestant*
- *Has antiviral and antibacterial properties*

DRAWBACKS

- *Makes the breath smell*
- *May induce migraines*
- *Occasionally causes contact dermatitis*

Herbalists and naturopaths regard garlic as something of a miracle food and use it as a remedy for dozens of complaints, ranging from asthma to arthritis. Garlic's reputation has some basis in truth, and the bulb's healing properties – as an antiviral and antibacterial agent – are now backed up with scientific evidence.

Garlic can be eaten raw in order to reduce nasal congestion as well as to help to relieve the other symptoms of a cold.

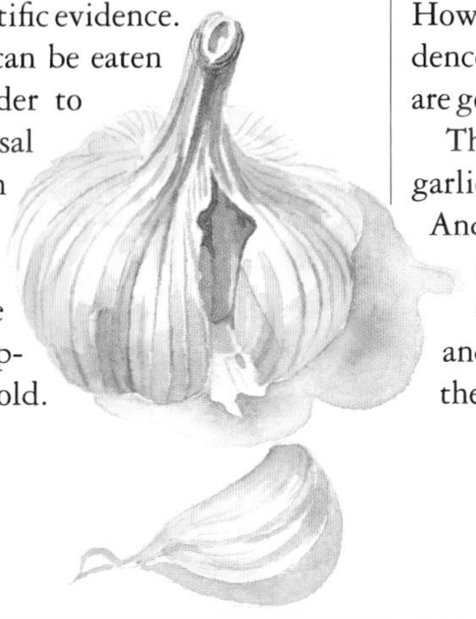

The medicinal properties of garlic are the result of the sulphur compounds it contains, including those that are responsible for the pungent odour released when a bulb is crushed. There is some dispute as to whether garlic offers the same health benefits when eaten cooked as when taken raw, as many of the volatile components are lost through cooking.

In several studies scientists have shown that the compounds in garlic are good for the heart: they lower BLOOD PRESSURE, suppress CHOLESTEROL production in the liver, reduce harmful cholesterol and raise levels of the beneficial high-density lipoproteins in the blood. In Germany, garlic is processed into a drug for lowering blood cholesterol levels. The recommended daily dose of fresh garlic is about 4g (⅛oz), equivalent to one or two small cloves.

Garlic can also inhibit blood clotting and increase the rate at which blood clots are broken down, but large amounts – ten or more cloves a day – may have to be eaten before any effect is noticed. Dried garlic preparations also have a slight effect in reducing blood pressure and blood cholesterol.

Animal studies have shown that the garlic compound allyl disulphide may also help to prevent the growth of malignant tumours. A 1991 population study conducted in Shandong, an area of China with one of the world's highest rates of gastric cancer, suggests that eating garlic on a regular basis may provide some protection. However, there is no convincing evidence that people who eat a lot of garlic are generally less prone to cancer.

The principal drawback to eating garlic is that it makes the breath smell. And in a few people it can trigger allergies; it can also induce migraine in susceptible people and, when handled, it can irritate the skin causing contact dermatitis.

Gastritis

The characteristic symptoms of gastritis are a burning sensation at the top of the stomach that can travel up into the chest, causing heartburn, nausea and flatulence. In its acute form, it is usually due to a sudden inflammation of the stomach lining. It often stems from an infection in the gut caused by the bacterium *Helicobacter pylori,* which can also cause gastric ulcers. Chronic gastritis is common among the elderly and may be linked to non-steroidal anti-inflammatory drugs used for arthritis. Other causes include excess alcohol, rich or spicy food eaten late at night, stress, or too many aspirin. About 1 in every 20 sufferers experiences considerable damage to the lining of the stomach, which may result in gastric ulcers.

As well as alcohol and spicy foods, gastritis sufferers should also avoid irritants, such as strong tea or coffee, and meat extracts. Regular and frequent small meals of bland food should bring some relief.

Many dieticians recommend an initial diet of water (to remove toxins from the body), bananas for energy and potassium, plain boiled white rice for low-fibre carbohydrate, apples for their cleansing action, and dry toast to provide bland bulk. All other foods should be avoided for the first 48 hours (see GASTROENTERITIS). Thereafter, camomile tea and LIQUORICE may help to soothe the stomach and to relieve some of the symptoms.

Case study

Imran not only enjoyed working in his uncle's restaurant but also loved eating the spicy food. But he ate irregularly, often preferring to drink instead. Recently, he had complained of stomach pain with wind. He suffered particularly at night and eased the symptoms by drinking milk. His doctor diagnosed severe stomach inflammation and advised Imran to stop drinking alcohol, avoid spicy food and eat regularly. After a month's course of medication and sticking to his new dietary regime, all of Imran's symptoms had gone.

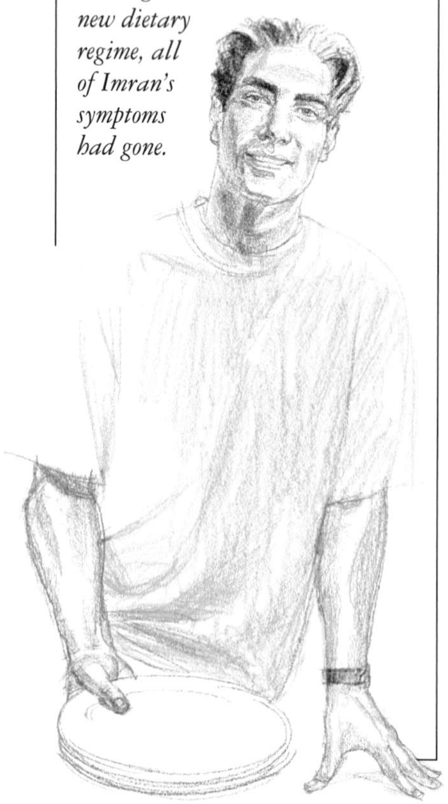

Gastroenteritis

TAKE PLENTY OF

- *Water to replace lost fluid*
- *Bananas, for potassium*
- *Boiled white rice and dry white toast for low-fibre carbohydrate*
- *Apples to cleanse the digestive system*

AVOID

- *All other food (especially dairy products) for the first 48 hours*

While gastroenteritis is often associated with DIARRHOEA and 'traveller's tummy', it occurs most often at home – usually as a result of poor HYGIENE or carelessness. Partly cooked meals, especially poultry, raw egg dishes and shellfish are the most common causes of bacterial and viral gastroenteritis. Another culprit is food that is not at its freshest. Dairy products and seafood may smell bad when they have 'gone off', but this is not necessarily the case for other foods. Therefore it is important to store food carefully, and always eat it before its use-by date.

Gastroenteritis is an inflammation of the lining of the stomach and intestines, often accompanied by acute diarrhoea and vomiting, stomach cramps and mild fever. An attack can last anything from 6 hours to three days. Symptoms can be caused by toxins produced by bacteria in the food or by inflammation of the intestines due to a virus or bacteria. Generally, food poisoning results in the more rapid onset of symptoms, which can strike within an hour or two.

Many types of virus can cause epidemic gastroenteritis, or intestinal flu. The virus can be transmitted through food handled by infected people, but it is mostly spread through personal contact or coughs and sneezes.

Bottle-fed babies are more likely to contract gastroenteritis than those who are breast-fed because they are not receiving the 'natural' immunity from their mothers' milk and because they are exposed to many more areas of potential contamination – the bottle, the teat, the formula and the milk or water used to prepare it.

Allergic reactions

Some people suffer a form of allergic gastroenteritis. Where there are no signs of acute FOOD POISONING or the condition cannot be pinned down to excessive smoking or drinking of coffee or alcohol, food ALLERGIES or intolerances could well be the cause of chronic and repeated attacks of gastric discomfort. Another cause of chronic gastroenteritis, which is common among young women, is the abuse of laxatives to keep their weight down.

THE BRAT DIET

Whatever the cause of an attack, take only fluids to begin with so as not to irritate the gut further. Oral rehydration solutions, which consist of dilute sugar and salt solutions, are better than water alone. They can be prepared by mixing equal volumes of fruit juice and water, or by dissolving eight teaspoons of sugar and one of salt with a litre (1¾ pints) of water.

A diet of bananas, boiled rice, apples and dry toast, known as the 'brat' diet, often helps to relieve discomfort. Bananas are a good source of potassium, which helps to regulate the body's fluid balance. Like rice, bananas are rich in the carbohydrates required to help to rebuild stores of energy, while apples are claimed to cleanse the digestive system. Dry white toast can help to settle the stomach and also provides carbohydrate for energy.

Eat small amounts of these four foods at regular intervals and, after 48 hours, introduce potatoes, cooked vegetables, especially carrots (which are kind on the stomach), and an egg. Gradually return to a normal diet. Leave the addition of dairy products until last because when the gut is inflamed it is more likely to develop an intolerance towards lactose, which is found in dairy foods.

FLUID INTAKE

For as long as you are experiencing diarrhoea take extra fluids in the form of a rehydration solution (two glasses for each bout) to replace lost fluids. To soothe the digestive tract, try sipping a cup of raspberry-leaf tea twice a day (except in early pregnancy) or up to three cups a day of ginger or cinnamon tea sweetened with a little honey.

GENETICALLY MODIFIED FOODS

BENEFITS

- *Longer shelf-life for fresh produce*
- *Foods that contain more protein and other nutrients*
- *Pest-resistant crops that grow in most climates and soils*
- *Higher yields and lower costs*

DRAWBACK

- *Risk of antibiotic resistance transferring to people or livestock*

There are ever-increasing demands for food across the world today. To meet these needs, scientists have been working on improving methods of food production and ways of increasing storage times. Genetic modification, better known as genetic engineering, is just one way of doing this. The technique involves altering the DNA in the genes of a cell, which determines that cell's hereditary characteristics. It can be used to speed up the process of selective breeding, so that scientists do not have to wait generations to obtain a result, which used to be the case with traditional breeding methods.

IMPROVING ON NATURE

Genetic engineering makes it possible to add just one hereditary characteristic – such as the ability to produce a substance that tastes bad to insects – which prevents pests eating crops. Another genetic modification might make crop plants resistant to a certain herbicide (used as a weedkiller). This enables farmers to spray a field with the herbicide, killing the weeds while leaving the crop unharmed.

Alternatively, certain hereditary characteristics can be suppressed. In California, for example, a tomato has been developed which contains a gene that delays softening, so that tomatoes can be ripened on the vine yet still be firm enough to withstand transport from the farm to the shop.

Genetic engineering is currently being used to develop plants and crops that can be grown in adverse conditions such as deserts, very cold areas, or places where sea water makes soil too salty for most agriculture. This could have an enormous beneficial impact on world food shortages.

Gene modifications can also produce crops of greater nutritional value. One gene, for example, makes grains manufacture more protein; another makes oil plants, such as the rapeseed, synthesise more unsaturated fatty acids. The results are 'healthier' foods.

Vegetarian versions of traditional cheeses, such as Cheddar, would not be possible without genetic engineering. All traditional cheeses rely on the enzyme rennet, obtained from calves' stomachs, to curdle the milk to make the cheese. Today, however, genetically modified micro-organisms are used to produce an identical non-animal enzyme.

ANTIBIOTIC RESISTANCE

For all the benefits genetic modification may bring, some people are still concerned that genetic manipulation of plants might cause potentially harmful bacteria, in the digestive tract of people or livestock, to become resistant to antibiotics.

This fear stems from the fact that scientists often incorporate an antibiotic-resistant gene (or tracer) into the genetic material being introduced to the plant to test the modification's success: if the modified cell survives antibiotic treatment, it means that it has become resistant to that antibiotic and has therefore also taken on the other characteristics of the newly added genetic material. So far, there is only limited evidence to suggest that antibiotic-resistant tracers can be transferred to disease-causing micro-organisms. All genetically modified products have to be scrutinised by several government committees before being released into the environment or entering the food chain.

Crossing natural barriers

The advent of genetically modified food is causing much controversy. Beneficial modifications can produce leaner animals with greater resistance to illness, or fish that provide increased amounts of nutritionally desirable polyunsaturated fatty acids. However, genetic engineering can have harmful side effects on the animals. In pigs, the incorporation of growth hormones has resulted in bone and joint problems, loss of coordination and damaged vision. Sheep that have been injected with genetically engineered hormones affecting wool growth become more vulnerable to the effects of heat stress. Many people are concerned about whether it is right to tamper with the genes of living creatures, and the suffering it may cause them.

Ethical questions have been raised in response to scientists' talk of experimenting with human genetic material to genetically modify dairy cows – enabling them to produce milk with the exact composition of human milk. Similarly, a controversial tomato modification, which uses genetic material from fish, is being researched. The aim is to produce tomatoes which can be successfully frozen. In simple terms, fish freeze well and tomatoes do not, so scientists are looking at ways of introducing relevant cell material from fish – in this case, flounders – to create a new breed of tomato.

Moral issues

The British Government's Food Advisory Committee recommends that all genetically modified foods containing genes that are described as 'ethically sensitive' should be clearly labelled under one of three categories:

- Contains a gene originally derived from a human.
- Contains a gene originally derived from an animal which is the subject of religious dietary restrictions.
- Plant or microbial material which contains a gene that was originally derived from an animal.

There is no doubt that genetically modified foods can offer many benefits in the future. However, ethical concerns, such as the power of scientists to 'play God', have to be considered alongside technological advancement.

Glandular fever

TAKE PLENTY OF

- *Fluids, especially citrus juices and water*
- *Small, light, nutritious meals*

AVOID

- *Alcohol, because inflammation of the liver is common*

Diet may not be able to alleviate the immediate symptoms of glandular fever (infectious mononucleosis), but it can help to cut short this viral disease which in rare cases can last for up to two years. After being diagnosed as having glandular fever, aim to give your IMMUNE SYSTEM the best possible chance of fighting the illness.

To make up for any fluid lost through sweating, drink lots of water – at least 1.7 litres (3 pints) per day. This may include diluted fruit and vegetable juices, which have the advantage of providing vitamin C, beta carotene, or other nutrients.

Some alternative practitioners recommend a short period of fasting (no more than 24 hours) at the onset of the illness, limiting yourself to fresh fruit and vegetable juices, herb tea made from peppermint and elderflowers, and plenty of water. However, most doctors agree that probably the best and safest remedy in the long term is a well-balanced diet, which can be made up of many small, light meals if the patient has a poor appetite. It is wise to avoid alcohol, as it can weaken the immune system and damage the liver, which is often inflamed.

Following a healthy, balanced diet should enable your body to recover from the illness. You may want to take daily supplements of vitamin C and vitamin B complex until you recover.

The kissing disease

A viral disease of children and young adults, glandular fever is caused by the Epstein-Barr virus. It is common in 15 to 25-year-olds, and is not highly contagious, although it tends to spread rapidly through schools and colleges. The virus is carried in the saliva of an infected person, hence its popular name of 'the kissing disease'.

The first symptoms are similar to those of tonsillitis: general tiredness, muscular pains, headache, fever, enlarged lymph glands and a white coating over the tonsils. A skin rash commonly appears if the antibiotic ampicillin is given for the 'tonsillitis'. The liver can become inflamed and, in the most severe cases, the spleen can become enlarged.

Recovery time varies greatly. Normally the illness lasts for a week or two, with repeated attacks of high fever, night sweats and a general weakness that leaves the sufferer utterly drained. However, it has been known for the symptoms to continue for up to two years after the original infection.

Gooseberries

BENEFITS

- *Useful source of vitamin C and soluble fibre*

Fresh and cooked gooseberries are both useful sources of vitamin C – a typical 100g (3½oz) serving provides around a quarter of the adult daily requirement. Only a small amount of vitamin C is lost in the cooking process.

Gooseberries are also a useful source of soluble fibre. They are low in calories (a 100g or 3½oz serving of fresh cooking gooseberries stewed with sugar contains 54 Calories), but because they can have a bitter taste they are often served with plenty of cream, which then turns them into a high-calorie dessert.

Goosegogs and honeyblobs

In *A Modern Herbal,* published in 1931, Mrs Grieve lists the many names gooseberries have been known by, including feverberry, carberry, feaberry, goosegogs and honeyblobs. The juice was once thought to 'cure all inflammations' and be 'greatly profitable to such as are troubled with a hot, burning ague'. The leaves were also regarded as being very 'wholesome' and corrective of 'gravel' (small stones formed in the urinary tract). *A Modern Herbal* recommends an infusion of 25g (1oz) of dried leaves to 600ml (1 pint) of water – a teacup to be drunk three times a day. The infusion was also said to be a tonic for 'growing girls' if taken before a period.

There are several varieties of gooseberry. Some have been bred especially for desserts and are sweeter-tasting as well as being larger than the varieties normally used in cooking. In northern Europe, gooseberries are used for jam, wine, tarts and even vinegar.

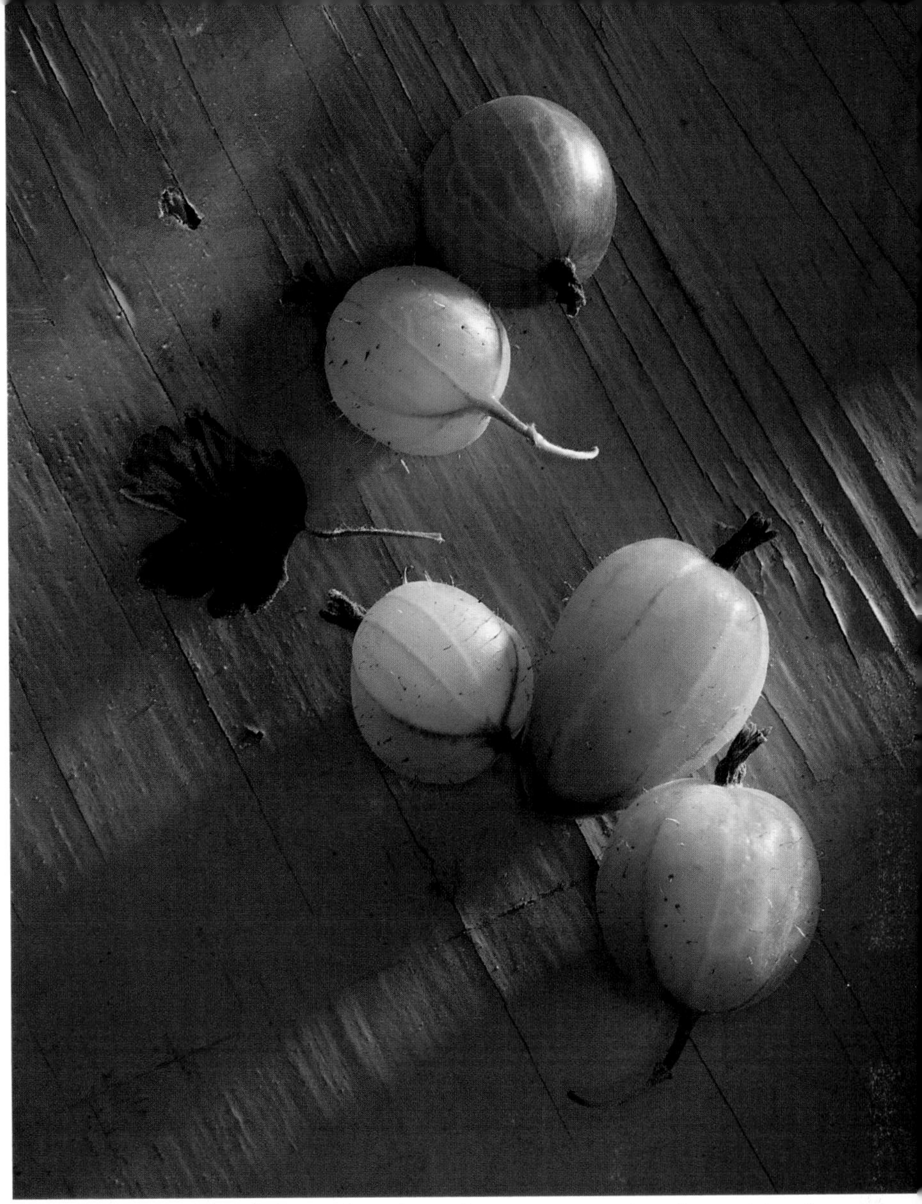

FORSAKEN FRUIT *Although the gooseberry has unfortunate connotations, its nutritional value should not be ignored; it is low in calories and is a useful source of vitamin C.*

Did you know?

The origins of the word gooseberry have nothing to do with geese, even though the acidic taste of gooseberries sets off the flavour of goose so well. It comes from the old English names for the fruit – groser, grosier and grozer – which are linked to the French *groseille,* meaning redcurrant. All these names go back to the Frankish *krûsil* – or 'crisp berry' in English.

Gout

TAKE PLENTY OF

- *Water, fresh fruit and vegetables*

AVOID

- *Excessive amounts of alcohol*
- *Offal, game, sardines and shellfish*
- *Aspirin-based drugs*

A type of ARTHRITIS, gout is caused by a defect in the body's ability to metabolise uric acid. The result is an accumulation of uric acid crystals in the joints, causing pain and inflammation. Typically a single joint is involved, most commonly the base of the big toe, although the knees, wrists and ankles can also be affected.

The precise causes of gout are uncertain, but there is often a family history. Overindulgence in food and alcohol does not cause gout, but these may trigger an attack. Gout is also commonly associated with OBESITY, especially with a build-up of fat in the abdominal cavity.

Symptoms and statistics

Although the big toe is a common place for it to start, the painful aching of gout can be felt in joints in almost any part of the body, but never in the spine.

Gout is often extremely painful and it is by no means rare. It affects 16 men in every 1000, but is less common in women (3 in every 1000), who rarely suffer from it before the menopause.

TREATING GOUT

Gout is diagnosed when a blood test reveals high levels of uric acid and a single joint is affected. Patients are usually prescribed drugs to increase the excretion of uric acid and so slow the formation of the crystals. Aspirin should be avoided as it causes retention of uric acid and interferes with the potency of the prescribed drugs. Anti-inflammatories, such as ibuprofen, can reduce the symptoms.

Controlling body weight, through a well-planned programme of exercise and diet, can also help to relieve gout; however, fasting can precipitate an attack. Gout sufferers should take plenty of fluids to help to prevent the build-up of excess uric acid crystals, which may also cause kidney stones. They should also eat plenty of fresh fruit and green leafy vegetables for potassium, which aids the excretion of uric acid by keeping the urine alkaline. Eating 225g (8oz) of fresh or tinned cherries a day can help to lower blood levels of uric acid. In traditional medicine, leeks are used to treat gout; CELERY is recommended for its anti-inflammatory action.

THE PROBLEM WITH PURINES

People who suffer from gout are generally put on a course of drugs, but they may also be advised to cut down on foods that are high in purines since high intakes of these foods can increase levels of uric acid in the blood, causing uric acid salts to be deposited in the joints. High-purine foods include offal, game, anchovies, sardines, poultry, shellfish and pulses. Low-purine foods include fruit and fruit juices, nuts, dairy produce, eggs and vegetables – with the exception of asparagus, cauliflower, peas, spinach and mushrooms.

FISH OILS

Research studies have found that omega-3 fatty acids can decrease the body's output of inflammatory compounds. Gout sufferers may find that fish-oil supplements, which contain omega-3 fatty acids, can offer some relief for painful swelling of the joints.

GRAPEFRUIT

BENEFITS

- *Rich source of vitamin C*
- *Contains pectin, which can help to lower blood cholesterol levels*

Half a grapefruit provides more than half of the adult daily requirement for vitamin C. Try to eat not just the juicy flesh but also some of the pulpy membrane that separates the fruit's segments, and a little of the white pith, too. Both contain a useful amount of pectin, a form of soluble fibre that may help to lower levels of blood cholesterol. Pink or red grapefruit are slightly higher in vitamin C than the yellow varieties.

Some experts believe that all citrus fruits have a role to play in protecting against cancer because the pulp and pith contain compounds known as bioflavonoids which are thought to neutralise cancer-causing substances.

GRAPEFRUIT DIETS

There is a popular myth that eating grapefruit helps you to slim because it has the ability to 'burn' fat. Some short-term diet regimes are based on eating grapefruit and little else – an unhealthy practice, since we all need to eat a variety of foods to obtain a full range of nutrients. Grapefruit are low in fat and calories, and eating them as part of a low-fat diet is fine, but no food has the ability to burn fat.

GRAPES

BENEFITS

- *Good source of potassium*
- *Black grapes are a source of antioxidants*

DRAWBACKS

- *Dust, yeast, pesticides and fungicides are often present on unwashed skins*
- *Black grapes may induce migraines*

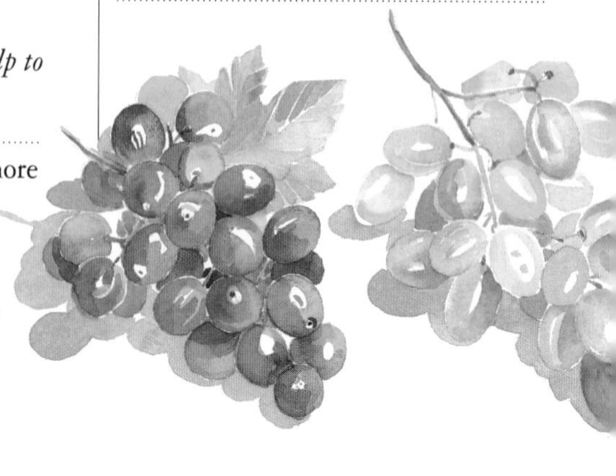

Offering grapes to people who are convalescing has become a tradition. Dessert grapes are a light, appetising food. They are sweet and relatively non-fattening: a handful weighing 100g (3½oz) contains around 60 Calories. Grapes are a good source of potassium, but otherwise provide few vitamins and minerals. Weight for weight, they contain one-twentieth the vitamin C of kiwi fruit.

Nevertheless, red and black grapes, as distinct from the green varieties, are high in bioflavonoids – antioxidants which are thought to neutralise FREE RADICALS – so they may help to protect the body against cancer and heart disease.

MIGRAINE INDUCERS

The polyphenols and tannins present in red grapes may trigger migraines in some susceptible people. The main problem with grapes, however, is contaminants on the skins, including yeasts, moulds and airborne pollutants, as well as pesticide residues. It is important, therefore, to wash grapes thoroughly before eating them.

SOUR ENDING

The term 'sour grapes' stems from Aesop's fable of the fox who tried to get at some grapes. When he realised they would always be out of reach, he went away saying, 'I see they are sour'.

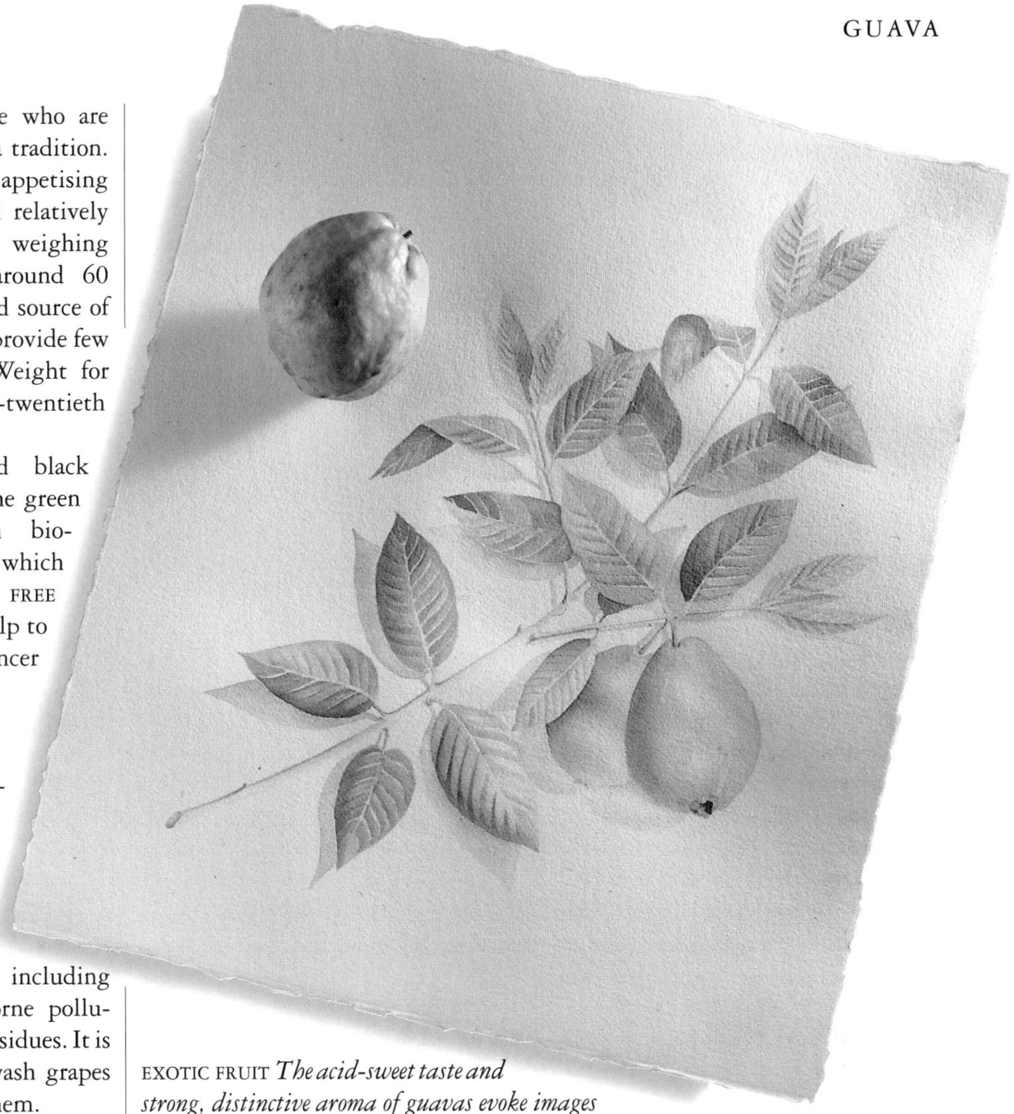

EXOTIC FRUIT *The acid-sweet taste and strong, distinctive aroma of guavas evoke images of a tropical paradise. The whole fruit is edible and rich in vitamin C.*

GUAVA

BENEFITS

- *Excellent source of vitamin C*
- *Good source of potassium and fibre*

Native to South America, guavas are grown commercially in many countries today. They are pear-shaped or round and are similar in size to a small apple. Their thin, tough yellow skin tastes slightly bitter, but the creamy, highly scented and juicy flesh is sweet. About half the fruit is made up of hard but edible seeds. These can be discarded, although they are as high in vitamins as the flesh.

Weight for weight, a guava contains more than five times as much vitamin C as an orange. One fresh 90g (3¼oz) fruit contains comfortably more than the recommended adult daily requirement of the vitamin. Even after losing almost 25 per cent of the vitamin in the canning process, tinned guavas in syrup are still an excellent source of vitamin C, which is vital for the production of collagen and healthy skin and tissues. Vitamin C is also an antioxidant, helping to mop up potentially harmful FREE RADICALS.

The flesh and seeds of a guava are a useful source of soluble fibre in the form of pectin. This fruit is also a good source of potassium, which can assist in regulating blood pressure.

Select greenish-yellow fruit that are just ripe and starting to lose their firmness. Once ripe store them in the fridge. Wash, cut in half lengthways and serve in the skin with a teaspoon.

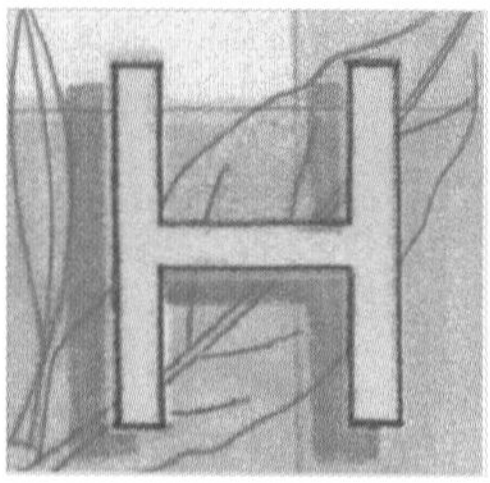

HAEMOPHILIA

Although haemophilia cannot be prevented, it can be controlled, with the right treatment. It is a hereditary condition, which mainly affects males, in which the blood does not clot properly, so that a cut or scratch, or an injury to the joints can lead to heavy bleeding and even death.

The most prevalent forms of haemophilia are caused by a deficiency in clotting factor VIII or IX (haemophilia A and B respectively), with A being about five times as common as B. Modern treatment seeks to control the condition by giving people regular infusions of a blood-clotting protein.

Because some donor blood containing factor VIII was contaminated with HIV in the early 1980s, several thousand haemophiliacs in the UK who received transfusions from affected sources became HIV positive. Today, however, all blood containing factor VIII/IX in Britain is free from contamination with HIV.

People with haemophilia have no specific dietary requirements. However, a lack of certain nutrients is known to increase the tendency to bruising and bleeding. Haemophiliacs may, for example, benefit from ensuring that their calcium intakes are adequate, because calcium promotes blood clotting. Nevertheless, the best advice is to follow a healthy balanced diet, so that the body receives adequate amounts of all the essential nutrients.

HAEMORRHOIDS

TAKE PLENTY OF

- *Apples, pears, beans, oats and cooked green leafy vegetables for their soluble fibre*
- *Wholemeal bread and brown rice for insoluble fibre*
- *Water*

CUT DOWN ON

- *Refined carbohydrates*

AVOID

- *Curries and other hot and spicy foods*

The most likely causes of haemorrhoids – itching or painful, swollen veins in anal tissue – are prolonged bouts of constipation or restricted blood flow to the abdomen caused by sitting for long periods. Obesity is another factor that frequently exacerbates haemorrhoids – more usually known as piles.

Straining to pass a bowel motion because of constipation is often the result of eating excessive amounts of refined foods which contain little or no fibre, and not drinking enough water or other liquids.

The condition often occurs during pregnancy, especially if there is a family predisposition to the problem.

HELP FROM FIBRE

To treat mild cases of haemorrhoids, eat plenty of foods that contain soluble fibre such as oats, fruit and vegetables, as well as whole grains and brown rice for insoluble fibre; and drink at least 2 litres (3½ pints) of water daily.

Following a diet which incorporates these foods may prevent people getting haemorrhoids in the first place. The soluble fibre found in oats is particularly good for treating constipation because it helps to ease bowel motions by creating softer stools. Hot and spicy foods, such as curries, should be avoided by sufferers as these usually exacerbate the condition and increase the discomfort of bowel movements.

In persistent cases, the bleeding that occurs may cause an iron deficiency which can lead to ANAEMIA. Good food sources of iron include liver (but not during pregnancy), pulses, nuts and dark green vegetables. Sources of vitamin C, such as fresh fruit, improve iron absorption.

If rectal bleeding is persistent, consult a doctor, as this can indicate cancer of the rectum. More severe cases of haemorrhoids are easily treated by surgery, usually on an outpatient basis.

HAIR AND SCALP PROBLEMS

EAT PLENTY OF

- *Eggs and liver, for vitamin A*
- *Dark green leafy vegetables, carrots and sweet potatoes, for beta carotene*
- *Vegetable oils, nuts and oily fish, for essential fatty acids*
- *Shellfish, red meat and pumpkin seeds, for zinc*

The condition of your hair and scalp is a clear pointer to your general well-being. Almost any illness or emotional stress can cause dull and lifeless hair, and your hair can therefore act as an early warning sign when you are out of sorts, or perhaps lacking in certain vitamins and minerals. But hair problems are also frequently caused by overexposure to chemicals (dyes, tints and perms being the main culprits), heat from electrical styling appliances and the wear and tear of too much brushing and combing.

GREASY HAIR

Healthy hair gets its shine from a thin coating of sebum – an oily substance secreted by the scalp's sebaceous glands near the root of each hair. If the

Case study

Jimmy had always had dry, scaly skin, which his parents treated with moisturising lotions. But when Jimmy's parents noticed that his hair was falling out they sought the advice of a dermatologist. He thought that Jimmy had a type of ichthyosis, which is usually incurable: all that sufferers can do is treat the scaling with ointment.

After many tests Jimmy's parents were told that his ichthyosis arose from a defect of vitamin A metabolism. The resultant scaling blocked the hair growth. This very rare condition meant that Jimmy could be treated orally with vitamin A drops and an ointment which reduced the scaling and allowed his hair to grow back thickly.

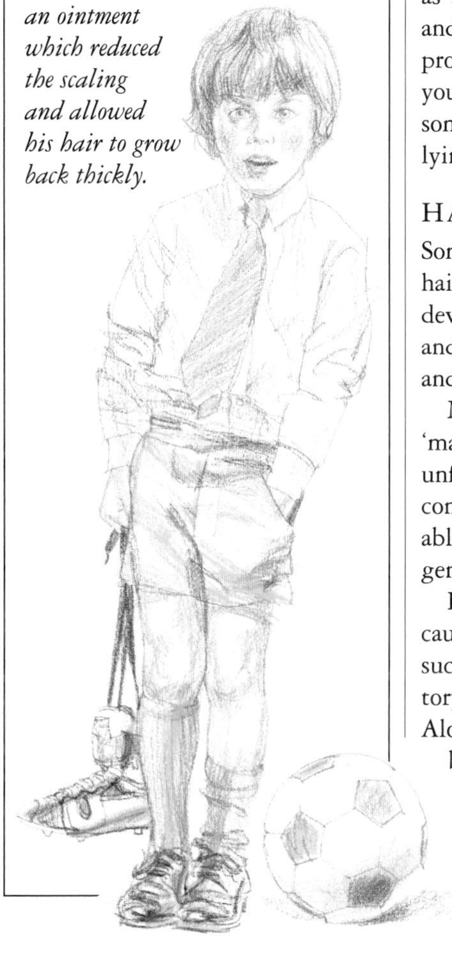

sebaceous glands become overactive and produce too much sebum, the result is lank, greasy hair. You should choose the mildest shampoo possible, and wash your hair as often as necessary. Frequent washing does not affect sebaceous secretion: it will not make greasy hair greasier or dry hair drier. Some alternative practitioners suggest that cutting down on sugary foods may help to prevent an oily scalp.

Dry scalp and dandruff

These problems may signal a zinc deficiency, so you should include zinc-rich foods such as shellfish (especially oysters), red meat and pumpkin seeds in your diet. Essential fatty acids also help to prevent dry skin and a flaking scalp: good food sources include most vegetable oils, nuts and oily fish such as sardines, herring, mackerel, trout and salmon. If dandruff and scalp problems do not respond to shampoos, you should consult a doctor as they can sometimes reflect more serious underlying health problems.

Hair loss

Some loss of hair is quite normal. A hair drops out because a new one has developed and grown underneath it, and healthy adults shed between 50 and 100 hairs each day.

Most excessive hair loss is due to 'male pattern baldness' which is, unfortunately – and despite the new concept of 'hair transplants' – untreatable, because it is largely due to genetic influences.

However, hair loss may also be caused by a variety of other conditions such as pregnancy, anaemia, circulatory problems and thyroid disorders. Alopecia areata is the appearance of bald patches which may regrow. As one patch regrows, another may appear. In roughly half of all cases stress is thought to be the main factor. People suffering from stress are often found to be short of B vitamins, which are essential for healthy hair. Good sources include wholegrain cereals, oily fish, yeast extracts, peas, natural yoghurt, eggs and milk.

A deficiency in vitamin A may also cause dull hair. Increase your intake by eating two or three eggs a week and a weekly portion of liver (although not if you are pregnant).

Ensure that your diet includes plenty of carrots, dark green leafy vegetables, sweet potatoes and dried apricots, all of which contain beta carotene, which the body's metabolism converts into vitamin A.

Diagnostic hair testing: a controversial science

Hair analysis is used by some practitioners to test for deficiencies of minerals in the body, and is even used by some companies to find out whether potential employees use illegal drugs. Strands of hair, cut into short segments, are washed and then subjected to 'f-tests' to confirm the presence, or absence, of specific substances.

Advocates of hair analysis say that the minerals in human hair correlate to those in the body. But individual testing is regarded by many scientists as unreliable and exploitative: mail order companies charge high fees for analysing locks of hair sent through the post, and then sell customers mineral supplements to redress their various 'imbalances'.

Scientists doubt the value of hair analysis, claiming that different laboratories often produce conflicting results on identical samples; no uniform definitions of ranges of mineral content exist, and air pollution, shampoos and bleaches also affect the results.

HEART DISEASE: HOW DIET CAN REDUCE THE RISK

Coronary death rates have been reduced through improved medical treatment and a better understanding of diet; nevertheless, heart disease still causes one in every four deaths in Britain.

Although coronary heart disease (CHD) is still responsible for more than a quarter of all deaths in Britain, improved treatments have resulted in a dramatic decline in the CHD death rate over the past decade. This fall has been most marked in people below the age of 45.

Nevertheless, Britain still has one of the highest rates of heart disease in the world. More than 300000 Britons suffer heart attacks each year. A disproportionate number of these people live in Scotland and the north of England where, traditionally, diets are high in saturated fats and low in fresh vegetables. This lends strength to arguments that the ANTIOXIDANTS present in fruit and vegetables may help in the fight against coronary heart disease.

COFFEE: OILS, NOT CAFFEINE, ARE THE CULPRITS

Heavy coffee drinking may cause high blood cholesterol levels and increase the risk of heart disease, but most medical experts agree that caffeine, long the suspected troublemaker, is not the culprit after all. Though caffeine temporarily raises both pulse rate and blood pressure, it has no effect on cholesterol levels. Instead, two substances – kahweol and cafestol – in the coffee oil, released during roasting, are blamed for raising cholesterol levels substantially. These are found in coffee that has been brewed by boiling, infusing or made in a cafetière; filtered or instant coffee can be drunk in moderation – even by people suffering from coronary problems.

PREVENTION STARTS YOUNG

Atherosclerosis – or furring up of the arteries – tends to develop over a period of 20 to 30 years, during which there are no symptoms. It is accelerated by smoking.

By the time they reach their 50s, many people have quite badly furred arteries on which plaques (fatty streaks on the walls of the arteries which have developed into fibrous growths) may have already built up, increasing the risk of a heart attack.

The ideal way to prevent atherosclerosis is to take plenty of exercise and to eat a healthy diet that is high in fibre and low in saturated fats (found in high-fat dairy products, fatty meats and hard margarines).

THE CHOLESTEROL FACTOR

High blood CHOLESTEROL levels are accepted as the main underlying cause of coronary heart disease, but such levels are determined by an intricate combination of genetic and dietary factors. In the West, one person in 500 has the misfortune to inherit the predisposition to extremely high blood cholesterol levels; and these people are 20 to 30 times more likely to develop heart disease at an early age than the average person.

Most people, however, bring about their own moderate increase in blood cholesterol levels, by consuming too many saturated fats, or by becoming obese. (Nonetheless, many people who have high blood cholesterol levels are not overweight.) If these factors are combined with smoking, the risk is further increased.

The risk posed by OBESITY can be reversed by losing weight, because weight loss is usually accompanied by a fall in blood cholesterol levels. This does not include crash dieting, where any loss of weight will be mostly fluid, and regained as soon as you resume a normal diet. The only effective way to lose weight healthily is to cut your intake of fat and refined carbohydrates and to take more exercise. It has also been found that people who maintain their body weight from early adult life, avoiding the fluctuations experienced by many unsuccessful dieters, do not show the same age-related increase in blood cholesterol.

CHOLESTEROL COMPLICATIONS

As people grow older their arteries become scarred and partly blocked by atheroma, a fatty substance made of scar tissue and plaques which contains quite large amounts of cholesterol. This condition, called ATHEROSCLEROSIS, progresses more quickly among people with high blood cholesterol levels, particularly if they smoke and have high blood pressure.

If one of the fatty plaques on the wall of a coronary artery ruptures, a blood clot, or THROMBOSIS, forms, blocking the flow of oxygen-laden blood to the heart. The risk of blood clots can be halved through the combination of a careful diet and medication. This means avoiding heavy, fatty meals, which increase the tendency of the

A jigsaw of contributing factors

An intricate web of factors influences the health of the heart. Some we can control – such as the food we eat, the habits we adopt and the exercise we take – others we cannot. For some people, high blood cholesterol levels are part of their genetic inheritance; there are external stresses in the work place; and all too often there is environmental pollution. These are some of the pieces of the jigsaw that determine the risk of heart disease:

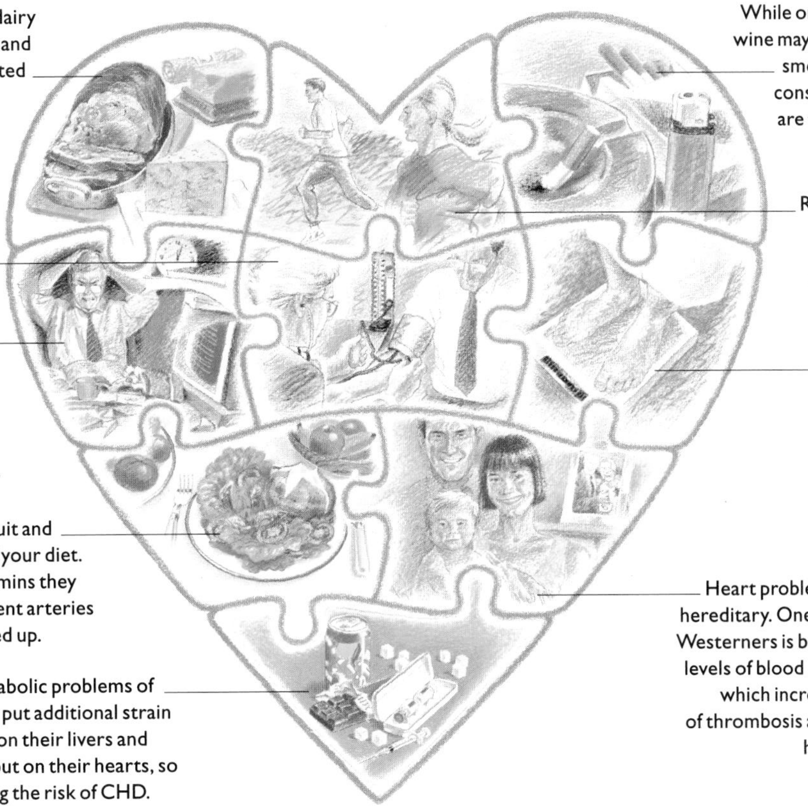
Fatty meats and full-fat dairy products such as butter and cream are high in saturated fats which raise blood cholesterol levels.
While one or two glasses of wine may benefit your heart, smoking and excessive consumption of alcohol are two habits to avoid.
Regular check-ups of your blood pressure may provide advance warning of potential heart problems.
Regular exercise not only keeps obesity and thrombosis at bay, but encourages blood circulation.
Stress and tension have long been recognised as major factors in raising the risks of angina and coronary heart disease.
Obesity is a major factor in increasing the risks of CHD. By reducing weight you will probably prolong your life.
Eat plenty of fresh fruit and vegetables as part of your diet. The antioxidant vitamins they contain help to prevent arteries from becoming furred up.
Heart problems are often hereditary. One in every 500 Westerners is born with high levels of blood cholesterol – which increases the risk of thrombosis and coronary heart disease.
The metabolic problems of diabetics put additional strain not only on their livers and kidneys but on their hearts, so increasing the risk of CHD.

blood to clot, and – in instances where people have already had a heart attack – taking half an aspirin twice weekly.

WHO IS MOST AT RISK?

Among the major factors known to increase the risk of heart disease are raised blood cholesterol levels, cigarette smoking, high blood pressure, obesity and diabetes. In both men and women, the risk of coronary heart disease rises rapidly with increasing age.

Heart disease tends to run in families, so that if either parent, a brother or a sister has suffered a heart attack before the age of 55, the risk to their immediate relatives is ten times greater than for members of families with no history of cardiac problems.

During their reproductive years, while oestrogen keeps their blood cholesterol levels low, women are less prone than men to atherosclerosis and heart attacks. After the MENOPAUSE, however, when women's oestrogen levels decline, and their cholesterol levels rise more quickly than those of men, women become increasingly vulnerable to CHD.

Some protection is afforded to women during the menopause and afterwards from hormone replacement therapy (HRT), which lowers blood cholesterol levels and thus reduces the risk of a heart attack. Nevertheless, statistically, older women are still more likely to die of heart disease than from any other single cause.

FOODS THAT HELP

Saturated fatty acids, which are found in hard fats (butter, some margarines, meat and cheese) increase levels of cholesterol in the blood. Replacing these with vegetable oils rich in monounsaturates (such as olive and rapeseed oils) or polyunsaturated fatty acids (such as sunflower, soya and corn oil) reduces

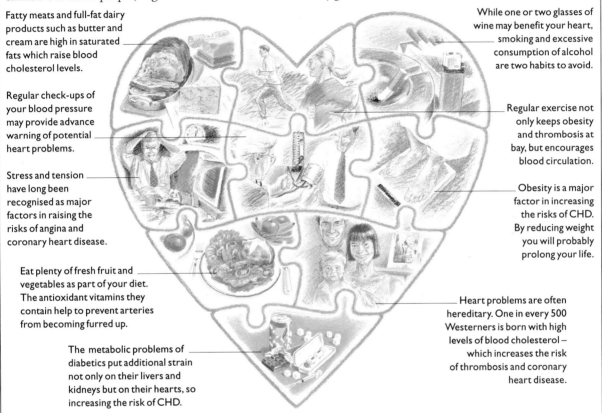

Case study

Bill, a 62-year-old council clerk, lived alone and had become rather set in his ways. Every morning he cooked himself a full breakfast of fried egg, bacon, sausages and fried bread before driving to work. One day Bill arrived at his desk and felt a tightness in his chest. As workmates turned to see what was wrong, he suddenly collapsed with a heart attack. Bill was treated at the local hospital and, fortunately, recovered quickly – it had been a mild attack. After six weeks he had a treadmill ECG test which showed that his heart was back to normal. However, his blood cholesterol level was far too high. The hospital dietician advised a regime to help lower it. This involved avoiding red meat and full-fat dairy products, and grilling rather than frying food. He was told to limit eggs to three a week, and to replace sweets, cakes and crisps with wholemeal bread and fresh fruit and vegetables. By following this advice, Bill has reduced the risk of another heart attack.

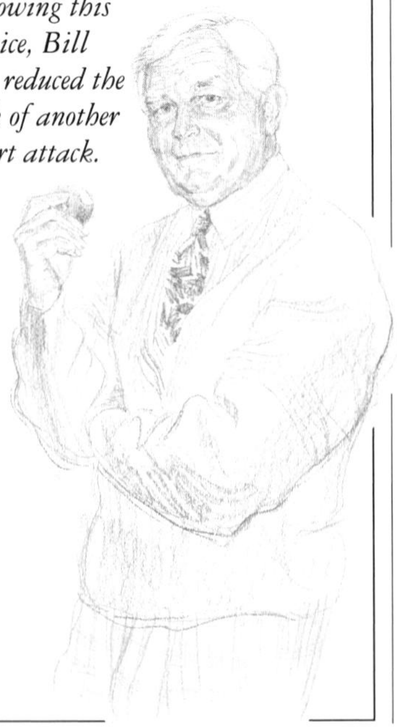

cholesterol levels. However, when liquid oils are hardened (by a process called hydrogenation) for commercial use, as in the making of biscuits or margarine, some of them are converted into trans fatty acids. Recent research suggests that these 'trans fats' may increase the risk of heart disease as well as raise blood cholesterol levels.

Foods rich in dietary FIBRE, especially the soluble type found in oats, beans and lentils, can help to lower blood cholesterol levels, though to a lesser extent than is achieved by reducing saturated fat or even dietary cholesterol, such as that found in egg yolks. Including garlic in your diet is said to lower blood cholesterol levels; for many people, garlic pills are a convenient way to boost their intake.

Recent American research seems to show that the more green vegetables you eat, the less likely you are to develop heart problems. Eating moderate amounts of nuts – especially walnuts and almonds – which are rich in polyunsaturated fatty acids, can also reduce coronary risk and can lower blood cholesterol.

Other fatty acids found in oily fish such as herring, mackerel, pilchards, salmon and sardines are thought to prevent the risk of THROMBOSIS. Eating oily fish twice a week will provide the equivalent of 1 g per day of omega-3, the fatty acid which helps to prevent blood clots forming in arteries. Fish oil supplements have the same effect.

A DAILY DOSE OF ALCOHOL?

Because alcohol dilates small blood vessels and increases the blood flow to the tissues, a moderate intake of up to three glasses of red wine a day can help to stave off coronary heart disease, especially in middle-aged and elderly men, even if they have already had a heart attack. Alcohol also increases the level of high density lipoproteins (HDLs) – protective molecules that transport cholesterol away from body tissues and artery walls. But too much alcohol increases blood pressure and can cause irregular heart rhythms, precipitating a coronary attack.

CAN GARLIC AND ONIONS REALLY HELP?

The belief that two of the most pungent vegetables – garlic and onions – can benefit the heart goes back for centuries. In Ancient Egypt, Greece and Rome both vegetables were used to treat heart disease; clay models of garlic bulbs were found in an Egyptian tomb of 3750 BC. But, while the pastes and infusions of the ancients were based on sympathetic medicine – which conceived the 'strong' vegetables as being good for the body's most important organ – recent medical research suggests a scientific basis for this old belief. Studies show that preparations based on raw onion or garlic juice help to reduce blood cholesterol levels and blood pressure.

ANGINA

Common among those in late middle age and the elderly, angina affects 2 million Britons each year. It is caused by the partial obstruction of the coronary arteries so that the heart muscle is not supplied with enough oxygenated blood. With age, these arteries become increasingly thickened and less elastic.

Angina is sparked by exertion or stress and is often an indication of a more serious underlying heart condition. It is characterised by discomfort or pain in the chest. This pain may radiate down either arm, across the chest and up to the neck. Lying down may aggravate it; for the fastest relief, sit or stand quite still. Prompt diagnosis is important: similar pain may also originate from disorders in the upper parts of the digestive tract such as gallstones or stomach ulcers. Smoking, high blood pressure and high blood cholesterol levels accelerate the artery-hardening process.

Angina patients with high blood cholesterol levels should cut down on saturated fats, and may be prescribed cholesterol-lowering drugs.

Fish, fruit and wine

Eating oily fish twice a week may help to prevent heart attacks in people with angina. This is because the fatty acids present in fish oil are thought both to prevent the thickening of arteries and to improve blood flow to the heart.

Some studies suggest that a lack of fruit and vegetables (which provide the ANTIOXIDANTS beta carotene and vitamin C, believed to help protect against hardening of the arteries) predispose people to angina attacks. It is wise to avoid eating heavy meals which can also lead to an attack.

Boost your intake of antioxidants by eating plenty of fruit and vegetables; try drinking a glass or two of red wine. Grape skins, which give red wine its colour, contain powerful antioxidants, and moderate quantities of alcohol may also help by causing tiny blood vessels in the body to dilate.

A HEALTHY RANGE *Nutritionists have discarded the old concept of dull, bland, foods being vital to the treatment of heart problems. Eat well, but sensibly, they say.*

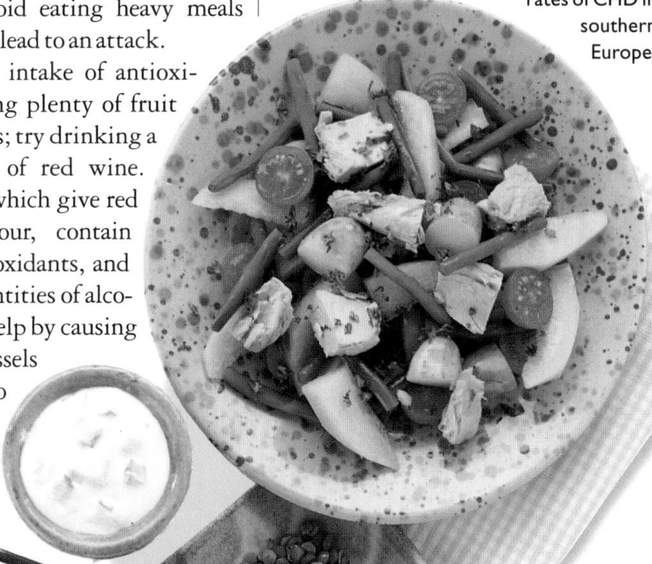

The Mediterranean diet, which includes salade Niçoise, undoubtedly plays a part in the low rates of CHD in southern Europe.

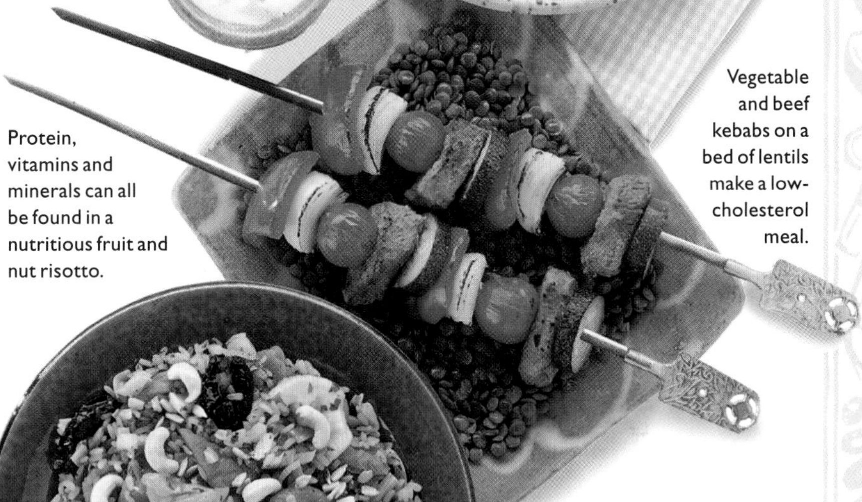

Vegetable and beef kebabs on a bed of lentils make a low-cholesterol meal.

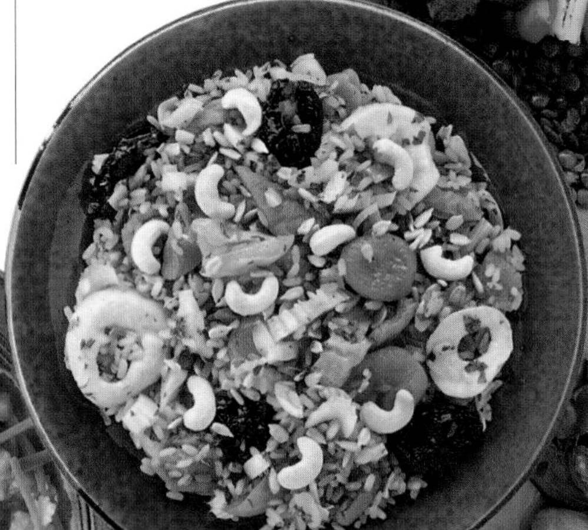

Protein, vitamins and minerals can all be found in a nutritious fruit and nut risotto.

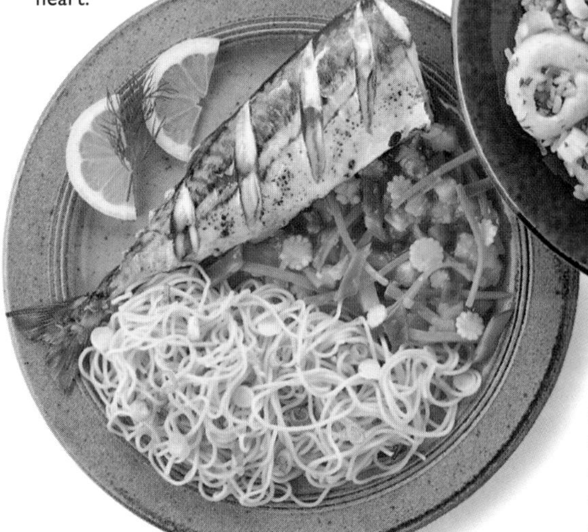

Mackerel, served here with hot sour sauce, is a source of omega-3 as well as the fatty acids vital to maintain a healthy heart.

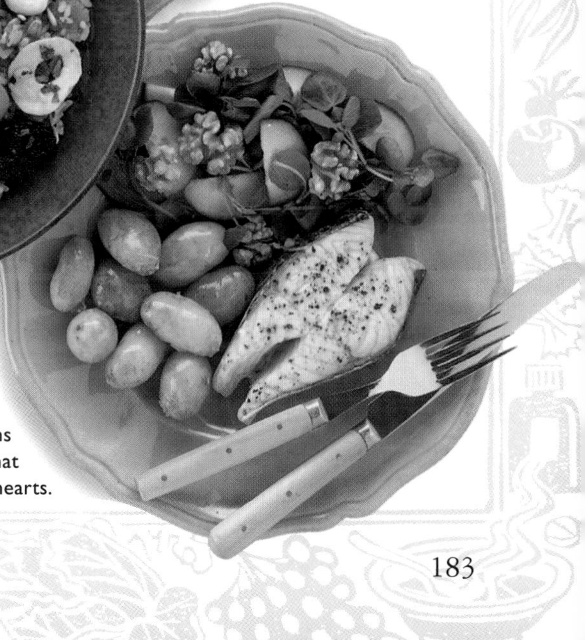

Grilled salmon with a cucumber, walnut and cress salad, is an appetising meal which offers the protein, vitamins and omega-3 fatty acids that are important to healthy hearts.

Hay diet

There is little or no scientific evidence to support the Hay diet, developed by an American, Dr William Hay, in the early 1900s. Dr Hay did not claim that his eating system would actually cure disease but felt it could remove obstacles to nature's own healing powers. He believed that many diseases and ailments such as arthritis, indigestion, allergy and skin disorders, were due to the wrong chemical conditions in the body, which in turn were caused by eating too much meat and refined carbohydrate, as well as by poor digestion and constipation.

Dr Hay believed that proteins and carbohydrates should not be eaten together because they require different conditions for digestion – an acidic environment for proteins and alkaline for carbohydrates. This underestimates the sophistication of the human digestive system which is normally capable of coping easily with both. The stomach contains acid which allows for protein digestion, whereas the small intestine contains alkali which allows carbohydrate digestion.

Dr Hay also recommended that the diet should include four times more of the foods that raise the level of alkali in the blood (vegetables, salads, most fruits and milk) than of the foods that raise its acid level (all animal proteins, most nuts, all the carbohydrate foods and citrus fruits). He considered this balance desirable as it reflects the ratio of acid and alkali normally excreted. In fact, the body has its own regulatory system which can generally counteract excessive acid or alkali intake.

The Hay diet may help those who try it simply because it encourages them to re-examine their eating habits and modify excesses. Many books claim that the Hay diet is a good method of slimming, but any weight loss is likely to be due to a reduction of calorie intake through eating fewer fats and having to restrict meals to one main type of food.

Some aspects of the Hay diet are in line with current healthy eating guidelines with their emphasis on eating plenty of fruit, vegetables and wholegrain starches and restricting fat intake. The carbohydrate intakes are likely to match the 50 per cent of total calorie intake that British Government guidelines currently advise, although this may contain a slightly higher proportion of sugars than is recommended. The belief that the human body cannot digest protein and starch together is not generally accepted by nutritionists and doctors. But the Hay diet may suit people with digestive disorders. Many people – including such famous advocates as Sir John Mills – have claimed the diet can relieve duodenal ulcers and that as well as being easy to follow it can improve quality of life.

The rules of the Hay diet

- Carbohydrates should not be eaten with proteins and acidic fruits.
- Vegetables, salads and fruits should form the bulk of the diet.
- Proteins, carbohydrates and fats should be eaten only in small amounts; refined and processed foods such as sausages should be avoided.
- Leave at least 4 hours between meals of different types of food.

Hay fever

EAT PLENTY OF
- *Blackcurrants and citrus fruit*

Unfortunately, nutrition does not have a major part to play in the management of hay fever – a seasonal allergy which is characterised by sneezing fits, a blocked or runny nose, a tickle in the

A typical meal plan for the Hay diet

According to the Hay diet the body cannot digest protein and starch together, so main food types are eaten separately. Carbohydrates include bread, pasta, rice, cereals, potatoes and sugars, while proteins refer specifically to animal proteins such as meat, fish, poultry and cheese. Acidic fruits include citrus fruits such as grapefruit and oranges.

BREAKFAST (ALKALINE) 8 AM

Plenty of fresh fruit; small carton of natural yoghurt sprinkled with wheatgerm or mixed nuts; herb tea; fruit juice.

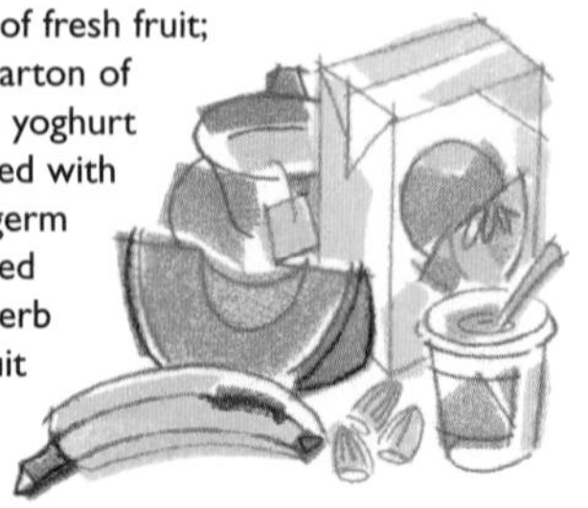

LUNCH (PROTEIN) 1 PM

Portion of meat, fish, eggs or cheese; fresh raw salad or cooked vegetables (not potatoes); followed by an apple or orange.

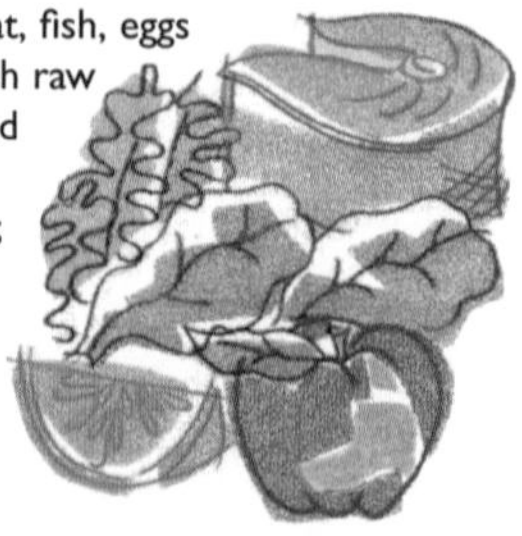

DINNER (STARCH) 6 PM

Jacket potato with butter or wholemeal bread and butter; cooked vegetables or salad; fresh figs with cream or fromage frais.

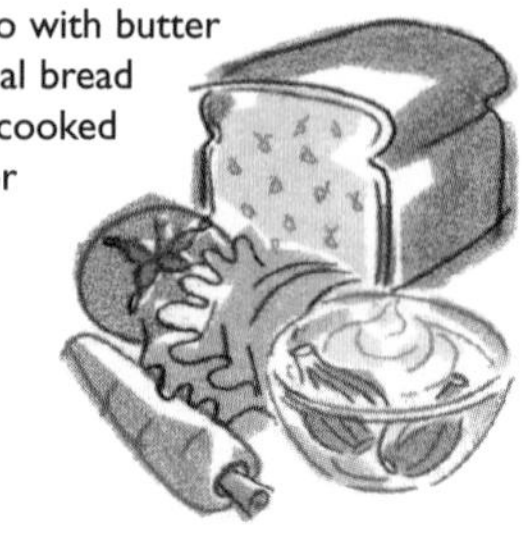

roof of the mouth and sore, itchy eyes. The symptoms are usually an extreme response to airborne pollens. In spring, the pollen allergens tend to come from trees, in summer from grasses, and in autumn from fungi.

Hay fever may be controlled in several ways. Avoiding the allergen by staying in an air-conditioned building during peak periods of pollen may help, but is not always practical. Over-the-counter or prescription medicines can help to reduce or eliminate symptoms. Desensitising injections are also effective for the most severe cases, when symptoms include wheezing similar to asthma.

Eating foods that have a natural anti-inflammatory action and are rich in vitamin C – such as blackcurrants and citrus fruits – may also help to relieve congestion.

Some naturopathic practitioners believe that by eating a tablespoon of locally produced honey every day for the three months leading up to the pollen season, you can acclimatise yourself to local pollens and therefore ease hay fever. However, the pollens responsible for hay fever tend to be from grass or trees and are not usually collected by bees to make honey.

HEADACHE

EAT PLENTY OF

- *Regular light meals to prevent low blood sugar levels*
- *Cold-pressed vegetable oils, avocados, nuts and seeds, for vitamin E*

CUT DOWN ON

- *Excessive caffeine in coffee, strong tea and cola drinks*
- *Alcohol*

Many people who suffer from recurrent headaches find that simple changes to their diet can offer fast and effective relief. Eating small, regular meals, for example, is a good preventive measure, as skipping meals is known to cause a drop in blood sugar levels, which in turn can precipitate headaches. If you often wake up with a headache, low blood sugar could be the culprit: try to maintain levels by eating a snack last thing at night, and again on waking in the morning.

Dehydration is another common cause of headaches, particularly in hot weather or following sport or excessive alcohol consumption; simply drinking plenty of water to replace lost fluids will often help to relieve these headaches. Try to avoid becoming dehydrated when exercising by sipping water during the activity.

Consuming excessive amounts of CAFFEINE may also bring on headaches by altering the blood supply to the brain. Doctors recommend that you drink no more than six cups of tea or coffee each day. Cutting down on caffeine can help people who suffer from recurrent headaches, but beware of eliminating caffeine too quickly from your diet, as this may cause withdrawal headaches.

Food allergies or additives used in certain processed foods can also be the cause of headaches. Chinese food eaten in restaurants can trigger short-lived headaches in some people. This is thought to be due to the fermented soya and fish sauces often used in Chinese cuisine. If you think that your headaches are related to specific foods, try keeping a food diary and cut out suspect foods one by one.

Many headaches are caused by tension – mental, physical or both. If your head is throbbing and you feel there is pressure behind your eyes and a tight band around your head, you probably have a tension headache. However, headaches can be caused by a range of conditions, such as poor liver or kidney function, low fluid intake or allergies.

Consult your doctor

- If a headache starts suddenly, and is accompanied by fever, a stiff neck, a rash or vomiting. This is especially important for children.
- If the type or pattern of your regular headaches changes.
- When ordinary painkillers do not help and the pain is severe.
- If your attacks become either more frequent or more severe.
- If your speech, memory or vision start to deteriorate.
- If your balance is affected, or you pass out.
- If you experience considerable weight loss or muscle weakness along with headaches.
- If you wake up with headaches which are made worse when you cough or sneeze.
- If your headaches are persistent.

Foods rich in vitamin E – avocados, cold-pressed vegetable oils, nuts and seeds – may help, because the vitamin neutralises the effect of toxic free radicals, which are believed to be involved in causing some headaches.

Other causes of headache include hangovers, worry, bad posture, strenuous activity, arthritis in the neck, whiplash injuries, grinding teeth or an uneven bite, long-distance driving, eyestrain, or wearing ill-fitting glasses that irritate the muscles of the forehead. Hormonal fluctuations before the onset of monthly periods, during pregnancy and at the menopause often trigger headaches in women.

Most headaches will respond to resting, drinking plenty of liquid and to painkillers such as aspirin.

HEART DISEASE

See page 180

HERBS FOR HEALTH

Herbs in the diet and herbal remedies are making a comeback as people rediscover the value of natural ingredients and natural cures and question the side effects of pharmaceutical drugs.

Herbal medicine can be viewed as the precursor of modern pharmacology; indeed, many of today's powerful drugs are derived from plants. Like drugs, however, herbs are not always as safe as some herbalists suggest. Nevertheless, there is much wisdom in the general approach of herbal medicine and there are usually fewer side effects. Furthermore, there are ailments, such as certain forms of ECZEMA, which appear to respond to herbal remedies where orthodox medicine has little to offer.

The medicinal value of herbs, known to earlier civilisations through a combination of keen observation, trial and error, is being rediscovered and confirmed by modern scientific tests. But while research continues to investigate the uses of new plants, many doctors and scientists still do not acknowledge the healing power of herbs, preferring instead to rely on 'tried and tested' pharmaceutical drugs. Yet our knowledge of herbs can be traced back to the Ancient Egyptians, whose priests routinely practised herbal medicine. A papyrus, dating from 1500 BC, lists hundreds of medicinal herbs – including many that are still in use today.

There have been many attempts by orthodox medical pressure groups to have herbal medicine banned. Only in 1994, it was feared that herbal remedies would be under threat due to a new European Commission directive prohibiting the sale of unlicensed medicines. However, as long as herbal remedies are not sold as medicines in Europe, they do not have to be licensed. Meanwhile, as more people begin to question the use of synthetic drugs, and their side effects, the interest in herbalism continues to grow.

THE HOME HERBALIST

Many herbs can be bought in the form of tea bags from health food shops and supermarkets, or you can make your own herbal drinks. Teas and infusions are the same thing; made from the flowers or leafy parts of the plant, they can be used as drinks or gargles. Use a teaspoon of dried herbs – or two teaspoons of fresh herbs – to a cup of boiling water. Pour boiling water over the herb and leave covered for between 5 and 10 minutes. Strain and drink while hot, without milk or sugar. Add a little honey if desired. For medicinal purposes, drink a cup three times a day. Decoctions, made by boiling roots or bark in water, can be prepared and used in the same way.

When using fresh herbs, flowers, bark or roots to make infusions or decoctions, you should wash them carefully first, in order to remove dirt or pesticide residues.

HERBS IN THE DIET

One way to use herbs for health is in your diet, and the following list gives both their culinary uses and alleged therapeutic powers. Generally, herbs have little nutritional value because of the small amounts consumed.

Basil The classic accompaniment to all tomato dishes and important in Italian cooking. A natural tranquilliser, basil is said to be a tonic and to calm the nervous system. It may aid the digestion and also ease stomach cramps. Basil tea may relieve nausea.

Bay An essential ingredient of the herbal seasoning *bouquet garni*, used in soups, casseroles and stews. Bay is used to stimulate and aid digestion.

Borage As a tisane, it is used against rheumatism and respiratory infections. Its leaves may be eaten in salads.

Chervil This winter herb has a unique flavour that is a little like parsley with a hint of aniseed. Medicinal uses include stimulating digestion.

Chives Primarily cultivated for culinary use, these tiny members of the onion family enliven potatoes, egg dishes, soups and stews. Chives can stimulate the appetite as well as help digestion during convalescence.

Coriander The pungent leaves are used in curries, salads and sauces. In herbalism, small fresh bunches are eaten as a tonic for the stomach and heart. Both seeds and leaves are used for strengthening the urinary tract and for treating urinary tract infections.

Dill Widely used in pickles, soups and fish dishes. Dill has proved itself to be effective in the relief of gripes and flatulence. Many babies are given dill in the familiar form of gripe water.

Fennel The feathery leaves, which taste like aniseed, are often added to sauces or stuffings for fish. Both the seeds and leaves can be used to aid digestion and help to prevent excessive wind, insomnia, nausea and vomiting.

PLANT POWER *Herbs owe their medicinal properties and flavours to the essential oils they contain. They should be picked before the midday heat for maximum pungency.*

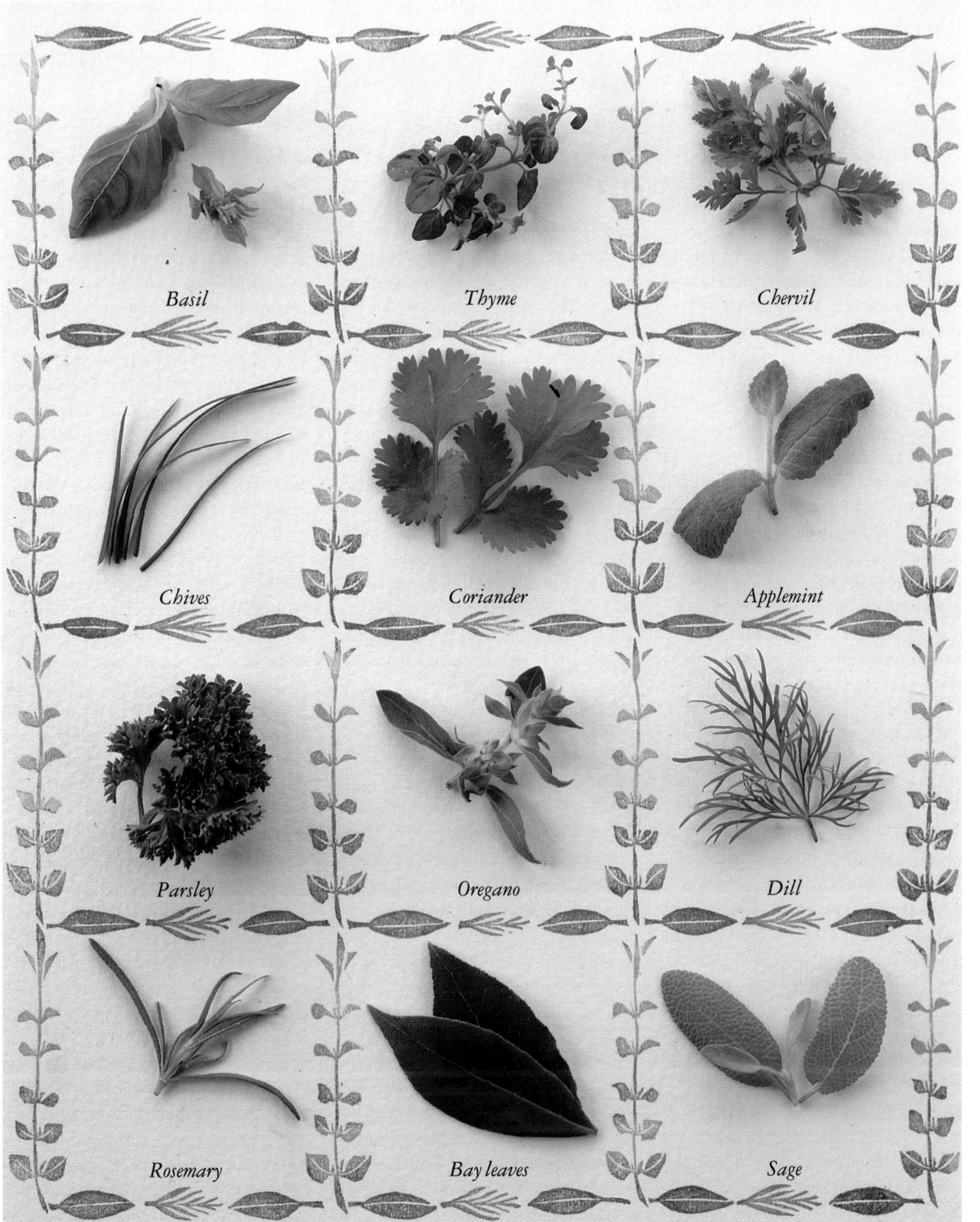
Basil
Thyme
Chervil
Chives
Coriander
Applemint
Parsley
Oregano
Dill
Rosemary
Bay leaves
Sage

Mint The leaves of many varieties are used in cooking – for savoury dishes such as lamb, and also desserts; subtle applemint will bring out delicate flavours. Mint aids digestion, and a hot infusion can help at the start of a cold.
Oregano Also known as wild marjoram, this herb is widely used in stuffings and pizzas. It is thought to aid digestion and relieve the symptoms of colds, coughs and flu when used as an infusion – but it must not be used medicinally during pregnancy.
Parsley This attractive and widely used herb is one of the most nutritious garnishes, containing useful amounts of vitamin C and iron. Fresh parsley also makes a good breath freshener; try chewing it after eating garlic.
Rosemary This herb is used with lamb and chicken dishes throughout the Mediterranean. It is said to act as a stimulant to both the nervous and circulatory systems, and may help to soothe the digestive system, relieving indigestion and flatulence. Drinking a weak infusion of rosemary may help with the relief of nervous headaches, neuralgia and colds. Rosemary also makes a good antiseptic gargle.
Sage Purple or red sage is used in stuffings with meats such as pork and venison. Herbalists claim that sage can aid the digestion of rich, heavy food and calm indigestion. Sage may also be used as a gargle to ease sore throats, and sage tea is recommended for indigestion, anxiety and excessive sweating.
Thyme This herb is used widely in cooking for its aromatic flavour, and in medicine as an antiseptic. An infusion can be used as a herbal gargle or expectorant for coughs and catarrh.

MYTH OR MEDICINE?

The Chinese and Indian cultures have always relied heavily on herbal medicine. In China, herbs still play a vital part in health care, and there are schools of herbal medicine and herbal dispensaries in most hospitals. The use of herbs is also part of an all-embracing traditional Indian system of healing known as ayurvedic medicine.
Ginseng The most famous medicinal plant of China, used for centuries as a cure-all and tonic for the body. Korean or Chinese ginseng (*Panax schinseng*) is said to stimulate the nervous system and strengthen the immune system. Its revitalising properties may help to combat physical and mental fatigue. Ginseng is considered to be an 'adaptogen'; which means that it will affect each person differently according to individual needs. For example, it may help to calm a stressed person or to stimulate someone who is tired.

Siberian ginseng (*Eleutherococcus senticosus*), the Russian relative of its oriental cousin, is also used in traditional medicine as a tonic to improve general health. Like Chinese ginseng, the Siberian variety appears to sedate or stimulate, according to the body's needs. Naturopaths claim that it can produce a state of increased resistance to both physical and mental stress, and help to reduce the harmful side effects of stress on the body.
Evening primrose The fatty oil obtained from the seeds of this herb, native to North America, is taken in the form of supplements. The active constituent of the oil is gamma-linolenic acid (GLA). Supplements are commonly used for the treatment of ECZEMA, premenstrual syndrome and painful breasts. There is some medical evidence that supplements benefit people with these conditions.
Aloe vera Two products come from the leaves of this fleshy succulent: aloe vera gel, used externally for minor burns and skin irritations; and aloe vera juice which is consumed. There is growing anecdotal evidence of the efficacy of aloe vera in both forms and claims have been made for the juice's help with arthritis, ME and eczema.

Herbal infusions and their uses

The herbal tea bags sold in health food shops and supermarkets have to pass rigorous quality and safety tests before they are made available to the public. Herbal teas make a good alternative to ordinary tea and coffee. It is best to stick to mild infusions of well-tried herbs. Pregnant women are usually advised to avoid herbal teas, with the exception of peppermint, lime and camomile, which are all said to relieve morning sickness. These are some of the more popular teas and their reputed uses:
Camomile Relaxing, calming tea, said to be helpful in the relief of anxiety and insomnia.
Elderflower May prove helpful for those suffering from colds and flu, as elderflower is said to ease catarrh and relieve sinus problems.
Fennel This tea has an aniseed flavour that may help to ease indigestion, wind and bloating.
Peppermint An after-dinner tea. Eases nausea and reduces wind.
Raspberry leaf Believed to soothe the digestive tract.
Rosehip Excellent natural source of vitamin C. When combined with hibiscus flowers, it has a pleasant lemony flavour.

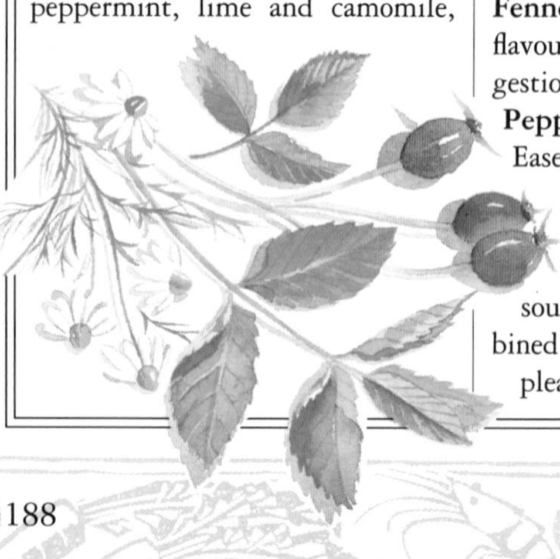

Drying your own herbs at home

A convenient way of storing herbs so that they are available all year round is to dry them. Stored in dark, airtight containers, they can be kept for up to 18 months. It is important to start the drying process as soon as possible after the herbs have been harvested. When the leaves or flowers have been separated from the main plant, they begin to decompose, losing their flavour and medicinal properties. The dried herbs will continue to lose their potency with time, and, for medicinal purposes, the fresher the herb the better.

Leaves, flowers and seeds should be dried in a warm, dry, dark, well-ventilated area – an airing cupboard for example – at temperatures of 21°-33°C (70°-91°F). Roots need temperatures of 50°-60°C (122°-140°F).

FROM LEAVES TO ROOTS

Make small bunches of herbs such as sage, oregano, thyme, rosemary, bay and lemon balm and hang with the stems upwards to dry. When the leaves have dried and are brittle, but not so dry that they crumble into dust, rub them off the stems and store. Lavender is also best dried on the stem, with a paper bag tied over the end to catch any of the flowers that may fall. Larger leaves, such as basil and burdock, should be spread out on muslin which has been stretched over a frame or cooling rack so that air can circulate freely. The flowers can also be dried in this way, but they usually take a little longer than the leaves.

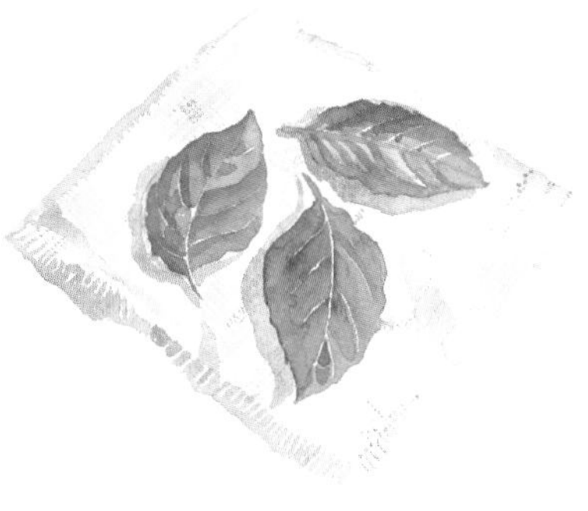

SWEET BASIL *Dry larger leaves as well as small flowers on a piece of muslin.*

Seeds such as fennel and dill are dried in a similar way to lavender. While they are still attached to the stems, hang the almost ripe seed-heads upside-down, with a paper bag over them to catch the seeds as they ripen and fall. Alternatively, you can place a large tray under the bunches to catch the dropping seeds.

When drying the roots, ensure that they have been scrubbed clean. Cut tough, large roots into small pieces and place them on a tray, turning them regularly.

When you come to use your dried herbs in cooking, always remember that when a recipe calls for a tablespoon of fresh herbs, you will only need a teaspoon of dried herbs, as their flavour is more concentrated.

FROZEN THYME CAPSULES

Most culinary herbs can be chopped finely and packed into an ice cube tray, which is then topped up with water and frozen. Each cube should hold about a tablespoon of herbs, which can then be conveniently added straight from the freezer to the saucepan when cooking.

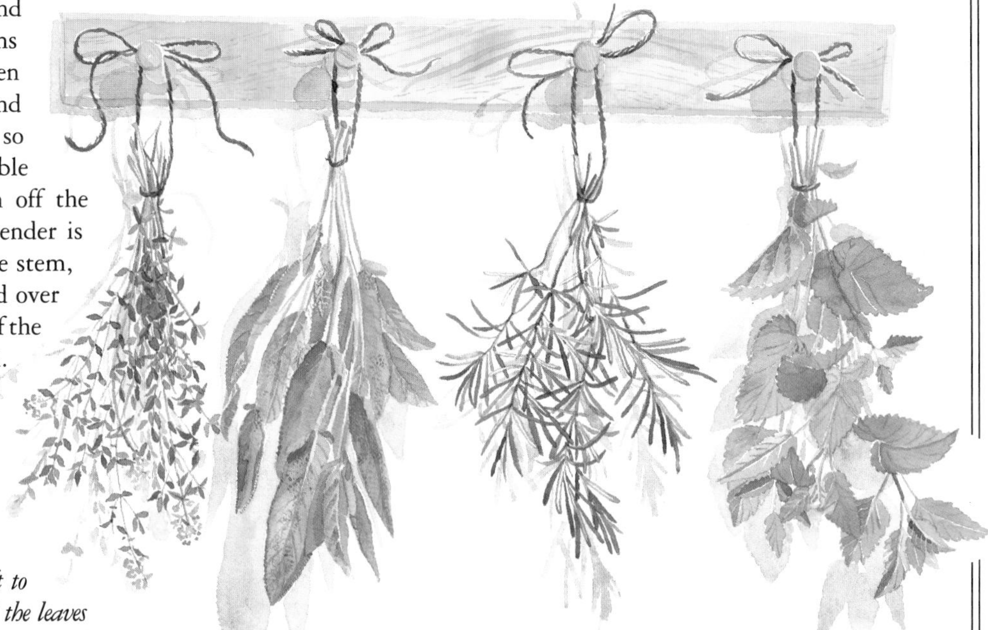

DRY YOUR OWN *From left to right: bunches of thyme, sage, rosemary and lemon balm are left to hang upside-down until the leaves are brittle enough to store in containers.*

Herpes

EAT PLENTY OF

- *Fresh fruit and vegetables*
- *Shellfish, lean meat, nuts and seeds for zinc*

CUT DOWN ON

- *Alcohol, caffeine and smoking*

The three most common forms of herpes all have the ability to 'lie low' in the body after the initial infection until they are reactivated. As a result, people often suffer from recurrent attacks. *Herpes simplex* type 1 (HSV-1) causes cold sores, usually around the mouth; *Herpes simplex* type 2 (HSV-2) causes genital herpes; and *Varicella zoster* virus (VZV), or *Herpes zoster*, is the virus that causes CHICKENPOX and may go on to give people SHINGLES in later life. All forms of herpes are infectious during attacks, but one type cannot usually cause another.

Most people will have been infected with HSV-1 at some time during their childhood, in which case recurrent cold sores or fever blisters around their mouth and nose may serve as nagging reminders of the primary infection.

HSV-2, which is predominantly a genital infection, is characterised by tiny, cold sore-like blisters. It is sexually transmitted and, like HSV-1, it is prone to flare up from time to time when the immune system is already being strained, for example during times of stress or illness, or just before menstrual periods. Exposure to sunlight or extreme cold can sometimes prompt an attack. HSV-2 cannot be cured, but the earlier treatment is given, the more likely it is to prevent or reduce the severity of an attack.

Chickenpox mainly affects young children and usually occurs in the late winter and spring. Following the primary infection, the *Herpes zoster* virus remains dormant for years in nerve tissue. In later life the virus may be reactivated, when it can reappear as shingles. With shingles, the virus multiplies and migrates along the nerve. The result is a severe, burning pain and a blistering rash that most commonly affects the shoulder and waist or one side of the face.

Boost your immune system

A well-balanced, nutritious diet is essential for maintaining general good health and resisting disease. To help to avoid a flare-up of a dormant virus, eat plenty of whole grains, fresh fruit and vegetables, as well as lean meat and fresh fish, which provide protein and micronutrients while being relatively low in saturated fat.

To give your immune system the best chance of fighting off an attack of any herpes virus, reduce your intake of alcohol and caffeine, which is found in tea, coffee and cola drinks. Cut down on smoking, or give up altogether. You should also try to make sure that you get plenty of rest and try to avoid stress as much as possible.

Zinc supplements have been found to inhibit the growth of HSV-1. Ensure a good intake of foods that provide this important mineral; nuts, sunflower seeds, meat and shellfish are all good to excellent sources.

In a clinical trial, a combination of vitamin C and bioflavonoids given at the first sign of a flare-up to a group of habitual sufferers of *Herpes simplex* was found to prevent the development of blisters in 24 out of 38 cases. Eating five portions of different fruits or vegetables a day should ensure that you have abundant supplies of these water-soluble vitamins.

Naturopaths believe that recurrent genital herpes is caused by a lowering of vitality. They aim to correct the imbalance with the amino acid L-lysine, found in lamb, chicken, fish, milk, beans, fruit and vegetables.

Cold sores

The virus that causes cold sores can be reawakened by excessive stress, or when you are fighting off a cold or another mild infection. Attacks can also be sparked off by increased exposure to ultraviolet radiation during beach or mountain holidays.

Women often suffer from cold sores just before the start of their periods. People taking immunosuppressant drugs as a treatment for cancer or after transplants can also experience continuous outbreaks.

There is no cure for cold sores, but they can be successfully treated with over-the-counter ointments. A balanced diet can also help by boosting the immune system and thereby reduce the risk of an attack. The most important nutrients for maintaining a robust immune system are vitamins A, C and E, and zinc. Liver (which should not be eaten during pregnancy) and eggs supply vitamin A. Blackcurrants, citrus fruits and peppers are excellent sources of vitamin C. The pith of citrus fruits is especially rich in bioflavonoids; these help to keep the skin in peak condition. Seed oils, wheatgerm and avocados provide vitamin E; lean meat, nuts and seeds supply zinc.

An attack of HSV-1 is usually preceded by numbness or tingling in the affected area. The liquid in cold-sore blisters is highly infectious, so contact should be avoided. To minimise the possibility of spreading infection, take care when using towels, pillowcases, facecloths, cutlery and crockery, and always wash your hands after touching a lesion.

Hiatus hernia

EAT PLENTY OF
- *Small meals*
- *Rosemary, sage, tarragon, fennel, dill and mint, which aid digestion*

CUT DOWN ON
- *Strong coffee and alcohol*

AVOID
- *Eating large meals late at night*
- *Foods that cause indigestion, such as fried foods*
- *Smoking*

This common condition occurs when part of the stomach forces its way into the chest through a weakness in the opening (hiatus) where the oesophagus passes through the abdominal cavity. As a result, the acidic juices in the stomach are allowed to flow back into the oesophagus. This can cause chronic heartburn (which is made worse by lying down), INDIGESTION, flatulence and a painful burning sensation in the back of the throat, but often there are no symptoms at all.

If you have a hiatus hernia, avoid large, heavy meals that over-distend the stomach. Instead, try to eat four or five small meals a day. Stop smoking, which increases the stomach's acidity. Cut out foods that can exacerbate indigestion, such as fried and fatty foods, as well as acidic foods such as pickles and vinegar, which may cause heartburn.

Drink water or soothing herbal teas, except for peppermint (not to be confused with mint). Along with alcohol and coffee, peppermint tea relaxes the oesophageal sphincter, which spurs the backward flow of juices from the stomach. Avoid fizzy drinks that cause burping, and foods that are very hot or cold because they can lead to irritation.

Do not lie down after eating, and try not to eat or drink anything for at least three hours before going to bed. The less there is in your stomach, the less uncomfortable you will be when lying down. Some alternative practitioners advocate adding certain herbs to foods when cooking because they can aid the digestion, particularly rosemary, sage, tarragon, fennel, dill and mint.

One practical step you can take to minimise any night-time discomfort is to raise the head end of your bed by about 7-8cm (3in), using bed blocks or a brick under both legs.

Hives

EAT PLENTY OF
- *Dark green leafy vegetables, and orange and yellow fruit and vegetables, for beta carotene*
- *Wheatgerm, offal, fish and pulses, for niacin*

AVOID
- *Foods containing tartrazine (E102)*
- *Any food to which you have an allergy or an intolerance*

Food ALLERGIES are often responsible for hives, which is characterised by a sudden outbreak of intense itching and a rash of red or white weals. The condition, which is also known as urticaria or nettle rash, is caused by the release of histamine into the skin, and is usually treated with antihistamines.

The reaction can occur anywhere on the body and sometimes there are additional symptoms such as fatigue, fever or nausea. You should seek medical advice if symptoms persist. If hives causes swelling within the respiratory tract and breathing becomes difficult, call an ambulance immediately as it could be an anaphylactic reaction – an extreme and potentially fatal allergy.

Attacks of hives are usually short-lived, disappearing within 72 hours, but the condition can become chronic if a victim is repeatedly exposed to an allergy-producing substance. Hives is often the result of insect bites or stings, or of skin contact with plants, such as primulas. Common food triggers for hives include shellfish, milk, strawberries, onions, garlic, parsley, beans, potatoes, celery, nuts, spices and some food additives, particularly tartrazine (E102), widely used as a yellow or orange food colouring. Other common triggers include drugs such as aspirin and penicillin; bacteria, animal hair, mould and viral infections.

Susceptible people, especially those sensitive or allergic to aspirin, may find that they react to foods containing salicylates – natural aspirin-like compounds. Foods high in salicylates include most fruits, particularly berries and dried fruits, some herbs and spices, and sweets made of peppermint or liquorice. Nuts and seeds also contain moderate amounts; low levels are found in meat, fish, pulses, grains, dairy products and most vegetables.

Hives can sometimes be caused by a combination of exposure to sunlight and eating certain foods. Buckwheat, for example, which is popular with health-food enthusiasts, is well known to have this effect. Beta carotene, the pigment in dark green leafy vegetables and orange fruit and vegetables such as spinach, carrots and apricots, seems to be especially helpful in relieving hives caused by exposure to sunlight.

If you regularly suffer from hives, try excluding any food or drink you suspect of provoking the complaint from your diet, but first consult a doctor or qualified nutritionist. It may also be worth including offal, wheatgerm, fish and pulses in your diet; all supply niacin, a B vitamin believed to help inhibit the release of histamine.

The treatment of hives usually involves antihistamine medication. In more severe cases, corticosteroids will be prescribed – which can be applied to the skin or taken by mouth.

Home cooking

The case for home cooking and making use of fresh ingredients rather than buying ready-prepared meals is a simple one: home cooking is usually less expensive and tastier, and it allows you to have control over what you eat. As long as care is taken over the choice of ingredients and how they are cooked, homemade meals are also usually more nourishing than their ready-made equivalents.

Pre-prepared meals are useful when time is short or when people unused to cooking have to fend for themselves. Carefully chosen CONVENIENCE FOODS are also a better option than unhealthy home cooking. Often, however, shoppers choose ready-to-eat meals which are high in fat and sugar and do not provide enough essential nutrients. In any case, lack of time need not be a problem: there are many cookbooks with simple recipes for dishes that can be made in half an hour or less.

Cooking on a budget

For anyone on a budget, home cooking is a less expensive option than ready-to-eat meals. There are none of the problems of portion-controlled packets, and you can also make extra and freeze the rest for later. Leftovers can be made into satisfying soups. Some of the cheapest foods, such as pulses, rice, pasta, potatoes and other vegetables, are also among the most nutritious and filling, allowing you to create substantial meals at little cost.

Healthy home cooking

Anyone can become adept at PREPARING, COOKING AND STORING food and deciding on menus. One of the advantages of cooking at home is that the home cook can be sure not only of the quality of his or her ingredients, but can also choose to cook them in the healthiest ways. Vegetables in pre-prepared meals are cooked, chilled or frozen, then cooked again when they are reheated for use. This sequence of operations leads to the loss of some important nutrients, particularly the B vitamins and vitamin C.

Good-quality fresh vegetables, on the other hand, prepared immediately before use and then microwaved, steamed or boiled for as short a time as possible, not only look more appetising and taste better, they also retain more of their nutrients. If the cooking water is then used for gravy or sauces, few of the nutrients are lost. If you do not have time to prepare fresh vegetables, frozen varieties can be just as nutritious. Properly cooked food can have as much as three times the nutritional value of food that has been cooked carelessly.

When cooking at home, it is also essential to be aware of the rules of kitchen HYGIENE. Never reheat foods more than once. Repeatedly reheating meat stocks, for example, can encourage the growth of bacteria and lead to food poisoning.

Cooking for special needs

Anyone who is a keen cook will be much more aware of what is in food, which is important when choosing a diet that is both satisfying and healthy.

Home cooking versus convenience foods

Replacing convenience foods with homemade meals can be healthier. The home-cooked menu below provides less fat, sugar and calories, and more protein and fibre. It supplies more of many micronutrients, except for B_2, calcium, phosphorus and zinc, and the same amount of iron and B_{12}.

A CONVENIENCE DAY	A HOME-COOKING DAY
BREAKFAST	
Toasted white bread with margarine and jam; cup of tea.	Homemade muesli; two slices wholemeal toast and butter; cup of tea.
SNACK	
Cappuccino and chocolate digestive biscuits.	Homemade flapjack and glass of unsweetened apple juice.
LUNCH BREAK	
Hamburger with French fries; one bar of chocolate; can of cola.	Homemade tuna and salad sandwich on wholemeal bread; banana; glass of fresh orange juice.
TEA TIME	
Cup of tea; jam doughnut.	Cup of tea with homemade fruit cake.
EVENING MEAL	
Supermarket heat-and-eat shepherd's pie with chips; frozen apple pie with two scoops of ice cream; fizzy drink or two glasses of beer or wine.	Homemade lentil soup; grilled chicken breast, jacket potato, broccoli, tomato side salad; strawberry and melon salad with ice cream; one glass of mineral water and one glass of wine.

COOKING FOR HEALTH AND PLEASURE *Cooking at home allows you to have complete control over what you eat, and it can also be fun.*

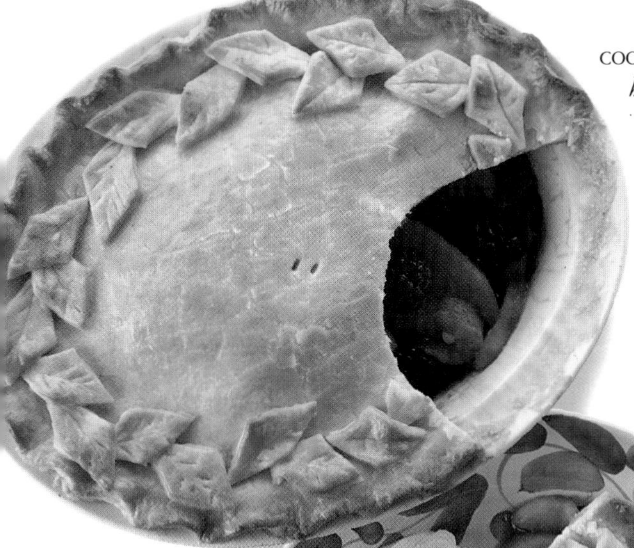

The tempting aromas of a freshly made blackberry and apple pie are hard to resist.

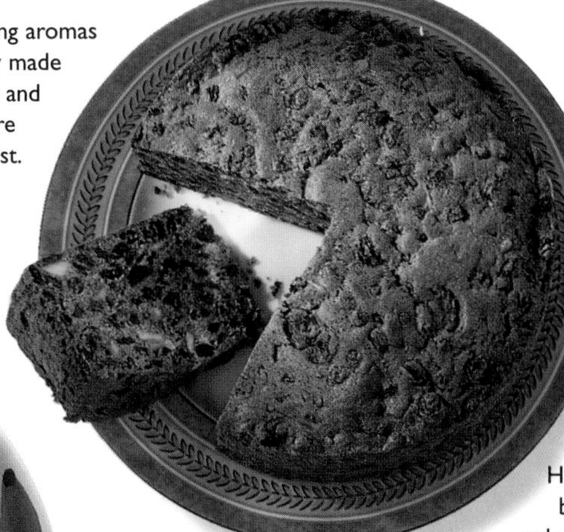

Home-baked cakes are often healthier than shop-bought ones.

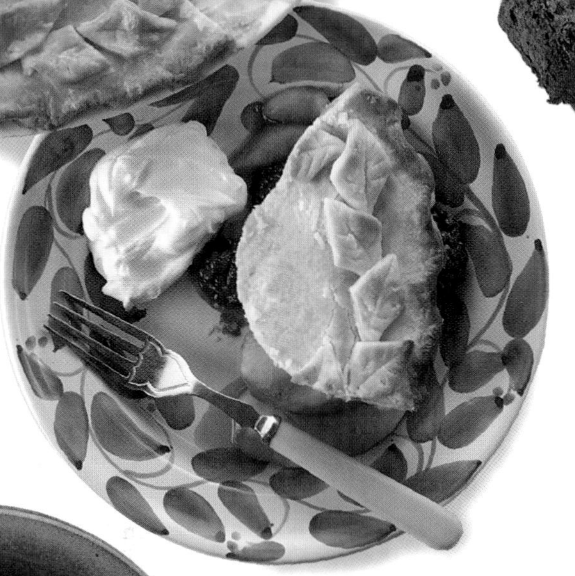

Not only is a home-made soup delicious and nutritious, it is also easy to prepare and cheap. If large amounts are made in one go, some can be frozen, or eaten the following day.

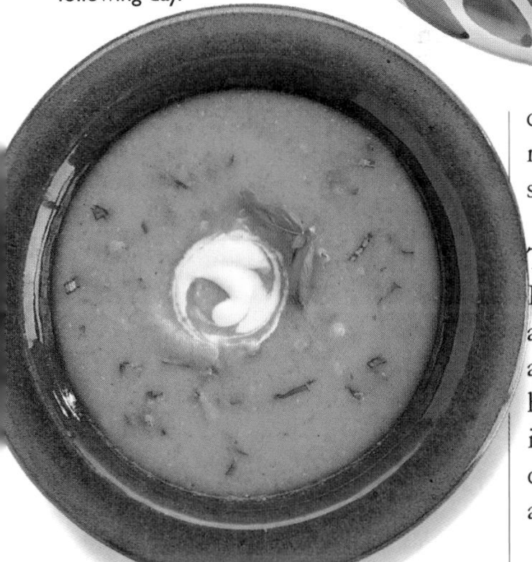

If a family member has particular dietary needs, menus can be tailored accordingly – something that cannot be done with complete ready-to-eat meals. This can be particularly helpful if you are cooking for anyone with a condition or illness that needs careful monitoring of food intake, such as a serious food allergy or heart disease.

THE PLEASURES OF COOKING

Eating is one of life's necessities and also one of its great pleasures. There are, of course, temptations for the home cook, especially when entertaining. Delicious soups end up laced with cream, and fish is served swimming in a rich sauce. Then the dessert arrives!

Cooking should be fun and relaxing and it is also a good creative outlet. Encourage children into the kitchen and allow them to experiment, make a mess and enjoy themselves (under supervision, of course). If they discover the pleasures of cooking early enough, they will have learnt a lesson for life.

HOMEOPATHIC MEDICINE

AVOID

- *Tobacco, coffee, peppermint, and any strong-tasting or smelling food and drink for 30 minutes before and after taking the medication*

Practitioners of this controversial system of medicine believe that illness is a sign of an inner disharmony. Their approach is 'holistic', concentrating on the whole person – mental, emotional, spiritual and physical.

Homeopaths regard a person's symptoms as a sign that the body is trying to heal itself. The principle behind the remedies – which are highly diluted extracts of natural substances – is that 'like cures like', in the way that vaccination with a small dose of a virus stimulates the body to produce antibodies against that disease. The theory is that if the substance were given to a healthy person it would produce the symptoms of a particular disease, but in someone who is sick the diluted homeopathic remedy will

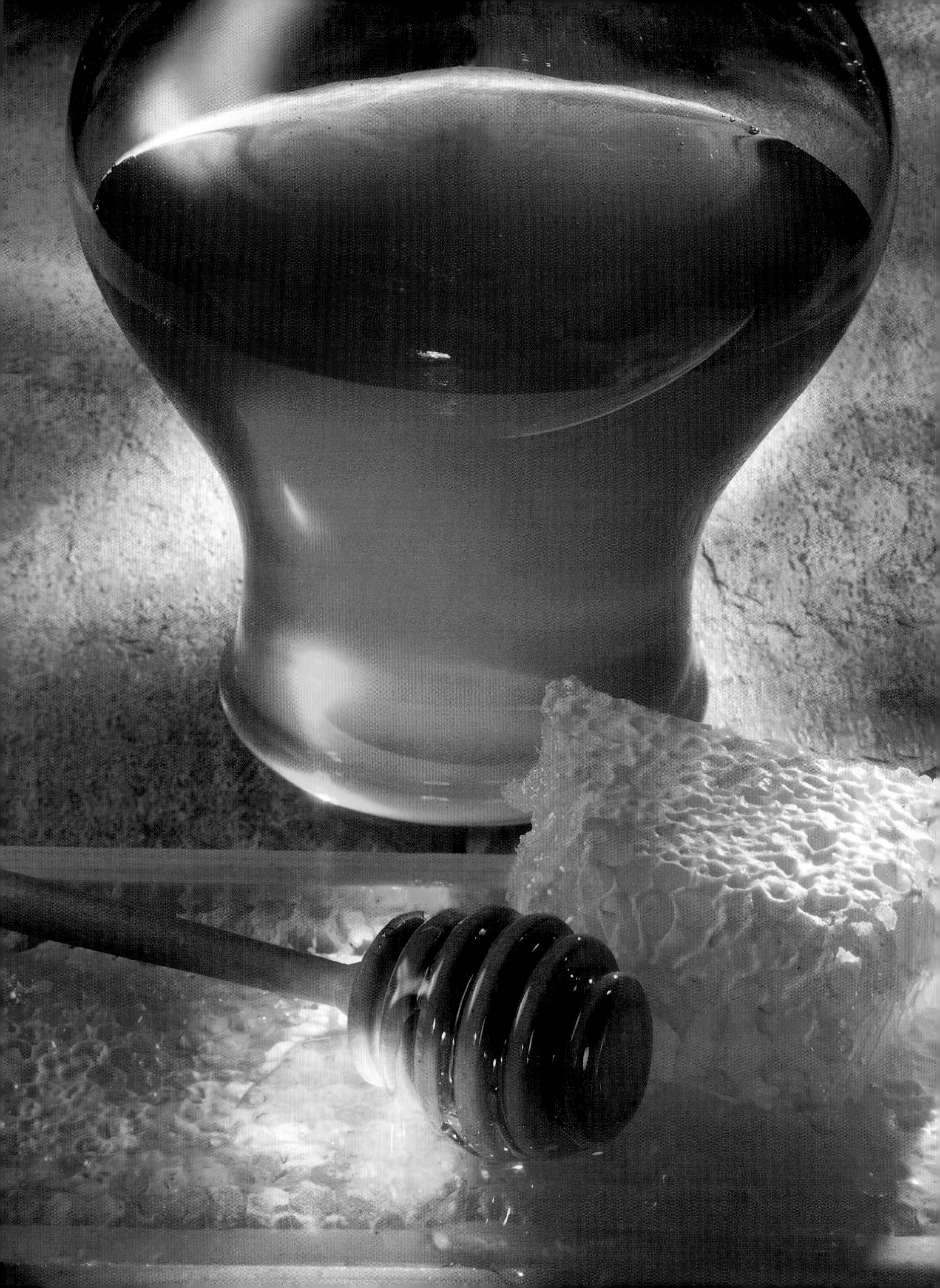

boost the body's ability to heal itself. Also, the more dilute the dose, the greater its effect; the remedies are prepared in a way that is said to make them more potent with each dilution.

The aim of homeopathy is to treat the person rather than the illness. When prescribing medication, practitioners will therefore take into account a patient's personality, feelings, habits, likes and dislikes, as well as any stress factors. As a consequence, two very different people suffering from the same illness will not be treated with the same remedy; similarly, the same remedy can be used for a range of symptoms, depending on the needs of the individual.

Because homeopathy is so tailored to the individual and people react differently to each remedy, it is difficult to lay down general rules. Whether or not certain foods and drinks can upset the effectiveness of the medication is the subject of debate. Some practitioners advise avoiding tobacco, coffee, mint and strong-tasting or smelling foods and drinks for 30 minutes before and after taking the remedies or even throughout the treatment.

HONEY

Lore and legend have endowed honey with unique nutritional and health-giving qualities. It has been hailed as an aphrodisiac and an elixir of youth. In reality, however, it supplies little more than energy in the form of simple carbohydrates.

Honey is produced by bees from plant nectar and is a mixture of water and two simple sugars: fructose and glucose. The clearer the honey, the higher the proportion of fructose, although honey will almost always granulate if it is kept long enough. Heating it will make it runny again.

LIQUID GOLD *Honey has been a much-prized source of sweetness since ancient times. It takes the nectar of one and a half million flowers to make a single jar.*

Honey supplies negligible amounts of nutrients, but its tiny nutrient content does make it a slightly healthier option than refined white sugar, which contains nothing but empty calories. In fact, weight for weight, honey contains fewer calories than sugar – 288 as opposed to 394 per 100g (3½oz) – because one-quarter of it is water. But when substituting it for sugar in recipes, it is worth remembering that because it is denser, one tablespoon of honey weighs more than one tablespoon of sugar, so that substituting by volume rather than by weight would give you more calories.

The flavour of honey depends on which flowers the bees have visited. Acacia honey is mild and suitable for cooking, while chestnut honey has a distinctive, almost bitter taste.

Honey can contain naturally occurring toxins from plants. Bees that collect pollen from rhododendrons, for example, can produce a toxic honey that can cause paralysis if eaten. There has also been some concern over pyrrolizidine alkaloids in honey made by bees that have foraged on ragwort.

MEDICINAL PROPERTIES

Honey still retains its reputation as a remedy for chest complaints, particularly for removing phlegm. It also has antiseptic properties – the Ancient Greeks and Romans believed that it could help to heal wounds – and it is claimed that it acts as a decongestant. Honey can also act as a mild sedative, in the same way as sugar.

A drink for sore throats can be made by adding two teaspoons of honey and the juice of half a lemon to a glass of hot water. All sweet foods stimulate the brain to produce endorphins, which are the body's natural painkillers. The sweetened liquid also encourages the production of saliva, which helps to soothe a dry and irritated throat.

Royal jelly

Worker bees produce royal jelly to feed the selected larvae that eventually become queens. Royal jelly is the richest natural source of pantothenic acid (although this is readily available from other foods) and is the only natural source of a most unusual fatty acid (10-hydroxy-2-decenoic acid), to which some of its alleged effects are attributed. It is recommended to help debility and fatigue. However, there is no scientific evidence to support these or any similar claims as yet.

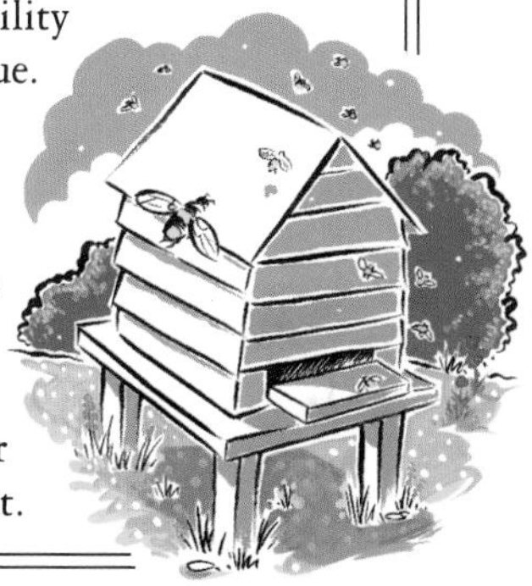

HONEY THROUGH THE AGES

Honey has featured in religious festivals throughout the world as a food fit for the gods. In Greek mythology, for example, young Zeus, having been rescued from his father, Cronus, was brought up in secret by the nymphs Adrasteia and Io, on a diet of milk and honey.

Long before beekeeping was introduced, Stone Age man valued honey from wild bees for its rarity as well as for its taste. In England, honey was the ordinary people's sweetener until the middle of the 17th century, while sugar was reserved for the nobility and the gentry. However, by the late 17th century, sugar was becoming the universal sweetener and honey the treat, hence the rhyme 'the Queen was in her parlour eating bread and honey'.

HYGIENE

Food hygiene is an essential part of maintaining good health. If the basic rules of hygiene are ignored or overlooked while buying, PREPARING, COOKING AND STORING FOOD, the consequences in terms of FOOD POISONING can be sudden and severe.

STORING YOUR PURCHASES

Unpack your food shopping as soon as possible. Store raw and cooked foods separately in the refrigerator, first wrapping or covering them in order to prevent cross-contamination. Packets and tinned goods should be kept in a clean, cool, dry place. Put the newest items at the back, bringing older ones to the front so that you use them first. Acidic tinned foods, for example tomatoes and pineapples, can be stored for 12 to 18 months; tinned foods with low acidity will usually keep for two to five years. Check the date on the can.

A CLEAN KITCHEN

In order to multiply, bacteria need food, warmth, moisture and time. Keep your kitchen clean and dry. Disinfect worktops often, especially after preparing raw meat or poultry. Tea towels should be changed daily, and dishcloths should be rinsed in diluted bleach or disinfectant and then aired after use. Empty rubbish bins frequently and disinfect them with diluted bleach. Keep pets away from food and kitchen worktops.

Keep food covered, do not leave scraps lying around, and wipe away any spillages. This will help to prevent insects such as flies spreading disease.

PREPARING FOOD

Always wash your hands in hot, soapy water before touching food. If you need to cough, blow your nose or sneeze, use a clean handkerchief so as not to spread germs, and wash your hands before touching the food again. If you have any cuts or infections on your hands, wear rubber gloves.

Defrost frozen food, especially poultry, thoroughly, preferably in the refrigerator. Be careful not to let the liquids from thawing meat or poultry drip onto other foods. Because moisture encourages bacteria, wash meat and poultry just before you need them. Vegetables need to be washed carefully as soil can contain listeria.

It is best to have a separate chopping board for raw meat, poultry and fish. Plastic boards are usually more hygienic than wooden ones. Never use the same knife for raw and cooked foods without washing it in between.

COOKING

Because chicken can harbour the salmonella bacteria, it must always be cooked thoroughly; it is done when the juices run clear. Pork should also be cooked through because of the danger of WORMS. Preheating the oven helps to ensure that it reaches a high enough temperature to kill bacteria.

Rice can contain *Bacillus cereus* and should therefore be eaten soon after cooking, or, if it is to be eaten cold, kept cool in the refrigerator.

Shopping for food

'Use by' and 'best before' dates are now required by law, but following a few other basic principles of food safety even while you are shopping can help to reduce the chances of problems such as food poisoning striking later.

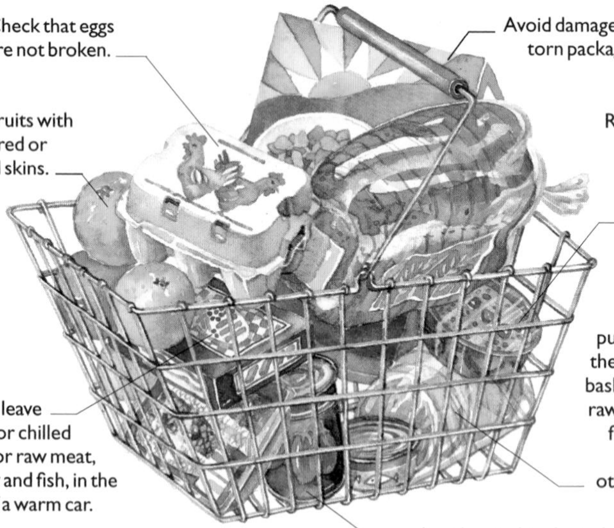
Check that eggs are not broken.
Avoid damaged or torn packaging.
Avoid fruits with punctured or bruised skins.
Refrigerate cook-chill foods as soon as possible.
Arrange purchases in the trolley or basket so that raw meat and fish cannot drip onto other foods.
Do not leave frozen or chilled foods, or raw meat, poultry and fish, in the boot of a warm car.
Avoid rusted or dented tins.

Taking food home

Make sure you are buying from a reputable source, especially if the foods will be eaten raw, as in the case of some shellfish. Look out for poor shop hygiene, such as overloaded chilled or frozen-food cabinets, or raw and cooked meat being stored next to one another. Pick up chilled and frozen foods last, so they have less time to warm up while you queue, and pack them together to keep them cold. If you shop during your lunch hour, only buy chilled produce if there is a refrigerator at work for storing it.

HYPERACTIVITY

AVOID

- *Food and drink containing additives such as tartrazine and benzoic acid*
- *Caffeine in coffee, tea and cola drinks*
- *Foods high in salicylates, such as apples, grapes, apricots, peaches and plums*

Over the past few years a great deal of medical and dietary research has been carried out to find cures for hyperactive children. It has been suggested that some synthetic food colourings, such as tartrazine (E102), and preservatives, such as benzoic acid, are to blame. However, there is still considerable debate as to the effects of these ADDITIVES and the number of children that are affected.

Nevertheless, some studies have found that children with behavioural and learning difficulties can show marked improvements once additives, which are present in orange squash, chocolate, bacon, ham, salami and other processed foods, are eliminated from their diet. Too much caffeine, found in coffee, tea, dark chocolate and some cola drinks, has also been blamed as a cause of hyperactivity, as has intolerance to certain foods (see ALLERGIES).

REFINED CARBOHYDRATES

Cakes, pastries, biscuits and confectionery should be eaten in moderation. This is because the body requires thiamin to help with the metabolism of refined carbohydrates. A low intake of the vitamin, resulting in too little reaching the central nervous system, is known to cause changes in behaviour. Thiamin is found in whole grains, brown rice, egg yolks and vegetables.

The possibility that sugar can contribute to hyperactivity in children is still highly controversial and many studies do not support these allegations. However, refined sugar lacks chromium, which is removed during the refining process, and chromium is needed for the metabolism of sugar. Without it, the body's insulin is less effective in controlling blood glucose levels, and this may therefore lead to, or exacerbate, hyperactivity and other behavioural problems.

PROBLEM CHILDREN

It is claimed that approximately 1 in 10 children shows some degree of hyperactivity, with 1 in 200 having severe problems. In these cases family life can be seriously disrupted. Hyperactive children are compulsive fidgets and suffer from poor concentration, never settling to a task. Their behaviour is unpredictable, so that they can suddenly become aggressive or tearful. Although hyperactive children are usually of average or above average intelligence, they often have learning difficulties, partly because of the problems they have concentrating. Some also suffer from ECZEMA or ASTHMA, and most find it difficult to sleep.

SALICYLATE FOODS

Salicylates, chemicals present in many foods, as well as in aspirin (acetylsalicylic acid), can trigger hyperactivity in some susceptible children. Salicylates occur naturally in most fruits, including apples, apricots, peaches, plums, berries and raisins. They are also found in potato skins, spinach, carrots and broccoli, as well as in peppermint and liquorice sweets. Curry powder, dill, thyme, oregano, turmeric and paprika are especially high. Nuts and seeds contain moderate amounts.

Fruits with a low salicylate content include bananas, peeled pears and papaya. Suitable vegetables include most beans (except for broad beans and green beans), cabbage, peas, lettuce and peeled potatoes. Poultry, meat, fish, eggs, cereals, pulses and dairy products are all low in salicylates.

Dos and don'ts for fridges and freezers

- Do keep the coldest part of the refrigerator at 0°-5°C (32°-41°F) – if necessary buy a refrigerator thermometer. Freezers should be kept at or below -18°C (0°F).
- Do clean the refrigerator regularly: take out all food, and wash all surfaces, including the shelves, with hot soapy water. A solution of bicarbonate of soda and warm water is a good cleanser and will not make the refrigerator smell.
- Do defrost fridges and freezers regularly to maintain efficiency. Wash the freezer and allow its temperature to drop to -18°C (0°F) before restocking.
- Do leave enough room for cold air to circulate in the refrigerator; by contrast, the deep freeze will function more efficiently if packed tightly (see FROZEN FOOD).
- Do keep raw meat, poultry and fish on the fridge's lower shelves, and ensure that they do not come into contact with cooked dishes or food that is to be eaten raw.
- Do use proper packaging such as freezer bags or plastic containers, which will prevent moisture penetrating the food and damaging it, and make sure you label them clearly with the date.
- Don't leave the refrigerator or freezer doors open, as the temperature within will rise rapidly.
- Don't put warm foods in the refrigerator or freezer; they will raise the interior temperature.
- Don't store eggs in the rack in the refrigerator door; keep them in the box or put them in a bowl so air can circulate freely. Three weeks from purchase is the maximum recommended keeping time.

HYPOGLYCAEMIA

CUT DOWN ON
- *Large, heavy meals*
- *Alcohol*

An important source of energy in the body, and the only source of energy for the brain, is glucose. This simple sugar is found in some foods, including grapes, and is one of the constituents of sucrose (the main component of cane sugar) and starch (found in potatoes and bread, for example). As they are digested, foods containing sucrose or starch release glucose into the bloodstream. Normally, insulin and other hormones maintain the right concentration of glucose in the blood for energy and brain function, but if the body cannot regulate its blood sugar levels this can lead to hyperglycaemia, when levels are too high, or hypoglycaemia, when levels fall too low.

The symptoms of hypoglycaemia include hunger, weakness, a cold sweat, palpitations, dizziness and confusion. If prompt action is not taken to raise sugar levels, the sufferer will lose consciousness.

CAUSES

Hypoglycaemia is most commonly seen in people with DIABETES, but it can be a sign of a LIVER DISORDER, because the liver helps to regulate blood sugar levels. It can also occur following severe physical exertion, as the result of stress, or after drinking too much alcohol.

There is also a condition known as reactive hypoglycaemia. In this case, the body produces too much insulin, causing levels of sugar in the blood to fall too rapidly. Chronic stress, missed meals and a diet high in refined carbohydrates can all contribute to reactive hypoglycaemia. Symptoms are most commonly experienced 2-5 hours after meals. If sugary foods are eaten in an attempt to boost blood sugar levels, the body again secretes too much insulin, and a vicious circle is set up.

AVOIDING HYPOGLYCAEMIA

Blood sugar levels can be controlled by making sure that you eat regularly and often – several smaller meals are better than three large ones. The main part of your meals should consist of complex carbohydrates such as whole grains, pulses, jacket potatoes and pasta, as well as fresh fruit and vegetables. Because these foods are broken down slowly, they provide a steady release of glucose into the bloodstream.

There is no need to cut out refined food and drinks containing sugar, such as honey, fruit juice and dried fruit, but these should be taken in moderation. Too much alcohol, which stimulates insulin production, should be avoided.

If you are diabetic and experience a hypoglycaemic attack, immediately take two to three glucose tablets, or four to five soft sweets, or half a can of a

Case study

During a morning surgery the local doctor was urgently summoned to the Greek deli, where Iannis, the owner's 29-year-old son, was behaving irrationally. Iannis had suddenly become aggressive and uncooperative towards his parents. He had also been staggering around as though drunk, but by the time the doctor arrived he had slumped into a chair and was sweating profusely. The doctor knew that Iannis was an insulin-dependent diabetic and that his symptoms might indicate hypoglycaemia (low blood sugar level). His mother said that Iannis, who was developing a cold, had not eaten any breakfast, although he had taken his usual morning dose of insulin. Taking the insulin without following it with some food had caused Iannis's blood sugar level to plummet, and this had triggered his unruly, 'drunken' symptoms. The doctor persuaded Iannis to drink a glass of sweetened milk and within half an hour he had returned to his normal self. He followed the milk with some bread, which provided slow-acting carbohydrates to stop his blood sugar level from falling too low again. The doctor then explained that because he still needed to take his insulin when he was ill, he also needed to maintain his calorie intake, even when he did not feel like eating. In the future, if he was unwell he might find it easier to have small, frequent snacks and drinks rather than full meals. Arrangements were made for him to see a specialist diabetic nurse, who would be able to tell him how, as a diabetic, he could best manage any episodes of illness.

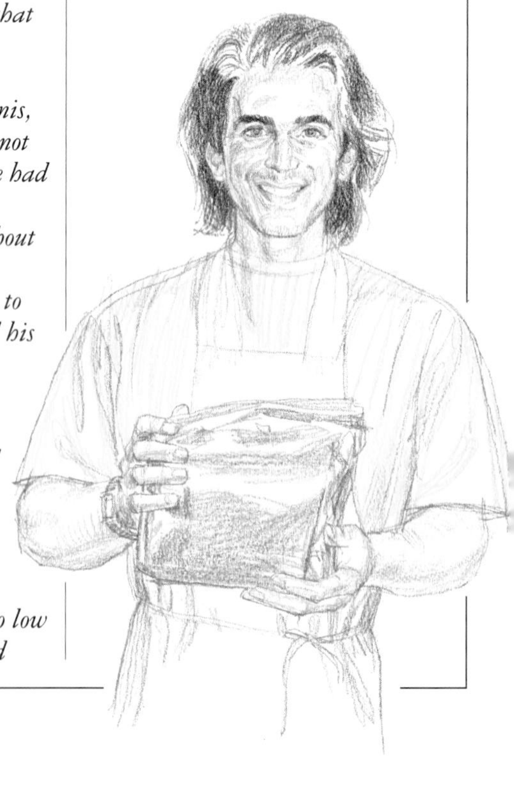

sugary drink. If your next meal is not due soon, follow this up with something more substantial, such as a glass of milk and biscuits or a sandwich. If you repeatedly suffer from hypoglycaemia before a meal, the meal time should be brought forward. Taking more carbohydrates before and after exercise is also essential. The amount needed will depend on your metabolic rate and the type of exercise. Always carry enough concentrated sugar with you in case you have an attack.

HYPOTHERMIA

TAKE PLENTY OF
- *Hot food, soup and warm drinks*
- *Small, frequent meals*

AVOID
- *Alcohol when a patient is waiting for medical attention*

Extreme chilling of the body caused by exposure to cold – whether indoors or outside – is dangerous and can often be fatal. Hypothermia, which is indicated by shivering, drowsiness and a slow pulse, is particularly common in elderly people who live alone in poorly heated homes, and in newborn babies kept in cold rooms at night. Premature babies and those suffering from illness are most susceptible; the signs are a bright red appearance, lethargy and a refusal to eat. Hypothermia can also affect anyone who is exposed to prolonged and extreme cold or damp, for example sailors, mountaineers and people taking part in winter sports such as skiing.

The situation becomes dangerous when the body temperature drops from its normal 37°C (98.6°F) to below 35°C (95°F) and the metabolism begins to slow down. Once the temperature drops to below 33°C (91°F), the shivering stops and the person will become confused and unsteady. Unconsciousness occurs at about 30°C (86°F), and the patient may die unless help is rapidly given. Anyone found in this state needs emergency medical treatment. Call a doctor or an ambulance immediately.

While waiting for medical attention, wrap the patient's head and body in blankets, or anything else that is suitable. Because warming up too suddenly is dangerous, avoid using hot-water bottles or any form of direct heat. It is safe to offer hot soup or a warm, sweet drink if the victim is conscious and capable of swallowing, but do not give any alcohol. Alcohol draws the blood away from vital organs to the skin, dilating the capillaries so that even more heat is lost.

PREVENTING HYPOTHERMIA

There are several steps that can be taken to stop yourself from becoming dangerously cold:
- Make sure you take plenty of warm drinks throughout the day.
- Try to eat at least one hot meal a day.
- Wear warm clothes. Several thin layers are more effective at trapping warmth than one thick one.
- Wear a hat to prevent body heat being lost through the head. Babies are especially vulnerable to this kind of heat loss.
- Try to keep active. Sitting in one position for a long time will only make you feel colder.
- Keep at least one room in the house warm – at a temperature of 21°C (70°F) – even if it means shutting off the rest of the house and living in that room only. Check for draughts and block any gaps.
- On cold nights, keep a Thermos flask with a warm, sweet drink by your bed.
- Plan ahead before you venture out for long periods in cold weather. Take weatherproof clothes with you even if the skies look clear. Wear wool rather than cotton. Eat well to keep your strength up and carry high-carbohydrate snacks in case of emergencies.
- Do not drink alcohol when out of doors in cold, wet weather. It decreases stamina and mental sharpness and also causes heat loss.
- If you are camping, make sure your tent is strong, waterproof and windproof. Carry a gas stove with extra gas, as well as a reliable fire starter.

Survival stories

In some situations, a bar of chocolate or a cheese sandwich can make the difference between life and death. In 1995, two students trapped by blizzards on Ben Nevis, in Scotland, survived for two nights by eating chocolate, sandwiches and energy tablets. They were suffering from both hypothermia and frostbite. Other mountaineers have also survived hazardous conditions with the help of energy-rich foods. One skier held out for three nights on a mountain thanks to a single Mars bar. Staying awake is vital, too. In 1994, a climber caught by an avalanche in the French Alps lived to tell the tale because he built a snowhole and moved about regularly to keep his circulation going.

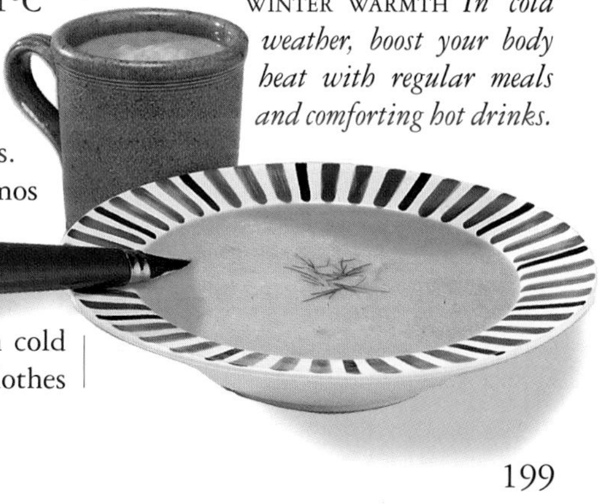

WINTER WARMTH *In cold weather, boost your body heat with regular meals and comforting hot drinks.*

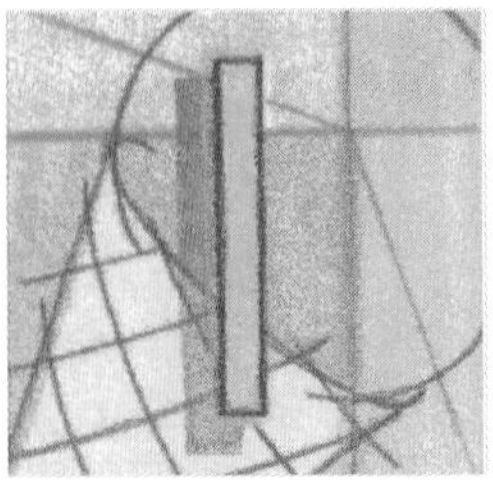

ICE CREAM

BENEFITS
- *Most varieties contain vitamins A, riboflavin and B_{12}*
- *Contains calcium*

DRAWBACKS
- *High sugar content*
- *Most brands are high in fat*

The nutritional value of ice cream depends principally on the levels of cream or milk it contains. Although cream and milk supply vitamins and calcium, they also supply a lot of saturated fat. Other ingredients include sugar and flavourings, to which stabilisers and emulsifiers may be added to improve the ice cream's durability.

Although ice cream has a bad reputation because of its high fat content, an average cone or scoop of ice cream may supply just 130-150 Calories. Besides tasting good, it generally contains vitamins A, riboflavin (B_2) and B_{12}, and provides calcium, needed for strong bones and teeth. Its protein content is similar to milk.

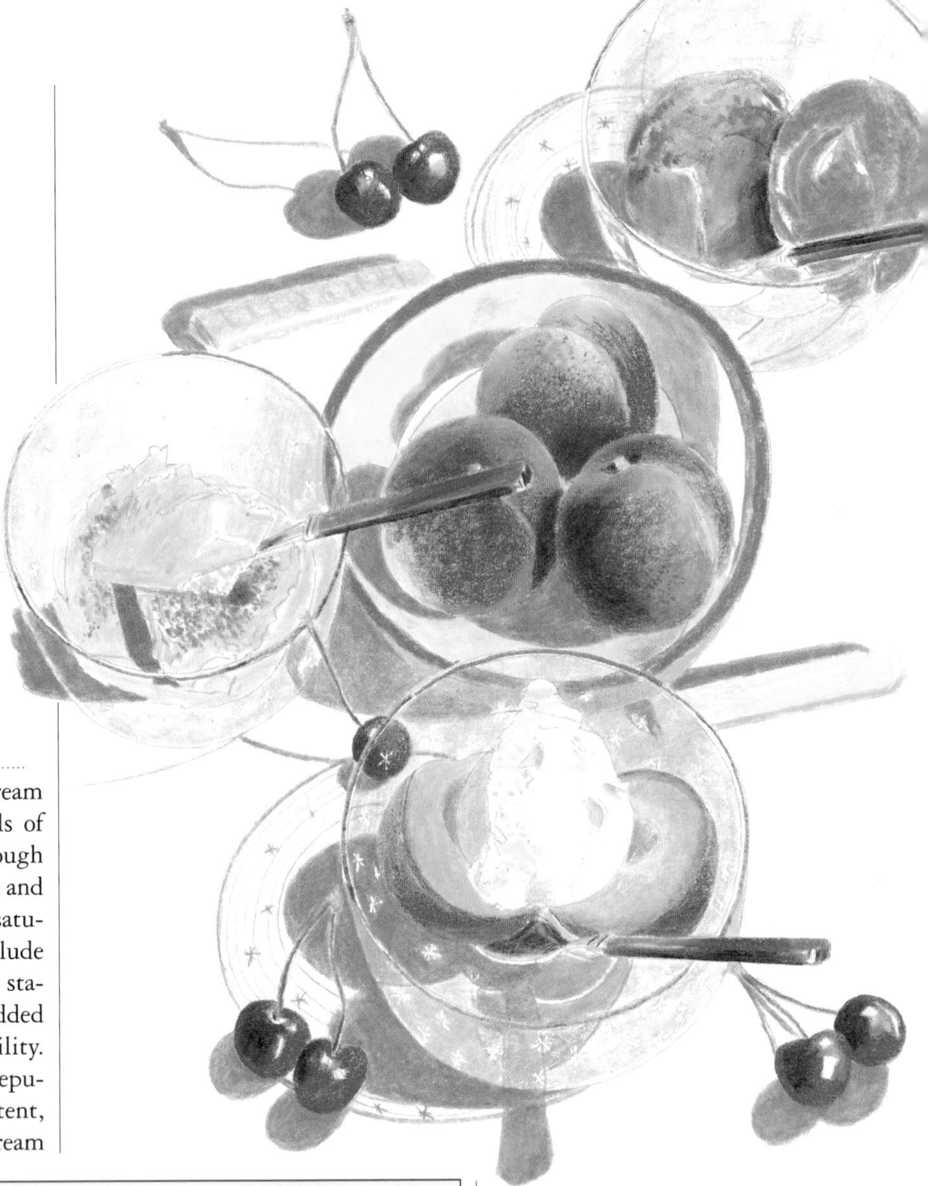

SUMMERTIME TREAT *An occasional scoop of ice cream will do no harm, and you can always combine it with some fresh fruit.*

What's in a 100g (3½oz) serving of ice cream

TYPE	ENERGY (Calories)	FAT (g)	PROTEIN (g)	CARBOHYDRATE (g)	CALCIUM (mg)
Dairy, vanilla	194	9.8	3.6	24.4	130
Dairy, flavoured	179	8.0	3.5	24.7	110
Non-dairy, vanilla	178	8.7	3.2	23.1	120
Non-dairy, flavoured	166	7.4	3.1	23.2	120
Reduced calorie	119	6.0	3.4	13.7	120

FAT CONTENT

Ice creams can be graded by their fat content with levels ranging from 5 to 15 per cent. Anything containing less than 5 per cent fat cannot be called ice cream and must be termed 'frozen dessert'. There are some frozen desserts available now which look and taste similar to ice cream but contain as little as 1 per cent fat.

'Premium' ice creams usually contain more fat, are less aerated than standard products, and use better-quality flavourings such as real fruit.

A dairy ice cream contains milk fat only; if other fats are used, the words 'contains non-milk fat' or 'contains vegetable fat' must appear prominently on the label.

Both dairy and non-dairy ice cream contain high levels of saturated fat which has been linked with heart disease. The latest recommendations from the Department of Health suggest that saturated fats should make up no more than 10 per cent of all calories consumed. It is therefore best to eat ice cream in moderation, or to choose the low-fat brands.

IMMUNE SYSTEM

EAT PLENTY OF

- *Protein-rich foods*
- *Citrus fruits for vitamin C*
- *Vegetable oils for vitamin E*
- *Spinach, sweet potatoes and carrots which supply beta carotene*

CUT DOWN ON

- *Animal fats, sugar, alcohol, caffeine and highly processed carbohydrates*

We need a steady and balanced intake of essential vitamins and minerals to keep our immune systems working properly to provide protection from infections and diseases. However, an immune system that is overactive may cause deterioration in people who are suffering from disorders such as ARTHRITIS and MULTIPLE SCLEROSIS. There are many factors that can have an adverse effect on the immune system: excessive intakes of alcohol and caffeine; ingestion or inhalation of heavy metals such as cadmium, lead and mercury; and tobacco smoke or other forms of pollution in the air. When pollutants or toxic substances are absorbed by the body, they threaten the effectiveness of the minerals and vitamins in food, and are sometimes described as antinutrients.

AN ALLY AGAINST CANCER

The immune system is known to play a role in preventing cancer. It is thought that a special type of white blood cells called 'killer' cells, which are part of the immune system, may identify tumour cells by the changes in their surface membrane. Other, 'helper' cells then assist the 'killer' cells to multiply and, when there are enough of these, they attach themselves to the tumour cell and destroy it.

THE ROLE OF DIET

To improve the body's natural resistance, the diet should provide ample amounts of vitamins and minerals, including ANTIOXIDANTS, and natural protective chemicals (bioflavonoids) found in plants. Antioxidants also help to neutralise any excess FREE RADICALS that are produced as part of the body's natural defence mechanism.

Fish, poultry, lean meat, low-fat dairy products, cereals and legumes (peas, lentils, beans) are all good sources of minerals. Foods such as cheese, eggs or liver, which supply vitamin A, and spinach, sweet potatoes or carrots, which are good sources of beta carotene, should also be eaten daily.

Vitamin B_{12} deficiency increases the risk of contracting diseases such as tuberculosis. This vitamin is found in meat, eggs, fish and fortified cereals.

Most fruit and vegetables supply vitamin C: moderately large amounts of this vitamin (up to 200mg daily) increase levels of immunoglobulin – blood proteins that act as disease fighting antibodies – which are produced by the immune system. Vitamin D (obtained from oily fish) and vitamin E (in olive oil, nuts, avocados and wholegrain cereals) are also vital to the immune system's effectiveness, as are essential fatty acids found in vegetable oils and fish oils.

One of the most common nutrient deficiencies which affects the immune system is a lack of zinc. Pumpkin seeds and lean beef are both a rich source of zinc, while oysters are an excellent source. A recent study among elderly people showed that a multi-vitamin and mineral supplement improved their immune responses.

IMPOTENCE

EAT PLENTY OF

- *Seafood (especially shellfish), offal, lean beef, nuts and other zinc-rich foods*

CUT DOWN ON

- *Alcohol*
- *Coffee, tea and cola drinks*
- *Smoking*

Physical or psychological and emotional factors are at the root of chronic impotence – the male's inability to attain or maintain an erection. Impotence is often a side effect of a wide variety of physical disorders including atherosclerosis, diabetes, thyroid disorders, ailments affecting the nervous system, urinary tract and genitals, or of prescribed drugs such as antihypertensives. It can be caused by STRESS, fatigue, anxiety, guilt, embarrassment or depression, and worsened by smoking, alcohol or caffeine. Men who suffer from impotence should therefore try to cut down on their intake of nicotine and caffeine (found in tea, coffee and some colas), both of which constrict the blood vessels and thus inhibit blood flow. Alcohol may help to shed inhibitions, but on the whole it is best avoided. If you must have a drink, limit yourself to one because alcohol reduces the strength of nerve signals. High intakes of alcohol also suppress the production of androgens (male hormones).

One recent US study suggested that men with high blood cholesterol levels run a greater than average long-term risk of becoming impotent. Cholesterol can partially block the arteries leading to the penis, reducing the blood pressure needed to maintain an erection. In 1993, the *Journal of the American Medical Association* reported that in half of the cases of men over 50 who had difficulty achieving or maintaining an erection, the problem was due to a partially blocked penile artery.

To reduce the threat of high blood cholesterol levels, the diet should be high in fruit, vegetables and whole grains, and contain moderate amounts of lean meat, and be low in saturated fats, found in butter, hard cheeses, the fat on meat and in poultry skin.

Zinc may help

Claims that zinc-rich foods, such as oysters, can act as potent aphrodisiacs are probably exaggerated. Yet a severe deficiency of the mineral can lead to impotence. The findings of a study on a group of impotent men, published in *The Lancet*, showed that taking zinc supplements improved potency and raised levels of the male sex hormone, testosterone, to normal.

Zinc has also been used to cure impotence in kidney dialysis patients. Ensure that you have a good intake of dietary zinc by eating plenty of seafood, offal, lentils, soya beans, nuts, eggs, meat and wheatgerm. Zinc supplements may also be useful at the first sign of any problem.

Indigestion

EAT PLENTY OF
- *Small, frequent meals*

CUT DOWN ON
- *Alcohol*
- *Strong coffee*
- *Fizzy drinks*

AVOID
- *Heavy or fatty meals late at night*
- *Smoking*

Almost everyone has indigestion from time to time. Excessive acid in the stomach causes discomfort and can reflux into the oesophagus – the tube that connects the mouth with the stomach. The result is heartburn and discomfort in the chest. Pregnant women often suffer because the uterus presses on the digestive tract as the baby grows. Overweight people are also susceptible because of pressure on their digestive tract.

Eating a healthy, fibre-rich diet, relaxing before and during meals, and regular exercise can all help to prevent indigestion. Mint tea is the traditional herbal remedy for indigestion and many people claim that it works. Put a mint tea bag or two teaspoons of chopped fresh leaves in a cup of boiling water, and sip slowly after meals. Be careful not to confuse the mild mint with peppermint which can actually antagonise indigestion.

Foods to avoid

Food culprits may include meat extracts, acidic foods such as pickles and vinegar, fried foods, hot spicy foods – especially those which contain chilli, and raw foods such as onions, cucumbers and peppers. Try to cut down on alcohol, strong coffee and fizzy drinks: alcohol increases stomach acidity; coffee causes irritation and fizzy drinks produce wind. Other common triggers are stress, rushed meals, not chewing food sufficiently, swallowing air and long intervals without food. Nicotine can actually increase the amount of gastric acid secreted. Although a healthy diet will not cure indigestion, avoiding the most common triggers of indigestion may prevent attacks from occurring.

Indigestion: the common culprits

Because some foods are less easy to digest than others, they can prompt bouts of indigestion among susceptible people. Some culprits are:

Raw salad vegetables such as onions, radishes and cucumber can be hard to digest.

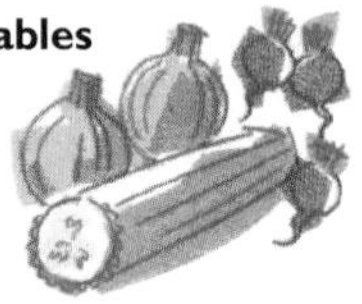

Too much liquid dilutes digestive juices, but a glass of wine aids them.

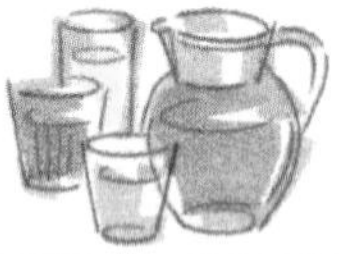

Hot spicy foods, such as curries, in large quantities tend to 'repeat'.

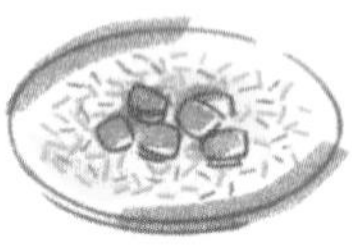

Fatty foods or fried foods can stimulate acid output in the gut.

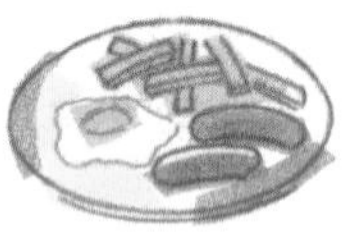

Strong tea and coffee are particularly hard to digest – especially with meals.

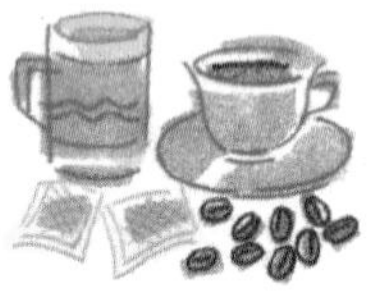

Unripe fruits are high in pectin making them hard to digest.

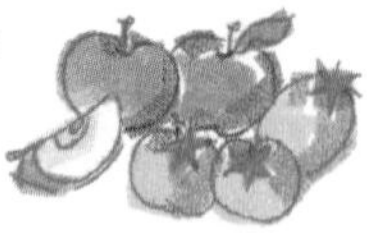

Cheese just before bedtime; its high fat content slows down digestion.

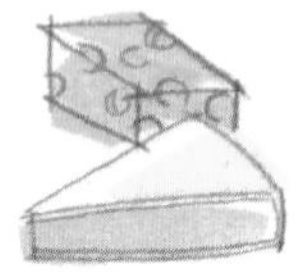

In some cases, however, indigestion is a symptom of other DIGESTIVE PROBLEMS. People with severe, recurrent indigestion, or those over 40 who suddenly begin to experience bouts of indigestion, should consult their doctor to exclude the possibility of some serious underlying disease.

LIFESTYLE

A few simple changes in your lifestyle may be all that is needed to prevent indigestion. For example, do not eat just before going to bed, and avoid irregular and hurried meals. Stop smoking and cut down on alcohol. Try yoga or some other form of stress-reducing exercise. Certain drugs, and the female hormone progesterone, can sometimes exacerbate indigestion. But if you suspect that a drug you are taking is doing this, always consult your doctor before you stop taking it.

INFERTILITY

EAT PLENTY OF

- *Shellfish, sunflower and sesame seeds, and nuts for zinc*
- *Citrus fruits for vitamin C*
- *Meat, offal and poultry for iron*
- *Brown rice, wheatgerm, pulses, oily fish, oats and fresh nuts for B vitamins*
- *Soya beans, almonds and wholemeal bread for magnesium*

CUT DOWN ON

- *Alcohol and tea*
- *Highly refined foods*

Failure to conceive may be caused by a range of medical problems in either or both partners. One common cause of infertility, however, is poor nutrition.

A survey of women attending fertility clinics in London revealed that half of them had been trying to lose weight by following diets that lacked vital nutrients. It is also crucial for women to maintain an optimum level of body fat – at least 18 per cent of body weight. If the level drops below this, hormone imbalances can occur which may result in a failure to ovulate and so, in turn, cause infertility.

At the other extreme, OBESITY can also lower a woman's chances of conception. Any woman concerned about her fertility should examine her daily diet. It should contain foods that ensure an adequate intake of zinc, magnesium, iron, folate, vitamin C and the essential fatty acids.

Some women who have been using the contraceptive pill for a number of years suffer reduced fertility for a few months after they have stopped. They may find it helpful to follow the advice provided here, with the addition of foods rich in manganese (oats, wheatgerm, chestnuts, rye bread and peas) which promotes the action of oestrogen, and vitamin B_6 (whole grains and green vegetables) which is also involved in oestrogen metabolism.

It is wise for both men and women to cut down on foods containing highly refined ingredients, such as white flour and sugar, because they often lack essential nutrients and take the place of more nourishing foods.

Drinking too much alcohol can interfere with the body's uptake of B vitamins and minerals such as zinc and iron, while drinking large amounts of tea can interfere with iron absorption.

Male fertility requires essential fatty acids (found in oily fish and polyunsaturated oils), vitamins A, B, C, and E, and zinc and selenium. These nutrients all play a role in the production of healthy sperm.

Many studies have demonstrated the link between healthy sperm and zinc; high concentrations of zinc are found in male sex glands and also in sperm. Healthy testicles also contain large concentrations of vitamin C. It has been claimed that high doses of vitamin C may cure a common cause of male infertility – the clustering together or 'agglutination' of sperm.

In one study at Texas University Medical School researchers gave 500mg of vitamin C twice daily for a month to a group of male patients. All the men in this study started with very low dietary levels of vitamin C. After three weeks, the percentage of sperm clumping together had fallen, on average, from 37 per cent to around 11 per cent which is well within the normal range for fertile men.

In many cases, however, the causes of infertility are not related to diet. In women there might be a history of infection, obstructions of the fallopian tubes, hormonal imbalances, failure to ovulate or even an allergic reaction to the partner's sperm. In men, impotence, insufficient, abnormal or weak sperm, prostate disease, previous illnesses such as mumps or orchitis (inflammation of the testicles) and injury are all possible causes.

DECREASING SPERM COUNTS

For whatever reason, there is alarming evidence from studies throughout Europe that sperm counts have dropped dramatically over the past 50 years. Among the factors blamed are alcohol, stress, and the increased use of chemicals in agriculture and industrial pollution. Britain's Ministry of Agriculture, Fisheries and Food is investigating the effects of 'oestrogenic' pollutants (present in river water and in plastic food wrapping) which can act like the feminising hormone oestrogen.

These compounds, which are used to make plastic more flexible, seem especially prone to 'leaking' into foods which contain fat, such as crisps, chocolate and even milk. They are also sometimes found in paints and cosmetics, from which they evaporate.

Scientists are looking at the possibility that these oestrogen mimicking compounds form part of a complex environmental cocktail of chemicals which may somehow be acting on unborn male babies, interfering with their ability to produce enough healthy sperm in later life.

A HISTORICAL PERSPECTIVE

Food and fertility have been linked throughout history. For fertility in general – and specifically for the birth of males – the Ancient Greeks prescribed dry foods such as pulses, cereals and nuts. Even today, there are some alternative practitioners who suggest that the mother's diet before conception can be tailored specifically to influence the sex of a baby. However, none of these diets has been shown to work using conventional methods of scientific study, and indeed, some – which involve increasing salt intake, for example – could even be damaging to the health of both the mother and her newly conceived child.

The Ancient Greek physician Hippocrates said that to be fertile, a man should not take a hot bath, nor should he be drunk. 'He should be strong, in good health, and should abstain from unhealthful foods.' His bride was advised to eat fruits with many seeds.

INFLUENZA

TAKE PLENTY OF

- *Fluids, especially diluted fruit juices*
- *Small, light meals*
- *Garlic, which has antiviral properties*

Loss of appetite is one of the symptoms of flu, along with a high temperature, coughing, shivering, headache, pain in the joints and excessive tiredness. Doctors generally advise people with influenza to rest, drink plenty of fluids and take paracetamol or aspirin regularly to relieve pain and reduce FEVER. Flu is a viral infection, and viruses do not respond to antibiotics, but where there is a risk of secondary bacterial infection causing bronchitis or pneumonia, they may be prescribed.

To prevent dehydration from perspiration, people with flu should drink plenty of fluid; a minimum of 1.7 litres (3 pints) a day. This can include fruit juice diluted 1:1 with water which contains sugars for energy.

Meals should be nutritious but small. Include plenty of complex carbohydrates, such as wholemeal bread and cereals, to supply energy, and try to ensure a good intake of vitamins.

Chicken broth is useful to introduce protein and B vitamins into the diet, and to replace any salt lost through sweating; it is easy to eat and comforting. Fish is also a good source of protein. Eat carrots, spinach and broccoli for beta carotene and plenty of fresh fruit and vegetables for vitamin C.

Folklore and flu

Elderberry wine and onion broth are reputed to ease the symptoms of flu, and there may be some truth in these cures, since both contain bioflavonoids which are known to help boost the immune system.

Another traditional cure is dried yarrow, peppermint and elderflowers taken as a tea. Several cups of yarrow and lemon balm tea a day may help to improve appetite.

GARLIC MAY HELP

Studies using extracts of GARLIC have shown that it may help to fight off flu. Garlic has both antiviral and antibacterial properties. It has long been used as a decongestant and is also said to ease sore throats, reduce fever and help the body to ward off infection.

IRRADIATED FOODS

Food manufacturers, growers and distributors are constantly looking for new ways to maintain the quality of fresh produce and extend its shelf-life. Irradiation is among the newest and most controversial of these methods to be introduced. In Britain only one company holds a licence, which permits it to irradiate herbs and spices. However, the application of irradiation for the preservation of highly perishable soft fruits and shellfish may soon become widespread.

Irradiation has attracted considerable suspicion. Some people worry that it makes food radioactive; in fact, none of the ionising radiation is retained. The dose is usually applied at low to moderate levels in order to reduce parasites or to inhibit ripening and natural spoilage.

At the highest dose approved in Britain, food is sterilised. This level of irradiation may be used in the hospital preparation of special diets for patients with weakened immune function. High doses are also used to remove contaminating bacteria from dried herbs and spices following the withdrawal of the chemical previously employed for this purpose. Exposing food to even higher irradiation levels would adversely affect its flavour and ultimately reduce it to a mush.

There is also concern because irradiation may result in the loss of some nutrients. Low to moderate-dose irradiation does not affect the mineral content or nutritional value of proteins, carbohydrates or saturated fats in foods. Losses of vitamins are insignificant when low doses are applied but at higher doses a food may lose up to half its vitamin A, vitamin E, vitamin K and thiamin content. Niacin, riboflavin and vitamin D

The effects of irradiation

The chart below indicates the levels of irradiation which are applied to different kinds of imported foods in order to extend their shelf-life.

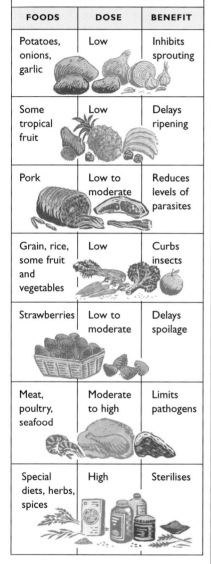

FOODS	DOSE	BENEFIT
Potatoes, onions, garlic 	Low	Inhibits sprouting
Some tropical fruit 	Low	Delays ripening
Pork 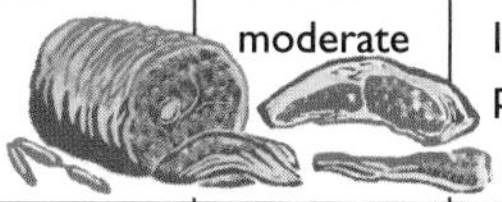	Low to moderate	Reduces levels of parasites
Grain, rice, some fruit and vegetables 	Low	Curbs insects
Strawberries 	Low to moderate	Delays spoilage
Meat, poultry, seafood 	Moderate to high	Limits pathogens
Special diets, herbs, spices 	High	Sterilises

appear to be relatively stable. For vitamin C, there is conflicting evidence; some studies indicate major losses and others none at all.

Some foods cannot be successfully irradiated because the process results in unpleasant changes in the look, taste or smell of certain produce. Irradiation can darken the flesh and adversely affect the taste of some meats; it oxidises unsaturated fats making them taste rancid and, in high doses, it can turn shellfish black.

How can you tell?

In many cases irradiated foods are indistinguishable in look and taste from unprocessed foods. This has led to concern that treated foods could be sold as fresh produce; fruits such as strawberries can look newly picked for several weeks after irradiation.

British regulations require the labelling of irradiated foods, most of which are currently imported as many countries now permit limited irradiation. However, it is feared that abuses could occur because there is, as yet, no simple and reliable means of detecting irradiation; the most likely indicator is when foods continue to look fresh well beyond their expected shelf-life.

Irritable Bowel Syndrome

TAKE PLENTY OF

- *Fresh fruit and vegetables, which provide soluble fibre*
- *Water – at least 1.7 litres (3 pints) a day*
- *Live natural yoghurt, which contains beneficial bacteria*

CUT DOWN ON

- *High-fibre breakfast cereals*

AVOID

- *Bran*
- *Foods that are known to produce wind, such as peas, lentils and beans*

Until very recently, bran was recommended as part of the treatment for irritable bowel syndrome (IBS). Some authorities now believe that, far from being a cure for the complaint, bran is in fact an irritant that can make the condition worse. Avoid bran and cut down on high-fibre breakfast cereals which may contain it. Gas-producing foods, such as pulses (peas, beans and lentils) can also exacerbate IBS and are best avoided.

High intakes of the sugar substitute sorbitol, and an intolerance to lactose (a sugar found only in milk) may also sometimes cause the illness. In cases where a food intolerance is suspected, an exclusion diet may be a useful pointer (see ALLERGIES).

In some cases, irritable bowel syndrome, which affects twice as many women as men, is completely unrelated to diet, and brought on by periods of STRESS. People with IBS may complain of a bloated stomach and bouts of diarrhoea alternating with periods of constipation. They may also experience intermittent sharp pains in the gut or a more continuous and generalised abdominal discomfort. However, because the symptoms are vague and there are no specific tests, IBS can be diagnosed only through the exclusion of other possible ailments.

The best treatment is the avoidance of stressful situations combined with sensible eating. The daily diet should include 18g of fibre obtained from ordinary foods – not concentrated bran or bran tablets. Most of this fibre should be in soluble form, found in apples, pears, dates and most other fruits and vegetables, as well as in oats, barley and rye.

Eat regular, moderate-sized meals and drink at least 1.7 litres (3 pints) of water daily. Include plenty of live natural yoghurt which will maintain a healthy balance of bacteria in the gut. When antibiotics are prescribed for other illnesses they have the side effect of destroying beneficial bacteria in the gut, which can cause symptoms similar to IBS. Eating live YOGHURT should help to counteract this problem.

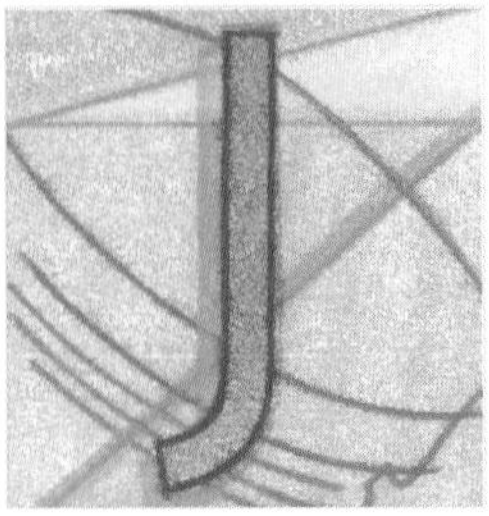

JAMS AND SPREADS

BENEFITS
- *Peanut butter is a rich source of niacin and a good source of protein and magnesium*

DRAWBACKS
- *Jams are high-sugar, low-nutrient foods*
- *Jams may prompt allergic reactions*
- *Savoury spreads are often high in sodium*

Nutritionally, jams and marmalade offer little more than concentrated energy in the form of sugar; one tablespoon contains around 40 Calories, although you can buy reduced sugar jams which contain roughly half the sugar and calories of normal jams. The fruit content of jams, which varies greatly between brands, contributes minute amounts of dietary fibre – in the form of pectin, seeds or fruit skins – and only tiny amounts of vitamins. The heat treatment involved in the boiling of preserves greatly reduces their vitamin C content.

Although in Britain, the USA and most of northern Europe, jams are used as spreads or as fillings for cakes or tarts, in many parts of the world they are served as separate sweetmeats, to be eaten on their own. Quinces have always been a mainstay of this tradition and it is from *marmelo,* which is Portuguese for quince, that the word marmalade is derived.

Like the fruits they are made from, many jams contain natural organic compounds called salicylates which can prompt 'allergic' reactions in susceptible individuals. In addition, many of the cheaper brands of jam contain artificial colourings, which may also trigger allergies in some people.

SAVOURY SPREADS

Meat and fish spreads have to contain at least 70 per cent meat or fish. They may contain added fats and cereals, as well as salt. Yeast and beef extracts contain high levels of sodium. But these spreads, though eaten in small amounts, are also concentrated sources of the B vitamins thiamin, riboflavin, niacin and folate. Some spreads made with yeast extract also contain added vitamin B_{12}.

Peanut butter is more than 50 per cent fat, but it is largely in a healthy monounsaturated form. Peanut butter is also a rich source of niacin and a good source of magnesium and protein. Peanuts can cause severe reactions in susceptible people (see ALLERGIES). Some wholefood nut butters are prone to contamination with moulds that produce aflatoxins, which are powerful carcinogens. However, most UK manufacturers monitor their nut products and the risk to public health is very low.

Natural setting

Pectin is fruit's answer to gelatin. Both are natural setting agents, but where gelatin is derived from proteins, pectins are a form of carbohydrate. Without pectin, jam or marmalade would be as runny as a dish of stewed fruit. Pectin becomes less effective as fruit ripens and will only make jams and jellies set firmly if there is a sufficient amount of sugar in them.

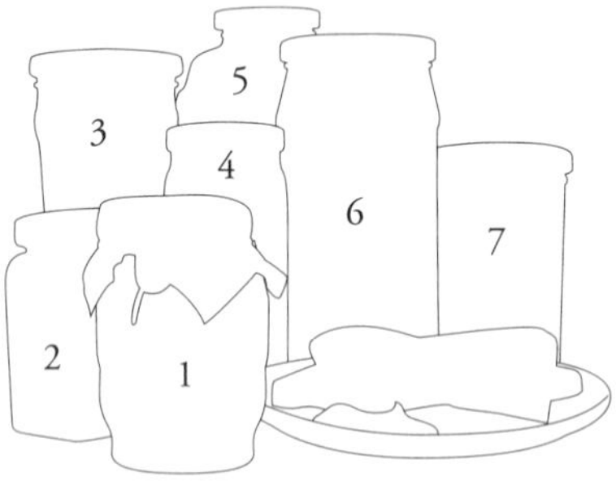

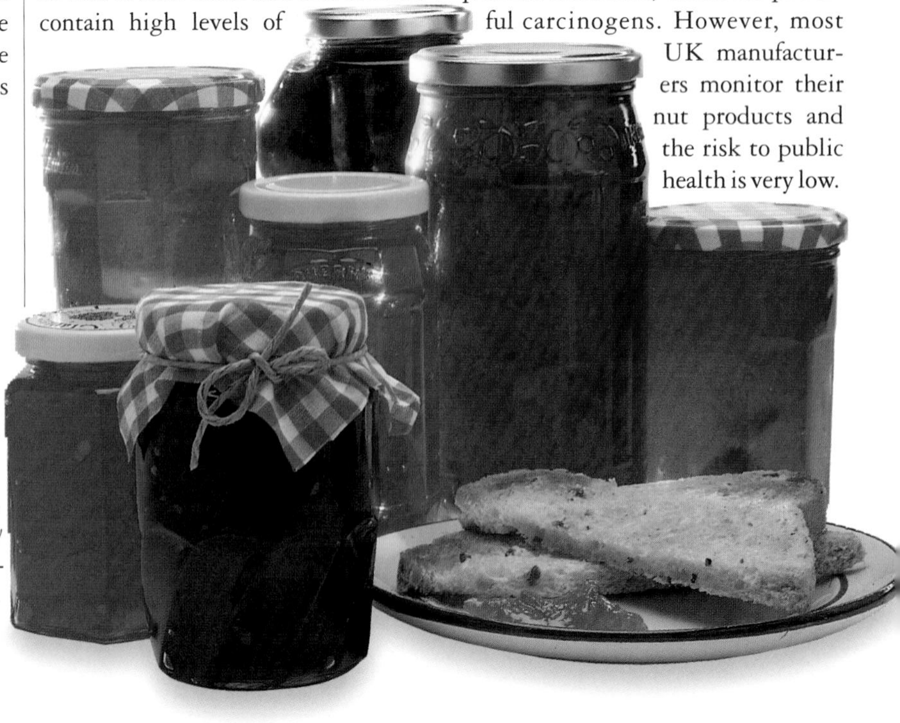

SUGAR AND FRUIT *When spread on thick slices of bread, without too much butter, jam can be part of a healthy snack. Blackcurrant (1), low-sugar strawberry (2), apricot (3), marmalade (4), blackberry (5), raspberry (6), strawberry (7).*

Jaundice

EAT PLENTY OF
- *Fish, poultry, offal and soya bean products for protein, iron and B vitamins*
- *Green cabbage and pulses for folate*
- *Oats and unsweetened muesli which are good sources of fibre*

CUT DOWN ON
- *Spicy and fatty foods*

AVOID
- *Alcohol*

The yellowing of the skin and the whites of the eyes, so characteristic of jaundice, is caused by the accumulation of the yellow bile pigment, called bilirubin, in the blood and is often the result of liver malfunction. The three main types of jaundice are: haemolytic due to breakdown of red blood cells; liver-cell, often caused by hepatitis or liver failure from CIRRHOSIS; and obstructive, due to the flow of bile from the liver being stopped by gallstones.

One rare form of haemolytic jaundice is known as favism, where an inherited defect in a particular enzyme causes red blood cells to be sensitive to a chemical found in a type of broad bean. It results in the destruction of red blood cells leading to anaemia.

Neo-natal jaundice

It is not uncommon for a baby to develop jaundice during the first few days after birth (this is especially true of babies born prematurely). This form of jaundice, known as physiological jaundice, is due to the liver being immature and unable to excrete bilirubin efficiently. The condition is usually harmless and clears up by the end of the first week.

There are other, more serious forms of jaundice affecting newborn babies, most notably a haemolytic condition where the mother's and baby's blood types are incompatible. Commonly, the mother's blood type is rhesus negative while the baby's is rhesus positive. Detecting an alien blood type, the mother produces antibodies which pass across the placenta to the foetus where they break down the red blood cells of the foetus. A blood transfusion may be needed before or after birth.

Jaundice and diet

In adults jaundice most commonly results from liver or gall-bladder disease where the capacity to remove bilirubin from the blood is impaired. Usually dead red blood cells are filtered from the blood by the spleen and liver, and broken down to form bilirubin which is excreted by the liver in the bile. In liver-cell or obstructive jaundice, the secretion of bile is hindered so bilirubin passes directly into the bloodstream, causing the tell-tale yellowy appearance of the skin.

Nutrients which can help to build red blood cells, vital in the case of haemolytic jaundice, include protein, iron and B vitamins. Fish, poultry, eggs, and dairy or soya bean products

Case study

Jean was an active and even-tempered 55-year-old when suddenly her temperament changed. She became aggressive, could not sleep at night – but dozed off during the day – and complained of an itchy skin, which gradually turned yellow. Her doctor quickly diagnosed liver disease complicated by hepatic encephalopathy – a condition which affects the brain as a result of liver failure. Jean was admitted to hospital and put on a protein-free, high-calorie diet. Tests confirmed that she had primary biliary cirrhosis. Doctors explained to her husband that the liver was damaged to the point where it could no longer break down toxic substances derived from proteins during digestion; these were accumulating in her blood, affecting her brain and leading to her bizarre behaviour. To both her husband's and Jean's relief, with treatment, she began to return to her old self. But as protein was gradually reintroduced to her diet Jean became more jaundiced and a build-up of fluid swelled her abdomen. Osteoporosis set off pains in her back and legs and, to her dismay, she also suffered several more episodes of encephalopathy. As her condition worsened, Jean was advised to have a liver transplant. Doctors pointed out that without it her chances of surviving for another year were less than 50 per cent; with it, she had at least a 70 per cent chance of survival. Five years after the transplant, she is deeply grateful to her donor and has seen some of her grandchildren go to school.

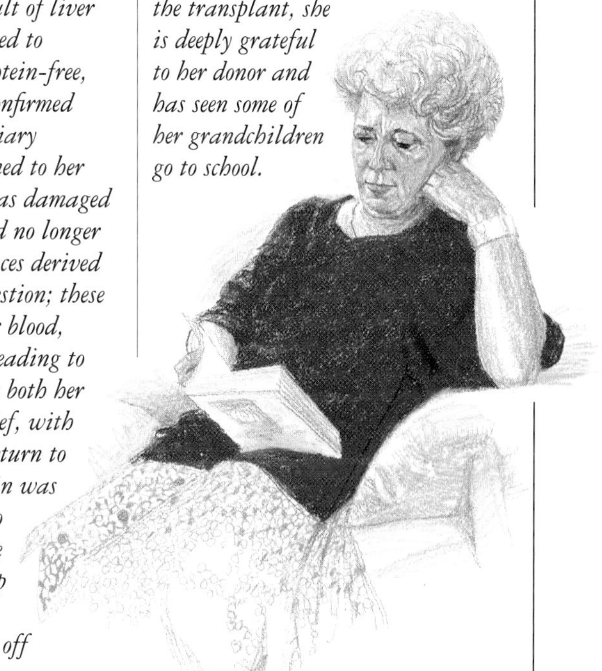

are good sources of protein, iron and B vitamins. You can also obtain iron from dried apricots, wholemeal bread and watercress. Other sources of B vitamins are wheatgerm, brown rice, yeast extract and nuts. An adequate supply of folate – found in green leafy vegetables, yeast extract and liver – is also needed for blood formation.

For all forms of jaundice, it is best to avoid all alcohol and spicy foods as well as keeping fat intake as low as possible, so as not to put undue strain on the liver. Stick to eating little and often, choosing a bland diet high in carbohydrates which will help the liver to recover. Oats and unsweetened muesli will help to avoid constipation, which often accompanies jaundice.

Around 20 per cent of middle-aged individuals have gallstones which tend to be more common among women. The chances of developing them are lessened, however, by avoiding obesity and eating a diet high in starchy foods.

JOINT PROBLEMS

EAT PLENTY OF
- *Oily fish and shellfish for essential fatty acids*
- *Fresh fruit and vegetables for beta carotene and vitamin C*
- *Avocados, nuts and sunflower seeds for vitamin E*
- *Whole grains, cereals and eggs for selenium*

AVOID
- *Obesity*

People who suffer from disorders which involve painful swelling of the joints should include plenty of oily fish, such as salmon, mackerel, herring, trout and sardines, in their diet. Several research studies claim that mild relief for joint problems has been obtained from fish oils, which contain omega-3 fatty acids. These seem to reduce the potency of the inflammatory compounds released by the body.

Those suffering from GOUT should take fish oils as a supplement rather than eat fresh fish, which may cause a gradual build-up of uric acid. When the blood contains excessive amounts of uric acid, crystals can form in the joints of susceptible people.

DANGEROUS DEFICIENCIES

There is scientific evidence that diets low in ANTIOXIDANTS – particularly the trace mineral selenium, and vitamins A, C and E – may predispose some people to joint problems.

To increase your intake of these nutrients, meals should include a weekly portion of liver (but not during pregnancy) for its vitamin A, and plenty of carrots, mangoes, apricots, sweet potatoes and cantaloupe melon; all of these are excellent sources of beta carotene, which the body turns into vitamin A. Red and yellow peppers, kiwi fruit, oranges, Brussels sprouts and cabbage are all rich sources of vitamin C, and avocados, nuts, sunflower seeds and olive oil are rich in vitamin E. Selenium is found in all fish and shellfish, as well as in meat, whole grains and cereals, eggs and brewer's yeast.

A common cause of joint problems, particularly of the hips and knees, is excessive body weight, which can also add to the pain. A study carried out in Sweden discovered that weight loss, together with the adoption of a vegetarian diet, relieved several of the symptoms of ARTHRITIS. As well as arthritis and gout, painful joints can be triggered by injury, overexertion and sometimes even infection.

PARTICULAR PROBLEMS

Bursitis is an acute inflammation of a bursa – a fluid-filled sac situated in parts of the body, such as joints, where friction would otherwise occur. The areas most often affected are the elbow and the knee (of which housemaid's knee is a well-known example).

When the protective sheath around a tendon becomes inflamed through overuse and strain, the condition is called tenosynovitis. This painful reaction usually affects the fingers and the tendons of the wrist.

Tennis elbow is probably the best-known example of inflammation at a site where tendons or ligaments join onto bones. It may be the result of playing tennis, but more frequently it is caused by repetitive manual tasks such as painting and decorating or housework. Golfer's elbow has a similarly painful effect, but occurs on the inside of the elbow joint.

Frozen shoulder, as its name suggests, is a chronic, painful stiffness of the shoulder joint. It may stem from injury or soft tissue problems, though it may arise for no apparent reason. At its worst, it is excruciatingly painful and allows only a restricted degree of movement of the affected limb.

Some painful joint disorders may need surgery or localised injections of steroids. However, all but the most serious problems can be treated quite successfully with massage, osteopathy, physiotherapy, chiropractic medicine, or acupuncture. A combination of these complementary therapies may be particularly helpful.

TENSION AND JOINTS

When muscles attached to a painful or displaced joint go into spasm, they can prevent the joint returning to its rightful position. STRESS can further exacerbate the problem, freezing up the muscles. Massage can help to release the tension; correct posture also helps. Make sure your chair is properly adjusted at work and, if you sit at a computer all day, find out how best to position the keyboard, screen and desk from your health and safety adviser.

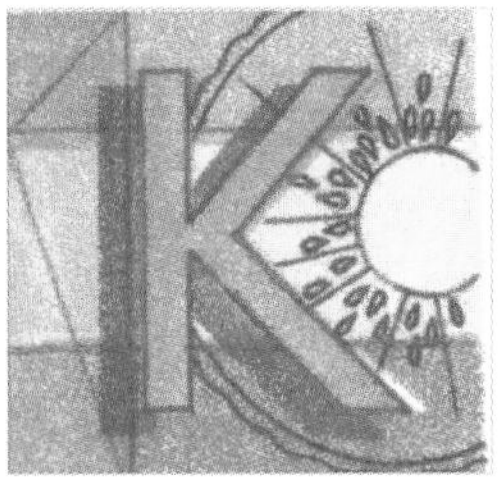

KALE

BENEFITS

- *Excellent source of beta carotene and vitamin C*
- *Good source of folate*
- *Contains iron and calcium*
- *Contains compounds that may help to protect against cancer*

This member of the cabbage family, also known as curly kale, collard and borecole, is native to Britain and the eastern Mediterranean region, where it has been cultivated for 2000 years. There are many varieties of both curly and smooth-leaved types.

Kale is an excellent source of two of the ANTIOXIDANTS – vitamin C and beta carotene. The body converts beta carotene into vitamin A, which is needed for good night vision, healthy skin and resistance to infection. A 100g (3½oz) serving of kale provides more than three-quarters of the recommended daily intake of vitamin A – and almost twice the recommended daily intake of vitamin C, which helps to maintain a healthy immune system.

Kale is a good source of the B vitamin folate, and it contains iron; both are needed for the formation of red blood cells. Because iron from plant sources is not so easily absorbed by the body as iron from meat sources, it is helpful to eat kale along with tomatoes, peppers or other foods rich in vitamin C, since the vitamin helps to boost iron absorption. Of all vegetables, kale is one of the richest sources of calcium – and it also supplies the mineral in a form that can be easily absorbed by the body.

Like Brussels sprouts and broccoli, kale contains compounds that may block the action of some carcinogens and so help to prevent cancer. Studies have indicated that high intakes of these vegetables are associated with a reduced risk of cancers of the stomach, bowel and colon. Kale also contains compounds known as indoles which stimulate liver metabolism, and so, indirectly, the breakdown and elimination of the female hormone oestrogen. High levels of oestrogen have been linked with hormone-dependent CANCERS, including breast cancer.

Studies on carotenoids (pigments which occur naturally in fruit and vegetables) has led Dr Walter Willett of the Harvard School of Public Health, a leading authority on nutrition and cancer, to cite kale as a highly potent anti-cancer food.

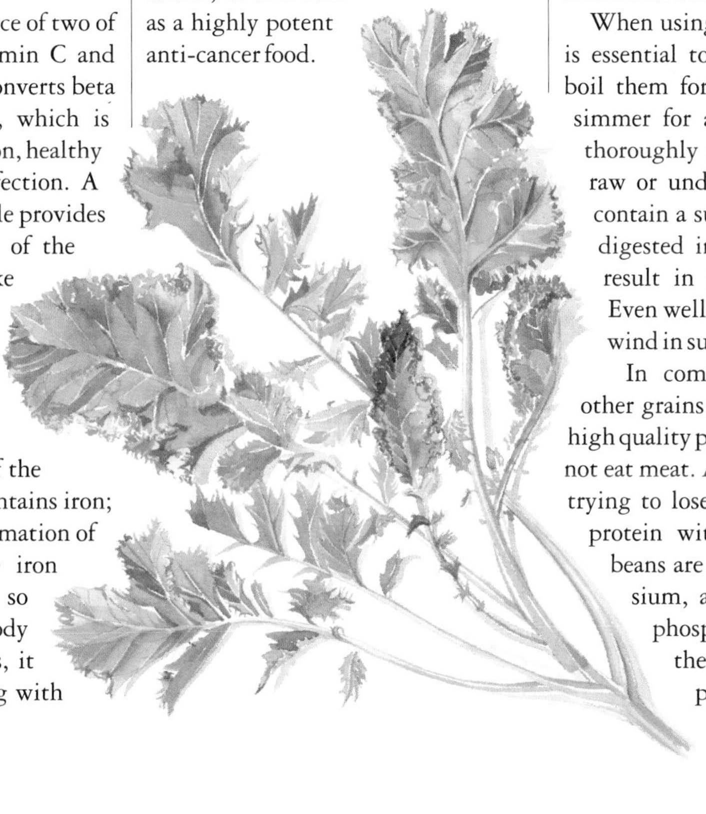

KIDNEY BEANS

BENEFITS

- *Good source of potassium*
- *Useful source of phosphorus, iron and folate*
- *Contain zinc*
- *Useful source of protein*

DRAWBACKS

- *Raw or undercooked kidney beans can result in severe food poisoning*
- *Fibre content may cause flatulence*

Most people think of the kidney bean as being the dark red variety that is used in the Mexican dish chilli con carne, but there are also black and white varieties available. Many dried beans are related to the common kidney bean, which they resemble (see also PULSES).

The red meaty beans are native to the Americas and were cultivated by the Aztecs. Named for their shape, kidney beans are commonly used in salads, soups and casseroles, and are sold either dried or canned in brine.

When using dried kidney beans, it is essential to soak them overnight, boil them for 15 minutes and then simmer for an hour or more until thoroughly cooked. This is because raw or undercooked kidney beans contain a substance that cannot be digested in the stomach and can result in severe food poisoning. Even well-cooked beans can cause wind in susceptible individuals.

In combination with rice or other grains, kidney beans supply a high quality protein for people who do not eat meat. And – for anyone who is trying to lose weight – they supply protein without fat. Red kidney beans are a good source of potassium, a useful source of iron, phosphorus and folate, and they contain zinc, which promotes wound-healing.

Kidney diseases

A number of major and minor disorders can affect the kidneys. Many require medical and dietary intervention; eating foods in the right proportions is a crucial part of the treatment.

Diet can play an important role in the prevention and treatment of minor kidney problems and, in more serious cases of renal failure, careful monitoring of food intake may help to allay the need for dialysis or kidney replacement.

Left untreated, infections such as recurrent cystitis, connective-tissue diseases and other conditions including high blood pressure, damage the kidneys and limit their ability to expel the body's waste products effectively. Kidney disease is also a major long-term complication of diabetes. Each of these disorders has specific dietary requirements.

Drinking as much water as possible is the best way to prevent one of the most prevalent renal problems – kidney stones – which, in Britain, may affect around 40000 people a year and is three times more common among men than women. To keep the kidneys healthy and free of stones, about 2-3 litres (3-5 pints) of fluid a day is recommended; anyone prone to the disorder should drink more to ensure that their intake exceeds all fluid lost in perspiration, urine and stools. Dehydration caused by heat, exercise, or as a result of vomiting or diarrhoea, may cause the substances that make up the stones to crystallise in the kidneys.

Symptoms – including acute pain which starts in the back, between the ribs and the pelvis, which gradually travels down to the groin area – persist until the stone is passed in the urine. Doctors suggest that any stones passed should be kept for analysis because the substances they contain will determine both the cause and the most suitable treatment.

The stones are usually deposits of calcium combined with oxalate or phosphate. Less common forms of the disorder are struvite stones which can be caused by urinary infections, and uric acid stones which occur in GOUT sufferers as well as leukaemia patients. The even rarer cystine stones are the result of a congenital abnormality and require a copious intake of fluids – 6.8 litres (12 pints) throughout the day and night – for life.

Cutting down on calcium (found in foods such as dairy products) will not prevent calcium oxalate stones as was once believed. Oxalate, which is made in the body and also obtained from some foods, is the prime substance involved in calcium oxalate stone formation, and more of it is absorbed when calcium is restricted.

Some experts therefore recommend cutting back on foods rich in oxalate, such as beetroot, chocolate, rhubarb, peanuts, spinach and strawberries, and possibly increasing calcium intake to discourage oxalate absorption. If a

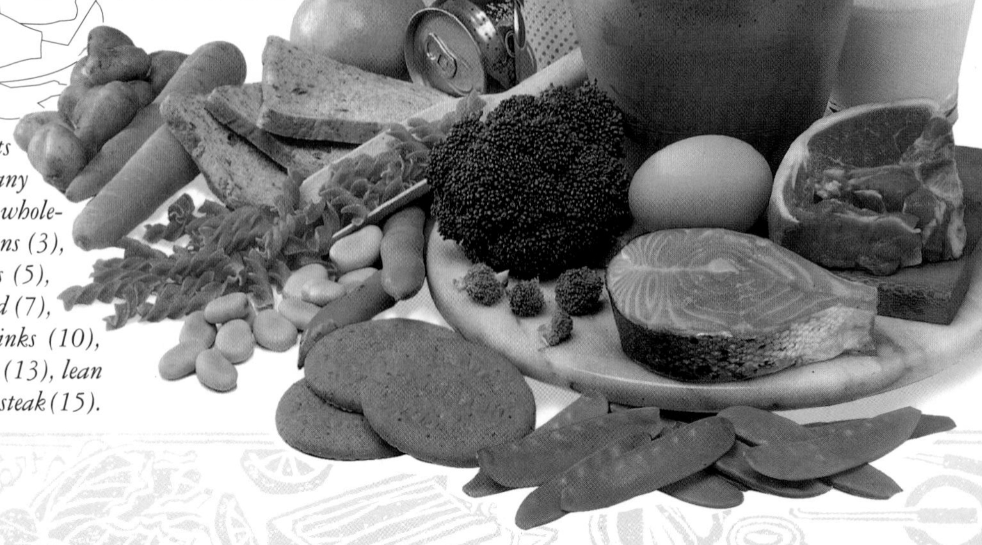

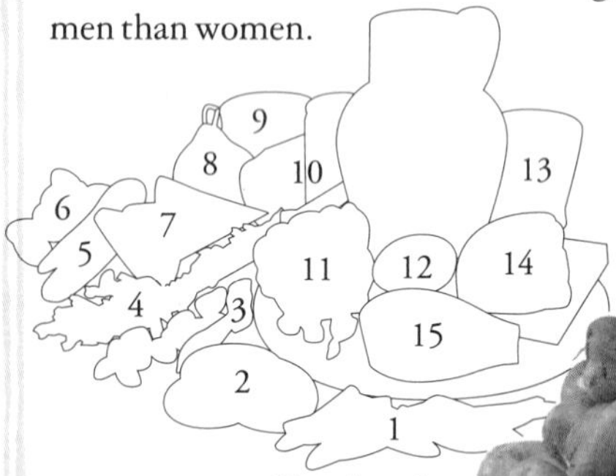

A TASTY CHOICE *Renal patients can select small portions of many foods such as: mangetout (1), wholemeal biscuits (2), broad beans (3), wholemeal pasta (4), carrots (5), potatoes (6), wholemeal bread (7), pear (8), tea (9), fizzy drinks (10), broccoli (11), egg (12), milk (13), lean lamb chop (14), small salmon steak (15).*

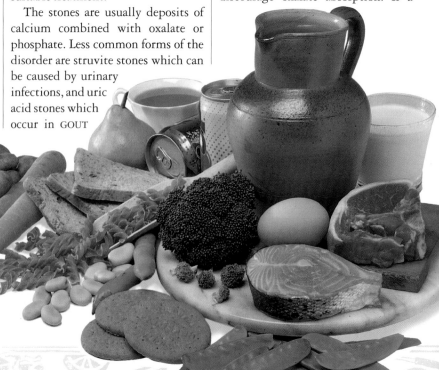

modified diet and high fluid intake does not eventually dissolve a renal stone, surgery may be required.

While stones passed in the urine are painful, those that remain in the kidney may be either symptomless or extremely dangerous. If they grow to a large size, a bacterial infection – due to an obstruction of the flow of urine – may occur, known as pyelonephritis; this is a common cause of renal failure.

A diet for renal failure

When the kidneys stop working they no longer filter out water and chemical compounds from the blood and then reabsorb or excrete them as required. As a result, toxic waste products build up in the blood, a condition known as uraemia, causing nausea, vomiting, drowsiness and, if untreated, death.

Kidney failure may be sudden: as a result of kidney disease, severe hypertension, serious infection, heart failure or haemorrhage. Appropriate treatment can prevent permanent damage. Renal failure may also result from slow damage to the tissue due to kidney disease, hypertension or diabetes.

If the progress of the disease cannot be controlled, dialysis or kidney replacement may become inevitable. But there is encouraging evidence that a carefully controlled diet can help patients to arrest deterioration and so postpone this type of treatment.

For patients who have maintained a healthy body weight, a daily intake of 35 Calories per kilo (nearly 16 Calories per pound) is recommended, half of which should be carbohydrates – mostly starches rather than simple sugars. It is vital, however, to take medical advice when deciding how to restrict and balance what you eat.

Restricting protein

Many renal patients benefit from diets that moderately restrict protein. This alleviates symptoms such as loss of appetite, nausea and vomiting, which occur because the kidneys cannot effectively excrete the chemical compounds produced when the liver metabolises proteins.

To reduce the load normally placed on the kidneys, dieticians often suggest eating small, precisely measured portions of foods such as meat, fish, eggs and milk that meet all the body's protein needs. These can be balanced and exchanged to provide varied menus in order to cater for vegetarian and ethnic tastes.

Patients may have to restrict their intake of salt and sodium, present in many processed foods, because failing kidneys cannot control the level of sodium in the blood. When sodium levels rise, thirst makes people drink to dilute the sodium to normal levels. Unhealthy kidneys are unable to excrete any excess sodium. Fluid is retained and swelling in body tissues (oedema) may result. Puffy eyes and ankles and, more dangerously, fluid in the lungs which can affect breathing, are common symptoms of oedema.

Potassium and phosphorus

In progressive renal disease, the kidneys' ability to expel excess potassium and phosphorus may also deteriorate. Potassium-rich foods may need to be restricted to prevent abnormally high potassium levels in the blood, which can lead to muscle weakness and affect the heart and other muscle tissue. Foods that supply potassium include avocado pears, bananas, pulses, seeds, dried fruit, chocolate, toffee and fudge. Instant coffee and powdered milk drinks also contain potassium. Although a high-fibre diet is generally recommended for renal patients to maintain healthy bowel function, wholegrain cereals, pulses, fruit and vegetables with a high potassium and phosphorus content should be limited. Many fresh fruits and vegetables are sources of potassium; patients on a low-potassium diet may eat some of them stewed and strained, as potassium is lost when they are cooked.

A carefully maintained balance of both phosphorus and calcium is essential for healthy bones. When the balance of these minerals becomes disturbed, a high concentration of phosphorus in the blood may occur which then lowers the calcium level, and can slowly lead to bone disease.

Restricting phosphorus can help to maintain a normal phosphate level and avoid calcium depletion. Drugs which encourage the body to excrete phosphorus may also be prescribed.

Many high quality protein foods such as meat, cheese, eggs and milk contain phosphorus, which further complicates the dietary equations.

The overall fluid intake is usually monitored and tailored to the individual patient's condition, since drinking too much may encourage oedema.

HELPFUL HERBS

The dandelion is well known as a traditional diuretic – hence its French name *pissenlit*, or its old English name 'piss-a-bed'. It is used, together with other herbs, to treat fluid retention resulting from kidney disorders. Diuretic plants such as the Cape gooseberry may help to dissolve renal stones. Rose tea is also said to be useful.

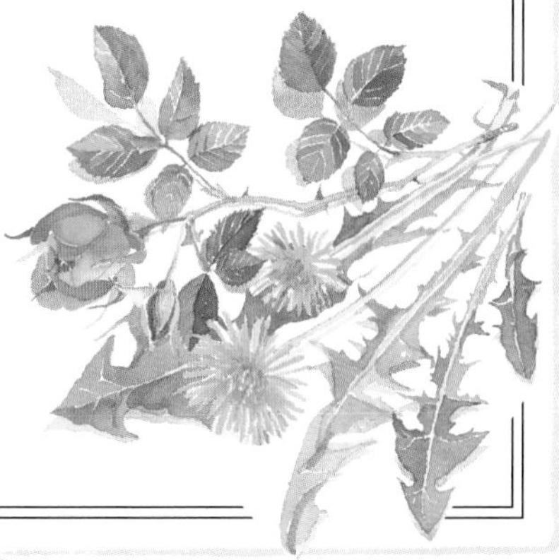

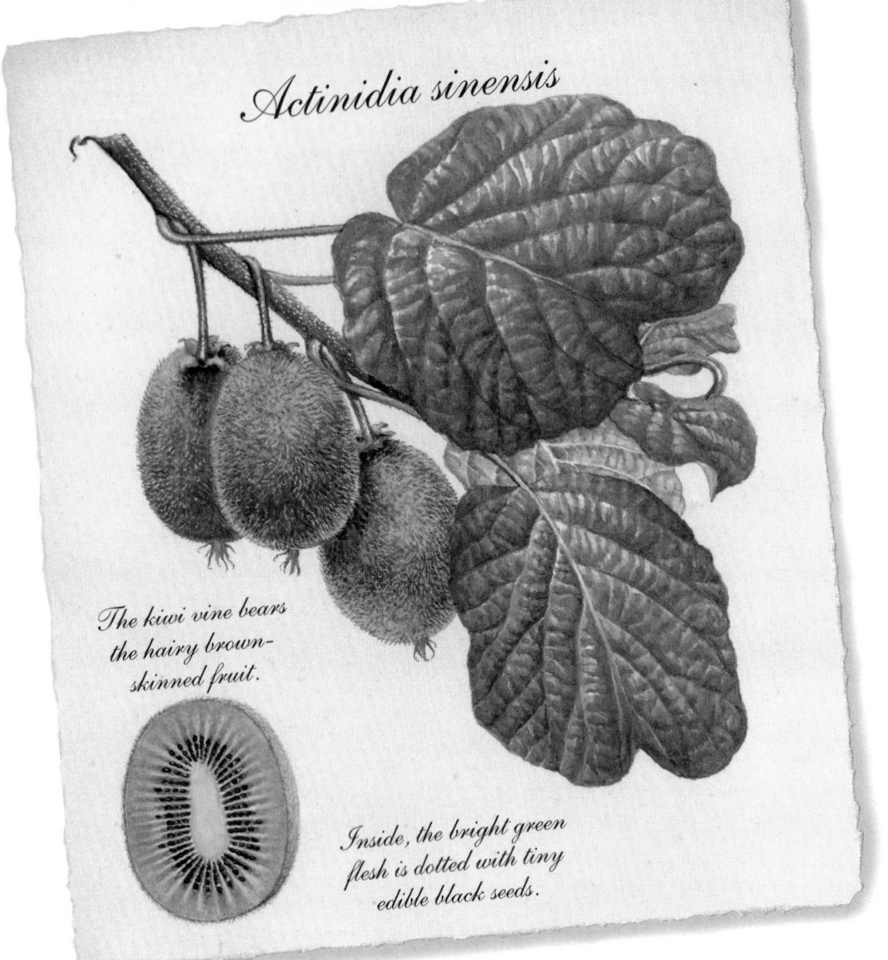
Actinidia sinensis
The kiwi vine bears the hairy brown-skinned fruit.
Inside, the bright green flesh is dotted with tiny edible black seeds.
DECORATIVE HEALTH *A kiwi fruit makes a useful garnish as its flesh does not discolour, and supplies as much vitamin C as an orange.*

KIWI FRUIT

BENEFITS
- *Excellent source of vitamin C*
- *Good source of potassium*
- *Supplies soluble fibre which can help to lower blood cholesterol levels*

This fuzzy-skinned, egg-shaped fruit originally came from China and it used to be known as the Chinese gooseberry. However, it was not popularised until earlier this century by growers in New Zealand and was eventually renamed after that country's national emblem, the flightless kiwi bird.

The fruit's bright green flesh is an excellent source of vitamin C. A single kiwi fruit supplies more than the normal daily adult requirement for the vitamin, which is essential for wound healing and a healthy immune system. Kiwi fruit are a good source of the mineral potassium which helps to counteract the high sodium content in a typical Western diet, and has been linked to healthy blood pressure.

The fruit also supplies useful amounts of soluble fibre which helps to lower blood cholesterol levels; when fats are digested, soluble fibre can bind to cholesterol causing it to be excreted as waste instead of being reabsorbed by the body.

The sugar content of kiwi fruit is around 10 per cent, with an average-size fruit supplying about 29 Calories. Its taste varies from sweet to tart. It is often used to garnish dishes and also adds an exotic touch to fruit salads.

KOHLRABI

BENEFITS
- *Good source of vitamin C*
- *May help to prevent cancer*
- *Good source of potassium*
- *Useful source of fibre*

Kohlrabi, along with cabbage, cauliflower, broccoli and Brussels sprouts, is a member of the cruciferous family of vegetables, which many experts believe may help to prevent certain forms of cancer.

The vegetable is a good source of both vitamin C, which is important for a healthy immune system, and potassium which, as part of a properly balanced diet, can help to keep blood pressure at normal levels.

Kohlrabi supplies useful amounts of dietary fibre in both soluble and insoluble form. Soluble fibre can help to lower blood cholesterol levels; insoluble fibre prevents constipation. Both types of fibre may also protect against certain forms of cancer by helping the body to expel carcinogens.

Plant chemicals in vegetables such as kohlrabi are now widely thought to provide extra protection. Indoles, for example, are thought to reduce the potency of the female sex hormone oestrogen and thereby lessen the risk of breast cancer. Other components such as isothiocyanates may combat cancers of the colon and rectum.

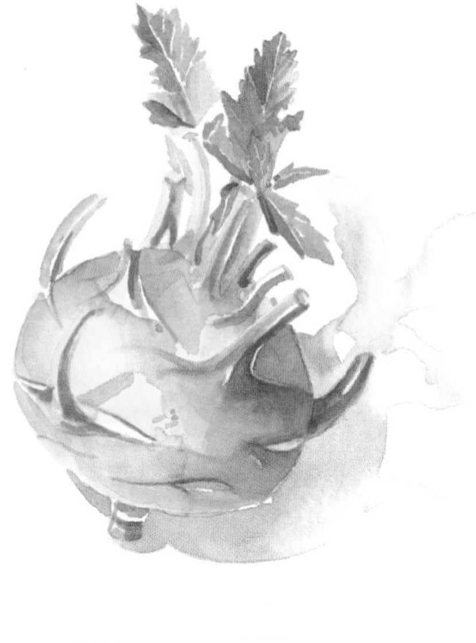

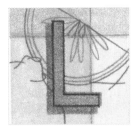

LABELS AND HOW TO READ THEM

The words and pictures used on food labels are governed by strict rules. For example, a carton of yoghurt made with artificial flavouring (but no real fruit) cannot bear a picture of fruit. The label must state if a product has been processed in any way, for example by pickling or smoking. It also gives the name of the product, its weight or volume, 'use by' or 'best before' date and a list of ingredients.

WEIGHT AND VOLUME

The weight is usually in grams (g) for solids, and either litres or millilitres (ml) for liquids. These figures can be useful for comparing value for money between the different products.

DATEMARKS

The term 'use by' is for foods with a short shelf-life. These should not be sold or eaten after the date on the label because of the risk of deterioration and FOOD POISONING. If food is labelled 'best before', it has a long shelf-life. While it may deteriorate in quality, most can safely be eaten for up to two months after the datemark.

INGREDIENTS

Packaged foods must list all ingredients in order of decreasing weight. Food additives are described by their function (preservative, stabiliser or colour), followed by their name or code. Some foods do not have to list ingredients – such as those that contain only one.

NUTRITIONAL INFORMATION

Where appropriate, packaging supplies nutritional information such as calories per serving or 100g. The vitamin and mineral content may be declared only if 100g (3½oz) or 100ml (3½floz) of the product contains at least 15 per cent of the Recommended Daily Amount (RDA), or if the food is purchased as single portions, such as individual chocolate bars or yoghurts.

Figures currently used in Britain for food labelling derive from a 1990 EC directive. There are two main criteria for nutritional information, RDAs and DRVs (Dietary Reference Values). RDAs are usually based on the amounts of nutrients needed by an adult male. DRVs are more accurate because they allow for age and sex.

Foods cannot make **statements** such as 'reduced calorie' unless they are much lower in calories than the usual version.

A **claim** such as 'made with fresh egg yolk' must be backed up by stating exact amounts in the ingredients list.

Ingredients are listed in order of weight. They help you to make comparisons between similar products, to establish value for money, and to avoid ingredients that you do not wish to eat.

Additives, either as a name or code (E) number, are listed after a word which describes their function, for example: 'stabiliser – carob gum', or 'colour – E102' (tartrazine). Flavourings must be mentioned on labels, but not necessarily by name.

UK manufacturers now provide more **nutritional information** concerning calorie content and levels of salt, sugar and fibre, for example. This is not yet required by European law, but is already a legal requirement in the USA.

Safe storage instructions such as 'refrigerate after opening' and 'consume within three days' should be observed to prevent food deterioration or bacterial growth causing food poisoning.

A **datemark**, stating 'best before' or 'use by' must appear on the package, whether printed on a label or lid, or indented into the base of a can.

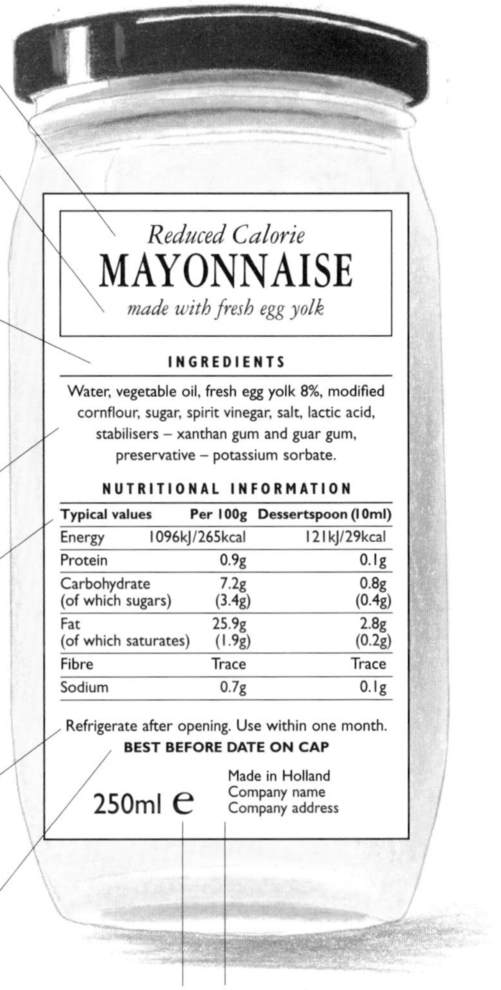

The large **'e'** indicates an average quantity in each bottle or pack, but the exact amount may be subject to slight variation.

The manufacturer's or supermarket's **address** is supplied, so that people can contact them if they wish to complain.

Lamb

BENEFITS

- *High in protein*
- *Rich source of most B vitamins*
- *Good source of zinc and iron*

DRAWBACK

- *Fatty cuts are high in saturated fat and calories*

Although it is often assumed to be the fattiest of all meat, lamb has a comparable fat content to beef and pork. Its saturated fat content can vary enormously, however, depending on age, breed and the cut of meat.

Like all red meats, fatty cuts of lamb should be eaten in moderation. High dietary intakes of saturated fat raise CHOLESTEROL levels in the blood, which in turn increase the risk of atherosclerosis and heart disease.

Because of the increasing awareness of the dangers of fats, particularly saturated fats, modern breeding techniques have produced lambs which are much leaner. Best-quality early lamb has fine grained, pinky brown flesh, with white fat. In the summer the meat is liable to be darker.

The importance of cut

Fat content varies with the cut and the cooking method. The leanest part is the leg; the fattiest is the shoulder and rack. A 100g (3½oz) serving of roast leg of lamb with the fat cut off contains 191 Calories and 8g of fat, while a 100g (3½oz) serving of grilled chops contains 277 Calories and 22g of fat.

Lamb is high in protein and rich in most of the B vitamins needed for a healthy nervous system. It is also a good source of zinc and iron.

Radioactive lamb

Since the Chernobyl disaster of 1986, when radioactive material was distributed over parts of the country, there has obviously been concern about the effects on the food chain, and the levels of radioactivity in sheep. However, fears that human health is still at risk from radioactivity in Britain are almost certainly exaggerated, and the likelihood of contaminated meat now reaching consumers is said to be minimal. The regular monitoring of sheep from affected regions has shown that the radioactivity is decaying over time, and more and more flocks have been found to be within safe limits. Any sheep that do not fall within these limits are clearly marked with paint, and it is illegal to slaughter such an animal for human consumption.

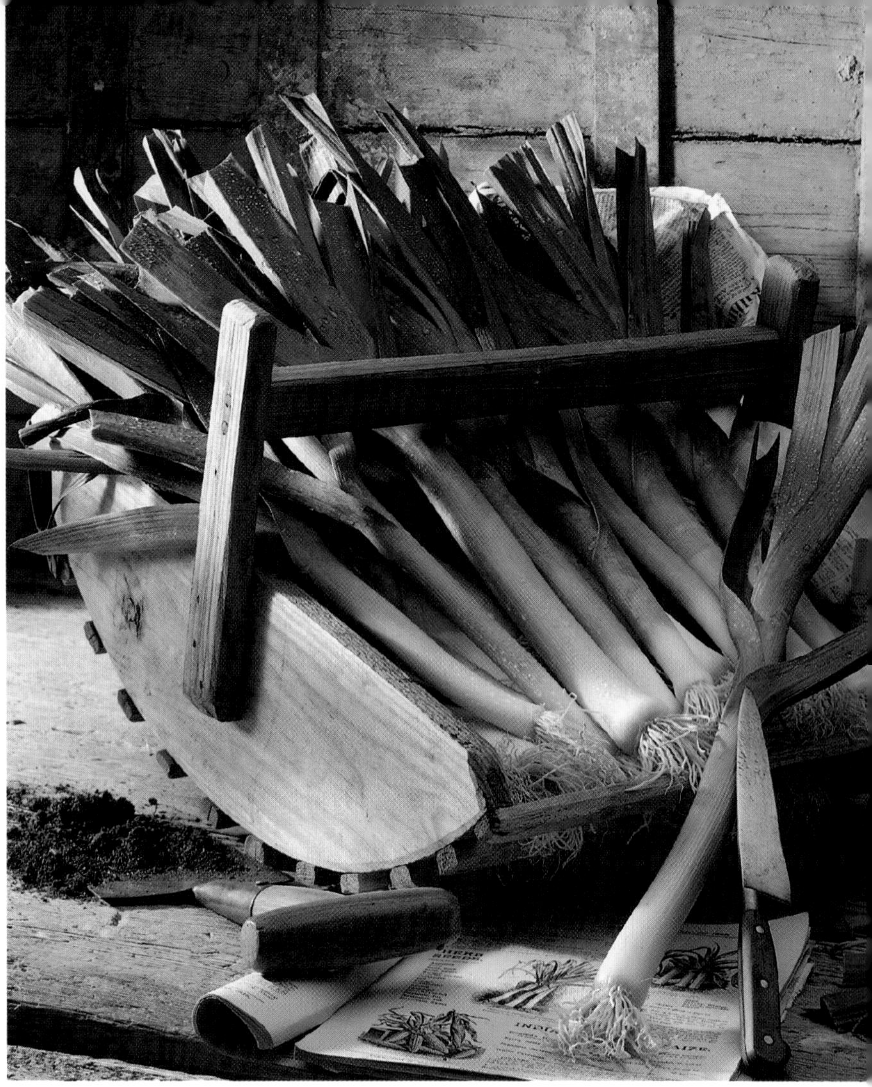

GARDEN FRESH *Leeks must be cleaned thoroughly before they are cooked as their layered structure means that they can retain a great deal of sandy grit or garden soil.*

Leeks

BENEFITS

- *Useful source of potassium and folate*

DRAWBACK

- *May cause flatulence*

In traditional medicine, leeks have been used to treat a variety of ailments, ranging from sore throats to gout and kidney stones. Because they contain potassium – one leek contains the equivalent of an eighth of an adult's daily needs of the mineral – leeks encourage the efficient functioning of the kidneys and are effective as a diuretic. They are also a useful source of folate, and one portion of cooked leeks contains almost a third of an adult's recommended daily intake.

As members of the same family, leeks share several of the properties of garlic and onions – including the risk of causing contact dermatitis in susceptible people. And the warning in Nicholas Culpeper's *Complete Herbal* (1653) that leeks are 'flatulent or windy' is well founded.

The Ancient Greeks, Romans and Egyptians valued leeks for their therapeutic properties: the Romans used them to cure sore throats, and Nero ate large quantities to improve his voice.

LEMONS

BENEFITS

- *Excellent source of vitamin C, which helps to maintain the immune system*
- *May help to relieve rheumatism*

DRAWBACKS

- *Lemon skins may be sprayed with fungicide and covered in wax*
- *High acidity can destroy tooth enamel*

When it comes to citrus fruits, most people enjoy eating oranges, tangerines and grapefruit; but lemons have such a sharp taste, that they are usually reserved for flavouring sauces and drinks. A squeeze over grilled fish or pancakes, a tablespoon or two in a salad dressing, or a slice in a gin-and-tonic is as much as most of us use.

But it is worth squeezing a lemon to make a fresh lemon-juice drink, as this is an excellent source of vitamin C and contains very few calories. Traditionally, a drink of lemon juice, hot water and a teaspoon of honey has been used as a remedy for colds. A low intake of vitamin C makes people more susceptible to infection, and honey helps to soothe a sore throat. Lemon

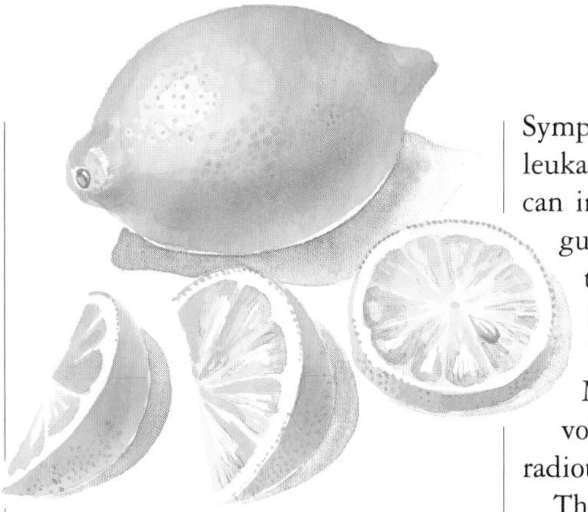

juice contains an oil which may help to relieve rheumatism by stimulating the liver to expel toxins from the body.

POTENTIAL PROBLEMS

Citrus fruits have been linked with MIGRAINE, and some people are allergic to them. As the juice from lemons is highly acidic, it can destroy tooth enamel. Lemons are normally treated with fungicide spray and wax, so before grating a lemon's skin, wash it thoroughly under a warm tap.

LETTUCE

See page 216

LEUKAEMIA

EAT PLENTY OF

- *Fresh fruit and vegetables, for vitamin C*
- *Whole grains, wheatgerm, molasses, nuts, pulses, fish and green leafy vegetables, for the B vitamins*

AVOID

- *Foods which may be contaminated with bacteria or viruses, such as shellfish, unpasteurised milk products and undercooked meats*
- *Smoking*
- *Alcohol*

In both its acute and chronic forms leukaemia is characterised by the overproduction of white blood cells. Symptoms of both acute and chronic leukaemia, a potentially fatal cancer, can include bleeding from the nose, gums, stomach and rectum, pain in the upper abdomen, anaemia, fever and an increased susceptibility to bruising and infection. Medical treatment usually involves either chemotherapy or radiotherapy or both.

Though no specific foods will cure leukaemia, the quality of a patient's life can be improved – and some of the illness's side effects held at bay – by adopting a healthy and varied diet. People with leukaemia should eat plenty of fresh fruit, vegetables and whole grains, plus a moderate amount of unsaturated fats and protein such as fish, lean meat and pulses.

Strawberries, blackcurrants, citrus fruits, guavas, broccoli, cauliflower and Brussels sprouts are all excellent sources of vitamin C, which decreases susceptibility to associated infections. To ensure a good supply of the B vitamins – which act together to make energy available from foods – sufferers should include wheatgerm, whole grains, brown rice, pulses and brewer's yeast in their diet.

Because leukaemia patients have a reduced resistance to infection, they must take particular care to avoid eating any foods which may be contaminated by bacteria or viruses such as listeria. Shellfish, game, raw eggs, unpasteurised milk products, soft-rinded cheeses, such as Brie and Camembert, and undercooked meats, particularly poultry, are all potentially hazardous and should be avoided.

Smoking should also be avoided as it can rob the body of nutrients. And because some drugs used to treat leukaemia can interfere with the metabolism of alcohol, it is best to abstain from drinking it altogether. Alcohol also depletes the body's reserves of vitamin C.

LETTUCE AND SALAD LEAVES

Although salad leaves are very low in calories, and more than 90 per cent water, they still provide nutrients including vitamin C, beta carotene, folate, calcium and iron.

The nutritional content of lettuce and salad leaves varies not only from species to species, but also according to the time of year, the plant's freshness, and even whether you are considering the inner or outer leaves. Because all salad leaves are low in calories, they can be helpful as part of a weight-reducing diet, provided that they are not coated in fatty SALAD DRESSINGS such as mayonnaise.

Most salad greens are a useful source of folate – an important vitamin for pregnant women, and those planning to become pregnant, as it helps to prevent birth defects such as spina bifida. Depending on how deeply pigmented the leaves are, salad leaves are also a useful source of the antioxidant nutrient beta carotene, which may help to prevent degenerative diseases such as cancer and atherosclerosis. Dark green outer leaves may contain anything up to 50 times as much beta carotene as the inner pale ones.

In herbalism, lettuce leaves are said to have a sedative effect, and a large bowl of fresh leaves is recommended to calm nervousness and induce sleep.

Lettuce is one of a number of plants, including CELERY, that accumulates nitrates. Within the European Union new safety levels for nitrates are being introduced because there is concern about the potentially harmful effects of high intakes of these chemicals.

Two very nutritious salad greens are SPINACH and watercress. Raw spinach is an excellent source of beta carotene; a rich source of folate and a good source of vitamin C. WATERCRESS is an excellent source of vitamin C and beta carotene; it also contains iron.

BENEFITS
- *Low in calories*
- *Useful source of folate*
- *Useful source of beta carotene*

DRAWBACKS
- *Often eaten with oily or creamy dressings which are fattening*

FAMILIAR LETTUCES AND SALAD GREENS

Butterhead Limp, bland-flavoured light green lettuce. For many years, it was the only lettuce to be widely available in the shops.

Chicory or Belgian endive Pale elongated tightly packed tapering leaves with a crisp texture and bitter flavour.

Chinese leaf or Peking cabbage Cylindrical shaped head with pale green leaf on broad crisp white ribs.

Cos or romaine Elongated leaves which are firm and flavourful: the main ingredient in Caesar salad.

Curly endive (also known as *chicorée frisée*) Curly frond-like ragged leaves. The outer leaves are bitter and the inner leaves have a milder flavour. Very popular in France.

Curly lettuce Tastes very similar to butterhead but has firmer leaves, with a slightly sharper taste.

Iceberg (also known as crisphead lettuce) Round, tightly packed pale green lettuce with a crunchy texture but bland flavour. A particularly useful source of folate.

Lamb's lettuce (also known as corn salad or *mâche*) Small velvety leaves with a delicate, nutty flavour. Often served on its own or with beetroot.

Lollo rosso Green leaves that have a distinctive reddish tinge around their frilly edges. They have a mild flavour and are popular as a garnish.

Oak-leaf lettuce (also known as *feuille de chêne*) Limp leaves with a reddish tinge and bitter flavour.

Radicchio Italian chicory that looks rather like a small cabbage with firm reddish-purple leaves. It has a crisp texture and a very bitter flavour.

Rocket or arugula Dark green dandelion-like leaf with a peppery flavour.

Spinach Salad greens that need washing thoroughly to remove any grit.

Watercress A member of the cruciferous family of vegetables, believed to be protective against some cancers.

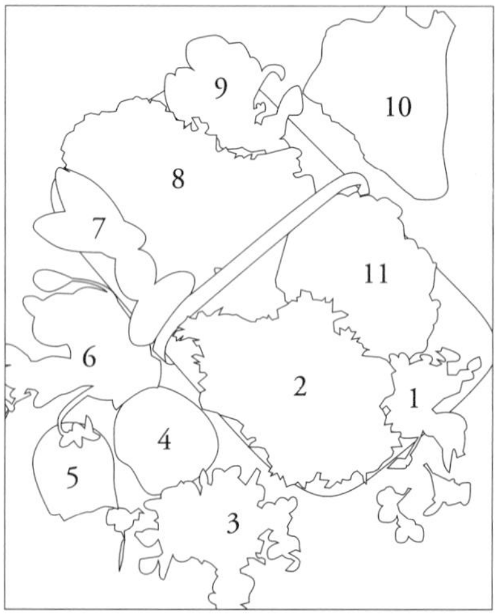

MIXED SALAD *A range of leaves makes an interesting, tasty green salad: watercress (1), curly endive (2), lamb's lettuce (3), iceberg (4), radicchio (5), rocket (6), chicory (7), curly lettuce (8), spinach (9), cos (10), lollo rosso (11).*

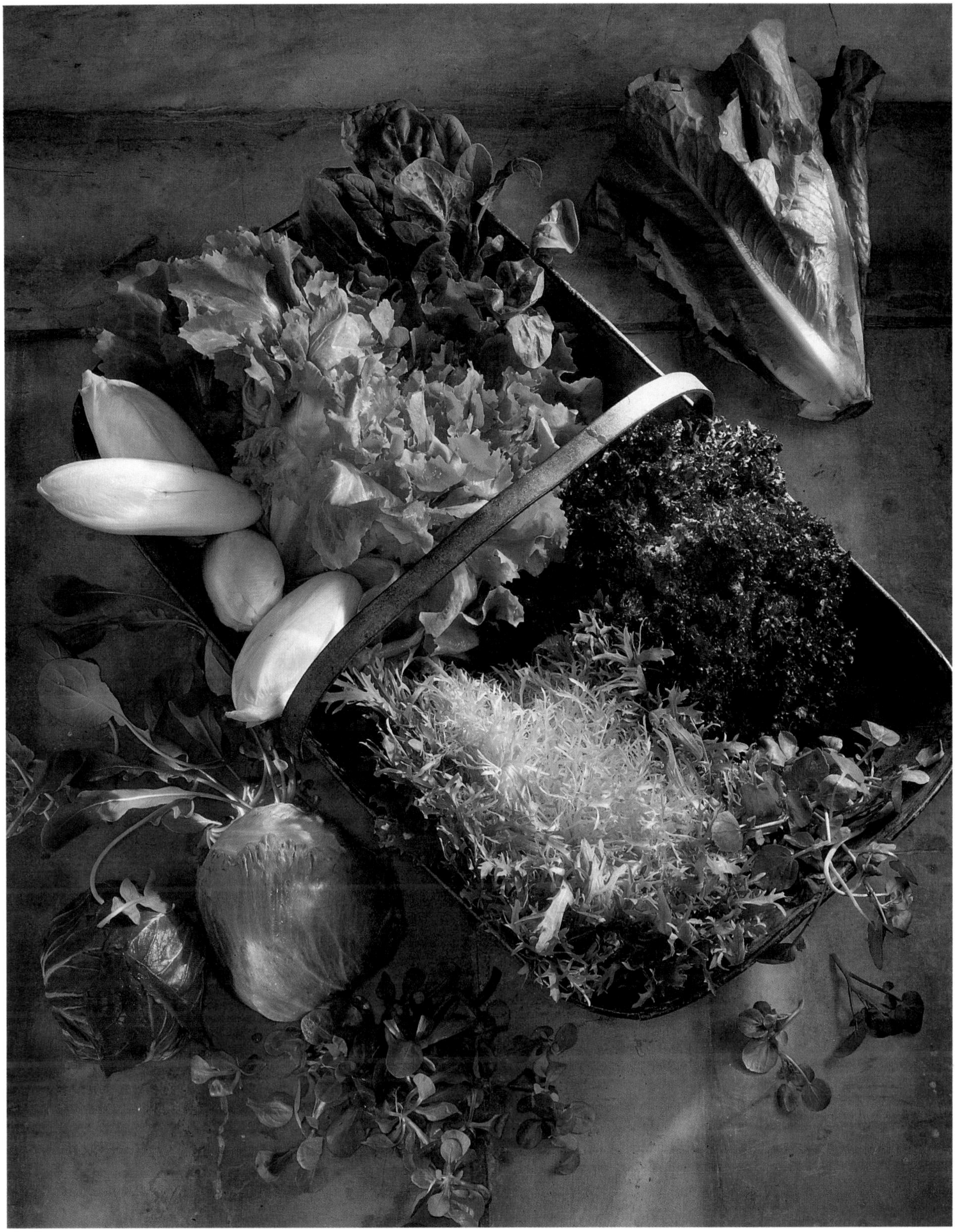

LIMES

BENEFITS
- *Excellent source of vitamin C*
- *A healthy alternative to salt and other seasonings*

In the mid 18th century the Scottish naval surgeon James Lind showed that scurvy, the former scourge of sailors, could be prevented by drinking the juice of limes, lemons or oranges. This is because the disease is caused by a deficiency of vitamin C, of which citrus fruits are an excellent source. Lemons and limes became essential rations for British sailors – hence the nickname 'limey', often used by Americans as slang for a Briton.

Like the other citrus fruits, limes contain significant amounts of bioflavonoids which act like antioxidants helping to protect the body against FREE RADICAL damage.

The juice of fresh limes, like that of LEMONS, is an excellent source of vitamin C and a small glass contains only 9 Calories. The juice is often used to bring out the flavour of other fruits, such as avocados and melons, while it also makes an excellent, tenderising marinade for meat. Dishes where lime juice has been used as a flavouring need little salt – which can be helpful if you are trying to follow a low-sodium diet.

Lime juice is a traditional ingredient in many Asian dishes and is used in pickles and salad dressings as well as in fish and meat dishes.

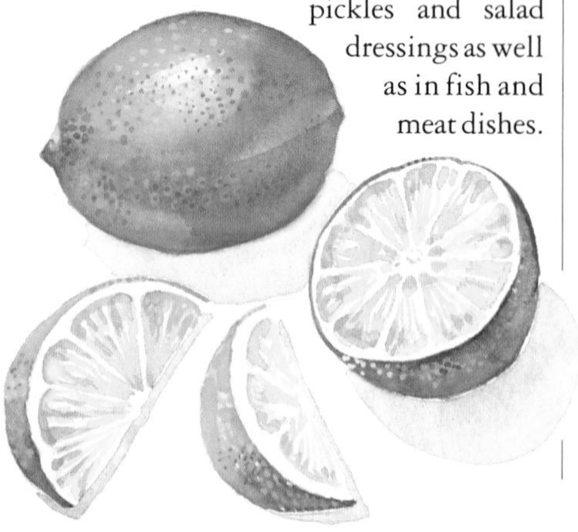

LIQUORICE

BENEFITS
- *May help to soothe ulcers*
- *An expectorant for respiratory problems*

DRAWBACKS
- *Can cause the retention of sodium and the depletion of potassium, which may result in high blood pressure*

In traditional medicine, liquorice has long been valued as a soothing agent for various internal pains. Chinese physicians have used it for thousands of years to treat everything from ulcers to constipation and vomiting.

The root and underground stem are dark, reddish-brown with a yellow, fibrous interior. Liquorice roots are crushed, boiled and then evaporated to make the many liquids, powders and lozenges that are used in medicines. The roots are also sold cut into sticks that can be chewed raw, and these are good for the teeth and gums. The sweetness in liquorice is due to the presence of glycyrrhizin – a compound that is 50 times sweeter than sugar. Nevertheless, research has shown that liquorice counters bacterial growth and plaque, helping to prevent tooth decay. The roots are usually available from good health-food stores as well as from herbalists.

Research has confirmed many of the medicinal properties claimed for liquorice; several active constituents have the power to soothe ulcers by protecting the stomach lining, and liquorice has been incorporated into some ulcer drugs. Certain types of liquorice confectionery, available from health-food stores, are recommended by herbalists to help to alleviate the symptoms of stomach ulcers.

Liquorice makes a good expectorant – increasing the production of sputum so that it can be coughed up more easily, and herbalists have long used liquorice in the treatment of bronchitis, catarrh and coughs.

People with high blood pressure should avoid eating liquorice as it can exacerbate the condition by causing the retention of sodium and the depletion of potassium in the body.

LIVER DISORDERS

TAKE PLENTY OF
- *Foods rich in vitamin C, such as citrus fruits and strawberries*
- *Vitamin B_{12}, found in liver and fish*
- *Folate, found in liver, green vegetables and fruit*

CUT DOWN ON
- *Saturated fats from fatty meats and full-fat dairy products*
- *Sugars*
- *Coffee and tea*

AVOID
- *Alcohol*
- *Heavily spiced foods*

A diet that is low in fats, alcohol and sugars is the key to maintaining a healthy liver. Protected by ribs, the liver is located in the upper right part of the abdomen. It is the largest organ in the body and performs more than 500 jobs, including at least 22 vital functions. The liver is the body's main detoxifier; it removes and neutralises poisons, drugs, nicotine and alcohol in the bloodstream.

Other functions include: storing glucose in the form of glycogen and maintaining blood sugar levels; manufacturing important proteins and breaking down excess amino acids (the by-products of protein digestion) into urea which is eliminated by the kidneys. It also manufactures bile which is stored in the gall bladder and passes into the duodenum – where it breaks down fats into tiny globules to make them more digestible. All of these functions are impaired by severe liver disease, most commonly caused by infections such as viral hepatitis or by drugs such as alcohol. Chronic inflammation of the liver leads to scar tissue being formed – the condition known as CIRRHOSIS. Another common liver problem is the failure of the liver to secrete bile because of stones forming in the gall bladder.

Although the liver has a remarkable ability to regenerate itself, the effects of persistent and long-term alcohol abuse may cause liver failure. Signs of chronic liver disease can include JAUNDICE, fever, loss of body hair, distension of the abdomen, and yellow fatty deposits in the upper eyelids.

To reduce the liver's workload, it is best to follow a diet that is low in fats, alcohol and sugars, and to cut down on tea and coffee. It also helps to avoid heavily spiced foods because they place an increased demand on the liver.

In the course of liver disease the vitamins B_{12} and folate are depleted. Animal liver is an excellent source of both vitamins (but not if you are pregnant). Fish and dairy products also provide B_{12}, and green vegetables and fresh fruit provide folate. High intakes of vitamin C, a powerful ANTIOXIDANT (found in fruit, especially citrus fruit), may also aid the recovery process by supporting the detoxification systems of the liver which are weakened when it is affected by disease.

Drinking beetroot, carrot or lemon juice may help to increase the flow of bile secreted by the liver, which in turn helps with the excretion of waste products from the body.

Anyone suffering from liver disease should avoid ALCOHOL. For protection against liver disorders, adults should follow the advice on safe limits: no more than 14 units per week for women and 21 for men.

Lupus Erythematosus

EAT PLENTY OF
- *Oily fish for omega-3 fatty acids*
- *Eggs, butter, milk and margarine for vitamin D*
- *Low-fat dairy products for calcium*

CUT DOWN ON
- *Salt*

AVOID
- *Alcohol, depending on your medication*
- *Obesity*

This incurable illness of the IMMUNE SYSTEM leads to the body's defence mechanisms attacking connective tissues, joints, muscles and any organs of the body, giving rise to inflammation, pain and organ damage. The illness often begins with headaches, extreme tiredness, aches and pains in the muscles and joints, and a skin rash: *Lupus erythematosus* means 'red wolf', describing the characteristic rash which can occur on both cheeks and over the bridge of the nose. Lupus can start suddenly, making the patient feel very ill, or it can gradually develop over months or even years. Some sufferers are sensitive to sunlight. Most victims of lupus are women.

No one really knows what causes lupus, but sufferers can help to manage their condition with drugs, and by following the advice of a dietician. The type of diet prescribed will depend upon the stage of the disease. For example, while some sufferers are advised to increase their intake of the mineral potassium, those with renal problems may have to restrict it.

Certain nutrients are vital to the proper functioning of the immune system: beta carotene (found in orange fruit and vegetables), vitamin C (in kiwi fruit) and zinc (found in oysters and other seafood). Studies show that eating plenty of oily fish such as herring and salmon can help to counter inflammation caused by lupus.

OBESITY is a factor that can exacerbate the condition, and keeping weight in check is central to controlling symptoms. This is particularly important for those patients who are prescribed steroids.

People with lupus are advised to avoid sunlight, so they need to obtain vitamin D from their diet: from eggs, butter, milk, fish oils, margarine and certain fortified breakfast cereals.

As many lupus patients develop kidney problems and high blood pressure, they should avoid foods that are high in salt. Drink at least 1.7 litres (3 pints) of water a day to keep the kidneys working properly, and to help to avoid infections of the urinary tract.

Helpful foods

Carrots and other orange coloured vegetables contain beta carotene. Eat three times a week or more.

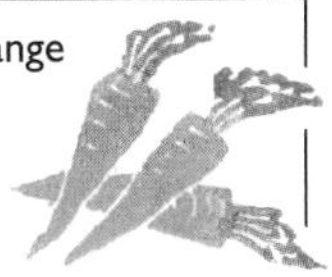

Oranges and other citrus fruits provide vitamin C and potassium. Try to eat them once or twice a day.

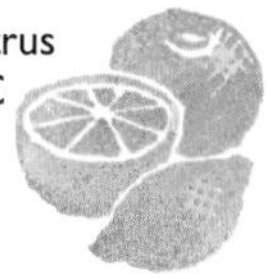

Fortified cereals provide vitamins B and D and calcium when served with milk. Eat daily for breakfast.

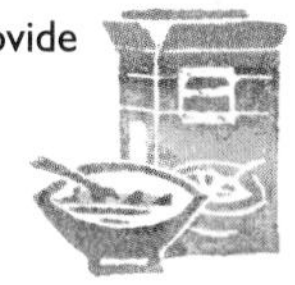

Poultry provides B vitamins and some zinc. Eat grilled or stir-fried without the skin three times a week.

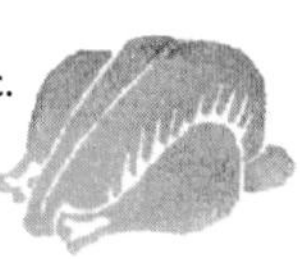

Sardines, or other oily fish, supply omega-3 fatty acids. Eat grilled or tinned three times a week.

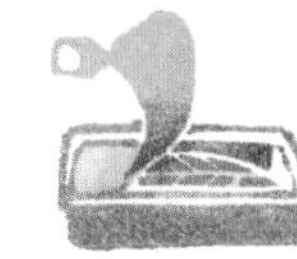

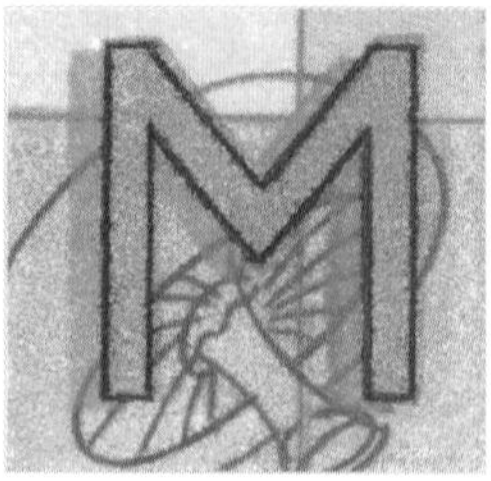

MACROBIOTIC DIET

BENEFITS

- *Low in calories and saturated fats*
- *High in fibre*
- *May help to reduce the risk of obesity, raised cholesterol, high blood pressure, constipation and some forms of cancer*

DRAWBACKS

- *Can cause anaemia*
- *Not suitable for young children or pregnant or breastfeeding women*
- *In its most extreme form, it does not supply adequate protein, vitamin B_{12}, vitamin D and iron*

In the 1880s a Japanese doctor, Sagen Ishizuka, claimed that he could treat many common health problems with a diet based on wholegrain cereals and vegetables, and published his ideas in two books. Early in the 20th century, the American-Japanese writer George Ohsawa tried the diet for himself and believed that it was responsible for curing his tuberculosis. He went on to develop a dietary system based on Ishizuka's ideas and called it macrobiotics – from the Greek words for 'large' and 'life'. He believed that the diet could increase energy and offer greater resistance to illness, enabling its followers to live life to the full.

Macrobiotics is largely based on the Chinese philosophy of two opposing yet complementary forces of nature – 'yin' and 'yang'. Yin is the female force, representing darkness, the cold and tranquillity, while yang is masculine and represents light, heat and aggression. People who are predominantly yin tend to be calm, relaxed and creative; predominantly yang people tend to be active, alert and energetic. The health and harmony of both body and mind are said to depend on a balance between the two forces, and the macrobiotic diet therefore needs to be tailored to the needs of the individual by a macrobiotic nutritionist.

According to macrobiotic philosophy, foods also contain the yin and yang qualities. Certain foods are predominantly yin or yang and should be balanced. For example, foods with a high yin content include sugar, tea, alcohol, coffee, milk, cream, yoghurt and most herbs and spices, while foods

The macrobiotic larder

There are seven levels of macrobiotic diet. The less extreme levels are mainly vegetarian (although some may contain fish), consisting of large amounts of unrefined cereals and small amounts of seasonal and locally produced fruit and vegetables. The most extreme, now rarely followed, consists of brown rice only which has led to several deaths as it contains too few nutrients. A suitable macrobiotic diet can include the following foods:

Wholegrain cereals Brown rice, oats, barley, wheat, buckwheat, corn, rye, millet and products made from these such as wholewheat flour, bread and pasta; couscous; whole oat porridge.

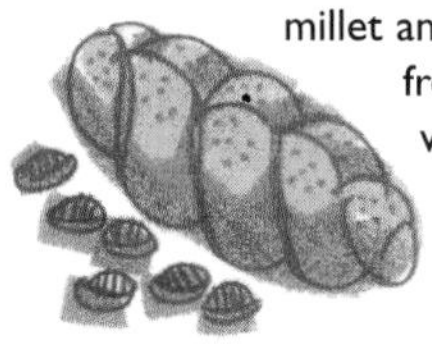

Fruit A mixture of fresh seasonal fruits, which should include some citrus fruit. To ensure freshness, buy frequently and, where possible, choose local produce.

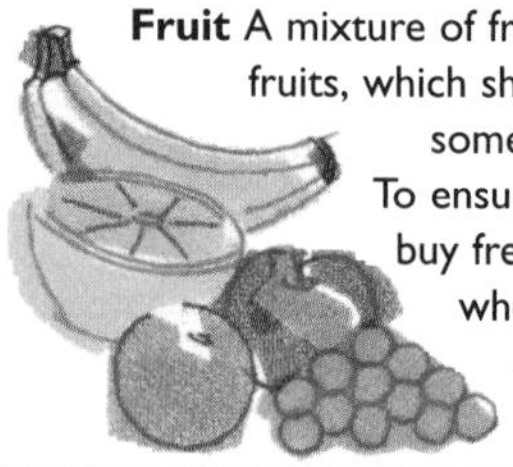

Vegetables and sea vegetables A wide variety of fresh vegetables is recommended. Seaweed is used to enhance the flavour and nutritional value of many savoury dishes.

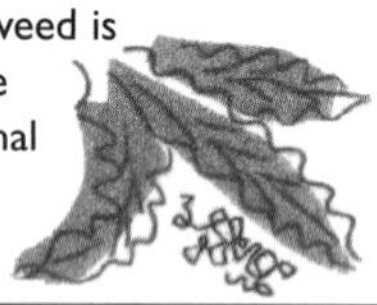

Legumes Lentils, chick-peas, beans, peas and soya products, such as tofu (bean curd).

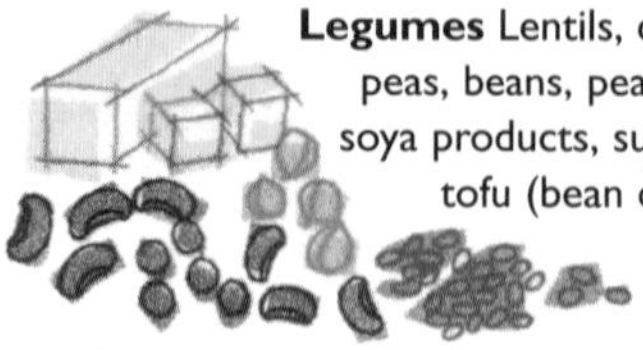

Soups Usually made with beans and lentils, and special oriental seasonings such as rich salty miso, made from fermented soya beans, and shoyu, a dark, soya sauce.

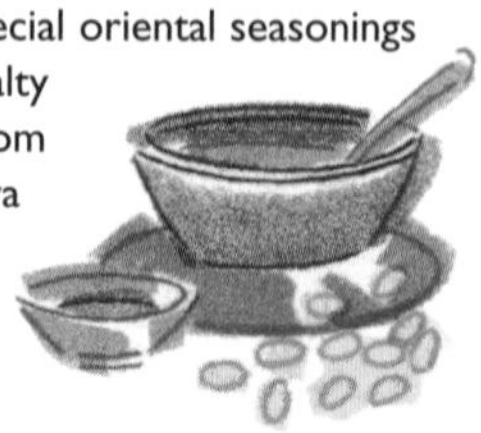

Seeds, nuts, flavourings and fish Sesame, sunflower and pumpkin seeds, peanuts, almonds, hazelnuts, walnuts, and dried chestnuts. In moderation, sea salt, ginger, mustard, tahini, cider vinegar, garlic, lemon juice and apple juice, can all be used to enhance the flavour of a dish. For non-vegetarians, three small portions of fresh seafood can be included every week. The yang qualities of fish and shellfish should be balanced by helpings of green leafy vegetables, grains or pulses in the same meal.

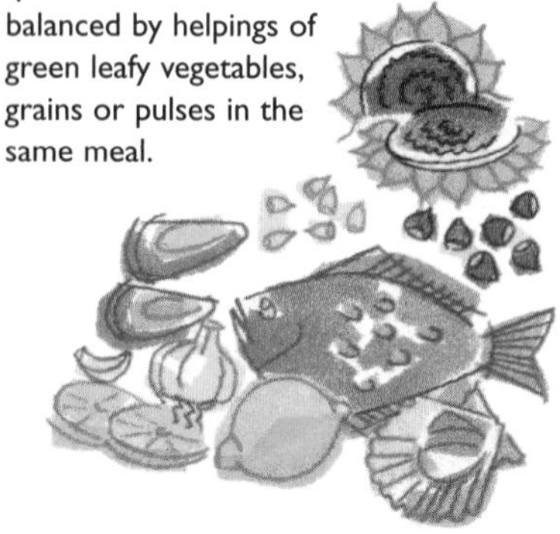

with a high yang content include red meat, poultry, fish and shellfish, eggs, hard cheeses and salt. Foods that are thought to contain a harmonious balance of yin and yang are: wholegrain cereals, fresh fruit, nuts and seeds, leafy vegetables and pulses (beans, peas and lentils).

Because the macrobiotic diet is low in calories and saturated fats, and high in fibre, it can help to reduce the risk of obesity, raised cholesterol, high blood pressure and constipation. However, you would get much the same benefits from a well-balanced VEGETARIAN diet, which is easier and safer to follow.

SOME DISADVANTAGES

At its most extreme, the macrobiotic diet does not supply adequate amounts of vitamin B_{12} for a healthy nervous system, iron for healthy blood, and vitamin D, which is needed for the absorption of calcium. As a deficiency in iron and B_{12} can lead to anaemia, supplements should be taken.

The macrobiotic diet should never be used by pregnant or breastfeeding women, people who are ill or anyone with special dietary requirements. It is also unsuitable for children. The bulky nature of the diet can lead to malnutrition in youngsters, and slow growth rates right through to adolescence.

MALNUTRITION AND DIETARY DEFICIENCIES

In the Western world, severe malnutrition is rare except in people who are chronically sick or suffering from an eating disorder, such as anorexia nervosa, or absorption problems such as coeliac disease.

However, people who follow rigid exclusion diets, alcoholics and the elderly living alone are vulnerable. There are many different illnesses and symptoms in the West which are the result of poor nutrition. The daily intake of nutrients recommended by governments and health authorities is not always a reliable guide to healthy eating. The figures tend to vary from country to country and are usually defined as the amount needed to meet the nutritional requirements of the majority of the population. A more recent concept has been the introduction of Dietary Reference Values. These take both age and sex into account and are aimed at preventing diet-related disease rather than preventing nutritional deficiency.

The following list of VITAMINS and MINERALS, and good dietary sources, outlines the most common deficiencies in the Western world.

VITAMINS

Vitamin B_1 (thiamin) Found in pork, whole grains, potatoes, pulses and nuts. An inadequate intake can lead to appetite loss, swelling of the limbs, mental confusion, an enlarged heart, muscle weakness and nervous disorders. Alcoholics are vulnerable.

Vitamin B_2 (riboflavin) Found in milk, eggs, meat, poultry and fortified breakfast cereals. Signs of deficiency include cracked lips, bloodshot eyes, dermatitis and mild anaemia.

Vitamin B_{12} Found in meat, fish, poultry, eggs and dairy products. A deficiency is unusual but may occur in old people and also vegans. Symptoms include fatigue, pins and needles, loss of feeling in the limbs, megaloblastic anaemia, and possible degeneration of the nervous system.

Folate (folic acid) Found in Brussels sprouts, green leafy vegetables, liver and pulses. A deficiency can cause megaloblastic anaemia and wasting of the gut which causes poor absorption of other essential nutrients.

Niacin (nicotinic acid) Found in meat, nuts, peas and beans, poultry and fortified breakfast cereals. The symptoms of an inadequate dietary intake include fatigue, a pigmented skin rash, dermatitis and diarrhoea.

Vitamin C Found in blackcurrants, peppers, citrus fruits, potatoes and strawberries. An inadequate intake may cause sore gums, scaly skin, slow healing of wounds and increased susceptibility to infection.

Vitamin D Found in oily fish, fish liver oils and fortified margarine. A deficiency can cause muscle weakness, softening of the bones (osteomalacia), and may cause rickets in children.

Vitamin E Found in margarine, nuts, and vegetable oil. A deficiency occurs only in people who cannot absorb fat; symptoms include nerve damage and haemolytic anaemia.

MINERALS

Calcium Found in dairy products, green leafy vegetables, tinned sardines with bones and sesame seeds. A deficiency can result in muscle weakness, back pain, soft and brittle bones, fractures and osteoporosis.

Iron Found in liver, beef, sardines, dark green leafy vegetables, dried figs, dried apricots, whole grains and iron-fortified cereals. An inadequate intake can cause tiredness, shortness of breath, iron-deficiency anaemia and reduced resistance to infection.

Magnesium Found in wheat bran, whole grains, nuts, sesame seeds and dried figs. Symptoms of a deficiency include weakness, cramps and muscle tremors which lead to convulsions.

Potassium Found in dried fruit, sunflower seeds, nuts, avocados, beans, peas and lentils. Symptoms of a deficiency (most common in those with eating disorders) include weakness, confusion, apathy, extreme thirst, poor digestion and abdominal bloating, respiratory and heart problems.

Zinc Found in liver, oysters and other types of shellfish, red meat and nuts.

Deficiency is rare except in those with eating disorders. Symptoms include slow wound healing, retarded growth, and delayed sexual development.

DEFICIENT HOSPITAL DIETS

In Britain, reports have highlighted the many cases of malnutrition among National Health Service patients; an alarming number are neither diagnosed nor treated. Elderly, long-term patients are among those most at risk.

In a study of 500 patients admitted to a Dundee hospital in 1994, 200 were found to be undernourished, but fewer than half of these had any nutritional information in their medical notes. When discharged, 112 of the 500 were reassessed and an average net weight loss was recorded. Patients who had been undernourished on admittance had suffered the greatest weight loss during hospitalisation.

Experts argue that such scant regard for diet is indefensible on ethical and economic grounds; it is known that the incidence of bed sores in long-stay patients can be linked to vitamin C deficiency. Also, hip-fracture patients who receive vitamin and mineral supplements have fewer complications and need shorter hospital stays.

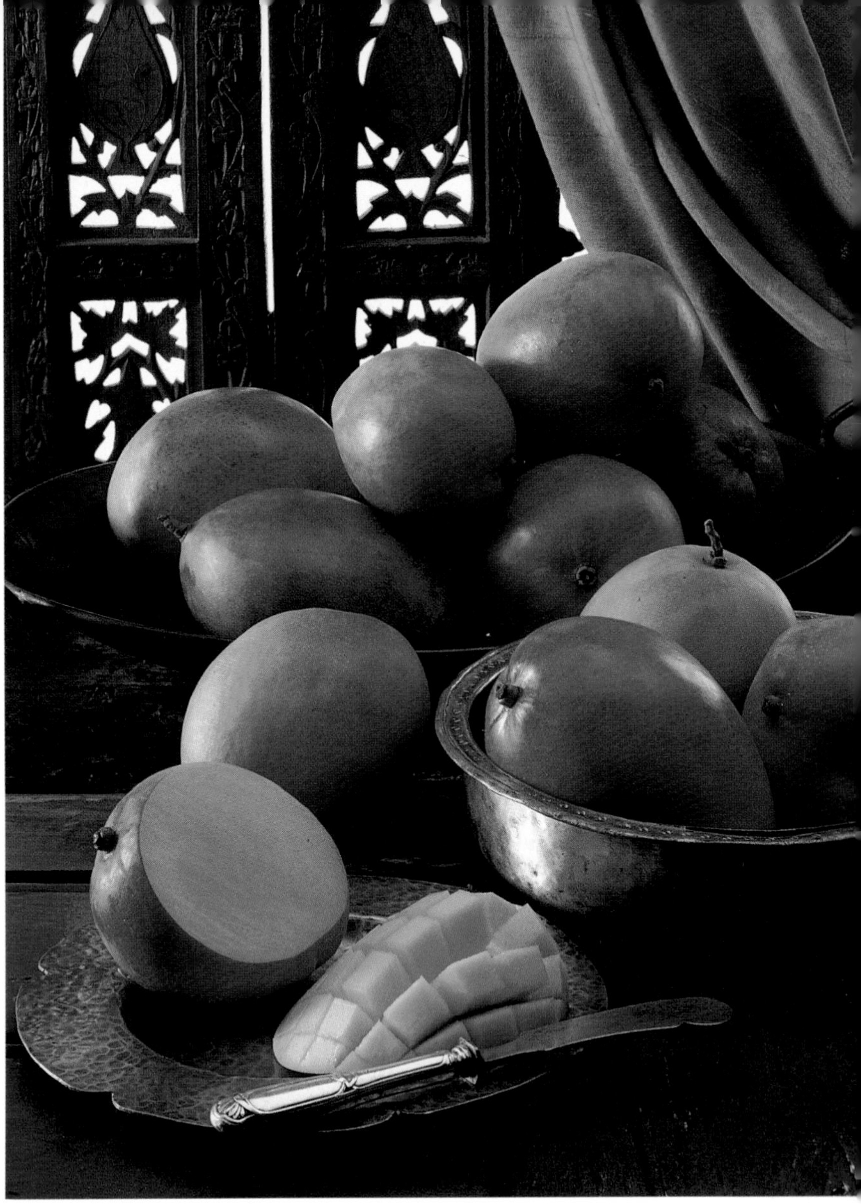

FRUIT OF THE TROPICS *The golden flesh of the mango beneath its tough skin is succulent and rich in beta carotene. Some varieties are as big as melons, others as small as plums.*

MALT EXTRACT AND MALTED MILK DRINKS

BENEFITS

- *Malt extract is a good source of phosphorus and a useful source of magnesium*
- *Milk drinks contain calcium and vitamin B_2 (riboflavin) and are a useful source of vitamin B_{12}*
- *Milk drinks help to induce sleep*

People who are ill or convalescing can often benefit from milk drinks based on malt. Malt itself is a sweet powder made from barley grains that have germinated for about a week. When it is dissolved in hot milk, the malted powder becomes an easily digested liquid food that provides vital calories for patients who have lost their appetite or who are, for any other reason, unable to eat.

Malted milk drinks, for example Ovaltine or Horlicks, supply useful amounts of vitamin B_{12}, vitamin B_2 (riboflavin) and calcium. They also help to induce sleep if taken last thing at night. However, they are high in sugar and can contribute towards tooth decay, although low-sugar varieties are also available.

Malt extract supplies phosphorus for healthy bones, and magnesium which plays a role in nerve and muscle function. It is made by soaking powdered malt in water, heating it, then reducing the liquid to produce a naturally sweet, dark brown syrup. Once given by the tablespoon to children as a blood-fortifying tonic, particularly after illness, malt extract is now used to sweeten and flavour foods.

MANGETOUT

BENEFITS
- *Excellent source of vitamin C*
- *Good source of beta carotene and potassium*
- *Supply useful amounts of fibre*

Mangetout contain significantly more vitamin C than garden peas because the pods – which are rich in the vitamin – are eaten as well, as the French name meaning 'eat all' implies.

An average 100g (3½oz) portion served raw in salads, or stir-fried, more than meets the recommended daily requirement of vitamin C (135 per cent when raw, 128 per cent if lightly cooked). Mangetout are also a good source of beta carotene and potassium and provide useful amounts of fibre.

Because the tiny peas in the small flat pods of the mangetout are immature, they contain much less protein than garden peas.

MANGO

BENEFITS
- *Rich source of beta carotene, which the body can convert to vitamin A*
- *Rich source of vitamin C*

A medium-sized fresh mango is a rich source of both beta carotene and also vitamin C. The ripe flesh of the fruit is easy to digest, and the beta carotene that it contains is readily absorbed by the body where it can be converted into vitamin A.

Vitamin C and beta carotene are ANTIOXIDANTS. Although the body can make its own, antioxidants supplied by foods boost defences and help to prevent FREE RADICAL damage, so reducing the risk of certain cancers.

However, mangoes are also quite high in sugar; a medium-sized fruit is about 14 per cent sugar. As they are also fairly acidic, they may contribute towards dental decay if eaten very frequently.

Mangoes have only recently begun to become popular in Britain. Native to India, they have been cultivated there for thousands of years but are now grown throughout the tropics.

EATING A MANGO

Preparing a mango is a messy process because its silky smooth, fibrous flesh is exceptionally juicy and slippery. The best way is to slice the fruit lengthways into two pieces, avoiding the stone in the middle, then to score the flesh into a crisscross pattern before turning each half inside out.

MARROW

BENEFIT
- *Low in calories*

There are few nutritional benefits to be gained from marrow. It consists of 95 per cent water, and contains only trace amounts of vitamins, fibre and nutrients. However, the vegetable can be a tasty component in a weight-reducing diet as an average 100g (3½oz) serving of its light green flesh contains less than 10 Calories.

Unlike orange-fleshed pumpkins and winter squashes, which are part of the same family, the marrow's flesh contains minimal beta carotene, although the skin, which can be eaten if it is not too tough, contains more.

Marrow seeds have been used in folk medicine for centuries, primarily as a diuretic and a treatment for tape worm when used with a purgative. Marrows were first grown in England in the 19th century and became a popular garden vegetable in Victorian times. Although giant marrows may be highly prized, smaller ones are tastier.

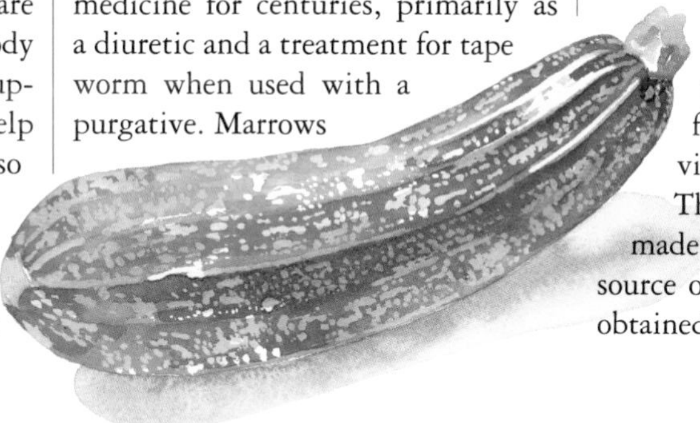

MAYONNAISE

BENEFIT
- *Rich in vitamin E*

DRAWBACKS
- *High in calories*
- *Raw eggs may pose a salmonella risk in fresh mayonnaise*
- *High in cholesterol*

In dietary terms mayonnaise, whether it is homemade or commercially produced, contains little protein or carbohydrate. Nevertheless, the egg yolks and vegetable oil with which it is made do supply vitamin E.

Use mayonnaise sparingly, however, since one tablespoonful of this popular accompaniment to salads and other cold dishes contains around 10g of fat supplying almost 100 Calories. Slimmers can use a 'low-fat' version (typically containing around 3g of fat and 50 Calories per tablespoon). Other low-fat alternatives include SALAD DRESSINGS that are based on low-fat yoghurt or fromage frais.

Most recipes for fresh, homemade mayonnaise recommend the use of cold-pressed olive oil which is composed of mainly monounsaturated fats. However, other OILS which have lighter flavours, such as safflower, soya bean or corn oil can be substituted for olive oil. These contain mostly polyunsaturated fatty acids, many of which are vital for healthy body function.

The raw eggs used in homemade mayonnaise can be a potential source of salmonella, unless they are obtained from a reliable source and consumed within their 'use by' date. Any raw egg products should be avoided by young children, pregnant women, elderly people and the sick; commercial mayonnaise producers use pasteurised egg yolk to avoid the risk. Egg yolks are also high in cholesterol and should not be eaten by anyone on a low-cholesterol diet.

Homemade mayonnaise should be covered and refrigerated until no more than 30 minutes before use. It can be kept in a refrigerator for several days.

MEASLES

TAKE PLENTY OF

- *Fluids including diluted fruit juices*
- *Light meals, including foods that supply vitamin A*
- *Fruits and vegetables that are rich in vitamin C*

A special diet will not cure measles but foods that supply vitamin A, such as eggs and most dairy products, can restore levels depleted by the disease.

The highly infectious virus, which often begins with a cough or cold, sneezing and sore, watering eyes, damages the mucous membranes and lowers blood concentrations of vitamin A. The characteristic rash appears three to five days later, usually just after the eruption of clusters of tiny white spots on the insides of the cheeks, called Koplik's spots; other symptoms include headaches, thirst and a raised temperature.

Research in developing countries, where measles is rife and often fatal, has shown that preventing a vitamin A deficiency reduces the disease's severity and the risk of eye complications.

The patient needs plenty of fluids; these can include fruit juices rich in vitamin C which help to maintain the immune system. They are more easily absorbed when diluted 1:1 with water.

MEDICINES AND DRUGS – THE LINK WITH DIET

Drugs can sometimes influence the body's ability to use certain nutrients. As a result, a person may have an iron deficiency, for example, even though their diet contains plenty. Similarly, certain nutrients can slow down or speed up the absorption of drugs. Some may alter the activity of the drug in the body or affect the rate at which drugs are broken down.

Certain drugs need to be taken with food and others between meals. Taking vitamin supplements is sometimes beneficial and sometimes harmful – depending on the drug being taken.

Dietary complications are seldom a problem when medicines are taken for a short time unless the patient is already malnourished. Nutrient-related side effects are much more likely during prolonged treatments for conditions such as hypertension or mental disorders and if over-the-counter medications are taken for extensive periods. Elderly people are especially vulnerable as they are often prescribed more than one type of long-term medication, and may follow an inadequate diet.

If you experience any unusual symptoms while taking either prescription or non-prescription drugs, consult your doctor or pharmacist. However, when prescribing or selling drugs, doctors or pharmacists ought to be aware of the most common problems associated with them and suggest any necessary precautions before you start taking the medicine.

The following examples cover the most commonly observed interactions between medicines and nutrients. You may not recognise the name or type of drug you are taking because many different proprietary and generic names are used by manufacturers for the same kind of medication. If in doubt, seek advice from your doctor or pharmacist.

FOR THE DIGESTIVE SYSTEM

Antacids These are used for treating indigestion, heartburn and stomach ulcers. Those that contain aluminium (usually in the form of aluminium hydroxide) should not be taken on a continuing basis because they reduce the body's ability to absorb phosphorus. If the diet is low in phosphate (derived from phosphorus), using these drugs long-term can lead to softening of the bones (OSTEOMALACIA). Meat, fish and eggs supply phosphate.

Laxatives Regular use of strong laxative drugs, known as purgatives, is harmful because excessive loss of water from the body can lead to dehydration and to low levels of potassium in the blood. Furthermore, the accelerated bowel function reduces the absorption of almost every type of nutrient.

Mineral-oil laxatives such as liquid paraffin have a similar effect and their use is declining; they also interfere with the absorption of vitamins A, D and K as well as beta carotene. Since vitamin D is essential for the absorption of calcium, excessive use of this medication can increase the risk of OSTEOPOROSIS in elderly people and post-menopausal women.

If constipation is a problem and requires medication, it is preferable to use a bulk laxative (such as bran, psyllium seeds or ispaghula). Better still, remedy the cause of constipation by eating a fibre-rich diet which includes green vegetables, pulses, wholegrain cereals and stewed dried fruits; prunes and figs have a natural laxative effect.

FOR HEART AND CIRCULATION

Anticoagulants These are used to reduce blood clotting and are prescribed for certain forms of stroke, thrombosis and other problems to do with the heart and circulation. They include warfarin and similar drugs which act by inhibiting the role of vitamin K in the blood-clotting process. While receiving this treatment, which must be carefully monitored, do not take supplements of vitamins A or C as sudden high intakes of either nutrient can reduce the effectiveness of anticoagulants. High vitamin E intakes may have the reverse effect and can cause bleeding problems.

Drugs to control cholesterol levels (lipid-lowering drugs) Several types of drug are prescribed to reduce high levels of blood cholesterol, and other blood fats. One group, called bile-acid sequestrants (examples are cholestyramine and colestipol), act by binding cholesterol in the intestine to prevent it being reabsorbed into the bloodstream. As these drugs interfere with the absorption of iron and folate, oral supplements of the nutrients should be given to children who are prescribed these drugs. The effectiveness of this medication is generally enhanced by reducing saturated fats and cholesterol in the diet.

Treatment of the heart Drugs such as digoxin should not be taken at the same time as fibre-rich foods as they tend to bind with both insoluble and soluble forms of dietary fibre; this makes them less effective because less of the drug gets into the bloodstream.

For phenytoin, which is used to treat irregular heartbeat, see Anticonvulsants (overleaf).

TO TREAT INFECTIONS

Antibacterials and antibiotics A common problem associated with these drugs, which are used to treat bacterial infections, is that they can simultaneously destroy bacteria residing in the gut that produce small amounts of some B vitamins and vitamin K for use by the body. But as these types of medication are usually taken for short intervals, they are unlikely to affect the levels of vitamins in the body to any significant degree.

While taking a course of antibacterials or antibiotics, it is often helpful to restore the balance of the normal gut bacteria by eating a pot of live YOGHURT (preferably bio-yoghurt) twice a day. Check first with your doctor, however, because calcium-rich foods such as milk, yoghurt and cheese can interfere with the action of certain antibiotics, including penicillin, pencillamine, and tetracycline. The live yoghurt treatment may still be beneficial but it should be postponed until a few days after completing the course of antibiotics.

Although tuberculosis is no longer a serious problem in many countries, the antitubercular drug isoniazid is still quite widely used. It can cause drug-induced pellagra – a nutritional disease that is more commonly found in developing countries as a result of niacin deficiency. Symptoms include scaly dermatitis, diarrhoea and depression. Malnourished patients, the elderly and alcoholics are among the most vulnerable to this deficiency and should receive 10mg of niacin (vitamin B_3) daily, to compensate.

Nystatin, an antifungal drug often used for the treatment of yeast infections such as thrush, can inhibit the action of vitamins B_2 (riboflavin) and B_6. Both side effects can be minimised by eating plenty of foods rich in B vitamins such as whole grains, meat, eggs and dairy foods.

Antimalarials These drugs have been specifically developed for preventing or treating malaria. Of these, pyrimethamine may help to reduce absorption of folate and should not be taken by people such as pregnant women or the elderly, who might be susceptible to megaloblastic anaemia, a condition which can be due to a deficiency of

Case study

Grahame is a 50-year-old freelance photographer. He had been taking the diuretic drug thiazide, for mild hypertension, for five years. In recent months he had been feeling excessively tired but put it down to a particularly hectic series of commissions. However, when his workload eased, Grahame still felt exhausted, and his muscles were so weak that he could hardly lift his camera cases. Unsympathetic colleagues told him to pull himself together, but one suggested that he might be suffering from depression. Grahame decided to visit his doctor, who checked his blood electrolytes and found him to be deficient in potassium. She advised him to take potassium supplements in the form of tablets, and to eat foods that supplied plenty of potassium, such as dried fruits, nuts and seeds, bananas, and avocados. Within two weeks, Grahame felt stronger and more energetic. A blood test confirmed that his potassium levels were back to normal.

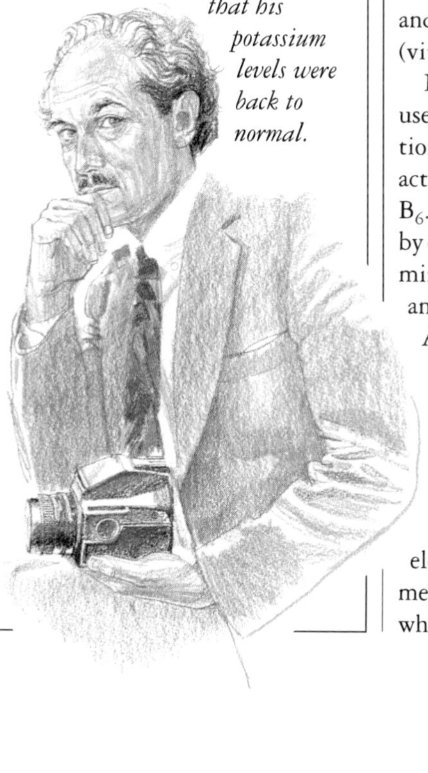

folate. To offset this, it may be helpful to take a folic acid supplement and to eat plenty of folate-rich foods such as green leafy vegetables and pulses.

For the urinary system

Diuretics These are taken to increase the output of urine from the kidneys, which is often necessary for treating fluid retention in the body, such as that associated with KIDNEY DISEASE. Some diuretics – the thiazide drugs, for example – may also be taken long term to reduce high blood pressure. The loss of minerals, such as potassium and calcium, is one of the inevitable effects of excreting high levels of urine. If the diuretic is known to cause a particularly high potassium loss, dietary supplements may be recommended. Losses of other micronutrients can be corrected by eating a diet that is rich in the particular vitamin or mineral, or by regularly taking multivitamins and mineral preparations.

For contraception

The Pill Early studies suggested that taking the Pill increased requirements for several vitamins and minerals but this view is no longer widely held. Indeed, the Pill may even increase the absorption of some nutrients such as iron and calcium. It also decreases blood loss during menstruation. When a woman decides to stop taking the contraceptive pill in order to conceive, it is most important that she increases folate intake to at least 400 mcg a day to reduce the risk of birth defects during a subsequent pregnancy. Doctors recommend a 400 mcg folic acid preparation daily for all women planning conception and for the first three months of PREGNANCY.

For muscles and joints

Non-steroidal drugs that are taken to relieve symptoms of rheumatoid arthritis and other similar complaints include sulphasalazine. It can reduce the body's absorption of folate, which is used for the production of white blood cells – an important part of the immune system. As a result, the body's defences can be weakened. This can be corrected by taking a folic acid supplement or eating folate-rich foods such as pulses or green vegetables.

The action of sulphasalazine is reduced by high levels of iron and calcium, so supplements containing these minerals should not be taken. High doses of vitamin C, which can cause kidney damage when taken with the medication should also be avoided. Those who are susceptible to salicylate should not take sulphasalazine.

Steroids These are widely used as long-term anti-inflammatory agents. However, prolonged use may sometimes cause DIABETES and raise blood CHOLESTEROL levels. Care needs to be taken to avoid weight gain and to follow a diet low in saturated fat.

For aspirin and methotrexate, also used for the treatment of arthritis, see Analgesics and Cytotoxic drugs respectively (below).

For the mind

Antidepressants Although they are now rarely prescribed, monoamine oxidase inhibitors (for example, phenelzine and tranylcypromine) can interfere with the way the body uses certain nutrients, potentially causing excessive amounts of amines to accumulate and constrict blood vessels. Dangerously high blood pressure may result. Details of the foods to avoid should be given in writing by the doctor and pharmacist; they include yeast extract, meat extract, cheese, lentils, soya sauce and red wines.

For the nervous system

Analgesics These are taken for pain relief. Aspirin is one of the most commonly used drugs in this group and is available in many forms. Aspirin has been shown, in some cases, to reduce the level of folate in the body when it is taken regularly over a long period of time. Taking extra folate in the diet may be advisable in such cases; offal, green leafy vegetables and pulses supply dietary folate.

Anticonvulsants These are prescribed for treatment and control of epilepsy and psychiatric disorders and are normally taken for many years. They include phenytoin – a drug also used to treat irregular heartbeat – which can reduce the levels of folate and vitamins D and K in the body; phenobarbitone, which can affect the body's ability to use vitamin D; and primidone, which interferes with the metabolism of folate.

It is therefore important to avoid any vitamin deficiencies by taking a supplement or by eating foods rich in these nutrients, such as oily fish, eggs, dairy foods and leafy green vegetables.

Drugs for Parkinson's Disease One of the most commonly prescribed drugs for the treatment of Parkinson's Disease is L-dopa (levodopa). Its action is impaired by the amino acid, phenylalanine, and by vitamin B_6. Hence it is important to avoid supplements of these nutrients.

Anti-cancer drugs

Cytotoxic drugs These drugs are used in cancer chemotherapy to limit the growth of abnormal cells. One of them, methotrexate, which is also used for the treatment of rheumatoid arthritis, can cause gastrointestinal bleeding and diarrhoea and interfere with the body's use of folate.

When prescribing this and similar drugs, doctors will monitor the condition of patients. They should not take folic acid supplements because high levels of the vitamin reduce the effectiveness of the treatment, which aims to provide just enough folate to support normal blood formation – but no more. However, patients will benefit from a nourishing well-balanced diet that can include folate-rich foods.

Effects of alcohol

Even moderate consumption of ALCOHOL is known to affect the function of the liver. Patients are often advised to avoid alcohol when they are taking a course of medication because it accentuates the toxic side effects of almost every type of drug and decreases the effectiveness of some, including the anticoagulant warfarin and the anticonvulsant phenytoin.

The opposite applies when the liver has been damaged by heavy drinking. The action of many drugs may be enhanced because the liver cannot break them down properly, so they are not being removed from the body as quickly as they should be.

ME (MYALGIC ENCEPHALOMYELITIS)

EAT PLENTY OF

- *Whole grains and pasta for complex carbohydrates*
- *Foods such as offal, leafy green vegetables and pulses for B vitamins*
- *Fresh fruit and vegetables for vitamin C*

CUT DOWN ON

- *Refined carbohydrates such as white flour and sugar*
- *Caffeine in tea, coffee and cola drinks*

AVOID

- *Alcohol*

Also known as post-viral fatigue syndrome, ME or myalgic encephalomyelitis is one of the most baffling ailments to emerge in recent years. According to doctors who have dealt with it, the most effective treatment is to give the body time to heal itself, and to help it to do so by adopting a healthier diet and a sensible lifestyle.

ME follows some form of viral infection or, occasionally, a vaccination. The range of symptoms includes muscle fatigue and pain, exhaustion, flu-like symptoms, mood swings, poor concentration, short-term memory loss, depression, and some digestive complaints. To help your body to cope with these problems, you need to eat a healthy, well-balanced diet that contains enough complex carbohydrates, vitamins and minerals. It is best to eat small, regularly spaced meals throughout the day to ensure that your body receives a steady flow of nutrients to help it fight the illness.

Plenty of complex carbohydrates such as wholemeal bread, pasta, oat-based products, potatoes and brown rice are absolutely essential. These energy providers are particularly important for sufferers of ME because the illness can often leave people feeling completely drained. Foods such as pasta, wholemeal bread and those containing oats provide a steady release of energy and therefore control blood sugar levels. They also contain fibre which helps to keep the digestive system running smoothly. Bread, cakes, sugar and glucose drinks provide a more immediate energy boost, but this is soon used up.

Unrefined foods such as whole grains are good sources of B vitamins, which are vital for normal functioning of the nervous system. Offal, leafy green vegetables, nuts and oily fish also supply B vitamins.

Protein is essential for maintaining good health and vitality. Make sure that you eat sources of good-quality protein such as meat, poultry, fish, dairy products or eggs every day. These are rich in micronutrients and also provide adequate amounts of all the amino acids essential for growth and healthy tissues. Proteins in individual foods from plant sources do not provide the ideal balance of amino acids that the body needs to make its own protein; however, people who are on a VEGETARIAN DIET achieve that balance by combining the proteins from various plant foods in their diet.

Eating plenty of fresh fruit and vegetables will raise your intake of vitamin C. A good intake of vitamin C is particularly important during times of stress and illness, when the body's store is rapidly used up.

It may be helpful for susceptible individuals to cut down on drinks that contain caffeine, such as tea, coffee and cola. Caffeine can exacerbate symptoms because it stimulates the nervous system. Alchohol may also worsen symptoms, especially fatigue. It can increase the liver's metabolism and raises the rate at which B vitamins and vitamin C are broken down.

Dos and don'ts

- Do obtain an accurate diagnosis, preferably from a doctor who has experience of the disorder.
- Do keep a diary of your progress, noting your symptoms and what foods or activities affect your mood and physical well-being.
- Do establish a sensible and balanced programme of treatment covering diet and pastimes that add interest to your convalescence but do not involve overexertion.
- Do try to relax and take plenty of rest during the day.
- Don't take alcohol as it acts as a depressant.
- Don't drink more than three or four cups of coffee a day, and avoid coffee at bedtime.
- Don't, unless essential, undergo an anaesthetic or vaccination.

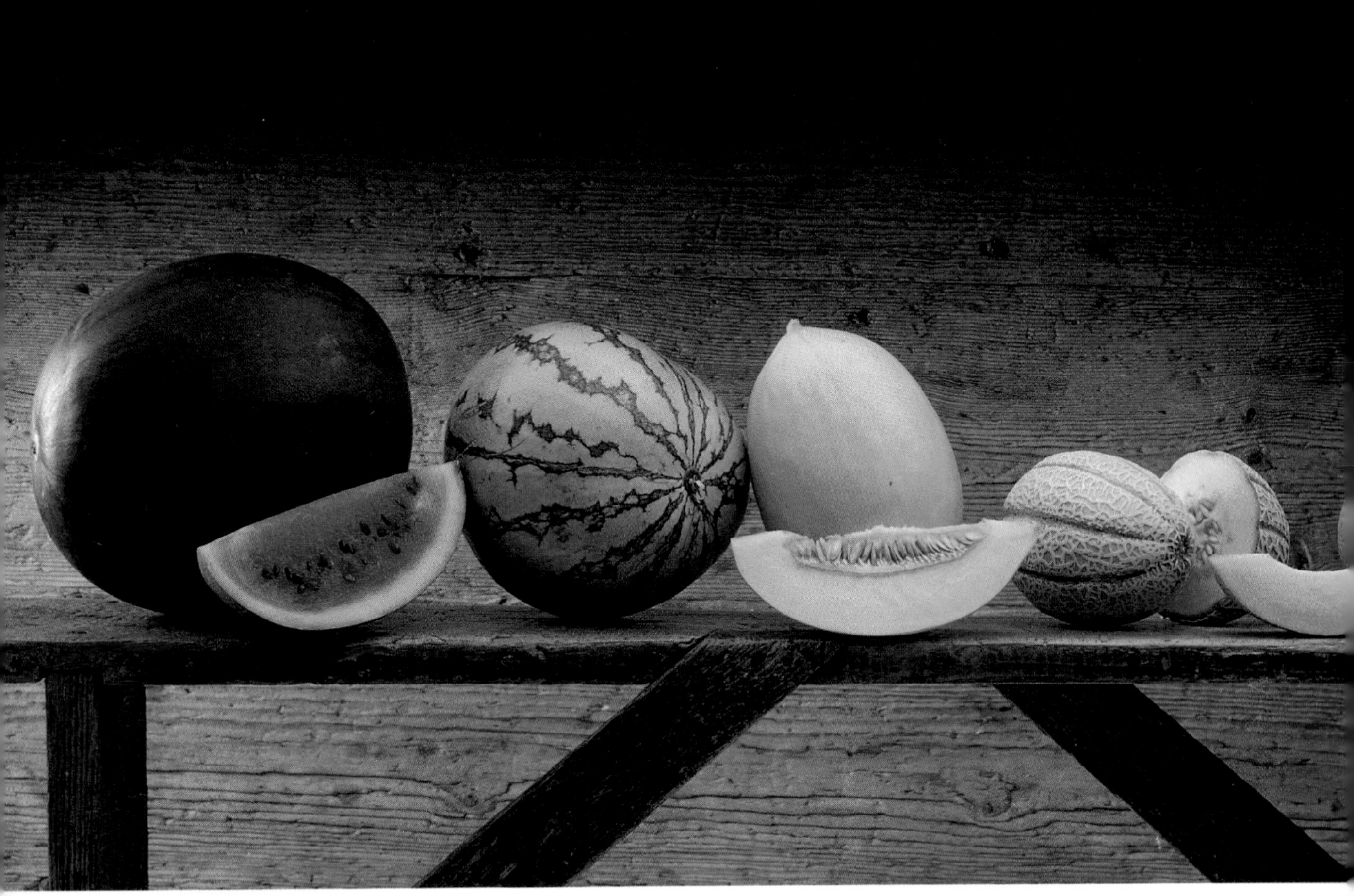

MELON

BENEFITS

- *Some varieties are good sources of beta carotene and vitamin C*

Orange-fleshed cantaloupe melons are among the most nutritious of the many varieties of melon. A 100g (3½oz) portion supplies more than half the recommended daily intake of vitamin C and is also a good source of beta carotene (which the body converts into vitamin A). Both of these are ANTIOXIDANTS which may help to prevent cancer and heart disease.

Melons with a lighter yellow or green flesh-colour, and also water melons, contain less vitamin C and they supply little, if any, beta carotene.

Melons are relatively low in calories – they contain between 19 and 31 Calories per 100g (3½oz), depending on the type. Their high water content may stimulate the kidneys to work more efficiently.

MENOPAUSE

EAT PLENTY OF

- *Dairy produce and green leafy vegetables for calcium*
- *Oily fish for vitamin D*

AVOID

- *Excessive caffeine and alcohol*
- *Obesity*

The period of time during which women stop ovulating is called the menopause. It usually occurs between the ages of 45 and 55 though the age of onset is extremely variable. For some women, the hot flushes, night sweats, mood swings and depression that can accompany the menopause are almost unbearable. Others have a much less traumatic time, and some view it as a positive, life-enhancing process.

Some symptoms are a result of hormonal fluctuations and imbalances, which also increase women's risk of HEART DISEASE and OSTEOPOROSIS, a disorder which results in brittle bones that fracture easily. Hormone replacement therapy (HRT) can counteract many of the unpleasant symptoms of the menopause, as well as reduce the risk of osteoporosis, and possibly heart disease, if it is taken for a long period. However, HRT also increases the risk of breast cancer and does not suit all women. Dietary changes may help too, but a link between diet and the relief of symptoms remains unproven.

However, it is known that your body's need for iron falls because you are no longer losing blood through menstruation. But you need more calcium to slow down loss of bone mass – some experts believe that menopausal women need at least 1000mg per day.

The best dietary sources of calcium are dairy products and green leafy vegetables. In order to absorb calcium efficiently, the body needs vitamin D. Oily fish are an excellent source of this vitamin, and tinned sardines also include edible bones which are rich in

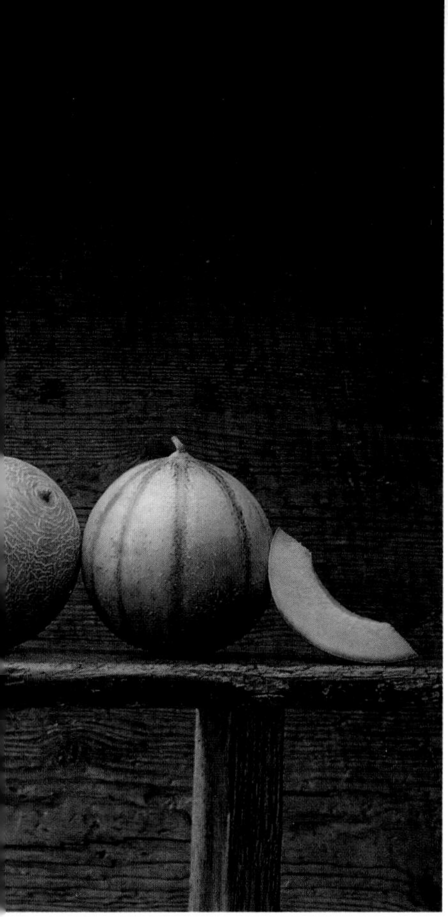

COOL AND REFRESHING *Popular varieties of melon include (from left to right): water melon, honeydew, and small, sweet cantaloupe, galia and charentais.*

calcium. Avoid eating raw BRAN, which inhibits calcium absorption, and cut down on tea and coffee, which promote the excretion of calcium.

Many women put on weight during the menopause. Excessive weight gain can lead to higher blood CHOLESTEROL levels which increase the risk of heart disease. To control body weight and blood cholesterol, select low-fat dairy foods and cut down on saturated fats, and do not drink too much alcohol.

Recent research has been investigating the possibility that substances from plants called phytoestrogens might help to reduce the severity of hot flushes and other symptoms of the menopause. Phytoestrogens, which mimic human oestrogen, are found in many foods, but are especially concentrated in soya beans and alfalfa sprouts.

MENSTRUAL PROBLEMS AND PMS

Several of the problems associated with the menstrual cycle can be helped by careful attention to diet. However, frequent or heavy blood loss, irregular bleeding or unusual levels of pain should be investigated by your doctor.

PREMENSTRUAL SYNDROME OR PMS

EAT PLENTY OF
- *Small, frequent meals high in carbohydrate and low in fat*
- *Supplementary evening primrose oil and vitamin B_6*
- *Foods containing vitamin B_6, such as meat, fish and whole grains*

CUT DOWN ON
- *Salt*
- *Caffeine in tea and coffee*

AVOID
- *Alcohol*

Premenstrual syndrome, or PMS, produces physical and mental changes which typically begin from mid-cycle onwards, or in the premenstrual week, and clear as soon as the period starts. Symptoms include backache, headache, water retention, cramps, breast tenderness, irrational behaviour, anxiety, depression and poor concentration.

PMS may be related to the production of the female hormones oestrogen and progesterone, which control the monthly cycle, and to a woman's sensitivity to changing hormone levels. As the condition has become more fully understood, most doctors have become increasingly sympathetic.

Some may suggest taking vitamin B_6 (pyridoxine) – which is involved in the breakdown of oestrogen in the liver – and perhaps evening primrose oil supplements. Sometimes hormones will be prescribed; many women find that their PMS symptoms disappear when they are on the Pill.

Researchers in both orthodox and alternative medicine agree that PMS symptoms can also be eased by diet. Studies suggest that a diet high in carbohydrate and low in fat is helpful.

Supplements of vitamin B_6 may help to counter premenstrual depression, lethargy, and water retention – characterised by a bloated stomach,

Helpful foods

Spinach and other dark green leafy vegetables for magnesium and vitamin B_6.

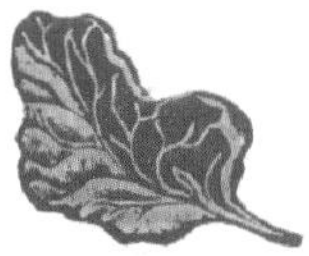

Wholemeal bread and whole grains for complex carbohydrates, vitamin B_6 and magnesium.

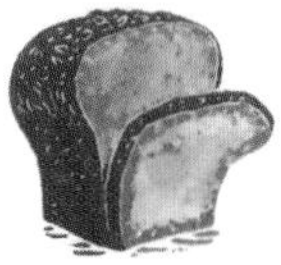

Eggs, wheatgerm or nuts for vitamin E which may reduce breast tenderness.

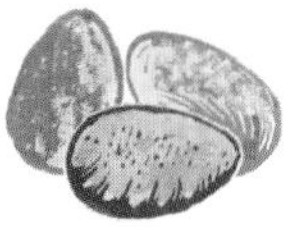

Red meat, poultry, liver (but not if trying to conceive), and offal for iron and vitamin B_6.

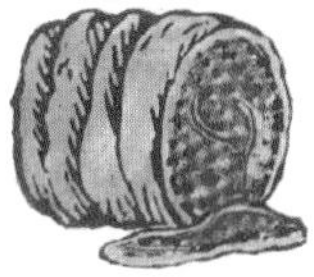

Oranges and other citrus fruits and juices for vitamin C; take with meals to help the body to absorb iron from other foods.

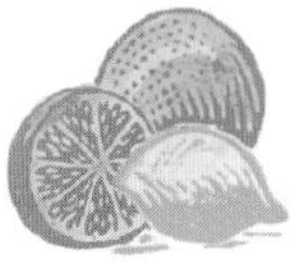

Cold-pressed virgin olive oil for vitamin E; use to dress salads and in cooking.

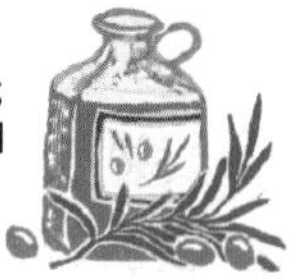

Shellfish and all forms of seafood, as well as nuts and dried fruit, for magnesium.

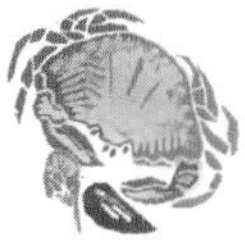

swollen fingers, toes or face, and tender breasts. It may help to increase intake of foods which contain useful amounts of this vitamin, such as meat, fish, whole grains and green leafy vegetables. Cutting down on salt can also help to reduce water retention. Eating foods high in vitamin E, such as cold-pressed oils and wheatgerm, may help to reduce breast tenderness.

Some studies have suggested that taking caffeine may exacerbate PMS. However, abruptly cutting out caffeine in coffee and tea can make things worse. Intake should be decreased gradually to minimise the likelihood of withdrawal headaches.

Some women who suffer from PMS have food cravings, especially for sweet foods. But after a sugar 'fix', they experience headaches, palpitations or fatigue. If these symptoms sound familiar, you could try eating small meals regularly to keep blood sugar levels stable. Finally, you should avoid alcohol, which exaggerates mood swings and behavioural changes.

DYSMENORRHOEA (PAINFUL PERIODS)

EAT PLENTY OF
- *Meat, wheatgerm and green leafy vegetables, for vitamin* B_6
- *Cold-pressed oils and eggs, for vitamin E*
- *Shellfish, nuts and dried fruit, for magnesium*

If painful periods start later in life they may have an underlying cause such as pelvic inflammatory disease, fibroids or endometriosis (the inflammation of the lining of the uterus), so it is wise to consult a doctor.

Painful periods often affect young women until their cycles settle down. Symptoms often ease after the birth of the first child or after going on the Pill. There is some evidence to suggest that vitamin B_6 and evening primrose oil can relieve symptoms. However the case for taking supplements is still unproven. Many women have found that increasing their intake of vitamins C and E, and the minerals calcium and magnesium can also help. This may be because the nutrients help to relax the walls of blood vessels, reducing cramping sensations.

Many foods, such as meat, whole grains, brewer's yeast and green leafy vegetables, contain vitamin B_6; while vitamin C is found in most fruits and vegetables. Vitamin E is found in cold-pressed oils, eggs, wheatgerm and sweet potatoes. Dairy products are rich in calcium, and shellfish and nuts are sources of magnesium.

AMENORRHOEA (MISSED PERIODS)

The most likely reason for a missed period is PREGNANCY. However, several other conditions result in missed or irregular periods, such as THYROID PROBLEMS, OBESITY and DIABETES. Exercising excessively, abrupt weight loss, emotional upheavals or severe stress, and even flying, can all interrupt the menstrual cycle. For example, amenorrhoea is a relatively common symptom of ANOREXIA NERVOSA, and it can also be a problem for young women athletes, especially distance runners and gymnasts.

Changing contraceptive pills, and low-dose mini-pills may also interfere with the normal menstrual pattern.

MENORRHAGIA (HEAVY PERIODS)

EAT PLENTY OF
- *Most meats, eggs and fish and other foods which supply iron*

Heavy periods tend to occur when girls first start menstruating or as the menopause approaches. They are also common in women who use the contraceptive IUD (coil). Intermittent bleeding throughout the month can have many causes, such as hormone imbalances or fibroids, so they should always be investigated by your doctor.

When women have heavy periods, they lose more blood than normal and can develop ANAEMIA. Even if you are not anaemic, it is sensible to eat plenty of iron-rich foods, the best sources are liver (but not if you are trying to conceive), kidneys and red meat.

Vegetarians can boost their iron intake by eating plenty of wholemeal bread, dark green leafy vegetables and dried fruits. Drinking diluted citrus fruit juices or eating fresh fruit with your meals is also helpful, because both contain vitamin C which the body needs to absorb iron.

METABOLIC DISORDERS

More than 3000 metabolic disorders sparked by enzyme defects can affect newborn babies, but fortunately most are extremely rare. Unless they are swiftly diagnosed and treated, however, any of these inherited diseases can lead to physical deformities or mental disorders. Only a few – including phenylketonuria (PKU), an inability to metabolise a vital amino acid – respond to treatment that involves following precise diets.

In Britain one in every 18000 babies is born with PKU – the most prevalent inherited metabolic disease. It is detected by the Guthrie test, which is performed on every infant in the first 6 to 14 days of life.

When the Guthrie test is positive, further checks for other possible enzyme defects are also carried out. As with most inherited metabolic diseases, the damaging effects of PKU can be reduced, or even prevented, if diagnosed and treated in time, though the underlying disorder will remain. PKU has been successfully treated for more than 20 years. However, if it is left untreated, it leads to severe mental retardation, convulsions, tremors, and reduced skin and hair pigmentation.

Treatment involves a diet that restricts the intake of the amino acid phenylalanine, which is found in many protein-containing foods as well as in the artificial sweetener aspartame. Because the amino acid is present in both breast milk and cow's milk, babies suffering from PKU are often fed on a special formula.

Other – and, fortunately, rarer – inherited metabolic diseases include:

Refsum's disease Caused by a defect in the enzyme systems responsible for the metabolism of phytanic acid, found in fish and dairy produce, Refsum's disease can manifest itself from the age of 4 to 20. Symptoms vary, but include night blindness and clumsy, uncoordinated movement. It is treated by a rigid diet designed to reduce or eliminate phytanic acid.

Maple-syrup urine disease This is a defect in the process of metabolising amino acids which are then excreted in urine which has an odour similar to that of maple syrup. The few children who survive are likely to suffer brain damage and must follow diets based on gelatine, gluten-free flour, butter, margarine, sugar and fruits.

Galactosaemia This disorder, caused by a defect in the body's ability to metabolise milk sugar (lactose) and its component galactose, can lead to the development of cataracts and eventual blindness as well as cirrhosis of the liver and mental and physical retardation. Treatment involves excluding milk sugar from the diet, so milks are specially treated. Only these specially treated milks can be used in food preparation and drinks.

Whenever these disorders are diagnosed sufferers should be referred to a specialist centre for treatment.

Migraine

TAKE PLENTY OF

- *Regular light meals to prevent a drop in blood sugar levels*
- *Ginger in cooking, or freshly grated with boiling water as a tea*
- *Oily fish such as salmon and mackerel*

AVOID

- *The four 'Cs': chocolate, cheese, citrus fruits and caffeine*
- *Alcohol, especially red wine and port*

Migraine is characterised by severe disabling HEADACHES. There are two types of migraine: the common type, or migraine without aura, typically accompanied by nausea, vomiting and visual disturbances; and migraine with aura, in which the attack is heralded by warning symptoms, such as flashing lights before the eyes.

Regular migraine sufferers try hard to identify possible 'triggers' for their attacks, such as food, hormones, the weather or stress. The most commonly cited dietary culprits include the four 'C' foods: chocolate, cheese, citrus fruits and caffeine. Alcoholic drinks, especially red wine and port, are frequently associated with migraine. Food ALLERGIES are also believed to precipitate migraine attacks.

A drop in the body's level of blood sugar may bring on an attack, so it is sensible for migraine sufferers to keep the level up by taking regular and fairly frequent light meals. Salmon, mackerel and other oily fish may help because they have a gentle anti-inflammatory action on the entire body; this is a long-term dietary change, and the benefit will not be experienced immediately, but after a period of two to three months.

Early warning signals of a migraine attack may include excessive hunger or thirst, exhaustion, or inexplicable mood swings. Then there may be an

Case study

Sally, a 30-year-old housewife, regularly suffered the debilitating blinding headaches associated with migraine. Invariably these attacks started with distorted vision, and a zigzag pattern in front of her eyes. This was followed within the hour by a severe headache which felt as if it came from behind her left eye; invariably, she vomited. Medication offered no real relief, but after several years she realised that her migraines occurred after she had eaten chocolate, or any food containing it. Sally has found that now she has eliminated chocolate from her diet, she no longer suffers from her migraine attacks.

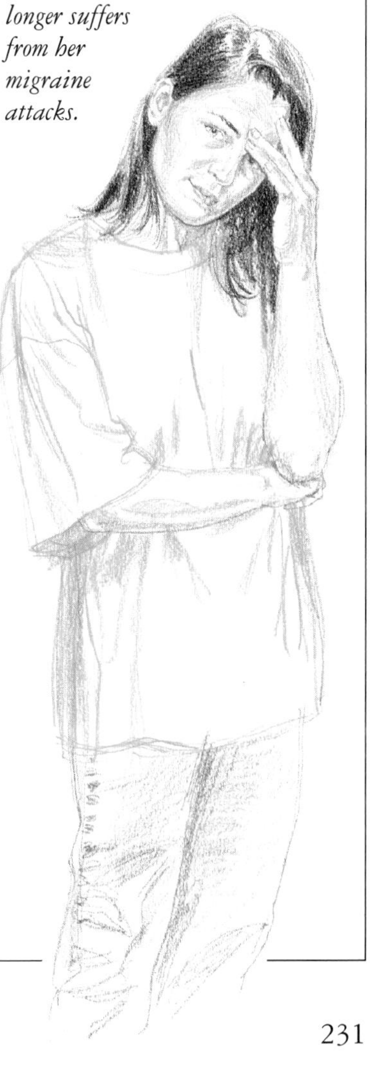

aura which alerts victims to an impending attack: a visual blind spot, flashing lights, zigzag patterns in front of the eyes and a dislike of bright light are all frequently cited.

These sensations may last from a few minutes to an hour, and may be followed by a severe, disabling headache, and often nausea and vomiting. Ginger, used in cooking or made into a tea by pouring boiling water over the freshly grated root, has been claimed by some alternative practitioners to help to relieve the nausea, and this has been backed up by some clinical trials.

Many migraine sufferers, however, do not experience visual disturbances: the characteristic violent throbbing headache of a 'common' migraine begins quite suddenly, with no warning. Attacks can last from a few hours to a few days, and are followed by a 'hangover' which usually leaves the sufferer feeling weary and washed out. To break the cycle of an attack, a hot compress on the nape of the neck, and a cold one – such as a wet flannel – on the forehead may sometimes help. Do not apply a hot compress, however, if you feel that heat may exacerbate the pain. Simply lying down on your back to stretch the joints and muscles, with a rolled up towel in the nape of the neck, is often a comfort.

The majority of migraine sufferers are women and, for many, attacks tend to coincide with menstruation which suggests a hormonal trigger. Another factor is stress, or more correctly, the aftermath of stress; Saturday morning migraines are a typical example. Despite these possible links, many attacks have no obvious trigger.

People who suffer from debilitating migraines regularly should seek medical treatment which usually involves taking prophylactic drugs that help to prevent recurrent attacks. An effective drug for halting an attack which has started is sumatriptan, in tablet form or, for more severe cases, as a self-administered injection. (This drug is, however, not suitable for pregnant women or heart patients.)

Herbal migraine relief

Feverfew is a herbal remedy for migraine; it cannot stop an attack which has already started but can help to reduce frequency, and in some cases prevent migraines occurring in the first place. Although feverfew is available in tablet form, alternative practitioners find the fresh leaves most effective: you can grow the plant on a window sill. A couple of leaves each day is the recommended dose, but eat them in a sandwich because nibbling on the raw leaves can cause mouth ulcers. Pregnant women should refrain from taking feverfew.

Soaking a towel or flannel in a cool infusion of feverfew, squeezing it out, and laying it across the forehead, may also be soothing.

MILK AND CREAM

BENEFITS

- *Provide high-quality protein*
- *Supply essential B vitamins as well as phosphorus and zinc*
- *Milk is an excellent source of calcium*

DRAWBACKS

- *Whole milk and especially cream are high in fat*
- *Unpasteurised milk is a relatively common cause of food poisoning*
- *Milk contains lactose, to which some people have an intolerance*

Few foods are more nourishing than milk. The calcium it supplies is easily absorbed; it is an important source of protein and provides other minerals and important vitamins. Pint for pint, skimmed milk contains half the calories of whole milk but retains most of the nutrients. In fact, because the fat is removed, skimmed milk contains slightly increased levels of the water-soluble B vitamins and minerals.

Both skimmed and whole milk contribute valuable amounts of thiamin (vitamin B_1), riboflavin (vitamin B_2), niacin and vitamins B_6 and B_{12}; they also supply phosphorus and zinc.

Fat-soluble vitamin A is lost when cream is skimmed off whole milk and must then be obtained from other food sources. Neither skimmed nor whole milk supply iron or the vitamins C or D, other than in trace amounts.

The benefits of goat's milk

Goat's milk is available in many supermarkets. It is nutritionally similar to cow's milk and can be used in the same ways.

It makes a good alternative for those who have an intolerance of cow's milk, such as children with eczema. And sufferers of gastric ulcers often find goat's milk easier to digest and lighter on the stomach. Goat's milk also freezes well.

BUILDING HEALTHY BONES

Milk is particularly important as a source of dietary calcium; most of the other nutrients it contains are easily obtained from other foods. Calcium ensures healthy strong bones and forms part of the structure of the teeth.

An adult requires a daily intake of about 700mg, which is contained in around 600ml (1 pint) of whole milk. However, calcium needs vary according to age and sex. Breast-feeding mothers need the most – 1250mg daily, or as much as would be obtained from drinking about 1 litre (1¾ pints) of milk.

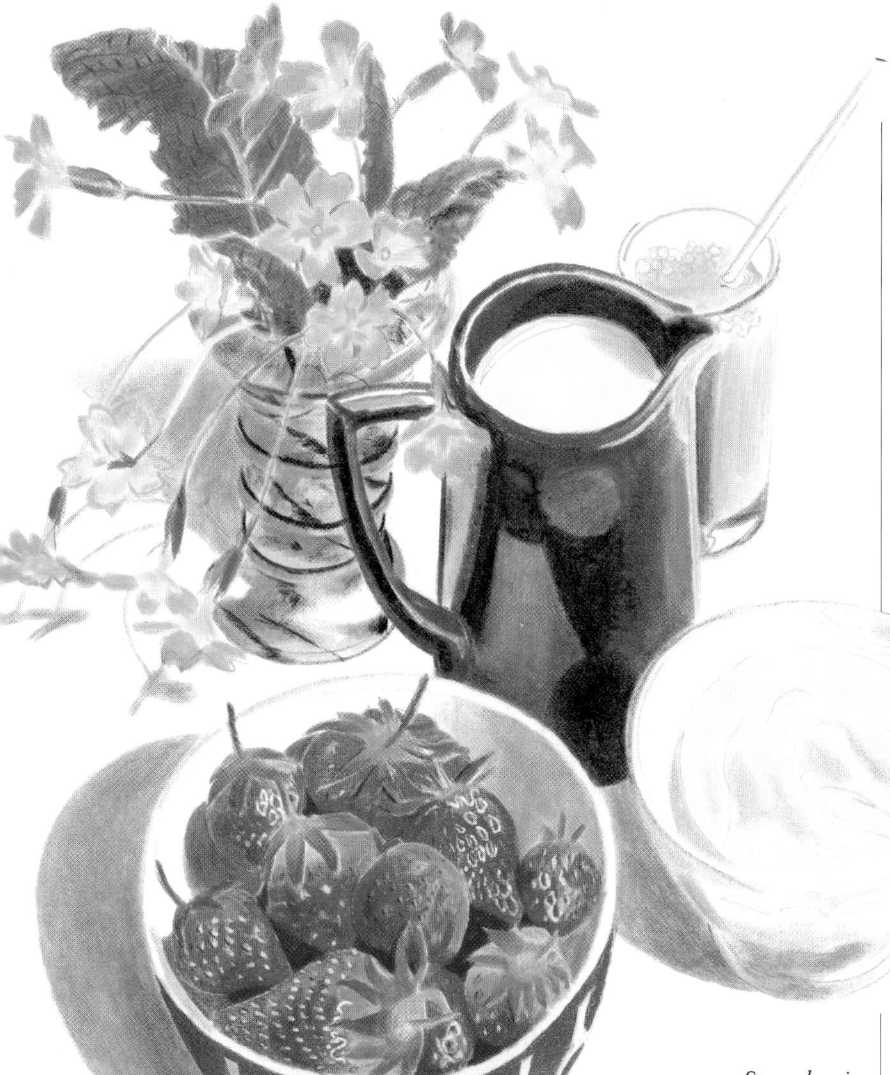

SUMMER TREATS *Strawberries and cream provide vitamins B and C. Milk shakes make fun and nutritious drinks for children, especially when made with fresh fruit.*

They are followed by teenagers who require a daily intake of between 800mg and 1000mg. Low calcium consumption in childhood and adolescence may result in less than optimal stores of the mineral (which the body normally builds up in the skeleton until the age of about 30). This may contribute to OSTEOPOROSIS in later life.

Only tinned sardines and pilchards eaten with their bones offer more calcium, weight for weight, than milk. However, an average 200ml (⅓ pint) glass of milk provides about 230mg of calcium compared with the average 70g (2½oz) portions of pilchards and sardines which provide 210mg and 385mg respectively.

Those who cannot tolerate lactose (milk sugar), or vegans who reject all dairy products, must find their calcium from other food sources, such as vegetables, pulses and nuts. The calcium from these foods is absorbed less efficiently than it is from milk.

Milk contains useful amounts of phosphorus, which is also essential for the formation of strong bones. Since vitamin B_{12} is normally obtained from foods of animal origin, milk is a valuable source of this vital nutrient for vegetarians. However, B_{12} is destroyed by boiling milk. Vegans have to take supplements or eat fortified foods.

The traditional pint of full-cream milk, now being replaced by 500ml cartons, is on average 3.9 per cent fat. Skimmed milk, however, contains only 0.1 per cent fat. It also supplies only half the energy value – there are 330 Calories per 500ml of whole milk, compared with 165 for skimmed; semi-skimmed milk, on average 1.6 per cent fat, contains 230 Calories. While skimmed milk is suitable for adults and slimmers, it should not be given to children under the age of five because of its low calorie, fat and vitamin A content.

TREATING MILK

Almost all milk that is sold in developed countries has been pasteurised by heating to kill off bacteria. The flavour is less affected than when milk is sterilised – a longer process using higher temperatures (up to 115°-130°C, or 239°-266°F, for 10-30 minutes) – which results in a cooked taste, a creamy colour, and the loss of about a third of the thiamin and half of the vitamin B_{12}. UHT (ultra-heat treated) or long-life milk has been heated to not less than 132°C (270°F) for at least one second. The ultra-heat treatment improves the milk's keeping quality but it has less of an adverse effect on its taste and nutritional value.

Homogenised milk is pasteurised first, and then has its cream distributed throughout so that it does not separate. Dried whole-milk powder contains all the nutrients of whole milk except thiamin and vitamin B_{12}. Dried skimmed-milk powder does not contain fat or any fat-soluble vitamins, but it does provide protein, calcium, zinc, riboflavin and vitamin B_{12}. Condensed milk supplies useful amounts of calcium, phosphorus and zinc, but its high sugar content makes it an unsuitable substitute for fresh milk.

LOW-FAT LUXURIES

A wide range of highly nutritious dairy products, which contain many of the nutrients but not the fat or calories of whole milk, is now available.

Fromage frais is much like natural yoghurt, but is less acidic, with a creamy taste ideal for topping baked potatoes. It can be used in dips as a healthy substitute for full-fat cream and mayonnaise. Fromage frais is widely available as a dessert with added fruit and other flavourings. According to brand and type, the fat content can vary – from 7 per cent to as little as 0.2 per cent – so read the label.

Quark is slightly coarser and more acidic than fromage frais. It is virtually fat-free, but cream may be added for a milder flavour and smoother texture.

Buttermilk is made from low-fat milk with added bacterial cultures to thicken it and to sharpen the taste. It is similar in nutritional value to skimmed milk, with less than 0.5 per cent fat. It is often used for baking and in low-fat spreads.

Smetana (or smatana) is a cultured product with a sharp taste suitable for both sweet and savoury dishes. Its 10 per cent fat content is not strictly 'low' but it makes a fair substitute for soured cream, which is 20 per cent fat.

NAUGHTY BUT NICE

All the different types of cream available supply useful amounts of vitamin A, calcium and phosphorus. But they are also high in saturated fat – the fat content varies from 13 per cent for half cream to 64 per cent for clotted cream – so use them sparingly.

Single cream will not whip, and contains 19 per cent fat. Double cream is thicker, contains 48 per cent fat and can be whipped. When it is homogenised to make it 'extra thick' it contains no more fat but will not whip easily. Whipping cream is lower in fat than double cream and can be whipped to about twice its original volume. Sour cream is made by culturing single cream with lactic acid-producing bacteria, to give it a tangy flavour.

Clotted cream is heated to just below boiling point, then cooled. Just two tablespoons contain more calories and almost twice the fat of 300ml (½ pint) of whole milk. (See also BUTTER, CHEESE and YOGHURT.)

Milk, nature's 'complete food'

Milk is sold in many different guises. It is useful to be able to compare the benefits and drawbacks of different products, for example their calorie and fat content. The calorie figures used in this chart are for 100ml (3½fl oz).

TYPE	CALORIES	FAT (%)	DID YOU KNOW?
Whole milk	66	3.9	Whole milk is known as a 'complete food' because it contains such a wide range of nutrients, especially protein, calcium, zinc, and vitamins A, B_2 (riboflavin) and B_{12}. It also has useful amounts of iodine, niacin and vitamin B_6.
Semi-skimmed milk	46	1.6	Like all milk sold in bottles, semi-skimmed milk can lose more than half its vitamin B_2 (riboflavin) if it is left in sunlight for an hour or two, as well as the small amount of vitamin C it contains.
Skimmed milk	33	0.1	Skimmed milk has half the calories of whole milk, but its vitamin (except vitamin A) and mineral content is just as high. Both skimmed and semi-skimmed milk can be frozen for up to a month, while whole milk tends to separate.
Condensed milk	333	10.1	Condensed milk is very nutritious, containing almost three times as much calcium as whole milk, but sugar makes up more than half its volume.
Single cream	198	19.1	Single cream and half cream will separate if they are frozen and will not mix again.
Whipping cream	373	39.3	Whipping cream is relatively high in fat, but once whipped, it appears to be light because half of it is air. Whipped cream can be frozen for two months.
Double cream	449	48.0	Double cream can be used for pouring, whipping and cooking. It can also be frozen for two months. Extra-thick double cream does not whip well.
Clotted cream	586	63.5	Clotted cream is not recommended for cooking – it tends to separate when heated. It can be frozen for up to a month, after which it may become buttery.

MINERALS

See page 236

MISCARRIAGE

To minimise the risk of miscarriage:

EAT PLENTY OF

- *Complex carbohydrates such as wholemeal bread and pasta*
- *Fresh fruit and vegetables, which provide fibre, vitamin C and folate*
- *Milk and dairy products*
- *Meat, fish, pulses, nuts and seeds*
- *Oily fish and seed oils, for essential fatty acids and polyunsaturates*

AVOID

- *Soft-rinded cheeses and unpasteurised dairy products*
- *Liver and liver products such as pâté*
- *Alcohol and cigarettes*
- *Herbal medicines and all drugs except under medical supervision*

The medical definition of a miscarriage is the expulsion of the foetus before the 24th week of PREGNANCY. Miscarriages are far more common than most people realise; it is thought that about three-quarters of all human conceptions do not result in the birth of a live baby. Often these miscarriages happen so early that the woman does not even know she is pregnant, but just seems to be having a heavier or later period than normal.

DIET BEFORE CONCEPTION

Potential parents should try to get fit before conception. Healthy babies tend to be produced by healthy parents who are neither markedly underweight nor overweight.

Both parents should eat a nutritious, balanced diet, make every effort to give up or cut down on smoking and ALCOHOL. Some form of regular exercise is also very important. Current thinking suggests that these lifestyle changes should be made at least three months – and preferably six months – before a baby is conceived.

ALCOHOL AND SMOKING

To increase the chances of a healthy baby, it is best to avoid all toxic substances. In women, alcohol is at its most dangerous in the earliest stages of pregnancy when foetal cells are dividing very rapidly. Unfortunately, this is when a woman is least likely to be aware of her pregnancy. It is therefore safest for women to avoid alcohol from the moment conception is planned.

Women who smoke have a higher risk of miscarrying and of their baby being underweight or even having a birth defect. But if a woman is an addictive smoker, her doctor may advise that the stress caused by trying to give up during pregnancy would be more harmful to her and her baby's well-being than continuing to smoke a few cigarettes. In these circumstances, pregnant women may find it useful to go to an anti-smoking organisation which helps people to give up.

DIET DURING PREGNANCY

It is generally accepted that a nutritionally poor diet during pregnancy increases the likelihood of miscarriage. During the first three months of pregnancy, when foetal cells are beginning to develop into rudimentary organs, the quality rather than the quantity of the mother's food is particularly important. Because at this stage the growing foetus is so tiny, a much larger calorie intake is not required.

What is needed is good nutrition: if the foetus lacks essential nutrients it may not develop properly and may be spontaneously aborted. A balanced diet should include plenty of foods which contain complex carbohydrates such as wholemeal bread, pasta and green vegetables; these supply energy, iron and zinc. Milk provides calcium, vitamins and protein, while lean meat, fish, eggs, pulses, nuts and seeds provide protein, iron, B vitamins and zinc. Oily fish and vegetable oils are good sources of essential fatty acids, and fresh fruit and vegetables will supply fibre, vitamin C and folate.

Keep to fresh, natural foods, and try to cut down on refined carbohydrates which may contain large amounts of sugar and saturated fats.

FOODS TO AVOID

Listeriosis, caused by the food-borne bacterium, *Listeria monocytogenes*, is a rare but serious infection. Should a woman become infected during pregnancy it could lead to miscarriage, stillbirth or severe illness in her newborn baby. High-risk foods include soft-rinded cheeses (such as Brie, and Camembert) and pâté – which should be avoided during pregnancy. Ensure that all meat, poultry and eggs are cooked thoroughly (to kill bacteria). Pregnant women and those trying to conceive should avoid liver as it is high in vitamin A, excessive amounts of which can cause birth defects.

Some studies suggest that caffeine (in coffee, tea and chocolate) should be restricted but many doctors advise that moderate amounts are harmless.

SUPPLEMENTS

The Department of Health advises that women should take a supplement of folic acid at least three months before conception and up to 12 weeks into pregnancy at a rate of 0.4mg per day. The link between a lack of folic acid and neural tube defects (such as spina bifida) is now well established; foetuses which develop such defects are more likely to miscarry. Many doctors prescribe supplements of iron and folic acid during the latter part of pregnancy to prevent anaemia. Most drugs and herbal medicines should be avoided during pregnancy.

MINERALS: VITAL NUTRIENTS ESSENTIAL FOR LIFE

We need a wide range of minerals to be healthy and we need them the right amounts. They strengthen bones and teeth, maintain a healthy immune system, and help vitamins to do their work.

Although the Western diet has improved in terms of nutrition over the last few decades, deficiencies in certain minerals, such as zinc, calcium or iron, are still relatively common. Nevertheless, fewer than two in every hundred people in Europe and North America are thought to suffer from deficiency-related illness.

Scientists have identified 16 minerals as being essential if the body is to function properly. For a mineral to be considered essential, it must perform at least one function vital to life, growth or reproduction. All told, these minerals make up only 3-4 per cent of the weight of the human body. Macrominerals, such as calcium, magnesium, sodium and potassium, are required in comparatively large quantities. Microminerals, such as iron and zinc, are needed in much smaller amounts; and some, such as selenium, magnesium and iodine, are required in such minuscule amounts that they are known as 'trace elements'.

The levels of some minerals found in foods often depend on the amounts present in the soil where plants were grown or animals grazed.

Various nutrients affect the body's ability to absorb minerals: vitamin D, for example, is essential for the uptake of calcium absorption; and foods which supply vitamin C help the body to absorb iron, particularly non-haem iron, which is found in plant foods as opposed to foods of animal origin. Other food components such as tannin (found in tea), or phytic acid (found in wheat bran and brown rice) can inhibit the absorption of calcium, iron and zinc. The body can maintain its own mineral balance over short periods. If the intake of minerals is low, it draws from stores laid down in the muscles, the liver and even the bones. If a mineral intake is too high, any excess is usually excreted so that there is little danger of the body being harmed, except by the overuse of supplements.

ALUMINIUM

While most minerals pose little threat to health, aluminium may be an important exception. Trace amounts of the mineral are found in all living organisms. However, scientists are still not sure if it has any biological function in the body. The mineral

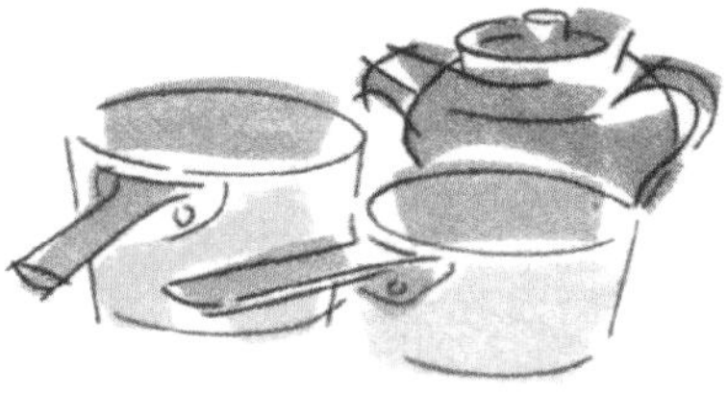

makes up some 8 per cent of the Earth's crust, yet plants – with the exception of tea – take up remarkably little of it from the soil. Most of the aluminium taken in by the human body is excreted rather than absorbed; the claim that excessive amounts in the diet can cause brain damage – and may exacerbate disorders such as ALZHEIMER'S DISEASE – remains contentious.

Aluminium is added to table salt to prevent the grains sticking together. Low levels of aluminium can also occur in tap WATER, because aluminium sulphate is used in its purification. Aluminium hydroxide is an ingredient in many antacid tablets used to treat indigestion, and the mineral may also be released into acidic foods, such as pickles or stewed fruit, which have been cooked in aluminium pans.

CALCIUM

A range of foods from milk and cheese, to sardines (eaten with their bones) and dark green leafy vegetables, contain calcium. It is a vital component of bones and teeth, which contain some 99 per cent of the body's total calcium. The other 1 per cent plays an equally important role in the body, both in cell structure and function, as well as in the blood, where it aids clotting.

Because of the body's natural regulatory systems, excessive calcium in the blood occurs rarely and only as a result of disease or through overuse of vitamin D supplements. If, however, the body needs more calcium than is supplied by the diet, it withdraws it from the bones.

During pregnancy, absorption of dietary calcium increases, so that no extra intake is necessary if the woman eats a balanced diet. The daily calcium requirement of 700mg could be supplied by three slices of Cheddar cheese and two glasses of milk, for example. However, pregnant women should avoid excessive intakes of tea, coffee, wheat bran and salt which either inhibit calcium absorption or promote

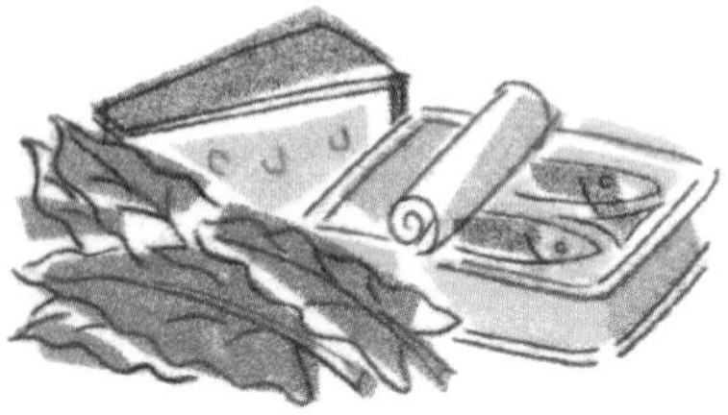

its excretion. Foods that contain oxalic acid, such as spinach and rhubarb, can also prevent the absorption of calcium.

Calcium is needed for the smooth functioning of nerves and muscles: supplements are used to treat muscle cramps, and problems of the back and bones related to ageing, such as ARTHRITIS, RHEUMATISM and OSTEOPOROSIS (the loss of bony tissue that results in brittle bones, particularly prevalent among post-menopausal women). Calcium deficiency often results from a lack of vitamin D and can lead to rickets in children – with the typical symptoms of bow legs, knock-knees and pigeon chests – caused by softening of the bones. In adults it can cause OSTEOMALACIA, characterised by aching bones, muscle spasms and curvature of the spine.

Chloride

This mineral acts with potassium and sodium to maintain the body's fluid and electrolyte balance. The highest concentrations of chloride in the body are found in cerebrospinal fluid and in digestive juices in the stomach. The main dietary source of chloride is table salt (sodium chloride). So if salt intake is restricted, chloride levels may drop. When dietary intake is low, the kidneys can reabsorb chloride efficiently, so a dietary deficiency rarely occurs. Excessive chloride losses can occur in the same way as sodium loss: through sweating, diarrhoea and vomiting.

Chromium

An adequate supply of chromium is particularly important in a diabetic's diet; as a vital link in the chain which makes glucose available to the body. Chromium increases the effectiveness of insulin by stimulating glucose uptake in cells. It also helps to control levels of fat and CHOLESTEROL in the blood. A deficiency of the mineral can lead to high blood cholesterol levels.

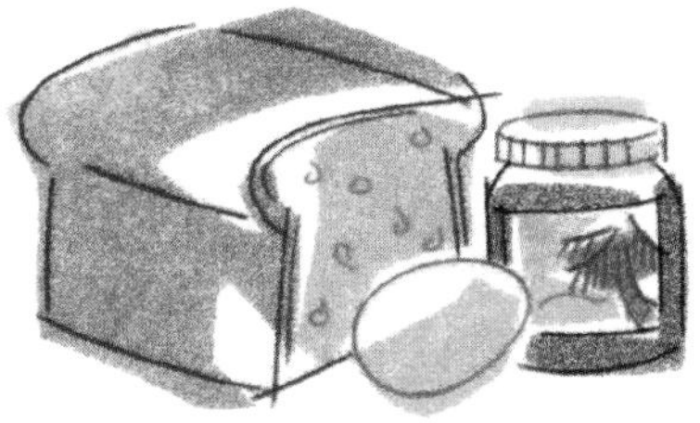

Good sources of chromium include brewer's yeast, wholegrain cereals, egg yolks, cheese and molasses.

Copper

A component of many enzymes, such as superoxide dismutase which helps to protect against FREE RADICAL damage, copper is vital in forming connective tissue, which supports and separates organs and is found in tendons, cartilage and bone. Copper is important for the growth of healthy bones and helps the body to absorb iron from food; a lack of copper can lead to iron-deficiency ANAEMIA because the mineral helps to make stored iron available for red blood cell production. Copper is also involved in the formation of melanin, the pigment which colours skin and hair. Liver, shellfish, cocoa, nuts and mushrooms

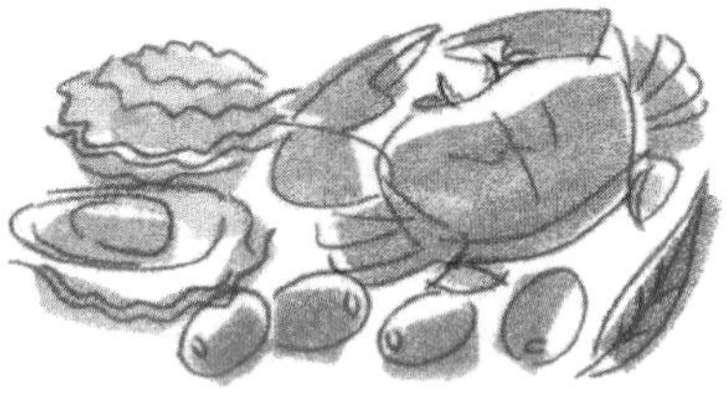

are all sources of the mineral, which is widely, but unevenly, distributed in foods. Deficiency is rare, usually occurring only in premature babies, infants who are malnourished or who suffer from chronic diarrhoea, or those with malabsorption problems.

Fluoride

Although a lack of fluoride can lead to childhood tooth decay, too much – either in the diet or from other sources such as swallowed toothpaste, tea and fluoridated tap water – can be harmful, causing fluorosis with its unsightly symptoms of mottled teeth with pitted enamel. Fluorosis may also cause excess bone formation, resulting in bones which are much denser than normal, but also less flexible – making them prone to fractures.

Although fluoride is not essential for life, it does play a role in the maintenance of healthy bones: fluoride combines with calcium to strengthen them. A deficiency, when associated with low intakes of calcium, may lead to osteoporosis. An adequate intake of fluoride, particularly in childhood,

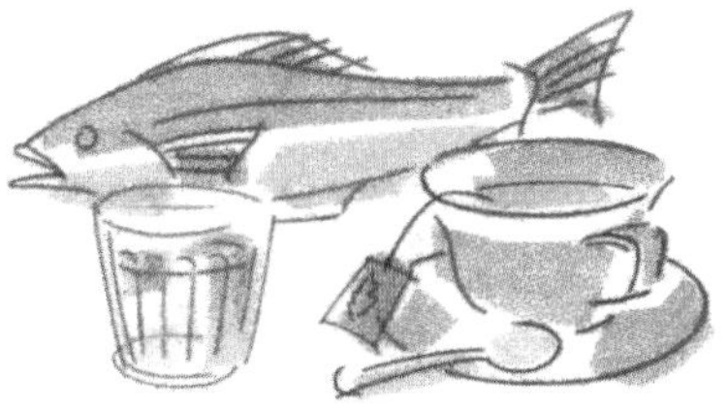

undoubtedly helps to prevent tooth decay. Levels of the mineral in drinking WATER vary from area to area, depending on the geology and source. Some water companies add extra fluoride to their supplies. Where levels are higher than 0.03 micrograms per litre (or more than 0.3 parts per million), children under two years old should not be given fluoride supplements. (Your local water authority can tell you if the supply is fluoridated.)

Differing levels of fluoride occur naturally in soils and affect the amounts found in crops, and in the meat of grazing animals. In Britain, tea is the main source of dietary fluoride as tea plants readily absorb the mineral from the soil. People who drink a lot of tea made with fluoridated water may have a high dietary intake.

Iodine

To many people, iodine and the smell of the sea are synonymous – and understandably so, for fish, seafood, seaweed, and the sea itself are the best sources of iodide, the mineral salt which derives from iodine. Fruit, vegetables and cereals also supply dietary iodine, but the amounts depend on the levels of the mineral in the soil where they are grown. Similarly, the meat and milk of grazing animals may also be a source.

Iodine is needed to make THYROID hormones which not only govern the

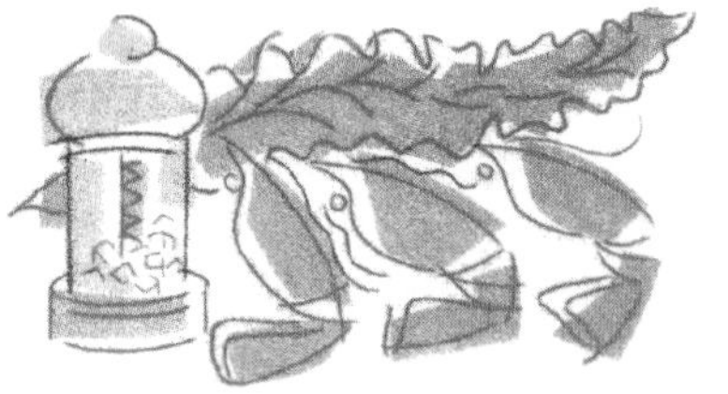

rate and efficiency at which food is converted into energy, but also regulate physical and mental development.

Mild iodine deficiency leads to a slightly enlarged thyroid gland (or goitre) and is most likely to occur in women of reproductive age. It is easily prevented by using iodised salt or eating seaweed, fish or seafood. Women with a severe iodine deficiency are at risk of bearing children deficient in thyroid hormone, who could suffer from a form of retardation known as cretinism unless treated from birth with thyroxine.

Coarsening of the hair and skin are often physical indications of hypothyroidism. This is not due to iodine deficiency, but is caused by the body developing antibodies against its own thyroid gland. Symptoms of this condition may include drowsiness, apathy extreme sensitivity to cold and muscle weakness as well as weight increase. Excessive intakes of iodine can cause hyperthyroidism.

IRON

Haemoglobin, the pigment in red blood cells which carries oxygen, via the bloodstream, around the body, cannot be produced without iron. A shortage of the mineral will quickly show itself in breathlessness, as the heart pumps faster and the lungs try to increase the body's oxygen intake. Iron is also required for the manufacture of myoglobin, a similar pigment which stores oxygen in muscles.

Iron-containing enzymes assist in the conversion of beta carotene (found in many deeply pigmented plant foods such as carrots, red peppers, apricots and cantaloupe melons) into the active form of vitamin A.

Other iron-containing enzymes are needed for the synthesis of DNA and RNA, and for the synthesis of collagen, which is essential for healthy gums, teeth, cartilage and bones.

Men and women have different requirements for iron. Indeed, women, from the onset of monthly periods until the menopause, need almost twice as much dietary iron as men. Lack of adequate dietary iron over a long period can result in iron deficiency ANAEMIA; symptoms may include chronic infections of the ears, gums and skin, excessive tiredness and lack of stamina, as well as a pale complexion. Strict vegetarians are often at risk from this type of anaemia.

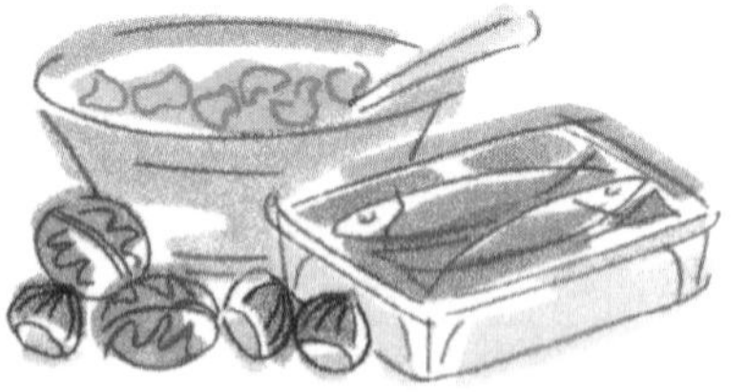

Offal, particularly liver and kidneys, is the best source of iron, although liver should not be eaten by women who are pregnant or trying to conceive because of the danger of excessive vitamin A intake. Iron is also found in other meats, sardines, egg yolks and dark green leafy vegetables.

About 25 per cent of the iron in meat (haem iron) is absorbed by the body, whereas people may absorb less than 10 per cent of the non-haem iron from plant sources such as vegetables, dried fruits, wholegrain bread or iron-fortified breakfast cereals. However, more of the iron from plant sources is absorbed if they are accompanied by food or drinks – such as peppers or orange juice – that contain vitamin C.

Iron poisoning is rare, possibly occurring most commonly in children who have found and eaten iron supplements, mistaking them for sweets. Others at risk from iron poisoning are people with haemochromatosis, a genetically inherited disorder which affects about 3 people in every 1000. In rare instances, the accumulation of iron in the body over a long period causes a form of iron poisoning called siderosis. This condition can be a result of numerous repeated blood transfusions, and has also been associated with long-term regular drinking of alcoholic drinks brewed in iron vats. Siderosis is characterised by a distinctive greyness of the skin.

If iron toxicity is suspected, seek advice from your doctor. Neither diets nor any particular foods are known to help the problem, although some experts suggest that giving a pint of blood weekly should help to reduce the levels of iron in the blood.

LEAD

The effects of long-term exposure to lead are insidious, and ingestion by mouth or from petrol exhaust fumes has been linked with behavioural problems and poor learning ability among children.

In older houses water supplies may be affected by lead from pipes, particularly in areas where the water is very soft. Even if the pipework in your house is made from copper, it may have been joined with lead solder. Water can absorb lead simply by standing in lead pipes overnight. The levels can therefore be significantly reduced if you allow the tap to run for a minute or two each morning before the water is used. And because lead dissolves more easily in hot water than in cold, always draw water for cooking – even for boiling potatoes – from the cold tap. Mains water should also be used both for drinking cold and for boiling to make tea or coffee.

MAGNESIUM

Magnesium's main role is as a constituent of bone. It assists in the transmission of nerve impulses and is also important for muscle contraction. It is an essential cofactor for about 90 enzymes which will function properly only when magnesium is present. Two such enzymes – cocarboxylase and coenzyme A – are involved in extracting energy from food.

Magnesium deficiency is rare, but diabetics, and people suffering from malabsorption syndromes, COELIAC DISEASE and some forms of kidney disease may have low body stores of the

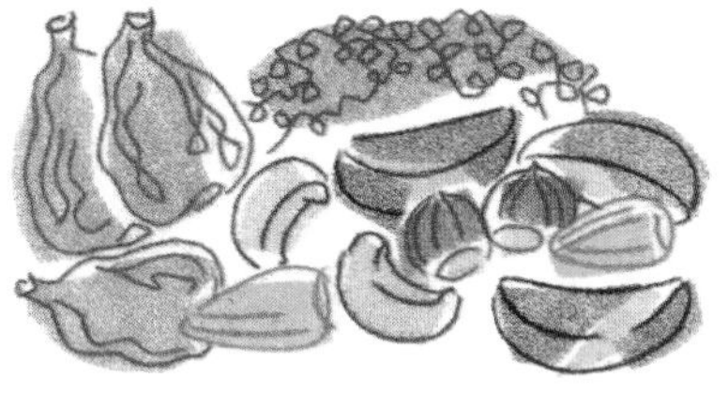

mineral. Levels may also be reduced in the short term when illness causes severe diarrhoea. This can lead to muscle twitching (tetany) or convulsions. Some studies in France have investigated a possible link between magnesium deficiency and cardiac arrhythmias (irregular heartbeat), but the link has yet to be proven in clinical trials. The body is very efficient at regulating magnesium levels. Usually, any intake of more than 2g a day is excreted unabsorbed. On the other hand, where dietary levels of the mineral are low, the intestine will absorb almost all of it, while at the same time the kidneys will conserve it more efficiently. Magnesium is found in a range of foods, and a reasonable balanced diet should provide all that the body needs. Important dietary sources are wholegrain cereals, dried figs, nuts, pulses and green leafy vegetables.

MANGANESE

Like many of the other microminerals, manganese has a broad range of functions. It is essential for activating

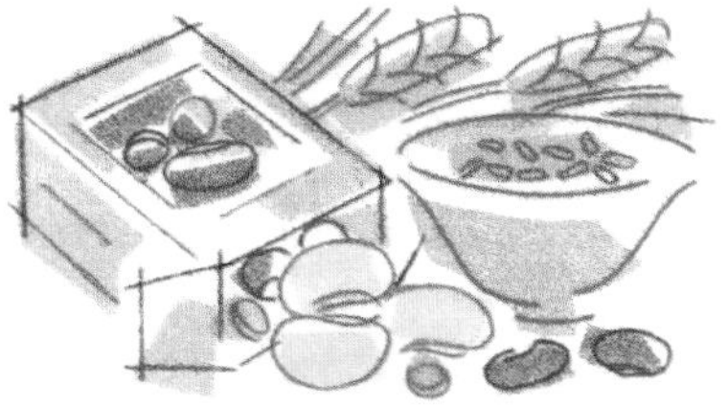

many enzyme systems – particularly those involved in the synthesis of cartilage. It is also a constituent of certain enzymes involved in the protection of tissues from FREE RADICAL damage. It is necessary to both thyroid hormone and sex hormone production, and is important in the manufacturing of cholesterol and in insulin production. It is also needed for storing glucose in the liver and for healthy bone growth.

The levels of manganese found in food – mainly in plant foods – depend on the amounts in the soil on which they are produced, but nuts, brown rice, wholegrain bread, pulses and cereals are particularly good sources.

Manganese deficiency is unknown in humans, although when artificially induced in laboratory animals it results in bone deformities. There are no documented health dangers from excess manganese in the diet.

MERCURY

Mercury is very poisonous, and long-term exposure to it causes brain damage: indeed, the expression 'mad as a hatter' dates from the 19th century when hatters used mercury salts to blacken top hats. Mercury has no essential function in the body. Apart from causing serious damage to the brain, excess mercury harms the colon and kidneys, and can lead to birth defects, loss of teeth, nerve degeneration and muscle tremors.

Recent concern that dental amalgams containing mercury could be harmful have been dismissed by the majority of doctors and dentists. In spite of claims that the material used in fillings was insoluble, some dentists have, nevertheless, gone on to develop mercury-free amalgams.

As little as 100mg of mercuric chloride can cause poisoning, but this is 200 times the amount contained in the average daily diet. However, shellfish – which have an exceptional capacity for accumulating mercury and cadmium – taken from contaminated waters off the shores of industrial countries, may contain dangerously high levels. Most countries have rigorous standards concerning permitted levels for heavy metals in fish and shellfish. The levels are routinely monitored and pose no risk, so there should now be no need to worry about the presence of heavy metals in tinned fish.

MOLYBDENUM

Without molybdenum many enzymes would not be able to carry out their function properly. For example, it is

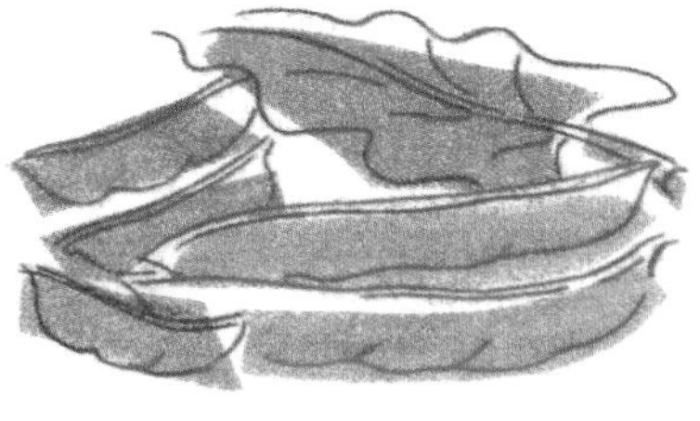

essential to the enzymes involved in the production of DNA and RNA, as well as those which are involved in producing energy from fat and in releasing iron from the body's stores. It is also needed for the production of uric acid. Molybdenum is found in tooth enamel, and it is possible that it may help to prevent tooth decay.

Liver is one of the best sources of molybdenum; it is also found in many plant foods, but the amount depends upon how much is present in the soil.

Required in only trace amounts in the diet, a deficiency of this mineral is virtually unknown. In rare cases it might be caused by an excessive intake of copper, when irregular heartbeats and reduced uric acid production may occur. Excessive intakes are also rare, but a high incidence of gout has been found in parts of Armenia where the soil is rich in molybdenum. High intakes of the mineral may also cause increased loss of copper in the urine.

PHOSPHORUS

Phosphorus compounds (phosphates) are major constituents in the tissues of all plant and animal cells. As much as

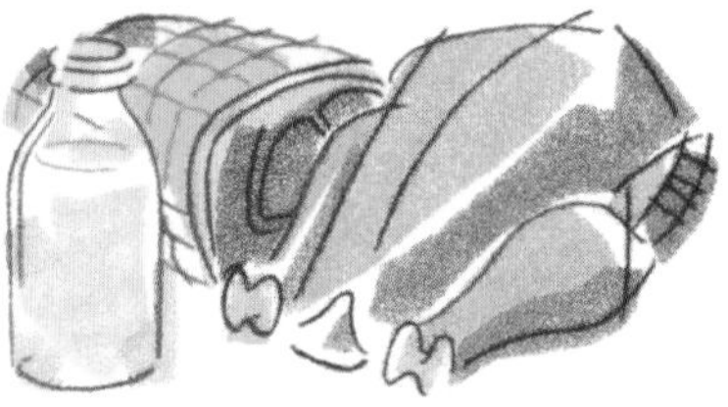

four-fifths of the body's phosphorus is found in the structure of bones and teeth – so although the process of laying down bone tissue is known as calcification, it actually involves large amounts of phosphate as well as calcium, and may be more accurately called 'mineralisation'. Phosphorus is essential to the release of energy in cells, and to the absorption and transportation of many nutrients. It also regulates the activity of proteins.

Phosphorus deficiency is rare, not only because the mineral is present in all plant and animal protein but because phosphates are added to cola-type drinks – to regulate acidity – and to processed meats and frozen poultry to retain moisture and so improve its texture. However, a deficiency can sometimes occur as a result of prolonged use of antacids.

The intake of phosphorus has an important influence on the body's calcium status: if there is too much phosphorus, calcium absorption may be reduced. High intakes of phosphorus increase the body's secretion of parathyroid hormone, which may upset the body's calcium balance by removing calcium from the bones – increasing the risk of OSTEOPOROSIS. The crucial factor is the balance, or ratio, between calcium and phosphorus in the body. This is usually easy for the body to maintain because foods rich in calcium tend also to be good sources of phosphorus.

A calcium-phosphorus imbalance can be triggered, however, by diets high in refined foods or fats, because these diets tend not only to be low in calcium, but may also contain large amounts of phosphorus. An excessive intake of phosphorus can also inhibit magnesium absorption.

POTASSIUM

Cells, nerves and muscles of the body would not function properly without potassium. It works with sodium to maintain the fluid and electrolyte balance in cells and tissues, to regulate blood pressure and to maintain a normal heartbeat. It helps to counteract the effects of excess sodium intake, such as oedema (fluid retention) and high BLOOD PRESSURE. It is also vital to the transmission of nerve impulses.

Blood potassium levels are carefully regulated by hormones and any excess intake normally acts as a diuretic, stimulating the kidneys to expel waste by producing more urine. However, people with kidney disease are unable to get rid of excess potassium, so they should avoid a high dietary intake of the mineral. This is because excessive levels of potassium in the blood can cause heart failure by inhibiting heart muscle contraction. Other symptoms of excess potassium are lethargy, paralysis and a slow heartbeat. Early signs of potassium deficiency are apathy, weakness, confusion and excessive thirst. It

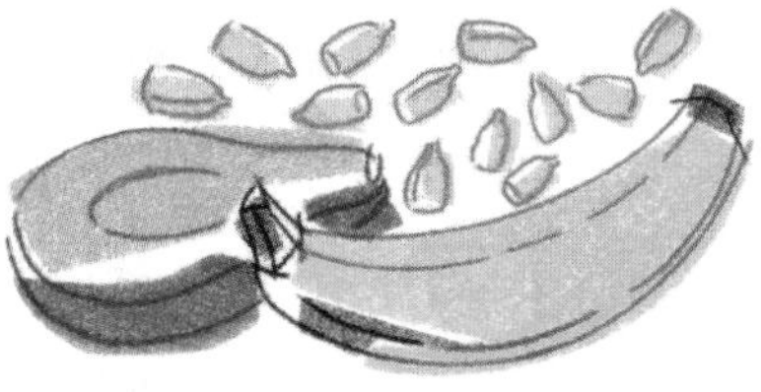

may also cause an abnormal heartbeat as well as other heart problems, and breathing difficulties.

Potassium is found in most plant foods, but especially good sources include avocados, nuts and seeds, pulses, whole grains, dried fruit, tomatoes, potatoes and fresh fruit – particularly bananas and oranges.

SELENIUM

Selenium (an ANTIOXIDANT mineral) is part of the enzyme, glutathione peroxidase, which is involved in protecting the body tissues against free radical damage. It also regulates the production of prostaglandins.

Without this mineral, normal growth and fertility would not occur, the liver would not function normally, and important hormone production would not take place. It has recently been discovered, for example, that

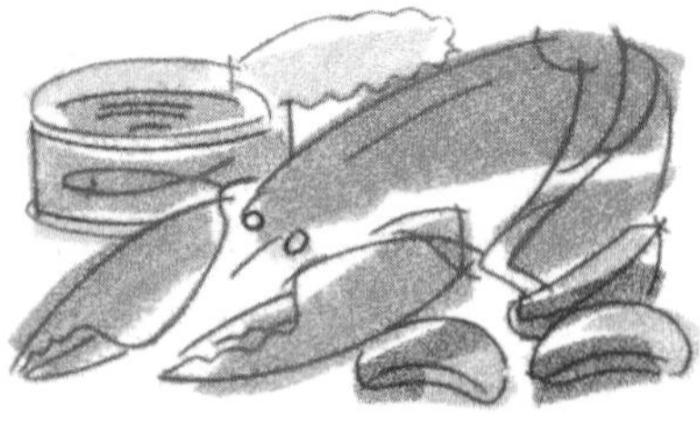

selenium is necessary for the formation of the active form of thyroid hormone. Its presence in the body is essential for healthy hair and skin and it is also needed to maintain normal eyesight.

As with many of the other microminerals, selenium levels in food are related to the amounts in the soil where it is grown. In some parts of the world, such as New Zealand, soil levels are so low that deficiencies are quite common, and the diet in the United Kingdom contains only just adequate amounts of this nutrient. In parts of China, Keshan disease, caused by selenium deficiency, is endemic: it tends to affect young children in whom it causes heart failure. Excessive intake of selenium is extremely rare, and there is little or no risk from the mineral in a normal well-balanced diet.

Selenium is found in offal and other meats, fish and shellfish, dairy products – especially butter – citrus fruit, avocado pears and whole grains.

SODIUM

Salt – or sodium chloride – was the first mineral identified as forming part of our diets – probably because it is easily detected by the taste-buds. Sodium is a major component of all body fluids and it is largely responsible for determining the body's total water content. Together with potassium, it is a key substance in regulating the balance of body fluids; for example, it controls the levels of electrolytes in blood plasma. Sodium also helps to regulate nerve and muscle function.

Most of the sodium in our diets occurs in the form of common table salt or sodium chloride. As sodium nitrite it is used in preserving ham, bacon, sausages and salamis, and it is also the main ingredient of monosodium glutamate, an additive used to enhance the flavour of many commercially produced foods.

Sodium deficiency is rare because salt is found in so many foods. However, since sodium is lost in significant amounts through sweat, people living in hot climates, or who take regular strenuous exercise, can be at risk of a deficiency. One of the first symptoms is cramp, which often affects the calf muscles. In more serious cases, a deficiency can lead to dehydration, causing low blood pressure,

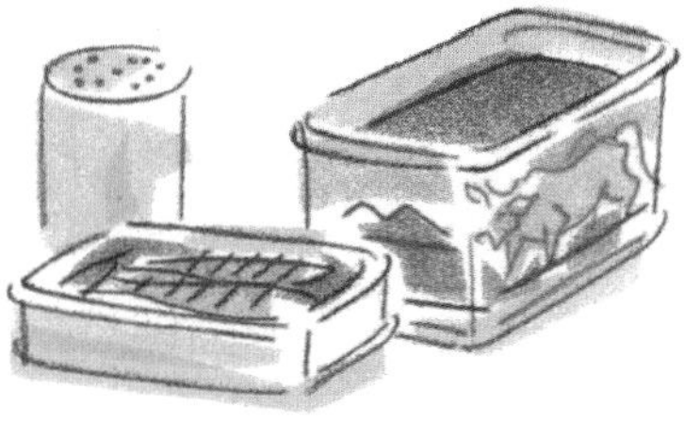

dryness of the mouth and vomiting. Normally, surplus intakes of sodium are excreted through the kidneys. However, in susceptible individuals, high intakes can lead to oedema (fluid retention) and high BLOOD PRESSURE. These in turn can cause heart failure, strokes or kidney failure.

SULPHUR

Sulphur is present in every cell of the body, and is especially concentrated in the skin, nails and hair. Most sulphur in the body is obtained as part of the protein intake, as it is an integral part of the sulphur-containing amino acids, cysteine and methionine. It is also a part of at least three B vitamins; thiamin, pantothenic acid and biotin. Inorganic forms of the mineral – sulphide, sulphates and sulphites – are not needed in the diet. Indeed, sulphites, used to preserve the colour of dried foods (such as apricots), can trigger asthma attacks in susceptible individuals. In its pure form sulphur acts as an antifungal and antibacterial agent, and is used in creams for treating skin disorders such as acne.

ZINC

Zinc is present in all the tissues of the body and is an essential component of a wide range of enzymes. It is also necessary for the maintaining and replicating of each individual's genetic material (DNA and RNA), and the body's ability to interpret this genetic information. Thus this mineral is vital for the normal growth of the body. It plays an especially important role in the development of the ovaries and the testes – a deficiency in childhood and adolescence impairs growth and sexual development. It is also needed for the efficient functioning of the immune system. Indeed, zinc is so important to the immune system that even a mild deficiency can lead to an increased risk of infection. The mineral is therefore especially important to the elderly, who may be particularly vulnerable to a wide range of infections.

Zinc is necessary for a healthy appetite and assists in our ability to taste foods. It is needed for night vision

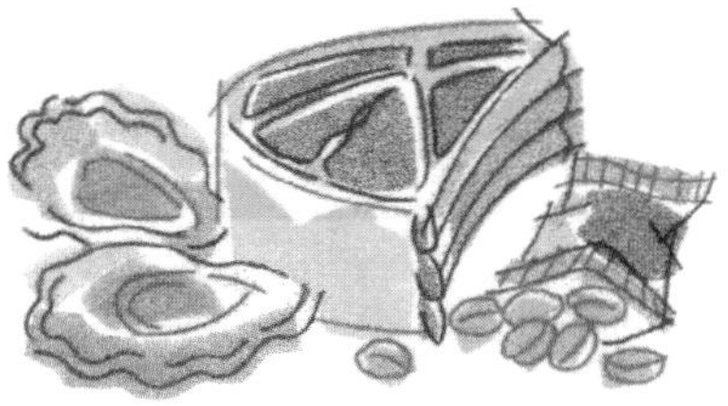

and the metabolising of alcohol, and is also required by enzymes involved in the destruction of FREE RADICALS.

The likelihood of zinc poisoning is remote, and tends to be restricted to people who regularly take large doses of zinc supplements.

A normal varied diet should supply all the body's daily needs, with the best source of zinc being shellfish – particularly oysters. Zinc is also found in grains, but is more easily absorbed from animal proteins such as meat, poultry, eggs or dairy produce. This is partly because the zinc in cereals is mostly found in the outer layers which are discarded during the milling process, and partly because the fibre in grains contains phytates, which are known to inhibit the body's ability to absorb several minerals, including zinc. Vegetarians and vegans may therefore need zinc supplements.

MINERAL	BEST FOOD SOURCES	ROLE IN HEALTH
MACROMINERALS		
Calcium	Milk and dairy products, tinned sardines with bones, green leafy vegetables, sesame seeds.	Builds bones and teeth and keeps them strong; vital to nerve transmission, blood clotting and muscle functions.
Chloride	Table salt (sodium chloride) and foods containing it.	Maintains the fluid and electrolyte balance in the body. Vital for stomach acid formation.
Magnesium	Wholegrain cereals, wheatgerm, pulses, nuts, sesame seeds, dried figs and green vegetables.	Important constituent of bones and teeth; assists in nerve impulses; important for muscle contraction.
Phosphorus	Present in all plant and animal protein, such as milk, cheese, red meat and poultry, fish and seafood, nuts, seeds and whole grains.	Helps to form and maintain healthy bones and teeth; needed to release energy in cells; essential for absorption of many nutrients.
Potassium	Avocados, fresh and dried fruit, seeds and nuts, bananas, citrus fruit, potatoes and pulses.	Works with sodium to maintain the fluid and electrolyte balance within cells, to keep heartbeat regular and to maintain normal blood pressure. Essential for the transmission of all nerve impulses.
Sodium	Table salt (sodium chloride), tinned anchovies, processed meats and yeast extracts.	Works with potassium to regulate fluid balance; essential for nerve and muscle function.
MICROMINERALS		
Aluminium	Not applicable: the ingestion of aluminium should be avoided where possible.	No known biological function in the body.
Chromium	Red meat and liver, egg yolk, seafood, wholegrain cereals, molasses and cheese.	Important for regulation of blood sugar levels; helps to regulate blood cholesterol levels.
Copper	Offal, shellfish such as oysters, nuts and seeds, mushrooms and cocoa.	Needed for bone growth and connective tissue formation. Helps the body to absorb iron from food. Present in many enzymes which protect against free radicals.
Fluoride	Toothpaste, tap water and tea.	Protects against tooth decay.
Iodine	Seaweed, seafood and iodised table salt.	Vital part of hormones secreted by the thyroid gland.
Iron	Offal, lean meat, sardines, egg yolk, dark green leafy vegetables and iron-fortified cereals.	Essential component of haemoglobin and many enzymes involved in energy metabolism.
Manganese	Nuts, cereals, brown rice, pulses and wholegrain bread.	Vital component of various enzymes involved in energy production; helps to form bone and connective tissue.
Molybdenum	Offal (especially liver), yeast, and pulses, whole grains and leafy vegetables, depending on soil.	Essential component of enzymes involved in the production of DNA and RNA; may fight tooth decay.
Selenium	Meat and fish, dairy foods such as butter, Brazil nuts, avocados and lentils.	Antioxidant mineral: protects cells against free radical damage. Vital for normal sexual development.
Sulphur	Protein from animal and vegetable sources.	Component of two essential amino acids which help to form many proteins in the body. Present in every cell.
Zinc	Oysters, red meat, peanuts and sunflower seeds.	Essential for normal growth, reproduction and immunity. Aids the action of many enzymes.

DAILY REQUIREMENTS		SYMPTOMS OF DEFICIENCY	SYMPTOMS OF EXCESS
MALE	FEMALE		
700mg	700mg	Muscle weakness, back pain, soft and brittle bones, fractures and osteoporosis.	None: surplus calcium is not absorbed by the body.
2500mg	2500mg	Deficiency does not occur on a normal diet.	None: excess chloride is excreted by the kidneys.
300mg	270mg	Apathy, weakness, cramps and muscle tremors (tetany) which lead to convulsions.	No reported symptoms.
550mg	550mg	Deficiency is rare but may be induced by prolonged use of antacids.	Excessive intake can affect the body's ability to use calcium and inhibit the absorption of magnesium.
3500mg	3500mg	Apathy, weakness, confusion and extreme thirst. In severe cases, there may be abnormal heartbeat and other heart and respiratory problems.	May cause lethargy, slow heartbeat, paralysis and heart failure.
1600mg	1600mg	Deficiency is rare but can lead to low blood pressure, dehydration and muscle cramps.	Fluid retention, high blood pressure which can lead to strokes; heart and kidney failure.
None.	None.	None.	Has been linked to Alzheimer's disease; may also cause hip problems in the elderly.
25 micrograms	25 micrograms	May cause glucose intolerance and raised blood cholesterol levels.	No adverse symptoms reported.
1.2mg	1.2mg	Deficiency is rare, and usually occurs only in premature babies or in infants with malabsorption problems.	High intakes are unlikely but could be toxic, causing liver and kidney damage.
There is no set dietary requirement.		Tooth decay.	Weak, mottled teeth, brittle bones.
140 micrograms	140 micrograms	Goitre; maybe coarse skin and hair; apathy.	High intakes can cause hyperthyroidism.
8.7mg	14.5mg	Shortness of breath, fatigue, iron deficiency anaemia, reduced resistance to infection.	Iron poisoning usually occurs when children mistake iron supplements for sweets.
1.4mg	1.4mg	No reported symptoms.	None: excess manganese is safely excreted by the body.
50-400 micrograms	50-400 micrograms	Deficiency is virtually unknown.	High intakes may induce copper deficiency.
75 micrograms	60 micrograms	Rare; could stunt growth, delay sexual development and reduce fertility.	Hair loss, skin depigmentation, fatigue.
There is no set dietary requirement.		Deficiency is unknown.	None.
9.5mg	7mg	Loss of appetite; in adolescents, impaired growth and development; poor immunity.	Remote unless inadvertently overdosing on self-administered supplements.

MOOD CHANGES AND DIET

EAT PLENTY OF

- *Carbohydrates (sugars and starches) for a calming effect*
- *Foods rich in B vitamins, such as brown rice, fish and green vegetables for a healthy nervous system*

CUT DOWN ON

- *Caffeine in coffee, tea and cola drinks*
- *Alcohol*

The coca leaf, opium poppies, certain mushrooms, alcohol and even nutmeg can produce sleep, elation, hallucination and freedom from pain. More surprisingly, everyday foods can affect people's moods quite profoundly. The link between food and mood is complex; nutritional deficiencies, adverse or allergic reactions (see ALLERGIES) and the level of glucose (blood sugar) in the bloodstream can all have an effect on a person's mental state.

CALMING CHEMICALS

The brain produces potent chemicals called neurotransmitters which are made out of nutrients from food. As a general rule, neurotransmitters are produced from amino acids, which are the building blocks of the proteins in the foods that you eat.

Some studies have shown that the manufacture and release of neurotransmitters in the body can be altered to some extent by certain foods, meaning that – in theory – diet can affect the way you feel and behave. Any specific cause and effect is difficult to define, as age, sex and any medicines you may be taking are factors that can also affect the chemical reactions of the brain.

An amino acid called tryptophan, found in protein-rich foods such as meat, milk and eggs, is a component of a soothing neurotransmitter called serotonin. Serotonin is needed for normal sleep, and some experts think that it may play a role in controlling certain types of depression.

It has been claimed that meals rich in carbohydrates (sugars and starches) help to increase the levels of serotonin in the brain, making a person feel calm and drowsy. People who suffer with SEASONAL AFFECTIVE DISORDER (SAD) often have a craving for sugary carbohydrates throughout the dark winter months. It is thought that in order to compensate for their feelings of irritability, moodiness and depression, SAD sufferers may unwittingly use carbohydrates to enjoy a temporary reprieve from their dark mood.

THE CHARMS OF CHOCOLATE

Chocolate appears to give an instant lift to the spirits and to act as an antidepressant. The so-called 'chocolate high' is due in part to a chemical in cocoa called phenylethylamine which occurs naturally in the brain, and is allegedly released at times of emotional arousal. Chocolate also contains the stimulants theobromine and caffeine, which increase alertness.

THE B VITAMINS

Deficiency in one of several B vitamins can also cause a change in mood. Vegetarians and vegans are prone to vitamin B_{12} deficiency, while alcoholics are prone to both thiamin and vitamin B_{12} deficiency. Rich sources of B vitamins include beans, brown rice, egg yolks, fish, nuts, soya beans, and wholegrain cereals, dairy products, poultry and brewer's yeast. Because vitamin B_{12} is found mainly in animal products, vegetarians and vegans may need to boost their intake of this vitamin by eating foods that have been fortified with B_{12}, such as soya milk, yeast extract and breakfast cereals, or by taking a regular supplement. Some women find that vitamin B_6 helps to relieve the symptoms of premenstrual syndrome (PMS). It is involved in the breakdown of the hormone oestrogen in the liver and may therefore have an indirect effect over mood, a lack of it leading to anxiety and nervous tension. Supplements may therefore help women who suffer with the irritability and tearfulness that can be part of PMS – though many doctors are sceptical about this claim. Good food sources of vitamin B_6 include brewer's yeast, yeast extract, wheatgerm, oat flakes, liver and bananas.

GLUCOSE AND MOOD SWINGS

Irregular eating patterns are a common cause of mood swings. If you go for long periods without eating any food, the brain compensates for reduced levels of blood glucose by using 'ketone bodies' for fuel – substances derived from the breakdown of fat. This reaction can cause a feeling of elation and wakefulness, and is one reason why fasting has become associated with the practice of meditation.

Eating a carbohydrate meal when you are tired is said to calm you down and induce sleep. Some people are very irritable on waking, and this is attributed to a low blood sugar level. Eating some carbohydrates is said to improve frayed tempers first thing in the morning. Some people become irritable about 2 hours after a carbohydrate-rich meal. This is also believed to be because their blood sugar levels drop below normal, due to too much insulin being secreted by the body.

AND ONE FOR THE ROAD

Many people drink to forget their worries, lose their inhibitions and feel more confident. Contrary to popular opinion, alcohol is not a stimulant, it is a depressant, and if you drink to excess it will slow down brain-cell function and reduce your powers of attention.

Case study

Joan was a lonely widow with no children whose best friend in life was her dog. Struggling to get by on her state pension, she lived on a staple diet of bread and butter – preferring to buy meat for her dog rather than for herself. One day, her health visitor, Sue, noticed that 67-year-old Joan had developed an ulcer at the corner of her mouth. After a lot of persuasion from Sue, Joan agreed to see a doctor. The first thing he noticed was Joan's pallor. He put this down to anaemia, but there was no evidence of blood loss to account for it and he was worried about the possibility of bowel cancer, given Joan's age. A blood test confirmed that she was actually iron-deficient – as suggested by the mouth ulcer – and fortunately a barium enema showed a normal bowel. A course of iron tablets soon resolved the anaemia, and meals-on-wheels now ensures that Joan enjoys a more healthy, varied diet.

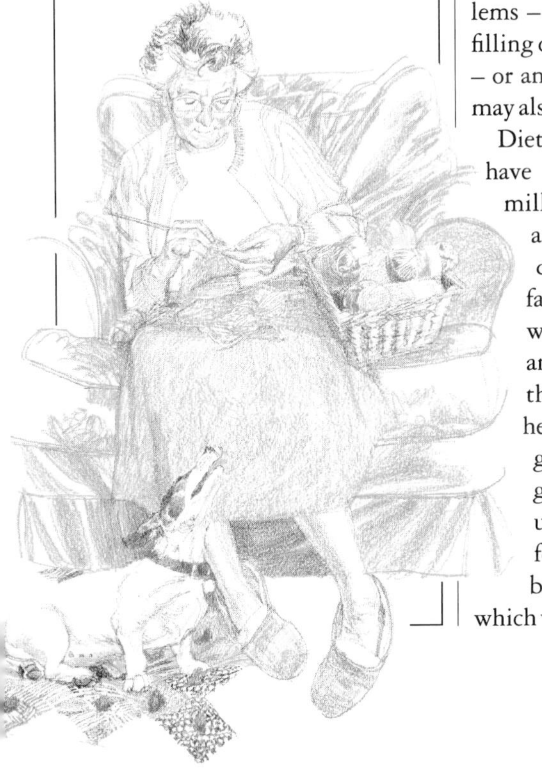

Mouth ulcers

EAT PLENTY OF

- *Dark green leafy vegetables and whole grains for their folate*
- *Milk and potatoes, for B vitamins*
- *Foods rich in zinc, such as shellfish and nuts*

AVOID

- *Salt and salty foods such as crisps*
- *Acidic foods such as pickles*
- *Boiled sweets*
- *Alcohol*

Painful white spots, called aphthous ulcers, can occur anywhere in the mouth. They usually have bright-red inflamed borders and may occur singly or in clusters. Recurrent ulcers can be the result of nutritional deficiencies (such as iron, in cases of anaemia), food sensitivities or allergies, or emotional stress. Mouth ulcers can also be symptoms of other illnesses such as coeliac disease and Crohn's disease.

Women who suffer from mouth ulcers may find that outbreaks coincide with their menstrual cycle. Other possible causes are dental problems – a jagged edge or a crumbling filling causing injury inside the mouth – or an infection, in which case there may also be a high temperature.

Diets that are low in the B vitamins have been implicated as a cause; milk, potatoes and whole grains are all good sources of B vitamins. A deficiency in zinc is another factor – good sources include wheatgerm, nuts, seeds, shellfish and eggs. Folate is needed to keep the cells lining the mouth healthy, and is found in dark green vegetables and whole grains. If you are suffering from ulcers, avoid salty and acidic foods, such as pickles, as well as boiled sweets and alcohol – all of which will only aggravate the problem.

Multiple sclerosis

TAKE PLENTY OF

- *Whole grains, cooked green leafy vegetables and fresh fruit, for fibre and energy*
- *Water, to avoid constipation*
- *Polyunsaturated fats from oily fish and sunflower, safflower, corn and soya oils*

CUT DOWN ON

- *Saturated fats (full-fat dairy products, fatty red meat)*

AVOID

- *Alcohol*
- *Smoking*

The causes of multiple sclerosis (MS) are still unknown and as yet there is no cure, although potential treatments are beginning to emerge. Some scientists and nutritionists believe the key to understanding MS lies with nutrition, but this view is controversial. Nevertheless, a balanced diet rich in nutrients and polyunsaturated fats can help sufferers to control some of the common symptoms and complications associated with the disease.

Symptoms

MS affects approximately one in 1000 people, and twice as many women as men, usually striking between the ages of 25 and 40. It is a chronic disease in which areas of the sheaths surrounding the nerve fibres in the brain and spinal cord become inflamed and eventually degenerate. It can affect the nerves involved in eyesight and speech and often leads to a gradual loss of sensation in the limbs, reduced muscular control and sometimes giddiness. People with MS commonly experience an unpredictable pattern of relapses and remissions, often over many years, with only one in five suffering severe disability. MS is not fatal, but some people with the disease may be more susceptible to other illnesses that can themselves be life-threatening.

NUTRITION AND MS

The relationship between nutrition and MS has been under investigation for the past 50 years. However, according to the International Federation of Multiple Sclerosis Societies, none of the dietary theories or regimens currently advocated by some scientists and doctors has been proven to have a significant therapeutic effect. Although some studies on the possible benefits of the omega-6 and omega-3 essential fatty acids (see FATS), used in the maintenance and repair of the central nervous system, have suggested that supplements might slow the progress of the disease and reduce the severity and duration of relapses, the effect is modest and is still undergoing investigation.

One of the diets that has received a lot of attention is the low-fat diet of Professor Roy Swank of Portland, Oregon, USA. He claims that patients following a diet low in saturated fats – less than 20g (¾oz) per day – and high in polyunsaturated fats had less frequent relapses, more energy and an increased life expectancy. Although its specific effects on MS remain to be proved, the Swank diet is at least a well-balanced one, in line with current recommendations on reducing intake of saturated fats and cholesterol, and is unlikely to pose any nutritional risks to MS sufferers.

This is not the case with some of the other unproven diets, for example the raw-food diet, vitamin and mineral therapies, and allergen-free diets that avoid certain substances on the basis that MS might be the result of an allergic reaction. Such diets could have harmful effects by reducing the intake of essential nutrients or increasing the risk of nutrient imbalance through megadoses of vitamins or minerals.

FIGHTING FATIGUE *Meals that are high in complex carbohydrates can help to overcome the chronic tiredness associated with MS.*

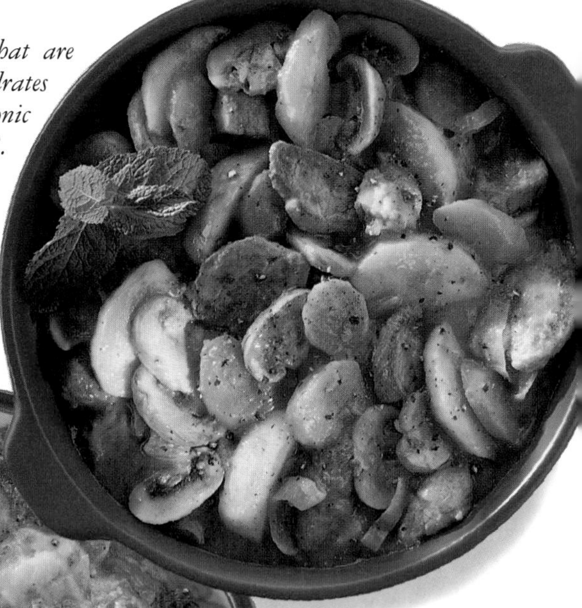

Trim all the visible fat from the meat for a healthier pork and apple casserole.

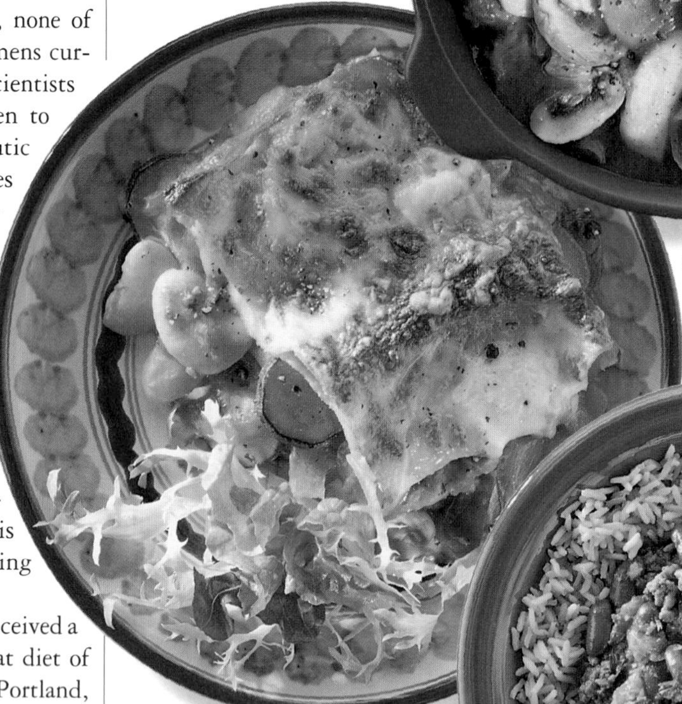

A vegetable lasagne shows how high-fibre and low-fat meals need not be boring.

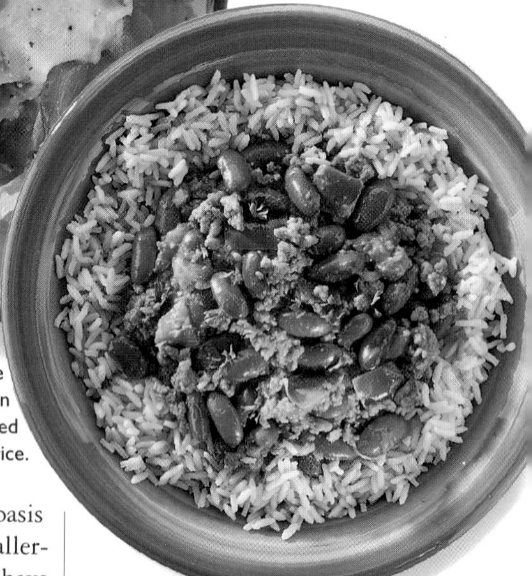

Chilli con carne made with lean mince and served with brown rice.

MANAGING SYMPTOMS

The main role of diet in MS is to enable people to manage common problems which include fatigue, incontinence and constipation and to help them avoid exacerbating other symptoms. Chronic fatigue is one of the most debilitating symptoms of MS. A nutritious, low-fat breakfast and plenty of complex carbohydrates such as jacket potatoes and brown rice at other meals will help to keep energy levels steady throughout the day. This can also help to keep weight under control as part of a calorie-controlled diet. Excessive weight gain can be a problem because of the decrease in energy expenditure associated with the condition, especially if sufferers also come to depend on convenience foods that are low in nutrients or eat too many 'comfort' foods which are often high in fat and sugar.

Excessive weight gain can further impair mobility and put a strain on the respiratory and circulatory systems, so it is important to control the intake of calories while ensuring that the diet is well balanced and provides a good intake of all nutrients.

ALCOHOL, INCONTINENCE AND CONSTIPATION

Alcohol can be drunk in moderation but some sufferers may find that it can temporarily exacerbate MS symptoms such as problems with speech and coordination. More importantly, it inhibits the vital conversion process of essential fatty acids, increases the level of saturated fat in the blood and depletes the body's supply of valuable nutrients. Smoking also depletes blood levels of vitamin C and can worsen the symptoms of the disease.

MS often affects the nerve fibres of the bladder, causing incontinence. This can indirectly affect the balance of the diet if sufferers severely restrict their fluid intake, especially if they cut down on vitamin and mineral-rich milk and fruit juices. Reducing fluid intake can often cause a dry mouth, which may lead to a loss of appetite and difficulty in swallowing. Long-term incontinence can also increase the risk of urinary tract infections such as CYSTITIS. CRANBERRY juice can be effective in helping to avoid this.

Fluid restriction can contribute to the common problem of constipation, especially when it is combined with decreased mobility and if the bowel is also affected. Plenty of water – at least 1.7 litres (3 pints) a day – and fibre-rich foods such as whole grains, cooked green leafy vegetables and fresh fruit will help to prevent constipation.

It is essential to remember that MS affects each individual differently and that relapses and remissions also play a key role in determining a person's dietary needs. People with MS should seek professional nutritional advice throughout the course of their illness.

MUMPS

TAKE PLENTY OF

- *High-calorie glucose drinks*
- *Light, easy-to-swallow meals*

Although vaccinations have greatly reduced the number of cases reported, mumps most commonly occurs in children aged between three and ten years old. It is a highly contagious viral illness, manifesting itself two or three weeks after infection by causing the salivary glands to swell which makes chewing difficult. Other symptoms include pain in the jaw muscles, a raised temperature and earache, which is often made worse by chewing and swallowing. There may be stomach-ache and vomiting.

In teenage or adult males, mumps can cause inflammation of one or both testes (orchitis). It can also cause inflammation of the pancreas, and so influence fat digestion.

Because chewing is painful, the illness requires a soft but nutritious diet. If the patient cannot eat, energy levels should be maintained with high-calorie drinks. Fruit juices may have to be avoided, however, as the citric acid they contain may sting the throat.

In general, a sensible, balanced diet is suggested, but food has only a limited role in the recovery process.

MUSCULAR DYSTROPHY

TAKE PLENTY OF

- *Lean protein such as skinned chicken*
- *Fibre from foods such as wholemeal bread, brown rice, vegetables and fresh fruit*

CUT DOWN ON

- *Snacks between meals*
- *High-calorie foods such as cakes, biscuits and fried foods*

There are more than 20 variants of muscular dystrophy, the generic term for an incurable progressive wasting disease which can affect different muscles and arise at different ages. All cases are hereditary.

A healthy diet and careful weight control are very important in all forms of muscular dystrophy so that already weakened muscles do not have the additional burden of carrying excess weight. Losing weight not only helps the sufferers to move more easily, but it also assists their carers, who may have to lift them. Moreover, in the later stages of the disease, there will be less strain on the weakened respiratory muscles.

To keep their weight under control sufferers should try not to eat snacks between meals, cut down on high-calorie foods and eat plenty of fibre. Fibre is not only filling but it encourages regular bowel habits, relieving the constipation often associated with the disease. Sufferers should not go on a crash diet, however, as this could cause muscle wasting and they should eat plenty of lean protein.

In all its forms, muscular dystrophy is characterised by the deterioration and wasting of muscle fibres, causing weakness in the legs and back which can make walking difficult. The most common form is Duchenne muscular dystrophy which occurs only in boys.

MUSHROOMS AND TRUFFLES

BENEFIT
- *Good sources of potassium and some trace elements*

DRAWBACKS
- *Mushrooms contain a variety of chemicals, including nitrosamines, which may be carcinogenic*
- *Mushrooms can accumulate heavy metals such as cadmium and lead*

Commercially available mushrooms and other fungi are good sources of potassium and trace elements. However, people tend to eat mushrooms in such small quantities – in terms of weight – that the contribution they make to the diet is much more to do with taste and texture than nutrition. They provide little energy, although their calorie content is increased significantly when they are fried.

Dried fungi have a more intense flavour than their fresh counterparts and they generally contribute more to the flavour than to the bulk of food. Most need to be soaked before use: rinse them first and then pour over enough boiling water to cover them, and leave to stand for half an hour. The soaking water can be used as a stock for soups or stews.

Fungi contain substances called hydrazines and nitrosamines, which have been shown to be carcinogenic in tests on laboratory animals and which may also be carcinogenic to humans. However, because people tend not to eat unusually large amounts of mushrooms, the levels of hydrazine ingested are infinitesimal and perfectly safe.

Nutritionally, there is little difference between wild and commercially cultivated mushrooms. But wild mushrooms usually have a more earthy flavour, and they colour sauces or stews with their dark juices. Both wild and cultivated mushrooms have a tendency to accumulate toxic heavy metals such as cadmium and lead if produced in manure (particularly if in a polluted environment).

If you want to try gathering mushrooms from the wild, be extremely careful. Some of the most toxic varieties look very similar to edible mushrooms. Ceps and chanterelles are very common in the wild, but pick them only if you are sure you have identified them correctly (see COUNTRYSIDE FOODS). If in any doubt, buy your mushrooms in the shops.

As people have become more adventurous in their eating habits, so the growers have responded by cultivating a wide range of exotic fungi. The following are now widely available.

Cep Fresh ceps look like glossy buns; dried ceps have a concentrated meaty flavour. The Italians call ceps *porcini*.

Chanterelle These trumpet-shaped golden mushrooms have a peppery, perfumed aroma and a firm texture.

Morel With its honeycomb cap, this fungus looks more like a sponge than a mushroom. It has a rich earthy flavour.

Oyster A fishy flavoured mushroom with a slightly chewy texture; almost always eaten cooked. It is popular in Chinese and Japanese cuisine.

Shiitake This richly flavoured tree fungus is usually sold in its dried form.

Fungi folklore

The Ancient Egyptians thought that commoners were not fit to eat mushrooms, and reserved them for the Pharaohs. The Romans served mushrooms at feasts, and believed that they gave their warriors unusual strength.

All over the world, many peoples have used mushrooms or fungi for their narcotic or hallucinogenic properties. The Dyaks of Borneo, for example, use the poisonous Fly Agaric as a stimulant.

On the continent, enthusiasm for wild fungi is so great that collecting them is a national pastime. There are close seasons and laws to prevent them becoming extinct.

In the Far East, herbalists recommend eating shiitake mushrooms for a long and healthy life.

ELUSIVE TRUFFLES

The gourmet fungi, essential in haute cuisine for their unique flavour, have defied all attempts at cultivation. Truffles grow underground, usually in the roots of oak or beech trees, and are sniffed out by trained pigs or dogs. The black or Périgord truffle and the white or Italian truffle are viewed as outstanding varieties by connoisseurs.

The pervasive, earthy scent of truffles is used to enhance various dishes. Because truffles are so expensive, they are eaten very rarely and in extremely tiny quantities, so their nutritional contribution to the diet is negligible.

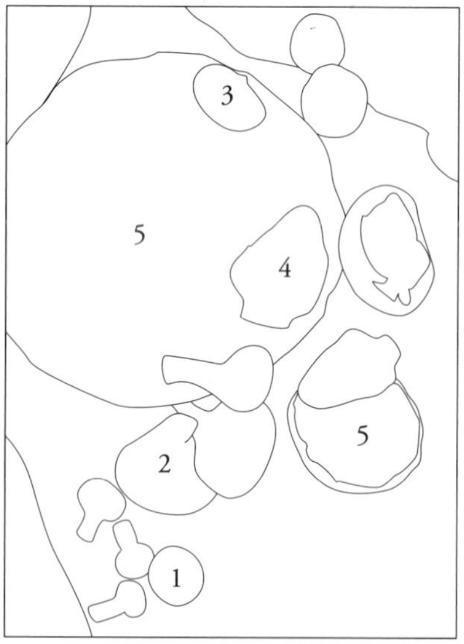

ALL SHAPES AND SIZES *There are now more varieties of mushroom available than ever before, including button (1), oyster (2), shiitake (3), morel (4) and field (5).*

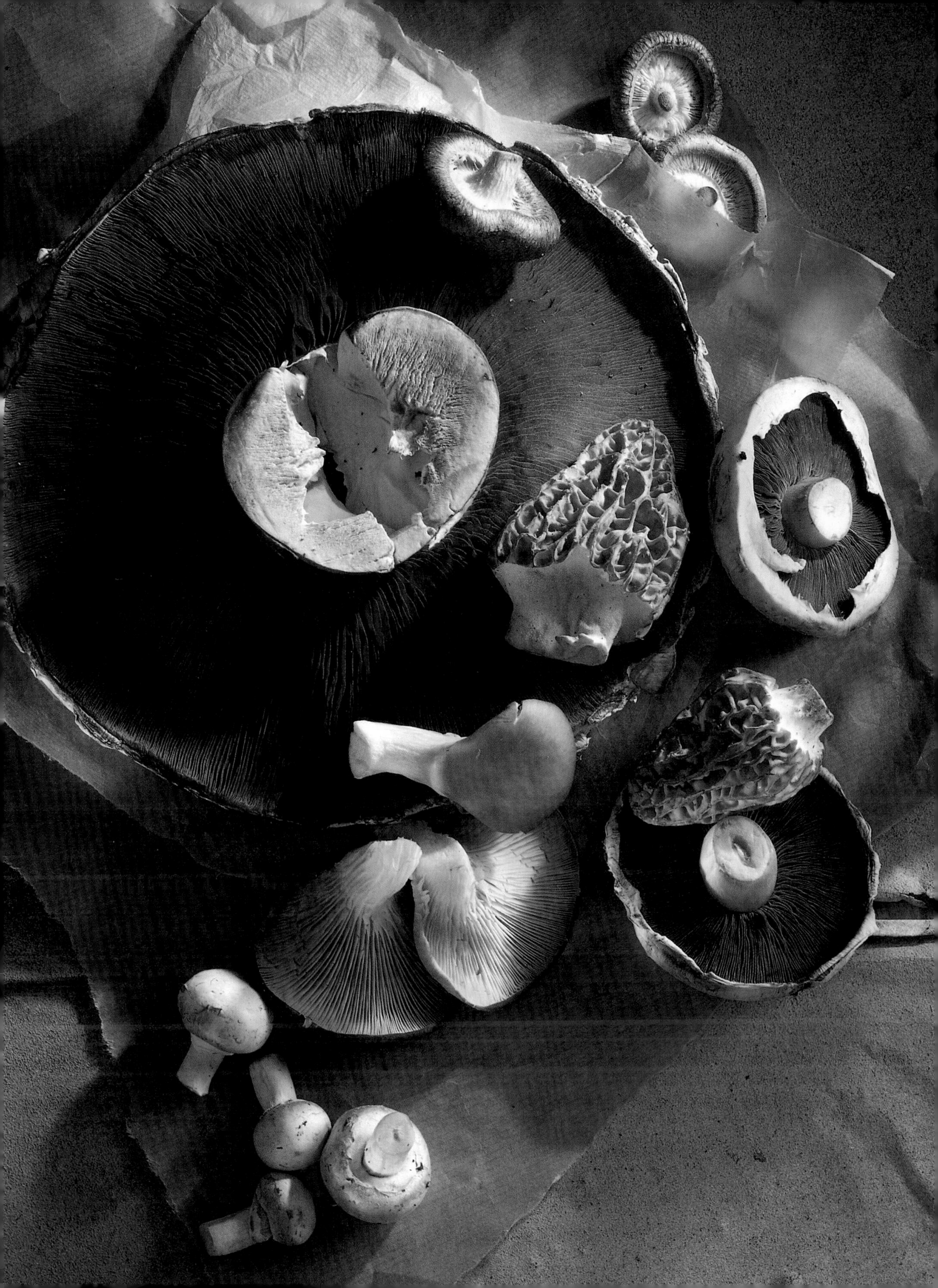

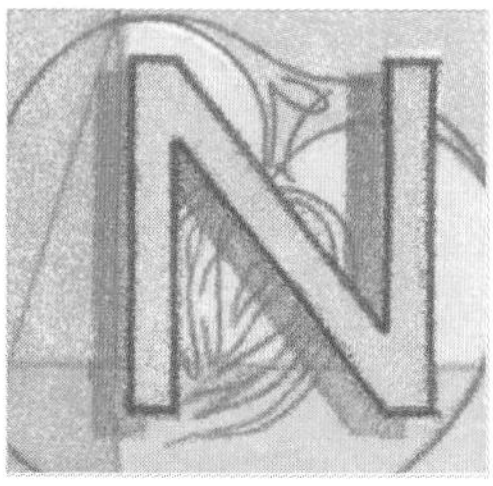

Nail problems

EAT PLENTY OF

- *Red meat and poultry, for iron*
- *Shellfish, fish, pulses, nuts and offal, for zinc and selenium*
- *Citrus fruit and juice, for vitamin C*

AVOID

- *Drinks which contain tannin, especially strong tea (which inhibits iron absorption) at mealtimes*

Healthy nails are strong, smooth and pink. They are made of a protein called keratin, and grow at an average rate of a millimetre a week. The state of your nails can indicate your general state of health. Like every other part of the body, nails need a supply of nutrients. However, the body prioritises its nutrient distribution and because nails are not vital organs, they are one of the first areas to be affected by nutritional deficiencies, whether caused by poor diet or illness.

Thin, spoon-shaped nails, especially on the thumb, characterise iron and zinc deficiencies in the diet. The nails may also become brittle and pale. Increasing iron intake will help to stave off iron-deficiency anaemia and improve general health as well as the condition of the nails.

Good sources of iron include red meat, fish and poultry, and green leafy vegetables. Because vitamin C helps the body to absorb iron from plant foods, try drinking citrus fruit juices with meals; and avoid drinking strong tea with meals, as the tannin it contains inhibits iron absorption.

Brittle nails and infections of the surrounding skin may indicate a lack of zinc in the diet. Eat plenty of zinc-rich food such as seafood, eggs, offal, meat, nuts, lentils and chickpeas.

Selenium deficiency can lead to wide bands, or ridges, developing on the nails, while too much can cause blackened nails. Shellfish and fish are both good sources of selenium, as are brewer's yeast, offal, grains and cereals.

The calcium myth

Many people believe that calcium-rich foods will make their nails stronger. In fact, the nails contain only very small amounts of calcium, and the mineral plays little or no part in strengthening them. The small white flecks on the nails, formerly thought to be caused by calcium deficiency, are now believed to be the result of a knock, overmanicuring or, in rare instances, a zinc deficiency. An improved intake of zinc – either through supplements or from dietary sources – often results in the disappearance of the unsightly white spots.

A diagnostic tool

Before surgery women are asked to remove their nail polish because when a patient's lips are covered by an anaesthesia mask, it is the nails that the anaesthetist will examine to ascertain whether the patient is getting enough oxygen. Pink nail beds indicate enough oxygen in the blood, but pale or blue ones show that the patient is not receiving enough oxygen.

A skilled diagnostician can also read the nails for signs of certain ailments. Pale, upward curving nails may indicate anaemia or zinc deficiency. Blue-tinged nails show that blood is not reaching the extremities – possibly a sign of circulatory disease and ridged nails show that the growth was interrupted, possibly by illness.

What triggers whitlows?

Whitlows (paranychia) are infections of the nail bed due to bacteria which usually enter the skin through a hangnail or other small injury. They usually respond to antifungal ointments. A balanced intake of vitamins and minerals will also help recovery.

Diabetics and those who are suffering from illnesses that stem from mineral deficiency are often predisposed to chronic whitlows. People whose hands are frequently immersed in water, such as kitchen staff, barmaids and nurses, are also prone to whitlows. To help to avoid this painful problem, always wear rubber gloves when washing up.

Water and soap may also be responsible for brittle or splitting nails. In this case the best treatment is to apply hand cream regularly, particularly after drying your hands.

Nectarines

BENEFIT

- *Rich in vitamin C*

The name nectarine comes from the Greek *nektar*, which is the drink of the gods in Roman and Greek mythology. Nectarines are sweeter than peaches, from which they were originally cultivated, and slightly more nutritious. One fresh nectarine contains almost enough vitamin C to meet the average adult's daily requirement. Vitamin C, which helps the body to absorb iron efficiently and maintain its immune system, is also vital to the production of collagen, which is an important component of the skin. Collagen helps to build scar tissue over wounds – an essential part of the healing process.

Nectarines have smoother skins than peaches, with none of the 'fur' that some people find unpalatable. The flesh, which tends to be firmer and may be pink, yellow or white, is often more intensely scented and flavoured than that of a peach. Nectarines contain slightly more energy – 36 Calories in an average nectarine compared with 30 in a peach of a similar size.

SUCCULENT SWEETNESS *Unlike their relative the peach, nectarines do not continue to ripen after they are picked; so only choose fruit that is already soft to the touch.*

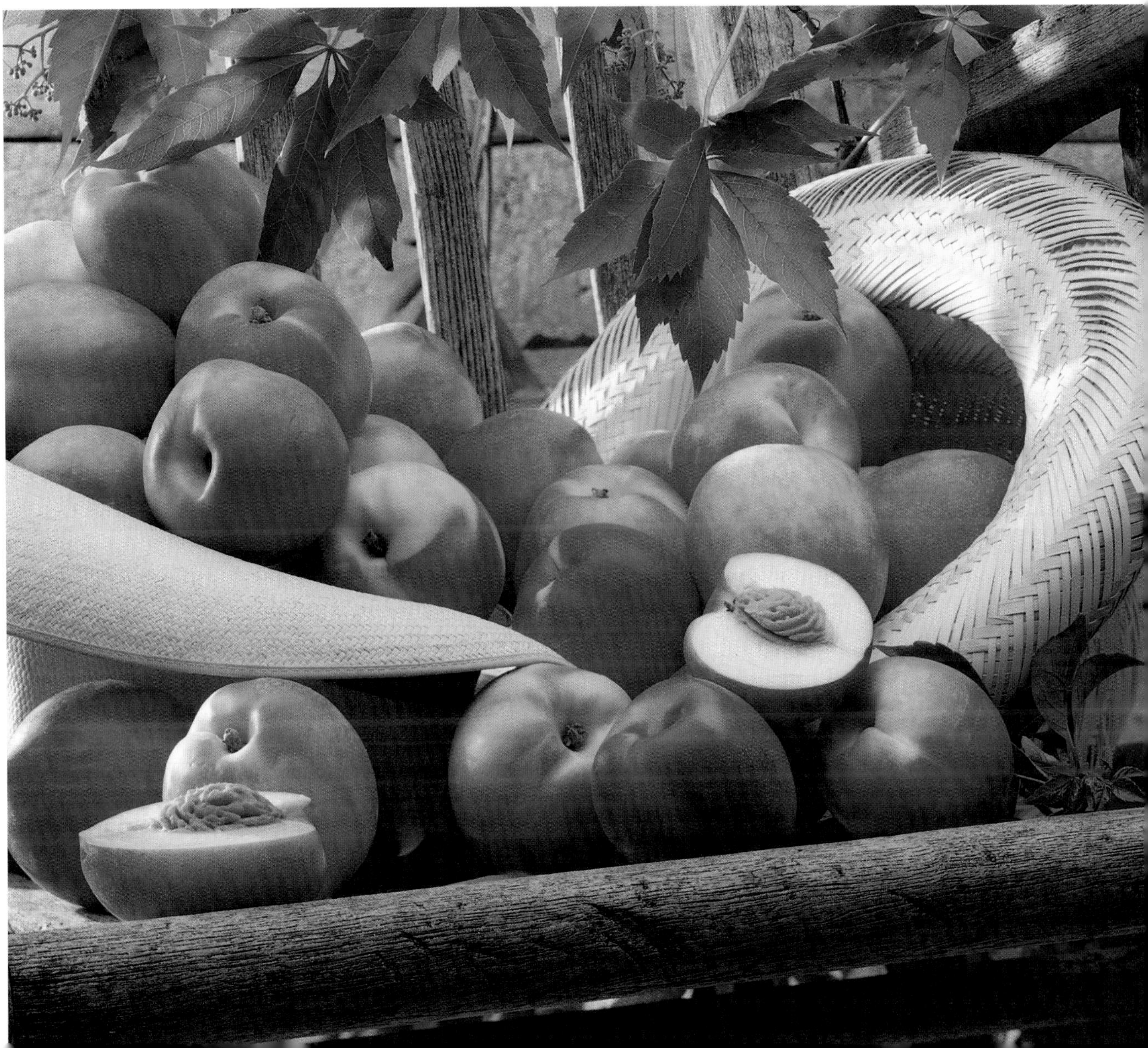

NEURALGIA

This is a painful condition, in which stabbing or burning sensations are felt along the course of a sensory nerve. It can occur as a result of the nerve being diseased, compressed or injured – perhaps as a result of a fractured bone or a slipped disc. Sometimes, however, there is no apparent cause at all.

Neuralgia can arise as a consequence of nerve damage caused by deficiencies of vitamin B_{12} and thiamin. It may also occur in patients with DIABETES. Vitamin B_{12} deficiency is rare except among vegetarians and vegans. Make sure your diet contains plenty of foods that are rich in B vitamins, such as wholemeal bread, brown rice, wheatgerm, nuts, pulses and green leafy vegetables. Thiamin deficiency can also cause nerve damage, however, it is unusual in the Western world – except among alcoholics.

SHINGLES, a common form of neuralgia, is an example of a diseased nerve. The herpes virus replicates in the nerve causing inflammation and results in a blistering rash following the path of the nerve. Pain is felt in the same region as the rash, and may even persist after other symptoms have disappeared. This is where a diet rich in anti-inflammatory vitamins may help. Eat plenty of safflower oil, nuts, olive oil and avocados for vitamin E, and citrus fruits for vitamin C and also bioflavonoids (antioxidants believed to have anti-inflammatory properties).

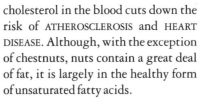

When the nerves at the back of the leg are affected, producing spasms of pain, the condition is known as sciatica, an example of a compressed nerve.

When the sensory nerves on the side of the face are irritated, the condition is termed trigeminal neuralgia, which usually occurs in spasms which often strike at a similar time each day – a phenomenon doctors cannot explain.

NUTS

BENEFITS

- *Excellent source of vitamin E*
- *Walnuts may help to reduce the risk of heart disease*
- *Useful source of the B vitamins thiamin and niacin*
- *Useful source of protein and minerals for vegetarians*

DRAWBACKS

- *High in calories*
- *Immature almonds can contain cyanide-producing compounds*
- *Peanuts are prone to contamination by moulds that produce carcinogens*
- *Peanut allergies can be fatal*
- *Danger of choking in children*

The daily consumption of 85 g (3 oz) of walnuts – when used in place of saturated fats as part of a low-fat diet – has been found to lower blood cholesterol, according to recent US research. Reduction of the levels of

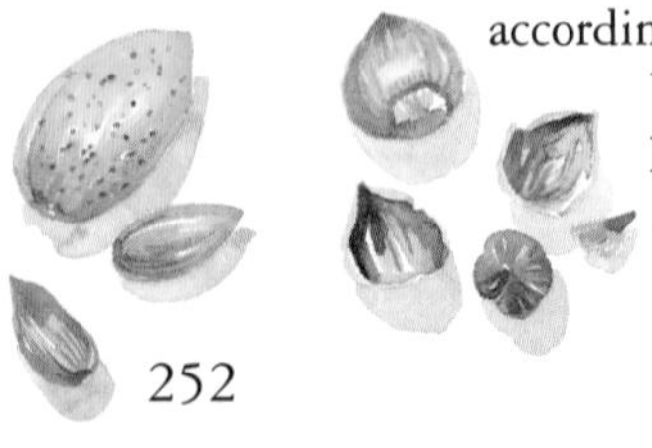

cholesterol in the blood cuts down the risk of ATHEROSCLEROSIS and HEART DISEASE. Although, with the exception of chestnuts, nuts contain a great deal of fat, it is largely in the healthy form of unsaturated fatty acids.

Unlike cereal grains, nuts are not closely related to each other biologically. Most edible nuts grow on trees, but peanuts (or groundnuts) are legumes like the soya bean and grow on long tendrils underground; their dry shells correspond to the pods of beans and peas.

Their high fat content makes nuts full of calories: most varieties contain more than 550 Calories per 100 g (3½ oz) – though the same weight of chestnuts contains only 170 Calories. Walnuts, peanuts and hazelnuts are especially rich in the essential fatty acids, which are vital for normal tissue growth and development.

For vegetarians, nuts can supply many of the nutrients usually obtained from animal sources. These include most of the B vitamins, phosphorus, iron, copper, potassium and protein. Like most other plant sources, nut proteins are only of moderate quality when compared with animal proteins – such as meat. They do not have the whole range of amino acids that the body needs to make its own proteins. Nevertheless, combining them with bread, grains and pulses (particularly soya beans and lentils) will ensure that your diet supplies a healthy balance of all the essential amino acids.

Nuts are also one of the richest vegetable sources of vitamin E, but both vitamin E and thiamin are destroyed when nuts are roasted.

NUT HAZARDS

Avoid eating almonds which have not fully matured as they can contain compounds which produce hydrogen cyanide, a poisonous gas which has a distinctive aroma of bitter almonds.

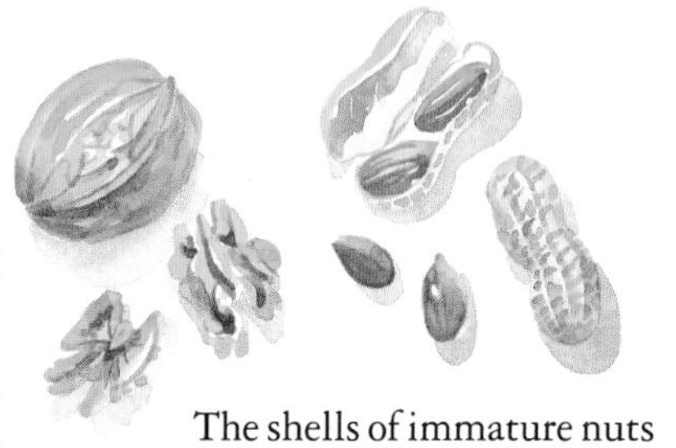

The shells of immature nuts may be slightly softer and are sometimes tinged with green, rather than the normal light brown.

Nuts should be stored in cool, dry conditions because they are prone to contamination with moulds. Some of these produce poisonous substances called mycotoxins, so never eat nuts with any trace of mould on the shell or kernel. In tropical countries, mouldy nuts may contain more dangerous mycotoxins – called aflatoxins – which cause liver cancer. These were identified in England in the 1960s when there was a large outbreak of liver disease in turkeys which had been fed on peanut meal. Peanuts are particularly prone to this form of contamination and, even though those imported into Britain are routinely checked for these moulds, it is safest to eat only peanuts that are sold in packets. Children should never be allowed to eat peanuts sold for use as birdfood.

Choking is one of the greatest hazards posed by nuts: for this reason, children under the age of four, who may not chew their food properly, should never be given nuts unless they have been finely ground.

Allergy alert

Nuts, especially peanuts, are one of the most common food allergens. In exceptional instances nut ALLERGIES can be fatal. Fortunately, such serious allergies are extremely rare, but people who are allergic to peanuts have to avoid all foods that contain even the tiniest traces of peanuts or peanut oil. Unfortunately, peanut allergy is normally a life-long condition.

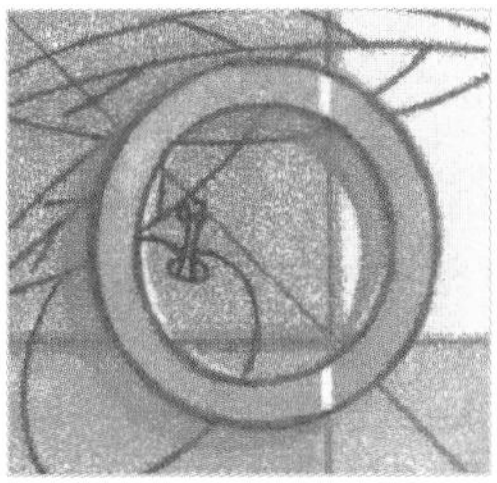

Obesity

EAT PLENTY OF

- *Complex carbohydrates, found in pasta, potatoes, brown rice and wholemeal bread*
- *Fresh fruit, vegetables, salads and pulses*
- *Lean meat, poultry (without the skin) and fish*

CUT DOWN ON

- *Fats of all kinds*
- *Alcohol*

AVOID

- *Full-fat dairy products*
- *Fatty and sugary snacks such as biscuits, cakes, crisps and nuts*
- *High-fat meats such as sausages, bacon and minced beef*

Obesity is the most common nutritional disorder in the Western world and is as prevalent in Britain as elsewhere. According to Department of Health statistics, between 1980 and 1993 the number of overweight British men rose from 33 per cent to 43 per cent, and of overweight women from 24 per cent to 30 per cent. In the same period, the proportion of clinically obese people rose from 6 per cent to 13 per cent of men and from 8 per cent to 16 per cent of women.

Doctors consider you to be obese if you are 30 per cent heavier than the normal acceptable weight for your height, sex and age. Health experts have drawn up standard tables that illustrate the acceptable range. Your GP should be familiar with these and may provide copies at the surgery.

Because weight is such an emotive issue, it may be useful to ask your doctor's opinion if you think that you or any member of your family may be seriously overweight.

There is no magic cure for obesity, but you can achieve a lower, healthier weight by increasing your level of physical activity and reducing your intake of calories – particularly those that are derived from fat.

Obesity can have devastating consequences for health and happiness. On an emotional level it can lead to a lack of self-esteem and depression because you cannot enjoy a normal, active life. Physical symptoms may include shortness of breath, aching legs and swollen ankles. The excess weight may damage joints, causing osteoarthritis, particularly of the knees and hips.

Seriously overweight people have an above-average chance of developing high blood pressure, diabetes, gallbladder problems and gout. They are likely to suffer more severe symptoms of disorders such as angina and arthritis, which will persist and worsen with age unless steps are taken to lose weight. Obesity has also been linked to atherosclerosis, heart disorders and certain types of cancer.

What makes people obese?

Obesity is normally caused by a combination of overeating and a lack of exercise. If you eat more calories than you burn off during normal daily activity, the surplus calories are stored as fat. This does not necessarily mean that you eat a great deal more than most other people.

However, if your diet contains high-calorie foods such as biscuits, cakes, crisps and pies, which may be packed with fat and sugar, even small portions can provide your body with more energy than it needs. This is likely to result in weight gain – unless you step up your level of physical activity to offset your calorie intake.

Why fat is the issue

Medical research has established that the fat-to-carbohydrate ratio of a diet is highly significant in controlling weight. People who consume the same number of calories are more likely to become obese if their diet is high in fat rather than in carbohydrates, which is why weight is lost more readily on a low-fat rather than low-carbohydrate diet. This is reflected in the British Government's 1994 COMA report, which recommends that around 50 per cent of our energy should come from carbohydrate foods and a maximum of only 35 per cent from fats.

Many obese people blame their weight on a slow metabolism, a hormone imbalance or on an inherited tendency to put on weight easily. But these are rarely the real reasons. Sometimes obesity seems to run in families simply because each generation is passing on bad, unhealthy eating habits. Often, people put on weight as they grow older because they continue with the eating habits of earlier, more active years when their energy output was higher. Others respond to emotional problems by excessive eating.

Women are more prone to obesity than men because their bodies are more efficient at storing fat; ideally, women should have 25 per cent of body weight as fat, and men should have 15 per cent.

The only sensible way to lose weight is by combining a low-fat diet with some form of regular physical activity. Obese people, however, should always begin with a course of gentle exercises such as brisk walking or swimming. (See DIETS AND SLIMMING.)

Offal

BENEFITS

- *Source of good quality protein*
- *Liver and kidneys are rich or excellent sources of iron and niacin and useful sources of zinc*
- *Liver is an excellent source of vitamin A and vitamin B_{12}*
- *Heart is an excellent source of riboflavin and vitamin B_{12}*

DRAWBACKS

- *High in cholesterol*
- *Liver contains such high levels of vitamin A that it may cause birth defects if consumed during early pregnancy*

Because it is rich in the B vitamins (especially vitamin B_{12}), iron and zinc, offal is a nutritious food that also offers good value for money. However, organ meats such as liver, heart and kidneys can be very high in cholesterol, and should be avoided by people on low-cholesterol diets.

Any edible parts of an animal – apart from the flesh – are classed as offal. These include the liver, kidneys, heart, brains, stomach (tripe), tail, tongue, feet and pig's trotters. Since the discovery of 'mad cow disease' or BSE (see BEEF), the British Government has banned the sale of some types of offal for human consumption: the brain, spinal cord, thymus gland (sweetbreads), spleen and intestines of cattle over six months of age; and the intestines and thymus gland of all calves cannot be included in food.

The Inuit and polar bears

Traditional wisdom has taught the Inuit people never to eat the livers of polar bears and seals. Less enlightened Arctic explorers have tried them, however, and fallen ill as a result. This is because the livers are extremely rich in vitamin A, which in high doses can be toxic. As it is fat-soluble, the body cannot excrete vitamin A, so any excess is stored in fatty tissue.

Liver

All types of liver are excellent sources of vitamin A, needed for healthy skin and resistance to infection, and vitamin B_{12}, necessary for red blood cell formation as well as a healthy nervous system. Liver also provides many other nutrients, including iron and zinc. But it should be avoided by women who are trying to conceive, or who are in early pregnancy, as high doses of vitamin A may cause birth defects.

Liver is a valuable food for anyone who is suffering from iron-deficiency ANAEMIA. However, because it is high in cholesterol it should not be eaten more than once a week.

The benefits of offal

Liver is an excellent source of vitamin A, riboflavin and vitamin B_{12}, a rich or excellent source of iron and niacin, depending on the type, a rich source of folate, and a useful source of vitamin B_6 and zinc.

Brains, a soft meat usually from lambs or pigs, are an excellent source of vitamin B_{12} and a useful source of niacin.

Heart is an excellent source of protein, riboflavin, niacin and vitamin B_{12}. It is also a rich source of iron and a useful source of zinc.

Kidneys are an excellent source of riboflavin and vitamin B_{12}, a rich or excellent source of iron and niacin, depending on the type, and a useful source of thiamin, zinc and folate.

Oxtail is an excellent source of vitamin B_{12}, and contains riboflavin and vitamin B_6, but is very high in fat.

Tongue, usually ox or lamb, can be high in sodium. Stewed sheep's tongue is an excellent source of B_{12}.

Oils

BENEFITS

- *Supply essential fatty acids*
- *Good source of vitamin E*
- *Increase the body's absorption of fat-soluble vitamins A, D, E and K*

DRAWBACK

- *Fattening if consumed to excess*

According to the experts, oils can be good for you provided that you use them moderately and choose those with the lowest level of saturated FATS. As oils contain around 160 Calories per tablespoon, adding a small amount of oil to food increases its calorific value significantly.

Vegetable oils are made from nuts, seeds and pulses, the most common being soya bean, peanut, corn, rapeseed, sunflower, safflower and olive. Blended vegetable oil is usually a mix of the cheapest oils – often soya bean and rapeseed. These oils are liquid at room temperature (22°C, 72°F), and are low in saturated fatty acids.

The different vegetable oils consist of varying ratios of monounsaturated and polyunsaturated fatty acids. Olive oil has a healthy image because it is high in monounsaturated fatty acids. These do not adversely affect blood cholesterol, and according to recent studies can even help to lower blood cholesterol levels. Polyunsaturated fats are necessary because they include the essential fatty acids the body cannot manufacture for itself. These are required for growth and development, as well as for specific functions such as blood clotting.

There are two families of essential fatty acids. The omega-6 family is derived from linoleic acid and is found in safflower and sunflower oil among others. The omega-3 family is derived from the similarly named linolenic acid. Sources include soya bean and rapeseed oils, and FISH, especially oily varieties such as sardines, herring, mackerel, trout and salmon.

Sunflower and wheatgerm oils are also particularly rich in vitamin E, which has antioxidant properties and is thought to protect cell membranes. Be sure to store vegetable oils in a cool, dark place, as they lose their vitamin E when they are exposed to sunlight.

A variety of speciality oils is now readily available, including walnut, hazelnut, sesame and almond oils. All are good sources of essential fatty acids. They are used mainly as salad oils or for flavouring purposes. Some are sold as 'cold-pressed' oils because the oil is pressed out rather than extracted by heat. It is often claimed that cold-pressed oils retain more vitamin E; however, they tend to keep less well than refined oils.

Unlike other vegetable oils, palm oil and coconut oil are relatively high in saturated fatty acids. Palm oil is about 45 per cent saturated fat, and coconut oil is more than 85 per cent.

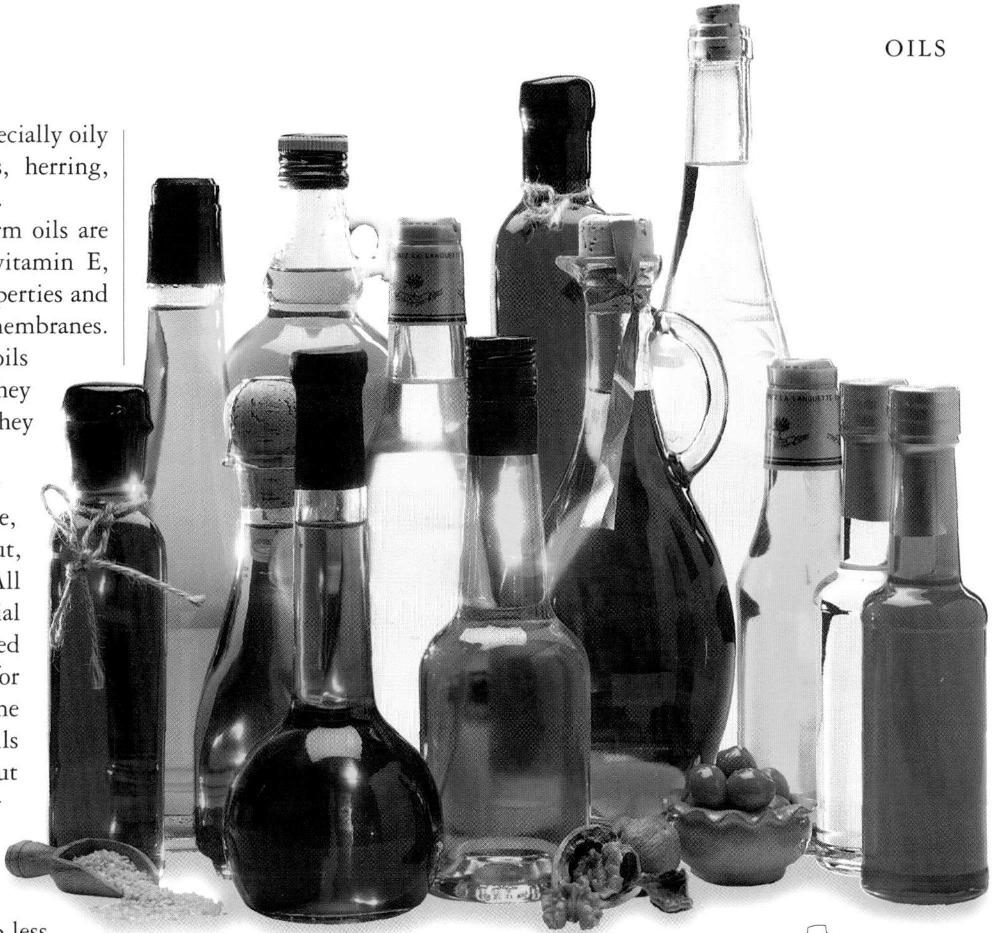

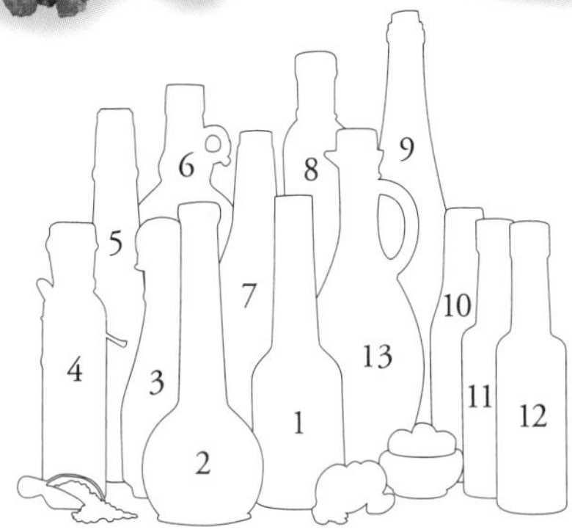

FLAVOURED OILS *While these oils tend to be expensive, they are usually healthier and more flavoursome than blended cooking oils. The range of oils now available includes walnut (1), cold-pressed extra virgin olive (2), olive and garlic (3), toasted sesame (4), olive (5), virgin olive (6), peanut (7), hot sesame (8), sunflower (9), hazelnut (10), garlic (11), chilli (12), and extra virgin olive (13).*

COOKING WITH OIL

Vegetable oils retain much of their nutritional value when used for frying, although extra virgin olive oil is not suitable for frying foods because heat impairs its flavour. Cooking oil should not be reused because constant reheating sets off a chemical reaction that can create FREE RADICALS.

It is healthier to fry foods in small amounts of oil that is predominantly polyunsaturated, such as sunflower or corn oil, or mostly monounsaturated, such as rapeseed, peanut or light or refined olive oil, than it is to use saturated fats such as lard, butter, beef dripping or solid vegetable fat. Many recent medical studies have linked the consumption of saturated fats with an increased risk of heart disease.

If meat is cooked in oil, there is some exchange of fat between the meat and the oil, which can decrease the saturated fat content of the meat. Meat does not take up fat readily, but if it is fried in a coating of breadcrumbs, this will absorb large quantities.

Fry at a high temperature (about 180°C, 356°F) where possible in order to seal food and minimise the uptake of fat. Wait until the oil is really hot before adding food. The amount of fat taken up depends on the surface area of the food and how much fat it absorbs. Large chips take up less fat proportionally than small ones. Kitchen paper can be used to remove excess fat.

Stir-frying – the technique used in Oriental cooking – requires only small amounts of oil, and, according to the traditional method, a little water too. As a result, stir-fried ingredients tend to absorb only small amounts of fat.

OLD AGE AND CHANGING NEEDS

Although energy demands are reduced as you get older, people still require meals which are nutritionally sound. A well-balanced diet is one of the best defences against the effects of time.

While ageing is inevitable, physical decrepitude is not. Many of the outward signs of growing old can be slowed – and life may even be prolonged – by maintaining a sensible approach to diet.

Elderly people may be poorly nourished for several reasons. They may have difficulty chewing, and as the body ages it no longer digests or absorbs food so readily. Those living on their own do not always bother to prepare nutritious meals. And, as time blunts the senses of smell and taste, so the appetite fades.

Make meals colourful and avoid slipping into preparing repetitive 'easy meals'. Attractive and varied food can revitalise a jaded appetite. Because age slows down physical activity – and sometimes leads to reduced mobility – energy requirements can decline by as much as 5 per cent for each decade after the age of 40, but the need for nutrients for repair and regeneration does not. In fact, US research now suggests that the body's demand for vitamins and minerals actually increases with age.

NUTRIENT DEFICIENCY

Both the body's metabolism and its ability to absorb food become less efficient with age, as less stomach acid and other digestive secretions and enzymes are produced. Also the effects of long-term bad habits, such as smoking, start to materialise. It is known that smoking and drinking alcohol, for example, can sap the body's stores of nutrients.

A reduced intake of vitamins B_6, B_{12}, D and folate, and of the minerals calcium, magnesium and zinc, is particularly common among the elderly. When the body's levels of these nutrients fall below the required daily level, health will almost certainly suffer.

Replenishing vitamin B_{12} can often help to reverse lapses of memory or problems of coordination and balance. This may be as simple as including plenty of fish, offal and pork, eggs, cheese and milk in your diet. But about 1 in every 200 elderly people in Britain, whose diets are low in vitamin B_{12}, lack the gastric secretions necessary for its absorption and may need injections to make up the deficit. Folate may also be lacking in the diets of the elderly due to a low consumption of

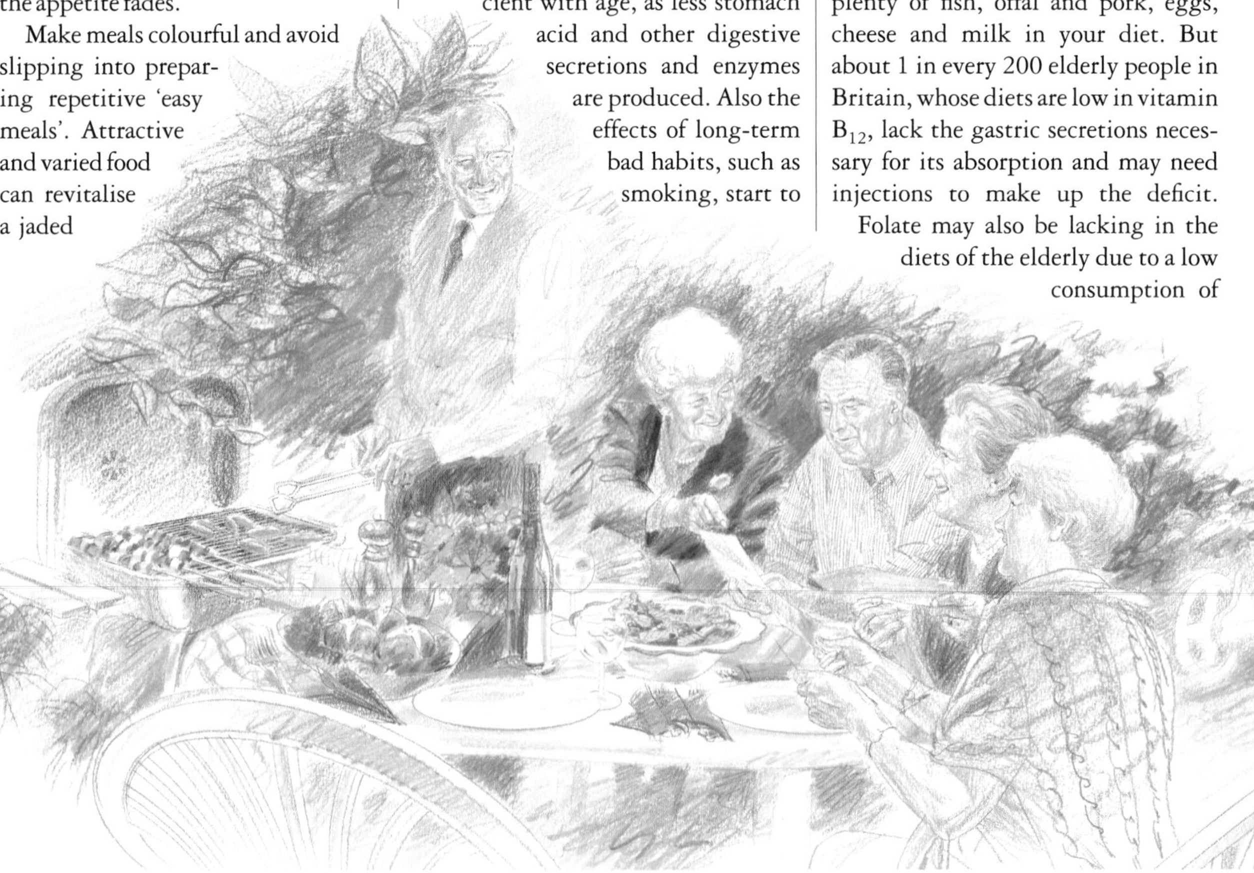

fruit and vegetables. And, since many elderly people may have only limited exposure to sunlight, a dietary source of vitamin D is needed. Vitamin D enables calcium to be properly absorbed – without enough calcium, bones become thin and fragile. Other than margarine or oily fish, there are few dietary sources of vitamin D and so it may be sensible to use a supplement.

After retirement, older people may feel they merit a few indulgences, such as cigarettes or an occasional drink. What is the point, their argument runs, in giving up such pleasures late in life? But smoking and excessive drinking deplete the body's stores of vital nutrients as well as stimulating the production of potentially harmful FREE RADICALS. The benefits of a moderate alcohol intake, and of giving up smoking, should not be underestimated. A good diet can also help by supplying the vital nutrients known as ANTIOXIDANTS – found in fruit, vegetables and most nuts – which can 'mop up' the free radicals.

Elderly people, worried about bladder control, may drink too little, but their need for fluid is much the same as in youth, and the risk of dehydration is as high. Sipping six to eight glasses of water a day should be sufficient.

Because excess weight can creep up as a result of a slowed metabolism and decreased energy needs, older people should exercise regularly. Obesity poses an even greater health risk in later life than it does in youth.

In old age, a balanced diet is as important as at any other stage in life. Choose foods supplying dietary fibre, such as bread, fruit and vegetables, to help to avoid CONSTIPATION and other DIGESTIVE PROBLEMS – which are quite common sources of misery in later life.

AN APPETITE FOR LIVING *A meal always tastes better when shared with friends. Try to eat a balanced diet, whatever your age.*

Nutritional needs of elderly people

As you get older and less active you need fewer calories – a fact often reflected in a smaller appetite and a lack of interest in food – but requirements for vitamins and other nutrients increase rather than diminish with age.

CARBOHYDRATES AND STARCHES	MEAT AND POULTRY
Whole grains, such as barley, brown rice and wholemeal bread, provide vitamin B_6, folate and other nutrients, along with insoluble fibre – which is essential for preventing constipation. Porridge made with milk, or fortified breakfast cereals, provide a simple, easily prepared and nutritious start to the day.	Offal, such as liver and kidneys, is an inexpensive and concentrated source of protein. Like all other meats, it supplies vitamins A, B_{12}, D, E, thiamin and folate, as well as iron and zinc. Poultry is particularly useful; the meat is an excellent source of easily digested protein, and the carcass can be boiled up to make a stock for soup.
VEGETABLES	DAIRY PRODUCE
Dark green leafy vegetables such as cabbage, kale and spinach are inexpensive, easy to cook and provide many important nutrients, including beta carotene, vitamins B_6, E and folate, as well as calcium, iron and magnesium. Root vegetables such as potatoes, turnips and parsnips are filling, cheap and also provide carbohydrate, fibre and vitamin C.	Milk, cheese and yoghurt are inexpensive sources of complete protein. They contain the vitamins A, B_{12}, folate, riboflavin and niacin, and provide calcium (vital for bone mass). Use about 250ml (9floz) of milk per day, on breakfast cereals or in drinks. Unless you have high blood pressure or raised cholesterol levels, you can eat about 250g (9oz) cheese per week.
FRUIT	EGGS
Citrus fruit, strawberries and tomatoes all provide valuable vitamin C. Apples and pears contain useful soluble fibre, which helps to lower blood cholesterol levels. Bananas are a good source of potassium and carbohydrate. Eat plenty of fruit, ensuring a joint fruit and vegetable intake of at least five 100g (3½ oz) servings daily.	Easy to cook, eat and digest, eggs are an excellent and inexpensive source of complete protein. They also provide vitamins A and D. However, because they also contain high levels of cholesterol, it is probably best not to eat more than three or four eggs a week.
DRIED BEANS, PEAS AND LENTILS	FISH
Pulses, a cheap source of protein, are best eaten with grain foods, such as bread, rice or pasta, which provide the essential amino acids to complete the chain of protein in pulses. Pulses are a good source of most B vitamins and fibre (both insoluble – needed to prevent constipation – and soluble, which may lower blood cholesterol levels). Baked beans on wholemeal toast provide a hot, nourishing meal.	All fish provides high-grade protein and B vitamins. Oily fish, such as mackerel and herring, are inexpensive and provide essential fatty acids, vitamin A and vitamin D. Tinned oily fish such as salmon and sardines offer most of the benefits of fresh oily fish with the added bonus of edible bones which are a good source of calcium.

OLIVES

BENEFITS
- *Good source of vitamin E*
- *Contain natural antioxidants*

DRAWBACK
- *High in salt*

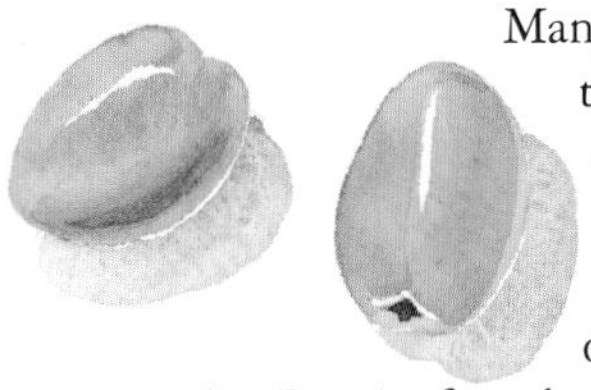

Many people used to think that olives were a high-calorie food because of the oil they contain. But in fact, both black and green varieties provide relatively few calories; a serving of ten olives contains between 30 and 40 Calories. Although olives are a good source of vitamin E, they are not consumed in large enough quantities to supply useful amounts to the diet. They also provide natural ANTIOXIDANTS. The oil derived from olives is high in monounsaturated fatty acids, which, unlike saturated fats, do not adversely affect blood cholesterol levels and may even help to lower them slightly.

Raw olives are so bitter and unpalatable that they have to be pickled in brine, or salted and then marinated in olive oil, to be enjoyed as a food.

Because olives are high in sodium, they should be eaten in moderation by anyone with high blood pressure.

ANCIENT AND SACRED

The olive tree has been cultivated for at least 5000 years. In Ancient Greece, it was sacred to the goddess Athena. The olive branch is traditionally a symbol of both peace and fertility; historically, an olive branch was a peace offering.

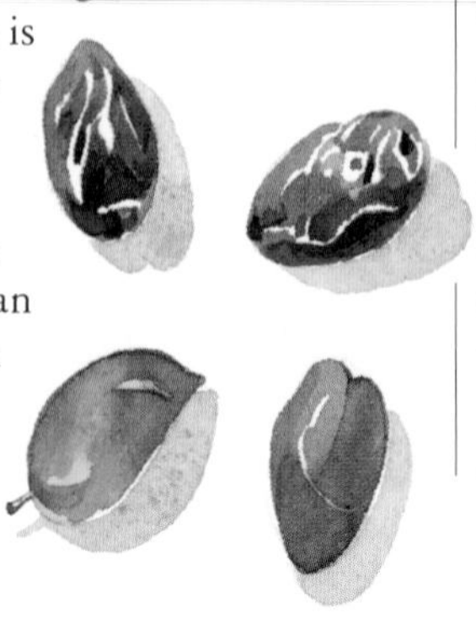

ONIONS

BENEFITS
- *May help to lower blood cholesterol levels and reduce the risk of coronary heart disease*
- *Prevent blood clotting*
- *May help to reduce the risk of cancer*
- *Used as a decongestant in traditional medicine*

DRAWBACKS
- *Can trigger migraine in susceptible individuals*
- *Cause bad breath when eaten raw*

Throughout history, onions have been revered as a natural cure-all. They belong to the same family as GARLIC – the allium family. While today's scientists agree that onions may have the power to prevent and treat certain illnesses, they have yet to discover the exact substances that have these remarkable healing powers; as a result, onions continue to be the subject of much research.

Experiments show that eating raw onions may help to reduce cholesterol levels because they increase levels of high-density lipoproteins (HDLs), special molecules that help to carry cholesterol away from body tissues and artery walls.

It has been claimed that onions, whether cooked or raw, protect against the harmful effects of fatty foods on the blood. They appear to contain a substance that helps to prevent the blood from clotting and may increase the rate at which clots are broken down. While these claims have not yet been proven, there is some evidence to suggest that this effect may help to prevent circulatory diseases such as coronary heart disease, thrombosis and a wide range of conditions associated with strokes and poor circulation. For this reason it may be worth including more onions in your diet: you could try combining mild raw onions with hamburgers, or, instead of an onion sauce, serve roast onions with lamb.

Researchers are also investigating the power of onions to protect against cancer, as it is believed that the sulphur compounds in onions may help to prevent the growth of cancer cells. Cooked onions have also been used to clear catarrh in traditional medicine. Eat the onions either roasted or boiled in dishes such as soups and stews.

Onions can lead to migraine in some people, however, and the sugars they contain can cause flatulence. Eating raw onions can also lead to bad breath.

HERBAL PANACEA

The sulphur compounds which give onions their flavour and strong smell led to the belief that the juices could prevent infection. In the Middle Ages, onions were used as protection against the plague. Some modern herbals state that applications of onion will remove warts and prevent acne, but there is no scientific back-up for these claims.

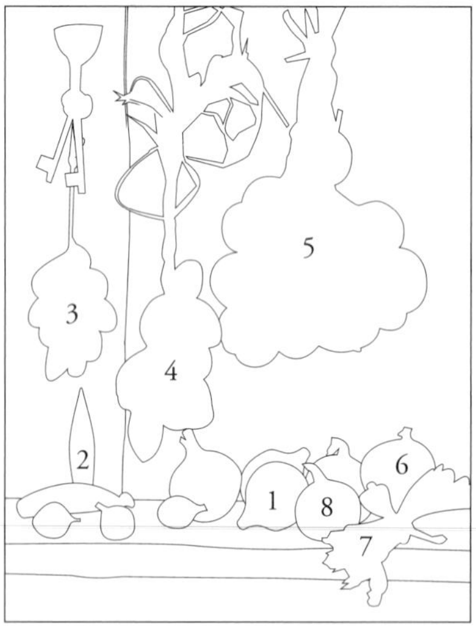

PUNGENT OR SWEET *The sharp flavour so characteristic of the onion family softens with cooking. Red onions (1), banana shallots (2), small onions (3), shallots (4), brown English onions (5), Spanish onion (6), spring onions (7), white onions (8).*

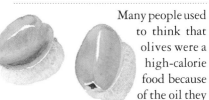

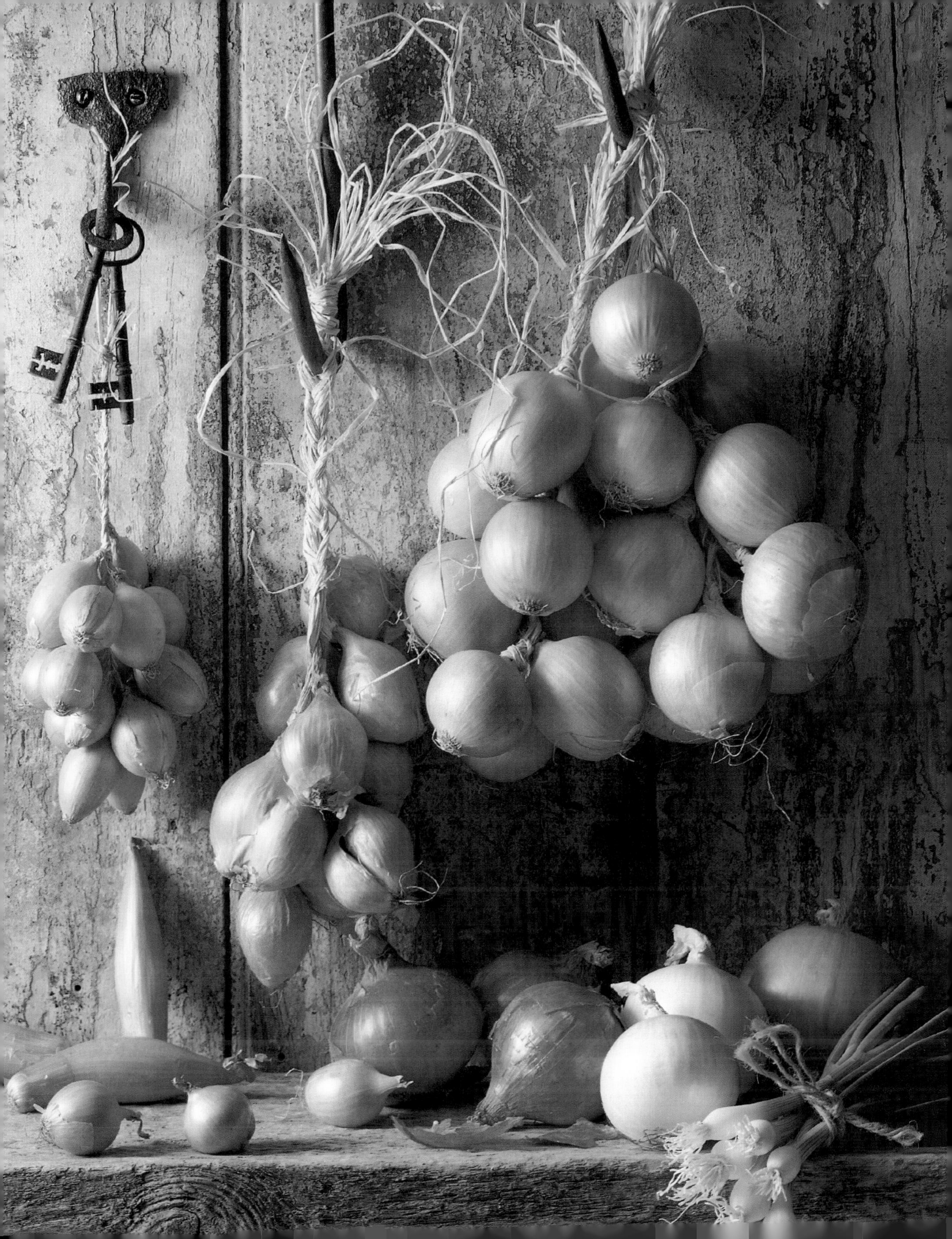

ORGANIC AND HOME-GROWN FOODS

Free from pesticides, additives and artificial growth hormones, organic food appeals to a public wary of chemicals. But most experts doubt whether organic food offers any nutritional benefits.

The production of organic food is governed by strict standards. For vegetables and cereals these standards are now laid down in an EU regulation while organic animal products are controlled on a national basis by the United Kingdom Register of Organic Food Standards (UKROFS).

KEEPING PESTS AT BAY

- Instead of using pesticides, grow plants and bright, scented flowers to attract insects that prey on the aphids that will damage fruit and vegetable crops.
- Plant aromatic summer savory to protect runner beans, fragrant buckwheat to keep pests off broad beans or pot marigolds to prevent whitefly from infesting the plants in your greenhouse.
- Surround your garden with a thick hedge to attract birds, which will eat up slugs and insects.
- Dig a pond which will encourage frogs and toads; they will also keep down the slug population.
- Leave a pile of logs to shelter beetles, which will prey on pests.
- A patch of nettles will attract ladybirds which feed on aphids.
- Fine-mesh or spun materials placed over susceptible plants will keep away carrot fly, cabbage root fly and cabbage white butterflies without affecting growth.
- A mulching material made of natural bark or wood chippings suppresses weeds and also contains nutrients that benefit the soil.

In organic farming the use of chemical fertilisers or pesticides is avoided; animals and poultry are raised in natural conditions on organically farmed land and must not be treated with antibiotics on a routine basis.

The notion of healthy food produced by natural means has impressed a public which has become nervous about the chemical pesticides and additives used in intensive farming and food production. The British Government is giving some support to organic farming to meet the consumer demand, while recognising that it is one option for a more environmentally friendly form of agriculture.

CAUSE FOR CONCERN?

During the 1980s, the government banned the use of 11 pesticides which were thought to be potentially carcinogenic or capable of causing birth deformities or gene mutations. The formulation and application of pesticides are now so advanced that the levels of pesticide residues in foods are generally much lower, and therefore less likely to cause any harm.

Yet there have been occasions when plant foods have been found to contain unusually high levels of pesticides. Recently in the UK high levels of organophosphates were detected in the skin of carrots. Although the levels were not considered high enough to pose a serious risk to humans, people were advised to top, tail and peel the carrots, to avoid the chemical.

Advocates of organic farming criticise many of the methods used in intensive animal husbandry, such as the old practice of feeding naturally herbivorous cattle with offal. It is believed that infected offal was the starting point of 'mad cow disease' (bovine spongiform encephalopathy, BSE), identified in 1986. Similarly, an outbreak of salmonella in chickens in 1975 may have been caused by feeding birds with salmonella-infected hens.

ETHICS VERSUS EVIDENCE

Despite the ethical arguments, there is still not much evidence to show any nutritional benefits from consuming organic food. However, one potentially dramatic endorsement is the claim that men who eat organic food have higher sperm counts than those who eat intensively farmed produce. Although research has been carried out which shows this effect, the results have been strongly contested. Further research is now being undertaken to examine whether there is indeed a link between declining male fertility and the huge growth in the use of agrochemicals over the past 50 years.

No significant nutritional difference between organic and intensively farmed produce has yet been proved. However, fresh home-grown fruit and vegetables are likely to contain more

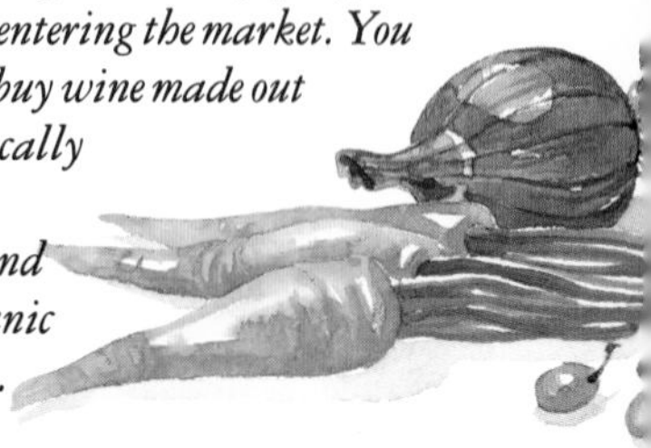

SPOILT FOR CHOICE *Consumer demand has led to a great variety of organic products entering the market. You can now buy wine made out of organically grown grapes, and even organic chocolate.*

vitamin C than food which has been transported and displayed for a day or two, as vitamin C levels begin to fall as soon as produce is picked.

SUPPLY AND DEMAND

Although many consumers would express a preference for natural, additive-free foods, organic food accounts for no more than 1 per cent of the produce bought in Britain, and an estimated two-thirds of organic food is imported. This is partly because shoppers who pay lip-service to the organic principle are still buying chemically treated fruits and vegetables that are cheaper and tend to look better than the more natural product. Many of the major food retailers have promoted organic food, but they have had little success as the majority of consumers are reluctant to pay more for inferior-looking fruit and vegetables.

Organic produce is more expensive to grow because yields are smaller. It spoils faster than chemically treated fruit and vegetables, so more has to be abandoned and therefore costs and prices rise. Because production is still limited, the British organic sector has yet to establish an effective distribution network – another key factor that drives up costs.

So the future for organic food is still not clear. There is some government support for organic agriculture in the form of an aid scheme for farmers. But the public still has to be persuaded to buy the produce. The large supermarket chains seem anxious to push the 'wholefood' image, but sometimes the products fall a little short of the organic ideal.

SOILS SUITABLE FOR GROWING YOUR OWN

Growing your own produce in a garden or allotment is the best way to ensure that the fruit and vegetables you eat are organic and pesticide-free. Although few people possess the area of land required to provide a varied year-round supply, a modest plot can still produce a satisfying yield.

To use the soil to best advantage, it is important to understand its nature and composition. Soils may be clay, loam, sand, chalk and peat but most are a mixture with one predominant type. As a rough guide, heavy clay soils drain slowly and can remain too sticky to work for a day or so after a lot of rain, but moderate loam soils can be worked on within a few hours. Light, sandy soils drain within minutes of a downpour and therefore need constant watering or mulching in dry weather.

A good natural farmyard manure made up of animal droppings and straw added to the soil will provide most of the chemical nutrients plants need. But an over-acid soil will need the addition of a layer of ground chalk or limestone to make it more alkaline.

Plants and crops need fertilisers while they are growing. Organic gardeners often prefer to use blood, bone and fishmeal rather than more easily absorbed non-organic products because this keeps bacteria in the soil active which in turn helps to promote healthy plant growth. The aim is to provide the key nutrients – potash, nitrogen and phosphates. Plants and crops also need magnesium, boron, manganese, iron and molybdenum, – trace elements, so-called because they are only required in extremely small amounts.

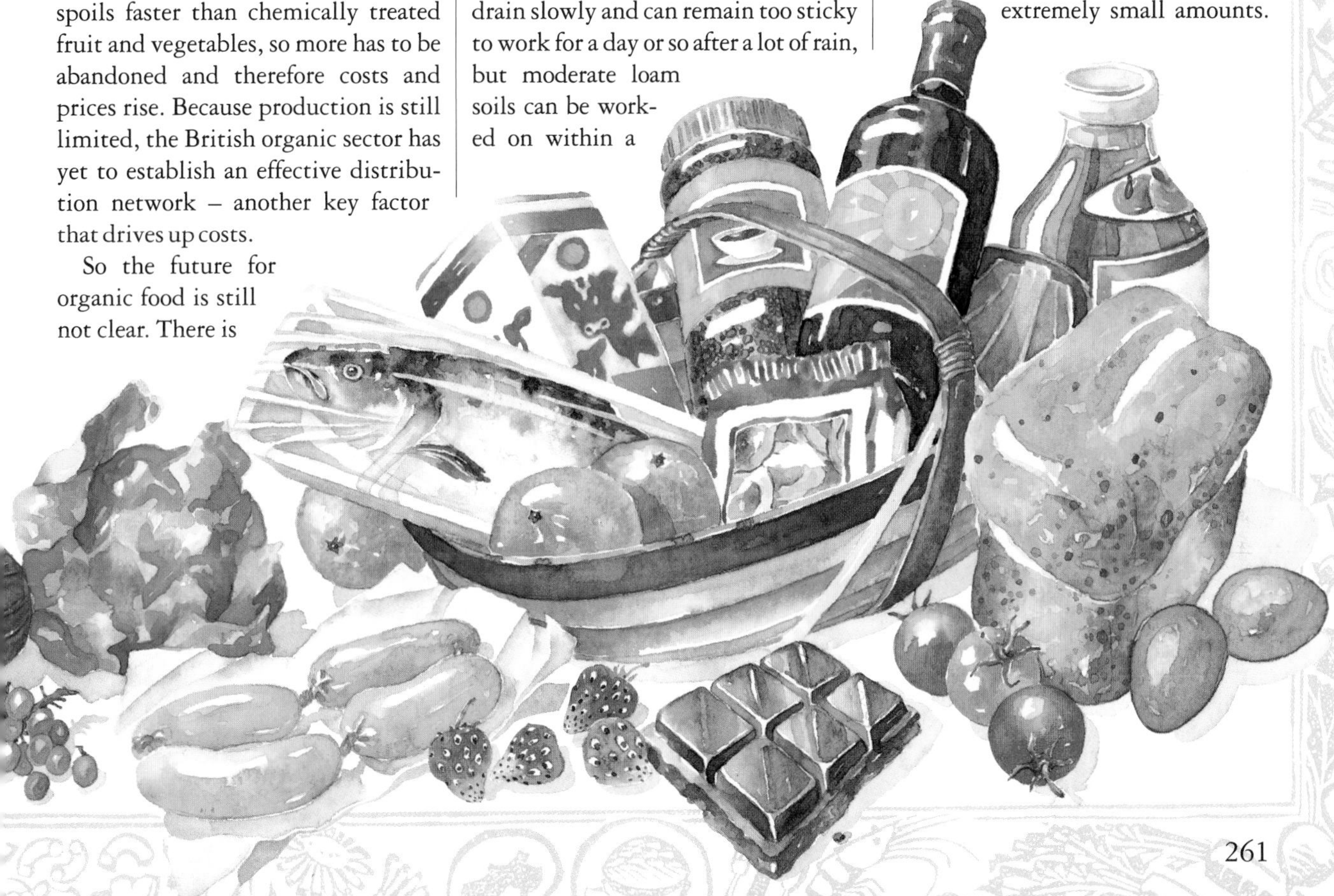

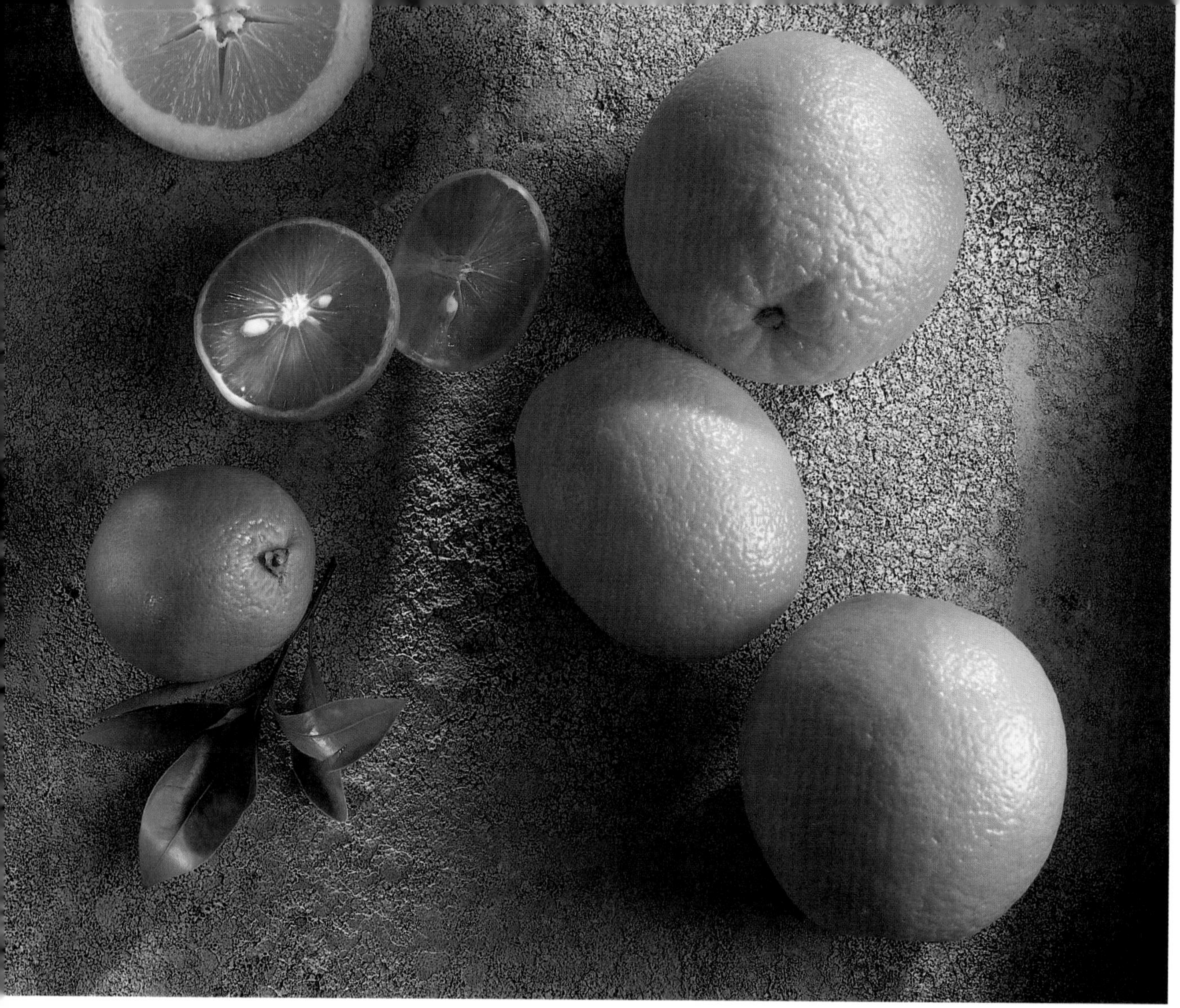

GOLDEN FRUITS *Originally from the Middle East, Jaffa oranges are now cultivated in sunny climates all over the world. The smaller blood orange is grown mainly in Italy.*

ORANGES

BENEFITS

- *Excellent source of vitamin C*
- *Contain thiamin and folate*
- *Contain pectin, which may lower blood cholesterol levels*

Most people associate oranges with healthy doses of vitamin C. They are right to do so: just one medium-size fruit supplies more than the adult daily requirement.

Vitamin C helps to make collagen, which is essential for healthy skin. It also helps to maintain the body's defences against bacterial infections. As an ANTIOXIDANT, it can prevent free-radical damage and may therefore help to ward off or inhibit certain cancers. Oranges also contain thiamin and folate, two of the B vitamins.

The nutritional benefits of oranges include the membranes between the segments. These contain pectin, a type of soluble dietary fibre found in most fruits, especially apples, lemons and redcurrants. High levels of pectin may lower blood cholesterol levels. The membranes also contain bioflavonoids, which have antioxidant properties. For maximum benefit, therefore, it is better to eat the fruit rather than just drink the juice. When a recipe calls for the zest of an orange, try to use unwaxed fruit if possible; otherwise, wash the fruit thoroughly to remove any wax or fungicides.

Some people are allergic to citrus fruits and may develop a rash soon after eating them. Citrus fruits have also been linked to migraines in some susceptible individuals.

Different species of orange include the Jaffa orange, the mandarin, the Maltese or blood orange, the seedless navel orange, and the bitter Seville orange, which is mainly used for marmalade. Candied peel, essential oils and pectin are among the by-products.

Organic food

See page 260

Osteomalacia

TAKE PLENTY OF
- *Oily fish, eggs and breakfast cereals fortified with vitamin D*
- *Sensible exposure of skin to sunlight*
- *Milk and dairy products, for calcium*

CUT DOWN ON
- *Wheat bran and foods containing phytic acid*

The adult form of rickets, osteomalacia, is relatively rare in the developed world today. Like rickets, it is usually due to a deficiency of vitamin D, although very occasionally it can be caused by a calcium deficiency. The body needs an adequate intake of vitamin D in order to absorb calcium and phosphorus from the diet. Both these minerals are vital for the development of strong, healthy bones. Without them, bones soften and are liable to become deformed and break easily.

Vitamin D is obtained mainly from the action of sunlight on the skin, but is also found in oily fish and dairy products and some fortified foods, such as margarines and breakfast cereals.

One cause of osteomalacia, therefore, is a lack of sunlight, for example in people with dark-pigmented skin who move to a less sunny climate. The risk is increased if they cover up their skin rather than expose it to the sun.

Vegetarians are at risk because vegetables contain little vitamin D. Some disorders of the bowel, such as coeliac disease, can lead to a deficiency because the vitamin may not be absorbed normally. Kidney failure and liver disease can lead to osteomalacia because the kidneys and liver cannot process vitamin D properly. The metabolism of vitamin D can also be affected by chronic alcohol abuse. The long-term use of antacids can lead to osteomalacia because they reduce the body's ability to absorb phosphorus, which influences the level of calcium in the body. However, such cases are rare and the diet would have to be very low in phosphorus (found in meat, fish and eggs).

High intakes of phytic acid, found in wheat bran, brown rice and pulses, may also add to the risk of osteomalacia by inhibiting calcium absorption. More than 3-4 cups of coffee a day, or a high intake of protein or salt, can increase calcium loss. Oxalic acid, found in spinach, rhubarb and chocolate, can also reduce calcium absorption.

Treatment of osteomalacia involves long-term vitamin D supplements prescribed by a doctor. Calcium-rich foods, such as milk and plenty of green leafy vegetables, may also help.

Osteoporosis

TAKE PLENTY OF
- *Foods rich in calcium, such as milk and dairy produce*
- *Food sources of vitamin D, such as oily fish and eggs*
- *Sensible exposure of skin to sunlight*

CUT DOWN ON
- *Foods rich in phytic acid, such as wheat bran, brown rice and nuts*
- *Foods containing oxalic acid, such as spinach, rhubarb and chocolate*
- *Alcohol*
- *Salt*
- *Caffeine*
- *Smoking*

There is mounting evidence to suggest that eating more calcium-rich foods, particularly during childhood and adolescence, is the most effective way of preventing, or at least minimising the extent of, osteoporosis. In this condition, which most commonly affects middle-aged and elderly women, the bones become weak and brittle, so that sufferers are more vulnerable to fractures, even after minor accidents. The areas most at risk are the hips, wrists and the spine. Other symptoms may include pain in the hips and back, loss of height and sometimes a stooped posture – as the bones of the spinal column become weak and compressed.

Who is at risk?

Throughout life, our bones are continuously being replaced. Cells called osteoclasts eat away at the existing bone, thereby releasing calcium into the bloodstream. At the same time, cells called osteoblasts form the new bone and deposit calcium into it. In young and healthy people, there is equal activity between the two types of cell, with the result that bone mass and structure are maintained. With age, however, we lose more calcium from our bones than is put back, and our bones lose density.

Women have a far greater risk than men of developing osteoporosis. They have less bone mass to begin with, and with the menopause they lose the hormone oestrogen, which slows bone loss. While postmenopausal women are most at risk, some younger women – marathon runners, gymnasts, dancers and anorexics, for example – can also suffer from osteoporosis. What they all have in common is a very low amount of body fat, irregular or non-existent menstrual periods, and low oestrogen levels. A low body weight increases the risk of osteoporosis because it puts less stress on bones, and stress increases bone density. Body fat also promotes oestrogen production.

Thinking ahead

Because the dietary levels of calcium during adolescence are of particular importance for maximum bone density and strength in adulthood, it is only sensible for parents to encourage their teenagers to include plenty of calcium-rich foods in their diet, such as milk and green leafy vegetables.

Vitamin D is needed by the body to absorb calcium. The main source of this vitamin is the action of sunlight on the skin, but it is also found in some foods, including oily fish and eggs, and in certain fortified foods such as margarine and some breakfast cereals.

The consumption of alcohol and salt should be limited because they can both hasten calcium loss. Heavy drinkers are particularly vulnerable because they tend to be both poorly nourished and accident-prone, which leads to correspondingly greater risks of bone loss and fractures. Caffeine consumption should not exceed 3-4 cups of coffee a day, as caffeine removes calcium from the bloodstream. The risk of developing osteoporosis is increased by smoking which interferes with oestrogen production.

Some drugs have also been associated with bone loss when prescribed in high doses; these include prednisone, used in the treatment of asthma, arthritis and other inflammatory diseases, and some antiseizure medicines.

Regular, but not excessive, exercise from an early age is another extremely important preventive measure. Bones respond to the stresses and strains involved in exercise by becoming denser and therefore stronger. People who have osteoporosis are also advised to take exercise because regular physical activity helps to prevent mineral loss from the bones and also improves strength, muscle tone and balance, which is important for the elderly because it reduces the chance of falling. Anyone who has been inactive for many years should start with a gentle form of exercise, such as walking or swimming.

Case study

At 47, Sheila had just reached the menopause and was anxious to avoid the many physical problems her mother had suffered. Sheila's mother, who had always disliked milk and cheese, had led a quiet life and very rarely left the family home.

In her mid sixties she had begun to develop back pain, which had greatly restricted her mobility. She consulted her doctor, who referred her to hospital where tests showed that she had osteoporosis (brittle bones). By the time she died, at the age of 78, she had suffered two collapsed vertebrae and a fractured hip. The doctor said that her condition was probably due to a combination of three factors: insufficient calcium in her diet; too little exercise; and reduced production of vitamin D in the skin because it was so seldom exposed to sunlight. Sheila's doctor explained to her that women are likely to develop osteoporosis after the menopause when their levels of oestrogen drop, because oestrogen regulates the amount of calcium in the blood. However, he added, making sure that her diet contained plenty of calcium could help to reduce this effect. Sheila took his advice and made sure she had a good intake of calcium from dairy products and green leafy vegetables.

She began a programme of regular exercise and also started taking hormone replacement therapy (HRT) to reduce the rate of bone loss. By modifying her lifestyle and boosting her uptake of calcium, Sheila knows she has minimised her risk of developing osteoporosis.

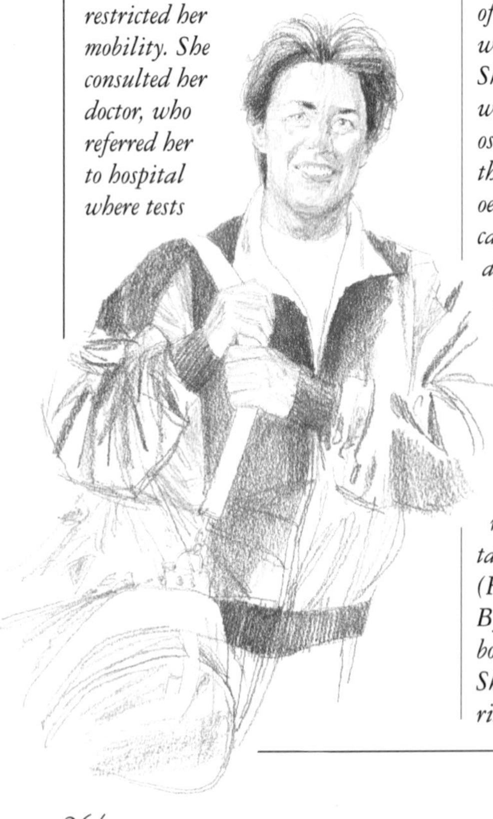

FIGHTING BACK

The treatment of osteoporosis aims to slow down or stop the bones from becoming weaker. People should cut down on smoking and alcohol, as they increase urinary loss of calcium.

Phytic acid, which is found in wheat bran, nuts, seeds and pulses, blocks calcium absorption, so people with osteoporosis should obtain their fibre from sources such as fresh fruit and vegetables. Oxalic acid, found in spinach, rhubarb, almonds and chocolate, for example, also reduces calcium absorption, so these foods should be eaten in moderation. A high intake of protein or salt can increase the loss of calcium from the body as well.

Many postmenopausal women can benefit from hormone replacement therapy, which replaces waning stores of oestrogen. Nevertheless, HRT can have its drawbacks, and any woman contemplating it should consider the balance of risks and benefits.

Daily supplements of calcium and vitamin D have also been shown to slow down bone loss and thereby reduce the incidence of fractures.

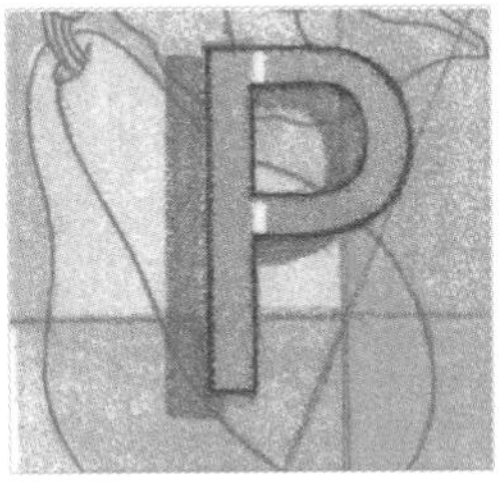

PALPITATIONS

CUT DOWN ON

- *Coffee, tea, chocolate and cola which all contain caffeine*
- *Smoking*
- *Alcohol*

Most people have experienced the occasional bout of palpitations – the awareness of the heart beating faster or irregularly during physical exertion or when they are particularly angry, anxious or scared. The sensation of thumping in the chest can be quite alarming, but sufferers should be reassured that palpitations are usually harmless. However, if they recur persistently, a doctor should be consulted. If abnormalities are suspected, the doctor will carry out diagnostic tests.

A rapid or irregular heartbeat can be caused by stress, an overactive thyroid gland, an excessive intake of caffeine or alcohol or an allergic reaction to food – some people report palpitations after eating soya sauce, for example. Lack of magnesium can also cause palpitations, so increase your intake of the mineral by eating green vegetables and whole grains.

Because nicotine stimulates the heart, smoking may also exacerbate the symptoms. Most cases of palpitations can be cured simply by reducing caffeine intake and by cutting down on drinking alcohol and smoking.

PAPAYA (PAWPAW)

BENEFITS

- *Excellent source of vitamin C*
- *Good source of beta carotene*

The sweet, juicy papaya is extremely nutritious. In common with other orange-pigmented fruits, it is a good source of beta carotene which helps to prevent damage by free radicals which might otherwise lead to some forms of cancer. Half a medium-sized fruit will provide an adult's daily requirement of vitamin C as well as supplying small amounts of calcium and iron. Papayas are an ideal food for invalids, because the flesh is easy to chew and swallow.

Papaya juice contains papain, an enzyme similar to the pepsin produced by the human digestive system to break down proteins. As a proteolytic enzyme (one that breaks down proteins), it is used in the food industry as a meat tenderiser. Medically, papain-containing ointment is used externally to remove the roughened skin from wounds. Papain also exhibits pain-relieving properties, and the US Food and Drug Administration (FDA) has approved its medical use in spinal injections to ease the discomfort of slipped discs.

Grown in many tropical regions, papayas have pink or golden flesh filled with seeds which are usually scooped out and discarded, even though they have a spicy flavour and can be dried and used as a peppery seasoning.

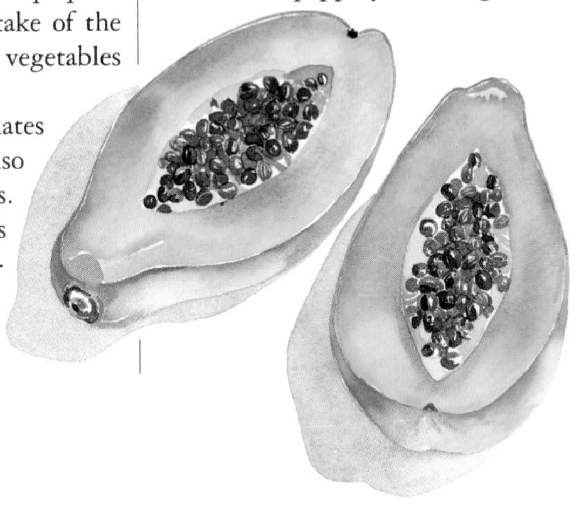

PARKINSON'S DISEASE

TAKE PLENTY OF

- *Fibre-rich whole grains, prunes, fresh fruit and vegetables to relieve constipation and to provide vitamins B, C and E*
- *Fluids – at least 1.7 litres (3 pints) a day*

Parkinson's disease is a progressive neurological disorder that is incurable; symptoms vary and not all people are severely disabled. Eating the right foods may help in the management of Parkinson's disease to a limited extent.

There are a number of problems that people with the disease can face when eating and drinking. These include trouble chewing or swallowing, because drug treatment can often result in abnormal tongue and mouth movements. Plenty of time should therefore be allowed for meals.

Patients with Parkinson's disease often lose weight, which may be due to reduced energy intake because of the difficulty in eating. Excess weight, however, can make the symptoms worse, because it places a further restriction on already limited movement.

In order to control their weight and improve health, people with Parkinson's disease should eat plenty of fresh fruit, vegetables and whole grains, with moderate amounts of protein and unsaturated fat, while cutting down on saturated fats and sugars.

AVOIDING CONSTIPATION

Patients should also eat foods that help to prevent CONSTIPATION, which is a common problem for people with Parkinson's disease. This means eating more fibre. Many people think of bran when they wish to increase their fibre intake; but although bran is high in fibre, it does not contain nutrients and can impair the body's absorption of some minerals. It is better to obtain fibre from fruit, vegetables and grains. This will help to speed food through the system; fruits such as figs, prunes, papaya and pineapple are especially valuable as they have a natural laxative effect. It is also important to drink plenty of fluids – at least 1.7 litres (3 pints) a day – to counter any tendency towards constipation. The best drinks to choose are water and fruit juice. Tea and coffee may have adverse effects on the nervous system, so only have moderate amounts of these.

MEALTIMES AND MEDICATION

A minority of people with Parkinson's disease find that too much protein interferes with the action of the drug L-dopa (levodopa), the main drug prescribed to help control the disease. The drug should therefore be taken between meals (at least 40 minutes before eating). Meals should contain moderate levels of protein, supplied by small quantities of protein-rich foods. When appetite is poor, as is often the case with Parkinson's disease, small helpings of food every 2-3 hours may be more appealing.

A MYSTERY DISEASE

The disorder affects a small part of the brain and is characterised by tremor, stiffness and slowness of movement. It progresses gradually and symptoms include a stooped posture, a rather expressionless face, speech problems, drooling and loss of dexterity. The cause of Parkinson's disease is still a mystery, but it is known that it occurs when a small group of cells in the brain fails to function normally. This is triggered by a shortage of dopamine, one of the chemicals that transmits messages between nerves.

Research has focused on either replacing or stimulating diminished supplies of dopamine with potent drugs, the main one being L-dopa.

PARSNIPS

BENEFITS
- *Useful source of starch and fibre*
- *Useful source of vitamins C and E*
- *Contains folate*

This sweet, starchy winter root vegetable makes a healthy alternative to potatoes. It is often overlooked as a source of fibre, which helps to maintain bowel regularity and may help to protect against cancer of the colon. Parsnips are a useful source of the antioxidant vitamins C and E and contain folate for healthy blood cells. Parsnips are at their sweetest a few weeks after the first frost: exposure to cold causes the starch they contain to start turning into sugar.

PASTA

See page 268

PEACHES

BENEFITS
- *Rich source of vitamin C*
- *Easily digestible*
- *Gentle laxative*

Fresh, ripe peaches are a tasty, low-calorie food. One average 100g (3½oz) fruit contains around 30 Calories and, if eaten unpeeled, provides more than three quarters of the daily requirement of vitamin C. The soft fruit is easy to digest and has a gentle laxative effect.

Weight for weight, dried peaches contain six times the calories of the fresh fruit. A 50g (1¾oz) portion of dried peaches supplies about two-fifths of the daily recommended amount of iron and a sixth of the potassium.

When canned, however, peaches lose over 80 per cent of their vitamin C content and, if canned in sugary syrup, are considerably higher in calories.

PEARS

BENEFITS
- *High in natural sugar*
- *A useful source of fibre, vitamin C and potassium*

A pear contains about 70 Calories, most of which are in the form of natural fruit sugars, so a pear provides a quick and convenient source of energy. Pears are also a useful source of vitamin C, although you would need to eat four or five fruits to meet the full daily requirement for an adult.

Because pears are among the least allergenic of foods, and well tolerated by nearly everyone, they are appropriate as a weaning food and also in exclusion diets. Pears make a useful contribution to potassium intake, which plays a part in regulating blood pressure. They are also a source of the soluble fibre known as pectin.

Dried pears are high in calories and a useful source of fibre. They contain iron and are rich in potassium. Eat them straight from the packet as a high-energy snack or reconstituted by soaking in water before stewing.

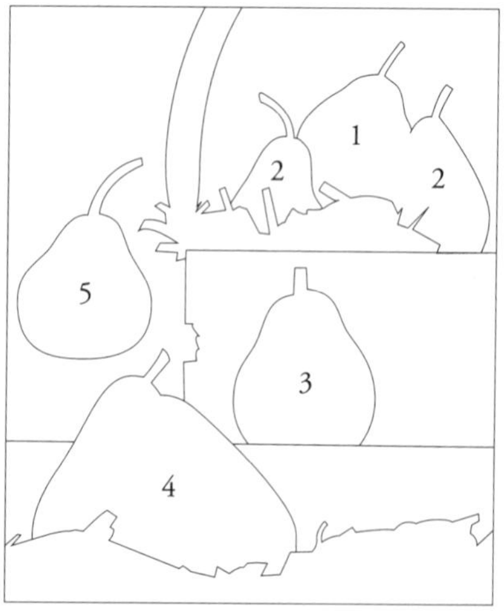

POPULAR PEARS *There are hundreds of varieties of pear, including Comice (1), Red Williams (2), Gold Williams (3), Conference (4) and Packham (5).*

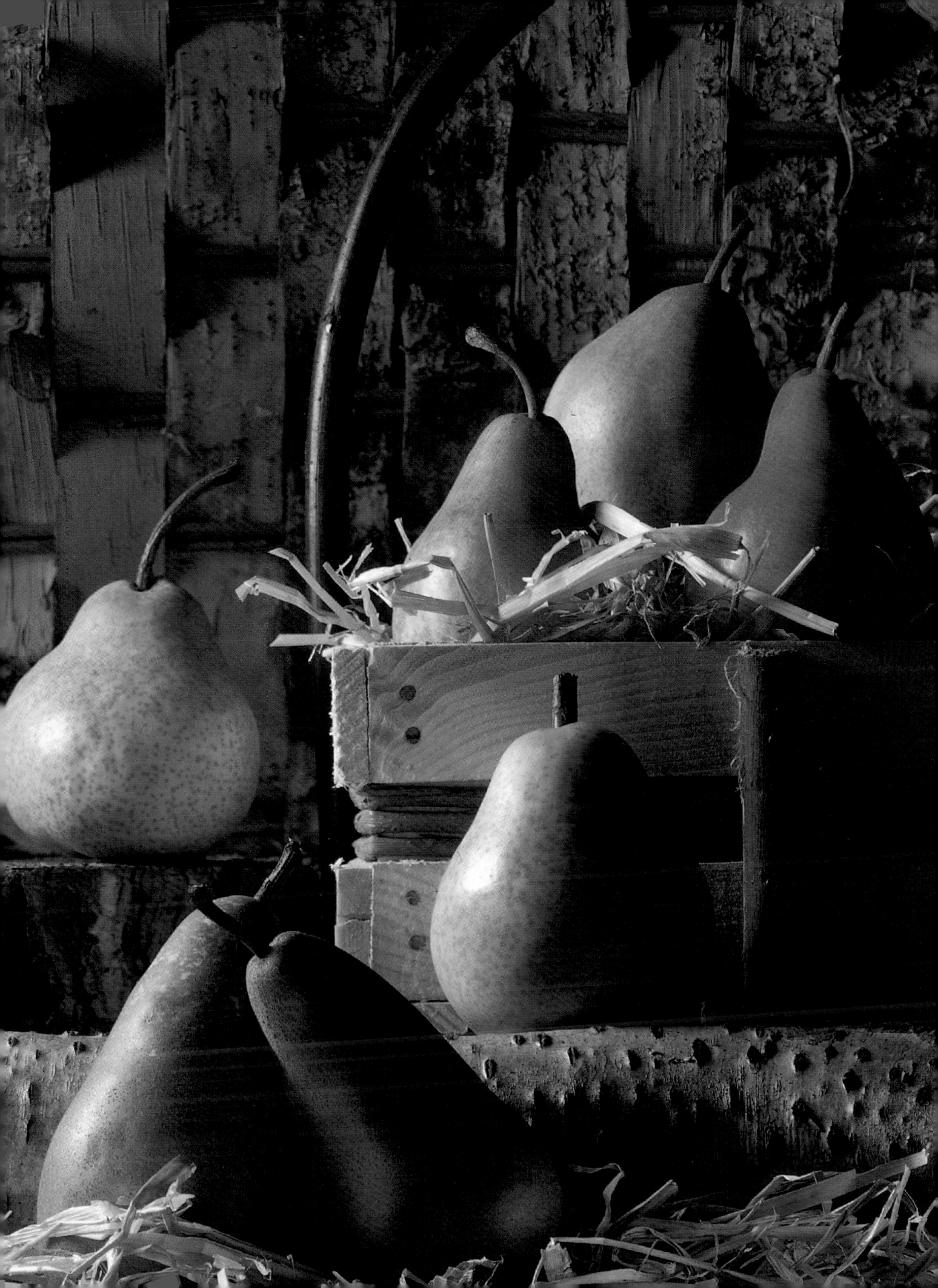

PASTA: A HEALTHY BASE FOR TASTY MEALS

Once dismissed as merely fattening, pasta has won much more than a reprieve; the benefits of complex carbohydrates are now well recognised and pasta dishes are enjoyed by almost everyone.

Pasta is one of the staple foods of the Mediterranean diet. The high consumption of pasta in Italy and some other parts of southern Europe almost certainly contributes to the low levels of heart disease in these areas. In Britain, people generally do not eat enough complex carbohydrates, such as bread and pasta. Instead, they fill themselves up on less healthy refined carbohydrates contained in cakes and sweets, or on fatty foods.

Pasta can be the base for an almost infinite number of quick and healthy main meals. Literally a paste or dough made with flour and water, it is used either dried or fresh. The complex carbohydrates it provides are broken down by the body and can be used to build up stores of energy, or glycogen. For this reason, many athletes eat a lot of pasta while preparing for endurance events such as marathon races.

Contrary to popular belief, pasta is not a high-calorie food and, if served with a simple tomato sauce, for example, or with other fresh vegetables, it can be included in a slimming diet. It is only when it is coated with butter and cheese, or served with a cream sauce, that pasta becomes fattening.

The dried white pasta that has become one of our great convenience foods is made with water and a coarse flour obtained from a high-protein (hard) wheat known as durum wheat. Even though the wheatgerm and bran are removed during milling, white flour still contains some fibre and resistant starch, which help to keep the digestive tract healthy.

Wholewheat pasta is made from 100 per cent wholewheat or whole durum wheat flour. It has a coarser, chewier texture than white pasta and is a better source of fibre and thiamin, the B vitamin needed to convert carbohydrates into energy. Wholewheat pasta provides about 10 per cent more calories and 5 per cent more protein than white pasta. Both types can be enriched with eggs. Other ingredients such as tomatoes or spinach, as well as various herbs, are sometimes added to flavour and colour the dough.

In South-east Asia, China and Japan, noodles are an integral part of national diets – whether served on their own or added to soups, salads and hot dishes. They are usually made from wheat, rice, mung-bean or buckwheat flour.

WHEN SAUCES ADD FLAVOUR

Simple pasta dishes can be transformed by one of several classic Italian sauces. Traditional ingredients include olive oil, garlic, onions, mushrooms, plum tomatoes, fresh basil and pine nuts. Among the most popular are *salsa al pesto*, made with extra-virgin olive oil, plenty of fresh basil, Parmesan cheese and pine nuts; *salsa pomodori,* also known as *Neapolitana*, made from a healthy combination of olive oil, onions, tomatoes and garlic; and *salsa alla Bolognese*, a tangy, beef-based sauce made richer by the addition of tomatoes and either white or red wine.

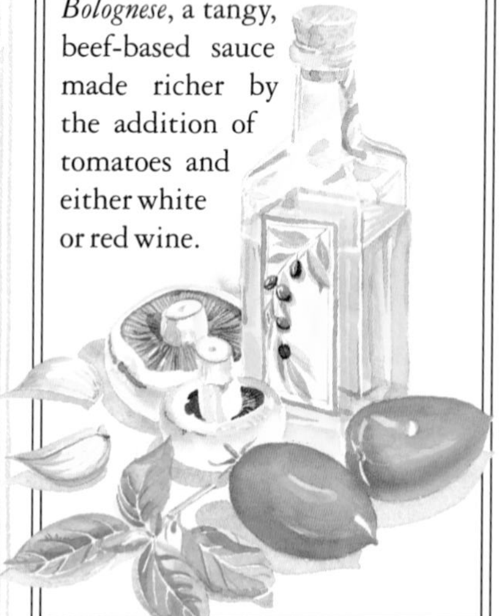

BENEFITS

- *Excellent source of complex carbohydrates for energy*
- *Useful source of protein*
- *Low in fat*

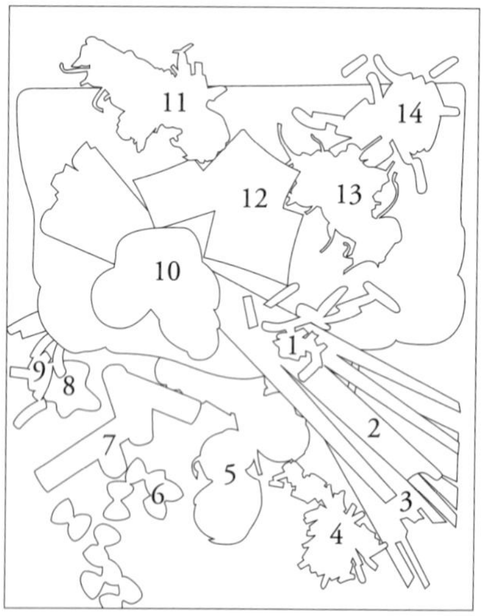

HEALTHY VARIETY *Pasta now comes in many different shapes, sizes and colours: fusilli (1), white (2) and wholemeal spaghetti (3), macaroni (4), tagliatelle (5), farfalle (6), cannelloni (7), semolina (8), rigatoni (9), vermicelli (10), egg noodles (11), ravioli (12), tortellini (13) and macaroni (14).*

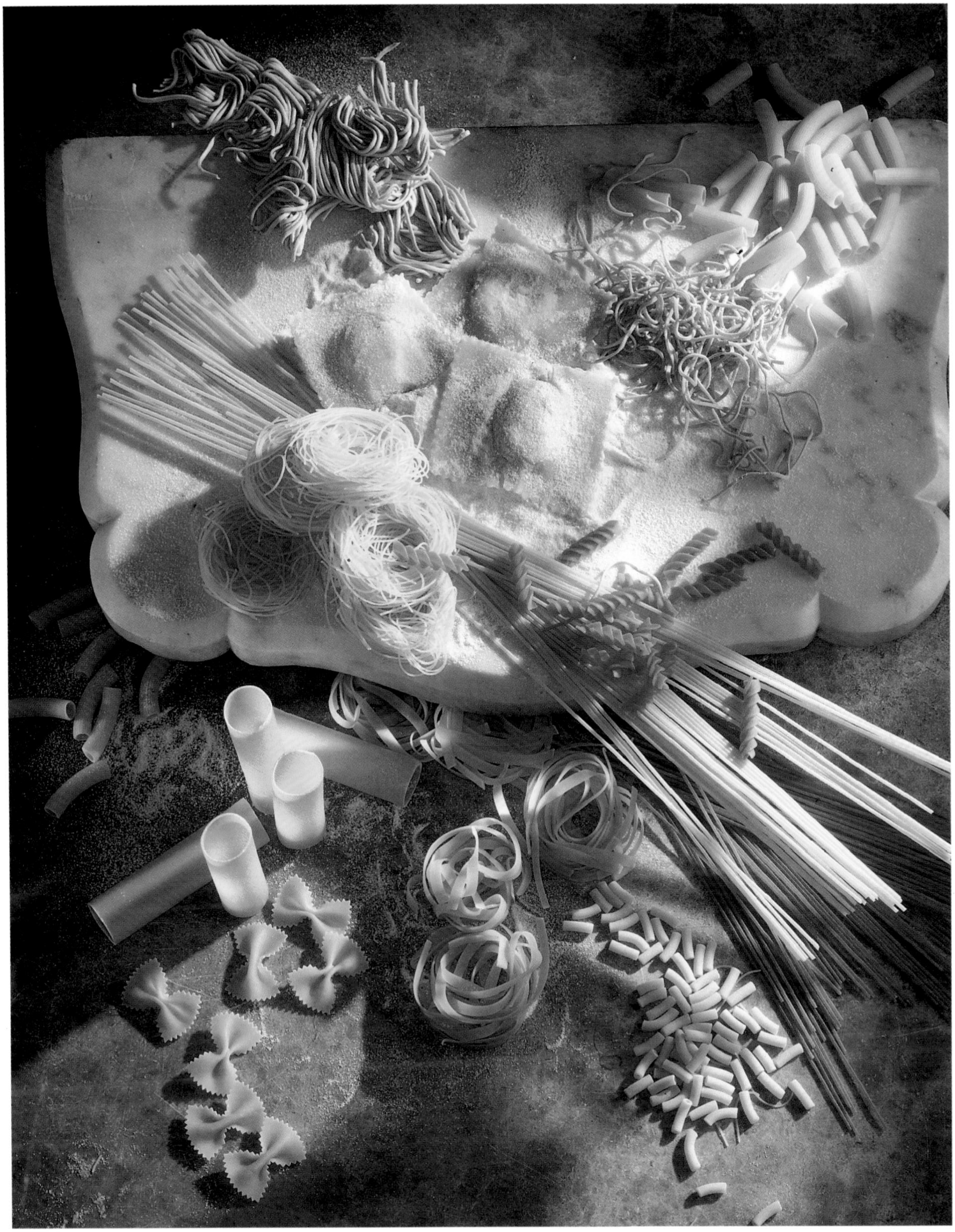

Peas

BENEFITS

- *Rich source of thiamin (vitamin B_1)*
- *Good source of vitamin C*
- *Contain protein, fibre, folate and phosphorus*

Because they are eaten while they are immature, peas contain proportionately less protein and more vitamin C than other PULSES. One serving of cooked peas (65 g, 2¼oz) provides 50 Calories and supplies a quarter of the vitamin C and half the thiamin required daily. Peas also supply folate, fibre and phosphorus.

As soon as the pods are harvested the natural sugar in peas begins to be converted into starch. As freezing usually takes place very quickly after the pods have been picked, chemical changes are minimal, whereas fresh peas may take several days to reach the greengrocer, by which time more of the sugar has turned into starch. This is why many people prefer frozen peas to fresh ones, finding them more tender. However, because they are blanched before they are frozen, peas lose some of their vitamin C and thiamin content.

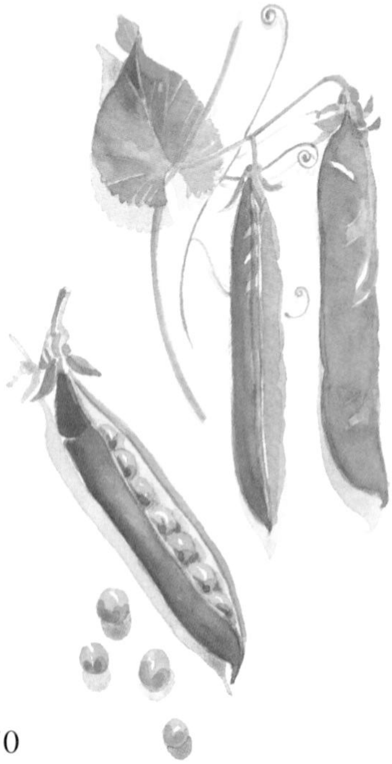

Further vitamins are lost when peas are boiled before eating. Tinned peas also lose much of their vitamin C content during the canning process and may contain added salt and sugar.

There are several types of peas now available. The traditional green pea has a pod that is not very palatable, but varieties such as the sugar snap or MANGETOUT should be eaten 'whole'.

Peppers (sweet or bell)

BENEFITS

- *Excellent source of vitamin C*
- *Useful source of beta carotene*
- *Good source of bioflavonoids*

Sweet or bell peppers are an excellent source of vitamin C, which is necessary for healthy skin, ligaments and bones. Weight for weight, green peppers contain twice as much vitamin C as oranges; red peppers contain three times as much, and are also an excellent source of beta carotene.

Beta carotene is an antioxidant and is converted into vitamin A as and when the body needs it. Peppers also contain bioflavonoids. Both beta carotene and bioflavonoids are thought to neutralise FREE RADICALS – possibly helping to protect against cancer.

Peppers change from green to red or to yellow, and become sweeter as they ripen on the vine. Most of the peppers we eat are green; they are fully developed but not completely ripe. The skin of green peppers in particular is waxy and may be difficult to digest, but it also gives peppers a long shelf-life.

Peppers make a delicious addition to salads and other dishes when charred under a grill and skinned; they lose few of their nutrients when served this way. They can also be grilled, skinned and puréed to provide a fat-free sauce to accompany meat, pasta or fish.

Peptic ulcers

EAT PLENTY OF

- *Vegetables rich in beta carotene and fruit containing vitamin C*
- *Zinc-rich foods such as whole grains, and seafood (especially oysters)*

CUT DOWN ON

- *Salt and soya sauce*
- *Spicy foods*
- *Caffeine in coffee, tea and cola drinks*
- *Alcohol*

Eating more vegetables and fruit, such as carrots, kale, red and green peppers, citrus fruits, apricots and kiwi fruit may promote healing of peptic ulcers, and protect against further damage to the gut wall. The helpful nutrients in these foods are beta carotene, which the body converts to vitamin A, and vitamin C. Foods rich in zinc, such as whole grains and seafood, can also help the healing process.

Peptic ulcers occur when the balance between the acidic digestive juices and the protective mucous membrane is disturbed: the lining of the digestive tract breaks down and ulcers are able to form. Some studies suggest that essential fatty acids (found in fish oils and seed oils) may help to protect against ulcers by increasing the production of prostaglandins (a group of compounds, one function of which is to protect the lining of the alimentary canal).

A study quoted in the *American Journal of Epidemiology* in 1992, linked large intakes of salt and soya sauce to a higher risk of gastric ulcers, a form of peptic ulcer usually found near the entrance to the duodenum (a section of the intestine just below the stomach).

The low-fibre diet, based on bland foods – such as poached white fish, milk and so-called 'sloppy' ingredients, taken as frequent small meals – which was formerly prescribed for people with ulcers, has been largely discredited after studies found that it was often ineffective. Modern advice puts more emphasis on letting people with ulcers eat normally. Large meals should still be avoided, however, as they can encourage the production of excessive acid. Sufferers may also find that chilli peppers, black pepper, mustard and other strong spices – such as those found in curries – may aggravate their symptoms.

Ulcers are relatively common in Britain, occurring in 1 in 10 men and 1 in 20 women. Symptoms range from discomfort to burning pain in the upper abdomen and, in severe cases, vomiting and weight loss.

THE ROOT OF GOOD HEALTH?

Liquorice root appears to be an effective herbal remedy for peptic ulcers, provided it has been treated to remove an acid which can raise blood pressure. The root, taken as a chewable tablet, has been shown to protect against ulcers caused by the harmful effects of aspirin, and other drugs such as ibuprofen, on the stomach lining.

THE BACTERIUM TO BLAME

Research reported in *The Lancet* found that a bacterium called *Helicobacter pylori* was present in the stomachs of people with ulcers. The symptoms usually disappeared after the bacterium was dispersed with antibiotics, which suggests that it is involved in forming ulcers. Domestic cats can carry the bacterium, and researchers are now trying to find out whether cats can pass it on to people.

Anyone who has an ulcer should avoid caffeine and alcohol which can increase the acidity of the stomach and so aggravate the condition.

PICKLES AND CHUTNEYS

BENEFIT

- *Most types of pickled fruits and vegetables retain their minerals*

DRAWBACKS

- *Often high in salt*
- *Pickled fish and meat may be linked with a higher risk of certain cancers*
- *Some types may trigger allergies*

Pickling is a traditional way of preserving fresh fruit and vegetables by discouraging the growth of microbes that would otherwise cause them to decompose. Although minerals are often retained in the process, many vitamins are usually destroyed. The

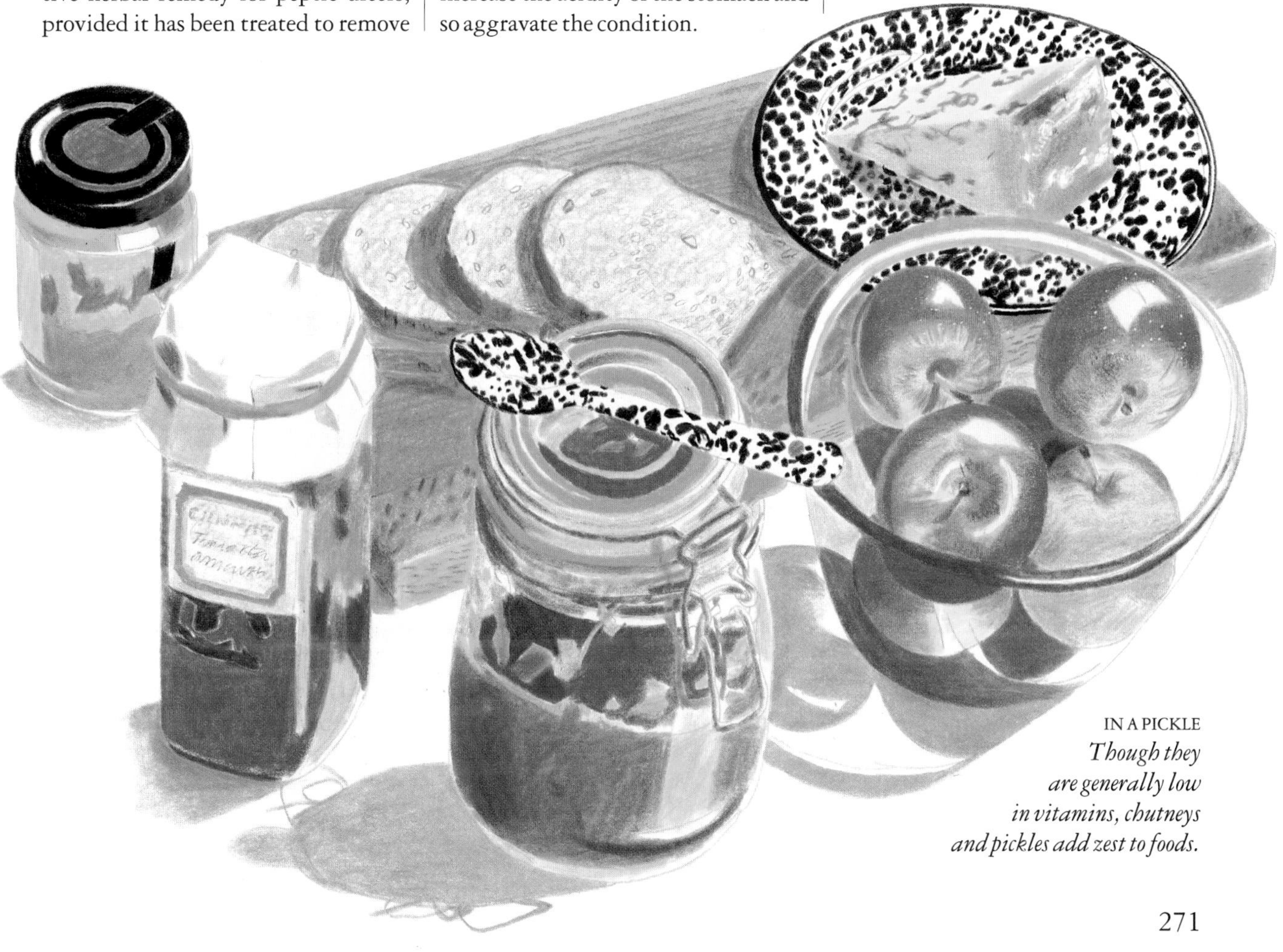

IN A PICKLE
Though they are generally low in vitamins, chutneys and pickles add zest to foods.

exception to this is sauerkraut (pickled cabbage), an unusual pickle which is a good source of vitamin C. A single 100g (3½oz) serving of sauerkraut supplies about a quarter of the adult daily requirement of the vitamin.

Sauerkraut and also dill pickles are fermented in a salt solution which is strong enough to prevent the growth of harmful bacteria but weak enough to allow some strains to proliferate, specifically those which produce lactic acid. It has been claimed that lacto-fermented foods have beneficial effects on the digestive system, but there is little evidence to support this claim.

More usually, pickles are prepared by adding hot or cold vinegar to the raw vegetables or by cooking them in vinegar. A third method, which causes loss of minerals as well as vitamins, involves treating vegetables such as cucumbers or gherkins with salt to reduce their moisture content and then preserving them in vinegar. In this method of pickling the sodium level of the food is much increased.

Unlike sauerkraut, most pickles, chutneys and relishes are eaten in small amounts, adding flavour to meals but few nutrients. Sugar is often added to chutneys, and fruit chutneys may consist of as much as 50 per cent sugar, although this figure includes sugars naturally present in the fruit.

Eating large amounts of salt-cured and salt-pickled foods has been linked by research with an increased risk of cancers of the mouth, oesophagus and stomach. The foods which may be particularly responsible for this include pickled fish and cured meats, which contain nitrates and nitrites that can turn into cancer-forming nitrosamines in the stomach.

People on low-salt diets should try to avoid pickles because of their high sodium content. Pickles, chutneys and relishes can also trigger allergies. Fermented foods may contain tyramine or histamines, while fruit and vegetable chutneys may contain salicylates: these are all potential allergens. When preparing homemade pickles do not be tempted to reduce the sugar or salt content too greatly, as this may enable the deadly bacterium *Clostridium botulinum* to proliferate and so cause botulism (see FOOD POISONING).

PINEAPPLE

BENEFIT

- *Useful source of vitamin C*

DRAWBACK

- *Can trigger allergic reactions in rare instances*

Traditional folk medicine credits the sweet, juicy flesh of the pineapple with various healing powers, with some apparent justification. The fruit does not, however, contain many useful nutrients. A standard 80g (3oz) portion supplies a quarter of the daily requirement of vitamin C, but other than that, it provides little in the way of vitamins and minerals.

Scientific interest has centred on the fact that the fresh fruit contains an enzyme called bromelain which breaks down proteins. Its action is so strong that people who work in pineapple plantations and canning factories have to wear protective clothing to prevent damage to their skin. Bromelain is sometimes used medicinally in concentrated tablet form for patients who have problems digesting protein.

Since bromelain's medical use was first investigated in 1957, some 400 papers have been written on its various applications. There are indications that it may help to break up blood clots and could therefore be useful in the treatment of heart disease. There is also some evidence that suggests it may help to combat sinus congestion and urinary tract infections. It might also augment the effect of antibiotics.

Bromelain has been used as an anti-inflammatory agent for the treatment of osteo and rheumatoid ARTHRITIS. And, because it is thought to accelerate tissue repair, it also has many applications for sports injuries, including bruises, blisters and sprains.

PINEAPPLE POWER

Prior to such research, fresh pineapple was used in folk medicine to treat a variety of problems. Gargling with the juice is a traditional treatment for sore throats, while eating pineapple has long been believed to help to relieve other disorders such as catarrh, arthritis, bronchitis and indigestion.

The canning process affects the vitamin C content only minimally, but it destroys the bromelain. Weight for weight, pineapple canned in its own juice, rather than in syrup, contains only marginally more calories than the fresh fruit – 47 Calories as opposed to 41 Calories per 100g (3½oz).

Pineapples do not become any sweeter after picking; good indicators of ripeness are a fruit that feels heavy for its size with fresh green leaves and, most important of all, a sweet, fairly strong fragrance.

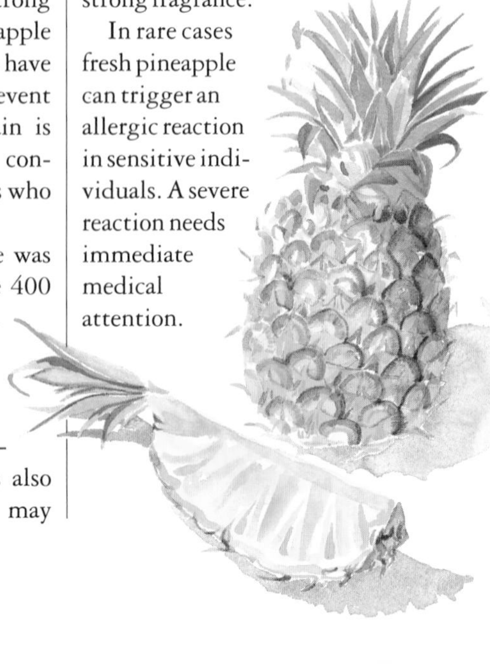

In rare cases fresh pineapple can trigger an allergic reaction in sensitive individuals. A severe reaction needs immediate medical attention.

PLUMS

BENEFITS
- *Contain vitamin E*
- *Good source of potassium*

There are more varieties of plum than any other species of stone fruit – about 2000 in all. Plums contain vitamin E, an ANTIOXIDANT that helps to protect cells from damage caused by FREE RADICALS, and may help to retard some of the effects of ageing, such as wrinkling. When plums are dried they are known as PRUNES. In this form, when most of their water content has been removed, they are a more concentrated source of nutrients, although only potassium and iron are present in really useful amounts.

Some health food shops stock plums pickled in brine, called *umeboshi*, which have long been used as a traditional medicine in Asia. There they are used to treat digestive problems, such as stomach upsets, nausea and CONSTIPATION.

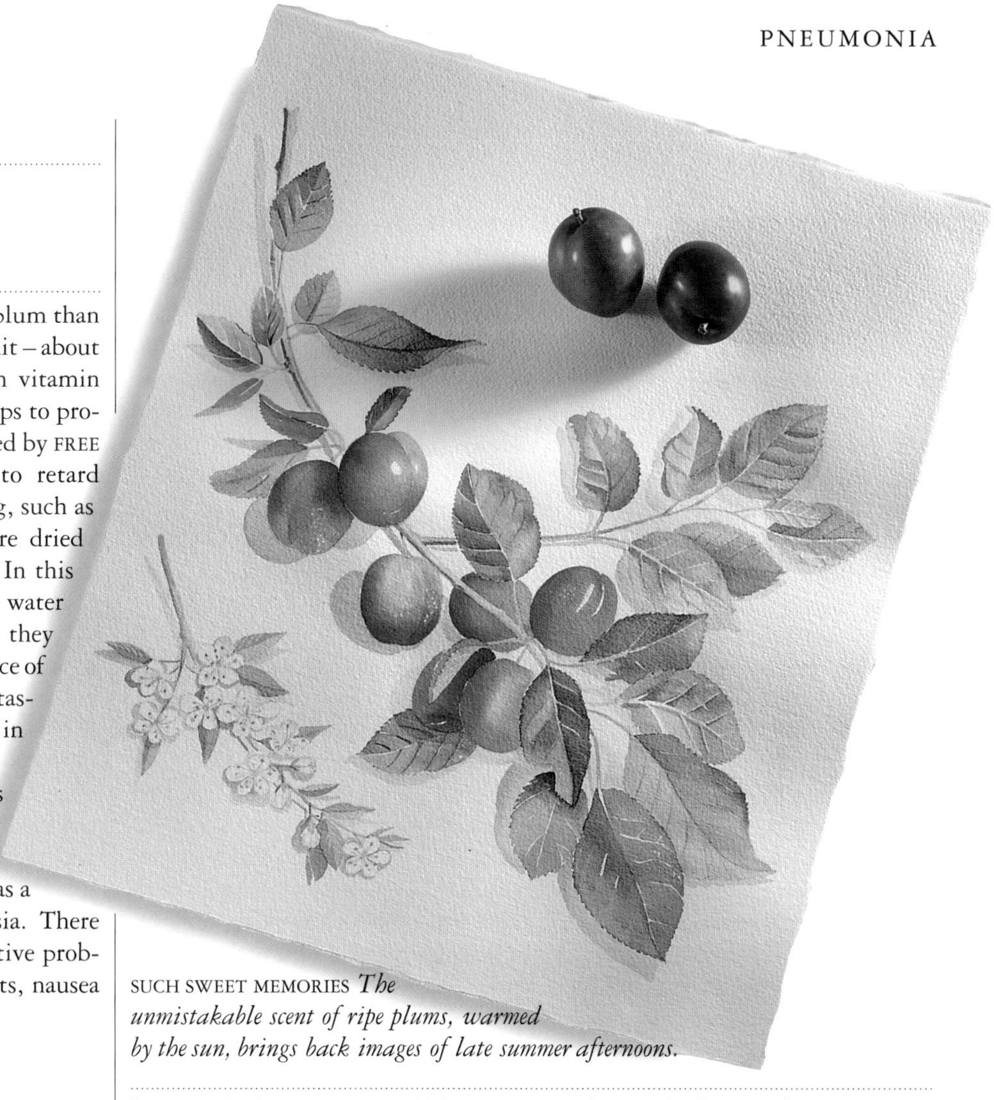

SUCH SWEET MEMORIES *The unmistakable scent of ripe plums, warmed by the sun, brings back images of late summer afternoons.*

PNEUMONIA

TAKE PLENTY OF
- *Fluids, especially fruit juices*
- *Fresh fruit and vegetables*
- *Oily fish, eggs and other good sources of vitamin A*

Diet can go some way to helping the medical treatment of pneumonia by maintaining the patient's fluid and calorie intake. Pneumonia is an acute lung disease where one or both lungs become inflamed and fill with mucus, often resulting in a cough, shortness of breath and chest pains. It may be caused by a virus, a bacterium or, in rare instances, by chemical irritants. If pneumonia is suspected, a doctor must be consulted. Diagnosis will be confirmed by a chest X-ray, and treatment will vary, depending on the cause. The FEVER accompanying this respiratory illness can take a heavy toll on the body's fluids and nutrients. Drink at least 1.7 litres (3 pints) of fluid a day, taken frequently in small amounts.

If your appetite is suppressed, fruit juices will help to provide energy until you feel like eating again. Thereafter, maintain your fluid intake along with the addition of light, nutritious meals. Fresh fruit and vegetables will supply vitamin C to boost the body's ability to fight the infection, while oily fish and eggs are good sources of vitamin A, which plays a vital role in maintaining the healthy membranes of the airways. Dark green leafy vegetables, especially spinach and kale as well as the orange-pigmented fruits and vegetables, such as cantaloupe melon and carrots, are excellent sources of beta carotene, the plant form of vitamin A.

FRUIT AND VEGETABLE FAST

With the onset of pneumonia, naturopaths sometimes recommend a fruit and vegetable fast followed by the gradual introduction of whole grains and protein into the diet. They may also advocate temporary elimination of dairy produce and sweet foods to decrease mucus production in the lungs. Such a specialised diet should only be followed for short periods and in consultation with your doctor.

POLLUTION AND PESTICIDES

We are exposed to a multitude of chemicals in our diet as well as from the environment. Though many are harmless, scientists are continuing to discover new threats to our health.

Many scientists believe that public anxiety over the pollution of foods is often unjustified. They argue that it is absurd for smokers, or heavy drinkers, to make much of this comparatively minor threat to their health. However, pollution is a problem, and one which is still increasing, as more and more contaminants enter the environment and the food chain.

PESTICIDES

There is much controversy over the agrochemicals used to protect crops from spoilage and pests, even though there are strict regulations controlling their use. During the 1980s, the British Government banned the use of 11 pesticides which were thought to be potentially carcinogenic or capable of causing birth deformities. Many experts point out, however, that cancer-causing agents which find their way into our bodies as a result of agricultural practices are insignificant compared with those occurring naturally in foods. Moreover, pesticide levels are strictly controlled, whereas toxic substances occurring naturally in foods are not.

Statutory limits have been established for the permissible levels of all pesticide residues in foods. The maximum residue levels (MRLs) are normally based on the amount that is low enough not to affect laboratory animals plus a safety margin, usually 100 times lower than the amount that causes no harmful effects in the most sensitive species tested. All pesticides have a 'harvest interval' – the time between the final application of the chemical and harvest of the crop. This is to ensure that by the time the crop reaches the consumer the levels of pesticide it contains have dropped to the appropriate MRL. The harvest interval varies for different crops and the type of pesticide applied.

ORGANIC OPTION

Anyone concerned about pollution and pesticides can buy fresh ORGANIC produce, grown by traditional crop rotation methods, using natural pesticides and fertilisers. However, some organic foods are expensive, and their availability can often be limited; it is

THE CHEMICALS APPLIED TO A RASPBERRY CANE *A residual soil-acting herbicide is applied in February to rid the site of weeds. Then from March until the end of August the crop is routinely sprayed every 10 to 14 days with a fungicide. If aphids are present in April an appropriate insecticide is applied. This is followed by an insecticide at the beginning and end of May to protect against the cane midge. In July, at first pink fruit, an insecticide is applied to protect against the raspberry beetle.*

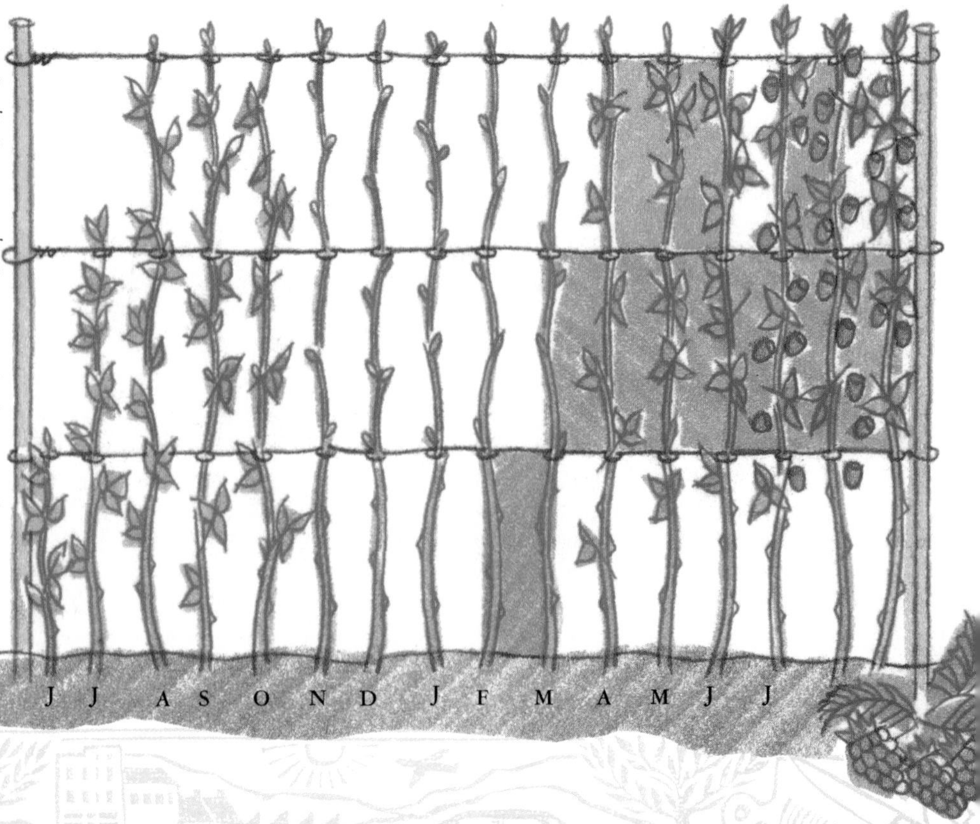

Pesticides: month by month. Pink indicates an insecticide, blue indicates a fungicide and green represents a herbicide application.

always important to ensure that you eat a wide range of fresh foods to supply plenty of micronutrients, particularly the antioxidant vitamins A, C and E, which may help to reduce the effect of various toxins.

The body can produce vitamin A from beta carotene, found in dark green vegetables as well as orange and yellow fruit and vegetables. Blackcurrants, oranges and broccoli are rich in vitamin C, while vegetable oils, wheatgerm and eggs are good sources of vitamin E. The benefits of eating at least five servings of fruit or vegetables a day far outweigh any known risk from accidentally eating small amounts of pesticide residues.

SKIN DEEP

Some pesticides are concentrated on the skins of fruit and vegetables, so that the intake will be greater if the peel is eaten. It is usually sufficient to wash fruit and vegetables, although you may wish to peel them.

Late in 1994 the British Government advised people to top, tail and peel carrots before eating them, after the discovery of 'unexpectedly high residues of acutely toxic pesticides in some individual carrots'. Routine tests on individual carrots detected much higher than expected residues of five organophosphate insecticides – used to combat carrot root fly – in about 1-2 per cent of the samples. In some instances, levels of the chemicals were up to three times the government's acceptable daily intake (ADI). The Ministry of Agriculture, Fisheries and Food promptly ordered farmers to reduce the number of insecticide treatments a year from as many as nine to three, and also stepped up its various monitoring procedures.

Citrus fruits – such as oranges and grapefruit – are often covered in a waxy coating, which seals in moisture and improves appearance. The wax may contain a fungicide to prevent mould growth, but it does not usually penetrate the rinds, and can be washed off in warm water.

THE FACTORY FARM

Surveys show that the public is more concerned about the potential harm caused by pesticides than about the use of antibiotics and growth hormones in livestock. However, it is alleged that the use of antibiotics in animals, along with the overuse of these drugs in human medicine, has led to the development of 'superbugs', or antibiotic-resistant bacteria.

Resistant micro-organisms in meat and poultry could harm meat-eaters by negating the effects of antibiotics which are used to treat infectious diseases. Also the law demands that livestock producers stop giving the drugs to their animals for certain periods of time before slaughtering (depending on the breed). The risk of accidentally consuming antibiotics should, in theory, be negligible.

The use of steroid sex hormones to promote growth and to fatten up livestock has been banned in the European Union since 1988. Unfortunately, there is evidence to suggest that this legislation has failed to stop the use of these hormones entirely. It is known that 'anabolic' drugs, which increase muscle and bone growth, are used illegally by unscrupulous producers who ignore the rules. There is little risk of this in British meat as the Veterinary Medicines Directorate has a statutory monitoring system. It is best to buy meat from reliable sources that have a record of providing 'clean' produce, or to eat organically farmed meat.

HEAVY METALS

Mercury, cadmium and lead are among the most poisonous chemicals which can find their way into the diet. The body is slow to excrete them, so they can build up in tissue to dangerous levels. Fossil-fuelled power plants are the main source of airborne mercury, but SHELLFISH and FISH from rivers and coastal waters polluted by industrial waste can be sources of heavy metals. The hazard to health is low from shop-bought fish and shellfish as the levels of heavy metals are routinely monitored.

The flesh of large, predatory fish such as shark, swordfish and the giant tuna are likely to have the highest concentrations of mercury. They should be eaten rarely and some specialists recommend that pregnant women avoid them altogether because traces of the chemical may injure the unborn baby. The meat from small tuna such as skipjack and albacore, sold in cans, is unlikely to contain mercury.

Large, freshwater fish, such as pike, may also contain excessive mercury. Anglers should check with the local water authority (under 'Water' in the telephone book) before eating them.

RADIOACTIVE FALL-OUT

Nuclear fall-out from Chernobyl, the nuclear power station in the former USSR where a reactor caught fire in 1986, caused serious radioactive contamination of British food supplies, notably of lamb in Cumbria. Restrictions were duly placed on the movement and sale of sheep from that region. As the radioactive particles break down the situation is improving, but monitoring continues, so that no lamb or mutton above the safe limit reaches the market.

As long as there are no more nuclear catastrophes and nuclear testing becomes less widespread, fall-out should be a diminishing problem. However, the risk posed by naturally occurring radioactivity, such as radon, remains.

PORK

BENEFITS

- *Excellent source of B vitamins and protein*
- *Useful source of zinc*

DRAWBACK

- *Cured pork (bacon and ham) is high in sodium and nitrites*
- *Risk of trichinosis if undercooked*

Pork is one of the leanest of all meats. However, many pork products – such as salami, sausages, spare ribs, belly of pork and streaky bacon – are high in saturated fat, excessive intakes of which are associated with high levels of CHOLESTEROL, hardening of the arteries and HEART DISEASE. Therefore, people wrongly assume that all pork is high in fat and thus incompatible with healthy eating.

In fact, lean pork is lower in fat than beef or lamb and is not much fattier than skinless chicken. For example, a 100g (3½oz) serving of lean roast leg of pork contains 7 per cent fat, while the equivalent serving of skinless roast chicken contains 5.5 per cent fat. In terms of protein and calories, there is also little difference between the meats, with the serving of chicken containing 25g (1oz) of protein and 150 Calories, and the pork supplying 30g (just over 1oz) of protein and 185 Calories.

Pork is an excellent source of B vitamins, especially vitamin B_{12}. It is also a useful source of zinc and contains iron.

The healthiest way to eat pork is to trim it of all visible fat before cooking, and to roast or grill it. It is extremely important to cook pork thoroughly as it can transmit tapeworm eggs, trichinosis or other parasites. The simplest way to tell if it is cooked is to insert a sharp knife or skewer – there should be no pink juices present. It is safer when cooking a joint, however, to use a meat thermometer to ensure that the internal temperature reaches 75°C (167°F), so that any bacteria (see FOOD POISONING) or parasites are destroyed. Trichinosis infestation is uncommon in Britain and the United States. However, when it does occur, it causes stomach pain, diarrhoea and vomiting within a few days of eating parasite-infested meat. A week or so later there may be severe muscle pain and difficulty in breathing. If left untreated, trichinosis can be fatal.

BACON AND GAMMON

Curing – the process of salting and sometimes smoking pork to produce bacon or ham – used to be an important way of preserving meat. Today, sophisticated refrigeration and freezing techniques have made curing less important as a preservation process, and pork is now cured largely because people like the flavour. The standard curing ingredients are salt, sodium nitrate and sodium nitrite. Among other ingredients which may be added are sodium ascorbate, which accelerates the curing process, sodium polyphosphate, which lets the cured meat retain extra moisture and gives it a juicier texture, and sugar, used to make sweet-cured meats. The cure may be flavoured with honey, molasses, juniper berries or spices.

Because of the curing process, products such as ham, bacon and gammon are exceptionally high in SODIUM, and should be eaten only in small amounts if you have high BLOOD PRESSURE or are following a low-salt diet.

Why is ham pink?

Cured ham, unlike pork, remains pink even when cooked. During the curing process, nitrites in the curing salt convert the oxygen-storing pigment (myoglobin) in muscle tissue into dark-red nitrosomyoglobin. Hence the deep purple-red of uncooked bacon and of some hams that are eaten raw.

The nitrosomyoglobin changes to its characteristic pink colour when bacon is fried or ham is boiled. If nitrites were not present in the curing salt, these cooked meats would have a greyish colour. Nitrites inhibit the growth of harmful bacteria, such as those that cause botulism. There is some concern that they may be harmful so the quantities added to food have to be regulated carefully.

POTATOES

BENEFITS

- *Useful source of vitamin C*
- *Contain starch and fibre*
- *Good source of potassium*

DRAWBACK

- *Green and sprouted potatoes can contain poisons*

People think of potatoes as fattening, but they are not. It is the fat that they are often cooked in, or which is added at the table in the form of butter or cream, that is the real culprit. Those trying to lose weight or stay slim should avoid fried potatoes and opt for boiled or baked potatoes instead.

Potatoes are a high-carbohydrate food which contain both protein and fibre. They also supply us with a significant amount of the vitamin C and potassium we need.

Their vitamin C content starts to drop almost as soon as potatoes are harvested so that freshly lifted potatoes contain the most. Frying or baking best preserves this water-soluble vitamin – though frying increases the calories. (Roasting usually uses less fat than frying.) Boiling leads to losses in the cooking water and mashed potato contains the least vitamin C. Vitamin loss also occurs via surfaces exposed to air, so the more potatoes are sliced, the lower their vitamin content will be.

Potato crisps are frequently labelled 'junk food'; and indeed they are high in calories, but they are also an excellent source of potassium and a good source of vitamin C. In fact, an average serving of 35g (1¼oz) of crisps provides just under a quarter of the recommended daily intake of vitamin C. Most crisps are made from sliced potatoes fried in vegetable oils and are high in salt – as they are sprinkled with it – but low-salt versions are available. Because of their large surface area they absorb about one-third of their weight in fat. Their saturated fat content depends on the oil used. Crisps cooked in palm oils are high in saturated fats, whereas those cooked in vegetable oil or hydrogenated vegetable oils are lower in saturated fat.

Properly cooked, chips are not only delicious but highly nutritious. However, they are also high in fat which is often saturated. Cooking chips in vegetable oil instead of animal fats will decrease their saturated fat content. Weight for weight, thinly cut chips contain more fat than thickly cut ones. Frozen chips also absorb fat readily, while oven chips, compared with deep-fried chips, are relatively low in fat. Oven chips contain about 5 per cent, ordinary chips 10 per cent and thin-cut chips 20 per cent fat. The fat content of homemade chips can be lowered after frying by blotting them on absorbent kitchen paper.

Green and sprouted potatoes contain alkaloids, called chaconine and solanine, too much of which can be acutely poisonous. Any potato which has patches of green on it should be discarded. Even when eaten in small amounts, solanine can cause migraine or drowsiness in sensitive people.

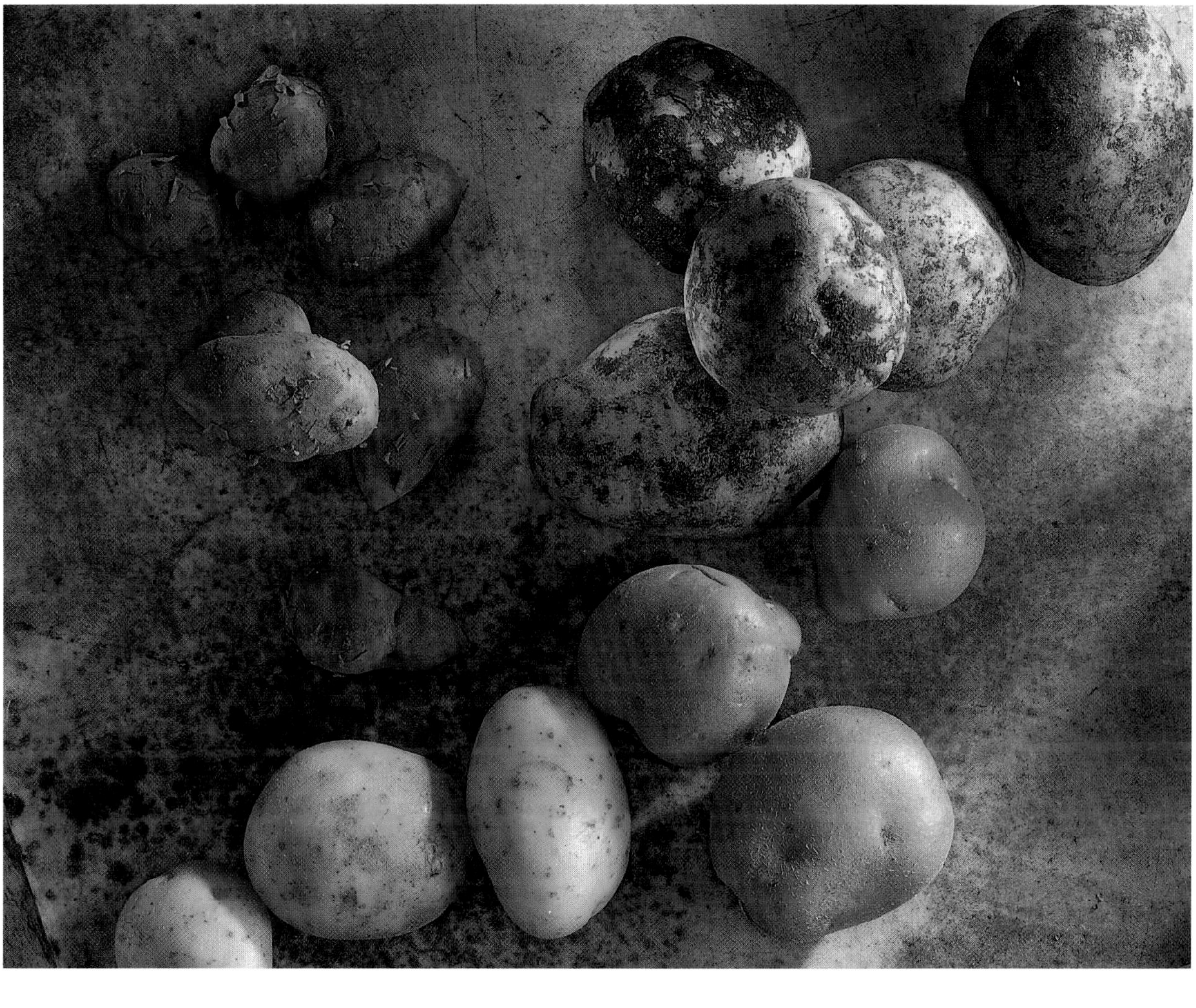

SKIN DEEP *The potato's best source of fibre and nutrients is the skin. Clockwise from top left are: Jersey Royal, King Edward, Romano and Maris Piper.*

Pregnancy: A Good Start

A healthy pregnancy begins even before conception. A woman's diet during the few months before she conceives can be as important for her baby's well-being as what she eats during her pregnancy.

The demands pregnancy makes on a woman's body are heavy, but the vast majority of pregnant women can fulfil their own needs and those of their babies by eating a normal healthy diet. A well-balanced, varied diet that is high in fibre-rich complex carbohydrates, fruit and vegetables, and low in saturated fats, will help a mother-to-be to stay fit and well and supply the foetus with all the essential nutrients for healthy development.

Ice Cream and Pickles

The popular myth of a pregnant woman longing for bizarre combinations of foods, such as ice cream and pickled onions, due to a physiological need is just that – a myth. There is no evidence to suggest that food cravings are a sign of any nutritional deficiency.

Nevertheless, food cravings are common during pregnancy, and according to one Canadian researcher, fruit and fruit juices, chocolate and dairy products top the list of foods most often craved, especially after the first three months. More likely still are aversions to specific foods or drinks, particularly to meat, fatty or spicy foods, tea, coffee and alcohol.

STRONG DESIRES *Fruit, cheese and chocolate are commonly craved foods.*

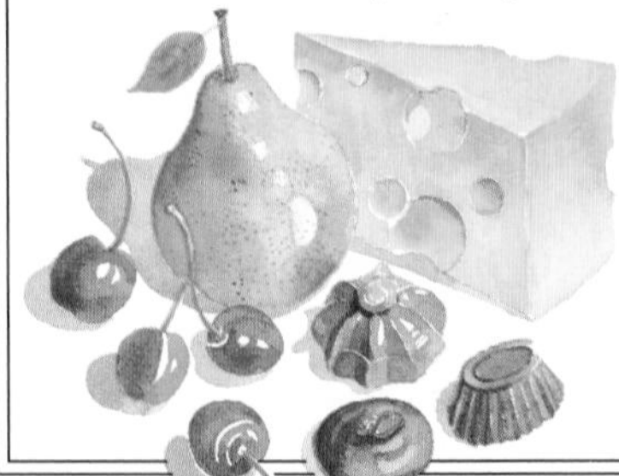

Preparing to Conceive

Studies suggest that a woman's diet for the three to six months before conception and during the first few weeks of pregnancy greatly influences the early development of the embryo. Excess alcohol, for example, is associated with birth defects and is therefore best avoided immediately before conception, and for the first 12 weeks of pregnancy. Thereafter, the odd glass of wine or beer – not more than one unit a day – is not considered to be a risk.

Research has also shown that high intakes of folic acid when trying to conceive and during the first 12 weeks of pregnancy significantly reduce the risk of giving birth to a baby with a congenital neural tube defect such as SPINA BIFIDA. Daily supplements from a doctor, together with plenty of folate-rich foods such as dark green leafy vegetables, nuts and pulses, will provide adequate folic acid.

A Normal Diet

A well-balanced diet will supply all the calories and nutrients for the health of both mother and baby, without causing the mother to gain excess weight. Slimming during pregnancy is not advisable, except under close medical supervision, as it may deprive the foetus of vital nutrients.

Energy requirements change very little throughout pregnancy. Some authorities estimate that towards the end of pregnancy, women may need an extra 200 or so Calories per day, but others argue that due to decreased physical activity, there is no increased calorie requirement in late pregnancy. Snacks such as fresh and dried fruit, toast, scones or plain biscuits can provide much-needed energy between meals and are a healthy alternative to sugary, salty or fatty foods.

There is no need for the mother to increase protein intake during pregnancy. She should keep her SALT intake within normal levels to reduce the risks of high blood pressure and toxaemia (a rare, but serious complication where seizures can occur).

Vitamins and Minerals

Ensuring a good intake of all vitamins and minerals is essential, but some are particularly important. Calcium, for example, helps the baby's teeth and bones to form, and is also vital for pregnant women under 25, whose bones are still increasing in density. Pregnant women need the calcium equivalent of about 600ml (1 pint) of milk daily (skimmed, semi-skimmed or whole). A small pot of yoghurt, or 25g (1oz) of hard cheese, will provide the same amount of calcium as 200ml (⅓ pint) of milk. Other food sources include bread, tinned sardines or pilchards eaten with the bones, sesame seeds and dark green leafy vegetables. Vitamin D helps the body to absorb calcium and pregnant women require an intake of 10mcg a day.

Zinc is essential for general growth and for the development of the foetal immune system. It can be found in lean meat, wholegrain cereals, cheese and nuts, but its absorption is inhibited by excessive intakes of bran.

Iron is needed for making the baby's blood as well as for maintaining the mother's own iron levels. Fortunately, the body's ability to absorb iron increases during pregnancy. As long as a woman starts off with adequate stores and eats plenty of iron-rich foods, such as meat, poultry, fish, eggs, green vegetables and dried fruit, neither she nor her baby will go short. Iron absorption is improved by including a good source of vitamin C, such as citrus fruit or juice, with meals. However, some women do develop anaemia in pregnancy despite an apparently adequate intake of iron from food, and need to take prescribed iron supplements.

Although liver is an excellent source of iron, it is also extremely high in vitamin A, excessive intakes of which have been linked with birth defects. Women who are pregnant, or thinking about becoming so, should therefore avoid all types of liver and liver pâtés. An adequate intake of vitamin A remains important, however. Suitable sources are brightly coloured fruit and vegetables such as apricots, carrots and red peppers. They contain beta carotene, which the body converts to vitamin A as it needs it.

Scientists have found that omega-3 fatty acids are especially important for the healthy development of the brain and eyes. Excellent dietary sources include mackerel, herring, sardines, salmon and fresh tuna.

Coping with problems

Morning sickness – a misnomer, as it can happen at any time of the day – can cause real misery until it subsides, usually after 12 to 16 weeks. It is best to eat little and often. This is also a good way of dealing with indigestion and heartburn, which are common during the later stages of pregnancy. Milk or yoghurt may help to relieve symptoms. Naturopaths claim that ginger tea may ease morning sickness.

Constipation can be another unwelcome side effect of pregnancy, largely because changing hormone levels have a relaxing effect on the intestines, so that food takes a long time to pass through. Drinking plenty of water and eating high-fibre foods should help. Dried fruits, especially prunes, are an excellent natural laxative.

Food safety

The bacterial infection listeriosis (see FOOD POISONING) is particularly dangerous for both pregnant women and newborn babies; and an unborn child infected through its mother may be stillborn. The listeria scare of 1989 resulted in doctors advising pregnant women not to eat Camembert or Brie, as well as other soft cheeses or pâtés, because of the danger of infection. As a precaution, ready-to-eat meals should be thoroughly reheated before eating. Ready-prepared salads and delicatessen foods, both of which are potential sources of bacteria, are best avoided during pregnancy. Because of the risk of salmonella, eggs should always be thoroughly cooked; mayonnaise-style dressings, sauces and puddings which incorporate raw or lightly cooked eggs should also be avoided.

Make sure that all meat is cooked through. Always wash your hands in hot water after handling raw meat to avoid infection with the parasite that causes toxoplasmosis. This may cause blindness if passed from a mother to her unborn child. The parasite reproduces in cats' intestines, so pregnant women should not handle cat litter and should wear gloves when gardening.

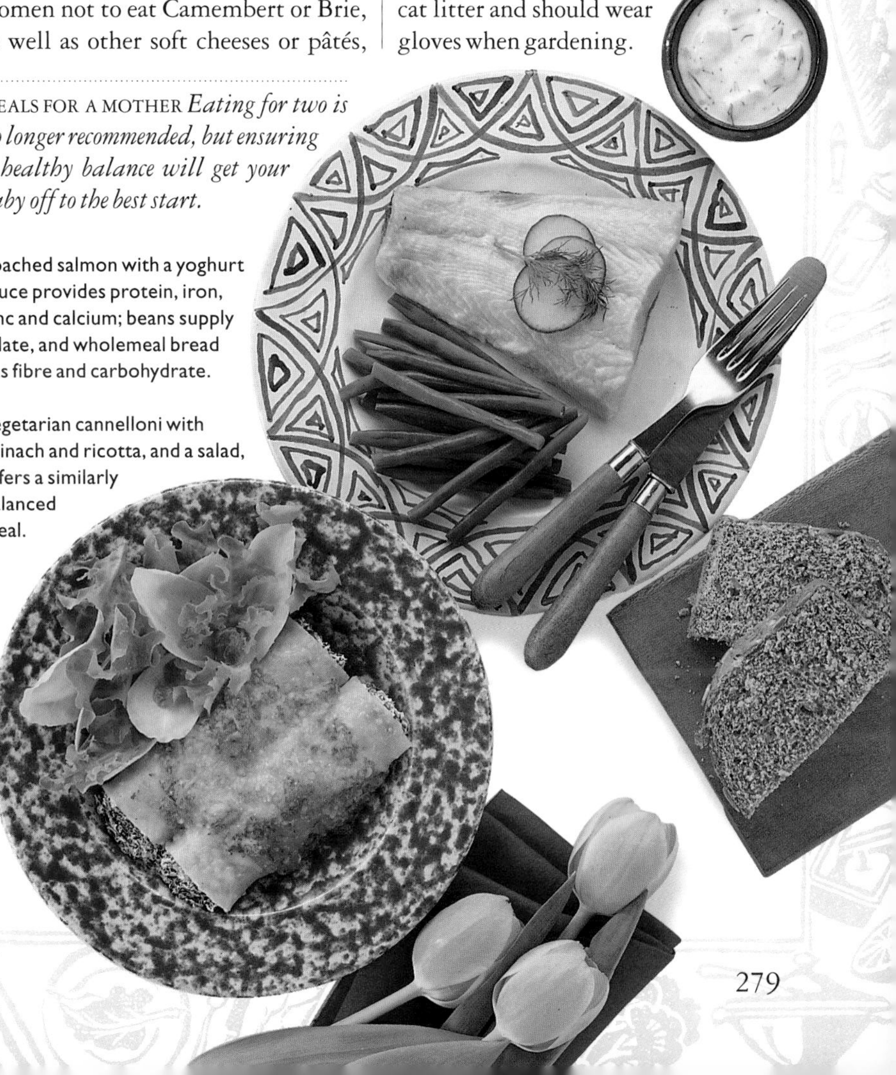

MEALS FOR A MOTHER *Eating for two is no longer recommended, but ensuring a healthy balance will get your baby off to the best start.*

Poached salmon with a yoghurt sauce provides protein, iron, zinc and calcium; beans supply folate, and wholemeal bread has fibre and carbohydrate.

Vegetarian cannelloni with spinach and ricotta, and a salad, offers a similarly balanced meal.

POULTRY

BENEFITS
- *Excellent source of protein*
- *Rich source of most B vitamins*

DRAWBACKS
- *Skin is high in fat*
- *Risk of food poisoning if undercooked*

Chickens, farm-reared ducks, turkeys and geese are classed as domestic fowl or poultry. They all contain protein that builds and repairs body tissue, plenty of B vitamins for a healthy nervous system and some zinc. Chicken and turkey liver (see OFFAL) are excellent sources of vitamin A, which is needed for healthy skin and resistance to infection, and vitamin B_{12}, which is vital for making DNA and RNA. Most of the fat in poultry is unsaturated and so will not raise blood cholesterol levels. While duck and goose are fatty birds, chicken and turkey are relatively low in fat (and most of it is in the skin so it can easily be removed). Skinless chicken and turkey breasts contain around 5 per cent fat, and so are recommended for people who need

Comparing the nutritional values of poultry (100g or 3½oz)

Poultry is a good source of protein, vitamins and minerals. Unless you are on a low-fat diet, there is no need to avoid poultry fat because it is relatively low in saturated fatty acids (which can cause problems with blood cholesterol levels). In any case, most of the fat is found in the skin and this can be removed quite easily, either before or after cooking.

ROAST MEAT	CALORIES	PROTEIN (g)	FAT (g)	VITAMINS	MINERALS
CHICKEN					
Meat and skin	216	23	14	Contains all the B vitamins, particularly niacin (around 85% of the daily recommended intake). However, there are only trace amounts of vitamin B_{12}.	Dark meat contains twice as much iron and zinc as light meat. Dark meat also contains useful amounts of phosphorus and potassium but light meat is an even better source.
Meat only	148	25	5		

TURKEY					
Meat and skin	171	28	7	Excellent source of vitamin B_{12} and a useful source of all the other B vitamins, especially niacin (93% of the recommended intake).	Good source of potassium and phosphorus. Contains over one-third more zinc than chicken – 100g (3½oz) roasted dark meat provides just under half of the required daily amount.
Meat only	140	29	3		
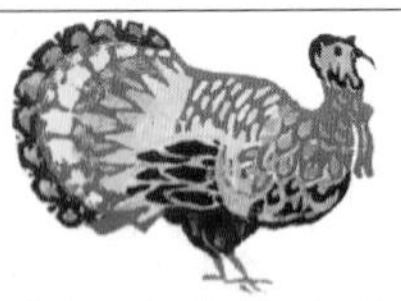					
DUCK					
Meat and skin	339	20	29	Good source of all B vitamins. Typical serving provides over twice as much thiamin and riboflavin as chicken.	Contains three times as much iron as chicken. Duck is also a good source of potassium and zinc.
Meat only	189	25	10		
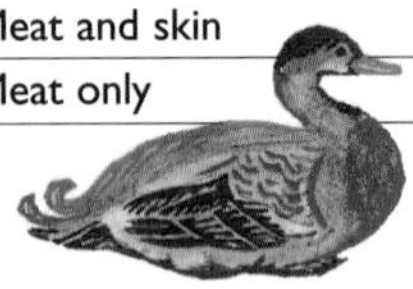					
GOOSE					
Meat only	319	29	22	A typical serving provides almost three times as much riboflavin as does chicken and almost twice as much vitamin B_6.	Good source of potassium and phosphorus. 100g (3½oz) contains one-third of the required daily amount of iron for women and over half for men.
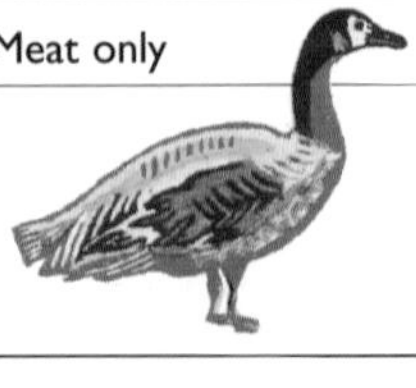					

a low-cholesterol or low-calorie diet. Curiously, studies in France have found that people who eat goose fat have low rates of heart disease.

Free range or factory-farmed birds?

The vast majority of chickens and turkeys are factory farmed. Most are kept in crowded conditions and need to be treated with drugs to prevent the spread of disease. The term 'free range' means that the birds have daytime access to areas where they can run freely and scratch for food, although the conditions may still be crowded.

Salmonella sense

Chicken is believed to be the most common cause of FOOD POISONING, mainly because it carries salmonella bacteria. Salmonella survives freezing but is destroyed by thorough cooking.

Pregnancy

See page 278

Preparing, cooking and storing food

See page 282

Processed foods

It is fashionable to dismiss commercial food processing – canning, freezing, pickling or smoking, for example – as harmful to the nutritive value of foods, but these processes have their benefits. Without these methods of food preservation, a large amount of food would be wasted and food poisoning would be much more prevalent. Many fresh foods start to deteriorate from the moment they are harvested, netted or slaughtered. Top-quality produce, that has been quickly processed at source, often has a higher nutrient value than 'fresh' foods that have been on display for a few days.

Heat treatment

Heat processing preserves food and extends shelf-life by arresting spoilage and by destroying harmful micro-organisms. It also makes the starches and proteins in food easier to digest.

Inevitably some vitamins will be lost during processing. Water-soluble vitamins, particularly thiamin (B_1), riboflavin (B_2) and C may be leached out during washing and blanching (a process which involves brief exposure to boiling water, steam or hot air).

UHT (ultra heat treatment), used for sterilising liquids before they are packed in cartons, helps to reduce vitamin losses while destroying bacteria. Pasteurisation involves lower temperatures, but the vitamin loss is similar. However, because pasteurisation lets some micro-organisms survive, these products have a shorter shelf-life.

Drying

Drying fruit by traditional methods, involving various evaporation techniques, typically causes losses of up to half of the vitamin C content, and up to one-fifth of the beta carotene. It also concentrates levels of sugar and fibre. Modern methods of drying result in better nutrient retention because the heat treatments used are less severe. In the case of freeze drying – where rapid freezing is followed by the removal of ice by low-temperature evaporation – minimal amounts of vitamin C are lost.

Freezing

The nutritional value of FROZEN FOODS is often very close to fresh equivalents. The main losses are the water-soluble vitamins from vegetables and fruit, which leach out during blanching, prior to freezing. Frozen foods cannot be kept for as long as TINNED FOODS since certain vitamins and unsaturated fatty acids tend to oxidise if exposed to air, even at sub-zero temperatures.

Fermented foods

Fermentation is used to make many foods, such as matured cheeses, bread, yoghurt, soya sauce and wines. Naturally occurring organisms may be encouraged to flourish or cultures may be added. Cultures are injected, smeared or sprayed on to cheeses, for example, to promote mould growth thus creating blue-veined cheeses with distinctive tastes and textures. Fermentation results in minimal nutrient losses; indeed, some nutrients, particularly the B vitamins, may actually be gained. In most cases, fermentation extends the food's shelf-life.

Milled grains

Milling grains, such as rice or wheat, to make polished rice or white flour, causes significant losses of both nutrients and fibre. This is because most of the vitamins and fibre are contained in the grains' outer layers, which are discarded during milling. To compensate for these losses and to provide extra micronutrients, many grain products are artificially enriched, or fortified.

Smoked, salted or pickled?

These days, many SMOKED, CURED AND PICKLED FOODS are processed merely because people like the flavours. Although not inherently unhealthy, such foods are often high in SODIUM. Some meats, such as ham, are preserved with nitrates and nitrites. Nitrites can react with protein constituents to form nitrosamines, which are thought to be carcinogenic. Because the smoke may contain carcinogenic substances, some experts suggest that eating large amounts of smoked foods may increase the risk of cancer.

PREPARING, COOKING AND STORING FOOD

The way food is handled before, during and after cooking can have a dramatic effect on its nutritional value. This is of particular importance if food is to play a part in overcoming an illness.

The top priority in any kitchen is HYGIENE; it is vital to prevent bacterial contamination and FOOD POISONING. The way in which food is prepared, cooked and stored will determine the extent to which food retains its valuable nutrients.

PREPARING

To avoid transferring the bacteria which naturally occur in raw meat and fish to other cooked foods, wash knives, chopping boards and your hands immediately after you have finished preparing each type of food. When stocking your fridge, place raw meat and fish in separate, covered dishes, and keep them on the lowest shelf so that they do not drip onto any other food. Harmful bacteria are inhibited at low temperatures, so ensure that the working temperature of your fridge remains at 0-5°C (32-41°F).

To minimise vitamin C loss from fresh fruit and vegetables, wash, peel, cut or grate them just before cooking or eating. Always use sharp knives for peeling and chopping vegetables as blunt utensils will tend to bruise the food, causing greater nutrient loss.

WATCH THE WRAP

It has long been recognised that plasticisers used in some types of cling wrap may be harmful. The government has warned that it is wise to avoid too great an exposure to plasticisers. It is best not to use these wraps in direct contact with fatty foods (such as cheese) since the toxins associated with the plasticisers are fat-soluble.

There is also a growing concern that exposure to chemicals which mimic the action of the female sex hormone, oestrogen, may be having a detrimental effect on male fertility. There are thousands of suspect chemicals, including some commonly used in plastic packaging. Research is now under way to determine exactly which chemicals are potentially harmful.

COOKING

Any form of cooking inevitably results in the loss of some nutrients. Water-soluble vitamins, such as vitamin C, are easily lost by leaching into the cooking water. These losses can be kept down to a minimum by steaming or microwaving or by making sure that food is not over-cooked.

Cooking is effective in destroying harmful bacteria, especially in meat. For example, the bacteria responsible for the most common form of food poisoning, salmonella, are killed off after an hour at 55°C (131°F) and after 20 minutes at 60°C (140°F). Cooking also destroys toxic substances which occur naturally in some plants, such as kidney beans, and it makes the starch in rice and potatoes digestible.

Some methods of cooking are considered healthier than others, either because they keep the fat content in food low, or because they involve less vitamin and mineral loss.

Grilling This is useful for all fish and tender cuts of meat, as well as fatty meats such as bacon, burgers and sausages. Grilling is a healthy alternative to frying because much of the fat from the meat drips into the tray below, although for low-fat meats grilling has little advantage over frying.

Barbecuing Similar to grilling, except that the heat source is below the meat, barbecuing is also useful for getting rid of the fat from meat. However, fat dripping onto the coals below can produce potentially carcinogenic substances in the smoke. To prevent this, clear the coals to each side, and leave a dripping tray directly beneath the meat. When meat is barbecued, most of its vitamins are retained.

Roasting One of the easiest ways of cooking large cuts of meat and poultry is by roasting. To prevent it from drying out, the meat can be periodically basted. Roasting poultry in its skin helps to retain moisture, but remove the skin before eating – this can reduce the saturated fat in a portion of chicken by 60 per cent.

Instead of cooking meat in a pool of fat, place it on a rack in the roasting tray so the fat can drain away. Some vitamins will be lost in the meat juices, but these juices can be used to make gravy. Roast vegetables are healthier if cooked in their own dish, rather than in the fatty dripping around the meat.

Frying Deep-fat frying is generally regarded as the most unhealthy of all cooking methods. This is true if the oil is not hot enough, because then the food will be deeply penetrated by fat. Chips cooked in hot oil take up around 7 per cent fat, but if frozen chips are added to hot oil, they take up to 20 per cent fat. When deep-frying is done properly, the outside of the food is sealed while the inside is effectively steamed. Vitamin losses are very low with this cooking method.

Stir frying This method of cooking meat, fish or vegetables needs little fat. The wok reaches high temperatures, and cooks the finely chopped meat and vegetables very quickly. Vegetables retain much of their crispness and nutrients, and do not absorb much oil.

Microwaving This is excellent for defrosting or reheating dishes and for cooking most vegetables and fish – which retain their moisture, colour and most of their nutrients (more than any other form of cooking). Remove any plastic packaging and do not cover food with cling wrap as the plastics can melt into the food at high temperatures.

Microwaves are not so good for cooking meat, however, as the texture tends to become rubbery and the meat does not always have a 'cooked' appearance. Combination ovens have been developed to enhance the appearance of microwaved food: meat is quickly cooked with microwaves and browned by conventional heating. A microwave does not always cook food evenly. For the food to be cooked through properly, change its position on the turntable halfway through cooking and ensure that standing times are observed. Some foods will explode in a microwave, such as whole eggs.

Steaming For nutrient retention, steaming comes a close second to microwaving. Broccoli, for example, can lose over 60 per cent of its vitamin C when boiled, and only 20 per cent when steamed. The only drawback may be the build-up of unpleasant-smelling gases with foods, such as Brussels sprouts, that contain a lot of sulphur.

Boiling In this method of cooking many water-soluble vitamins (particularly vitamins B and C) leach out and

The well-stocked refrigerator

The useful life of fresh foods can be extended by storing them at or below 5°C (41°F). Always transfer food to your refrigerator as soon as possible after purchase, but make sure that you do not pack things in too tightly, as the cold air will not be able to circulate to keep the contents properly chilled. Clean out your refrigerator regularly.

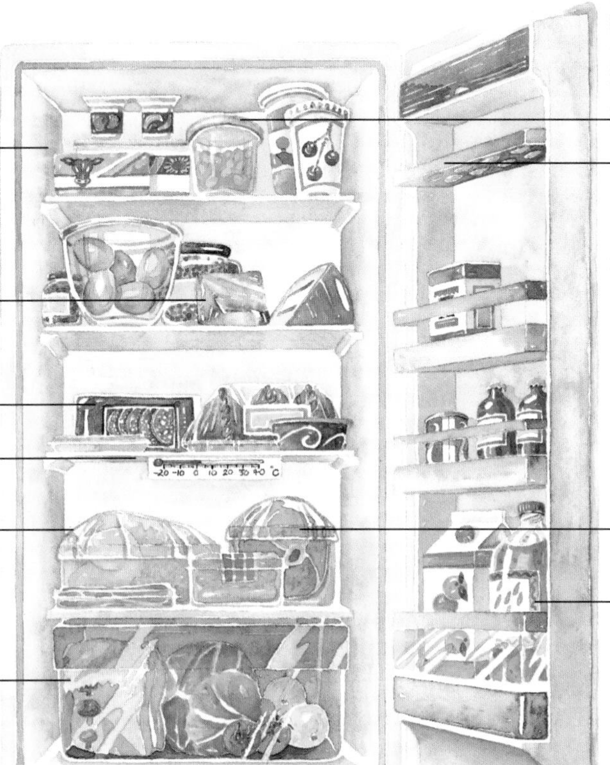

Keep dairy products such as butter and cream covered as they tend to absorb the flavours and odours of other foods in the fridge.

Store cheese in foil, not cling wrap. (Most cling wrap should not come into direct contact with foods that have a high fat content.)

Store cooked meats on a separate shelf to raw meats.

Keep the fridge at, or below, 5°C (41°F).

Raw meats should be stored on the lowest shelf so they will not drip onto anything. Remove giblets from poultry and store separately.

Store mushrooms in a paper bag so that they do not sweat. To retain their freshness, store salad vegetables in plastic bags in the salad drawer.

Once a tin of beans has been opened, empty the rest into an airtight container and store in the main section of the fridge.

Many old-fashioned fridges have ready-made egg trays in the door – but since eggs are perishable, they should be stored in the main part of the fridge, where they can be kept for up to 3 weeks.

Remove the polystyrene tray from meat bought in a supermarket as it slows cooling. Drain off fluids and cover loosely.

The door is the warmest part of the fridge. Only store items here that are either not likely to perish (cans of drink, bottles of beer, mineral water), or that will be used quickly (milk and orange juice).

are discarded with the cooking water – although you can make use of the stock in soups, sauces and gravy. Minimise the nutrient loss from vegetables by bringing the water to the boil before adding them to the pan or by boiling them in their skins and peeling them once they are cooked.

If scrupulously scrubbed, many vegetables can be cooked and eaten in their skins. Indeed, many people find that this improves their flavour. But be warned that the skins may contain pesticide residues, moulds and naturally occurring toxins. Adding baking soda keeps vegetables looking bright and fresh, but it will destroy vitamin C and increase the sodium content.

STORING AND PRESERVING

Several factors result in the spoilage of food: the growth of micro-organisms, enzyme action within the food itself, oxidation – when the oxygen in the air changes the appearance, texture and taste of the food – pests, and extremes of temperature. To delay and minimise such spoilage and so lengthen the life of food different methods of preserving and storing it are used.

Drying Removing the moisture from food makes it inhospitable to micro-organisms and halts many enzyme and chemical reactions which cause food deterioration. Drying is used for coffee and tea to fruits and pasta.

Drying under normal conditions can cause losses of vitamins, especially vitamin C from fruit and vegetables. This does not happen during freeze-drying, however, when the moisture is removed from the food at low temperatures while it is frozen. This process is expensive but very effective for drying meats, fish and quality instant coffee.

Freezing Keeping foods at or below -18°C (0°F) significantly slows down food spoilage. But each food group has a recommended maximum storage time beyond which it slowly begins to deteriorate. Nutrients are, in general, retained well. In some cases frozen vegetables may have a higher nutrient content than fresh ones, because they are frozen so soon after being picked.

There is a small reduction in the vitamin content of vegetables which occurs when they are blanched before freezing. The vegetables are blanched to halt the action of enzymes within the food, and so prevent spoilage. Some foods do not freeze well, such as milk, cream and sauces, mushrooms and cucumber. Freezing changes the structure of many fruits which is why they can lack firmness on thawing.

Irradiation This method of food preservation is the subject of much controversy, but IRRADIATED FOODS are not radioactive. Irradiation can be used for sterilising spices, extending the life of shellfish, strawberries and other soft fruits, preventing potatoes from sprouting and for destroying dangerous micro-organisms on poultry.

Canning Food is heated in its metal container to a high temperature for a particular length of time, depending on the food being tinned. It is then sealed. When buying TINNED FOODS check the use-by date which is usually stamped on one end of the tin and make sure the tin is not dented.

Additives The numerous chemicals added to foods can increase the shelf life from a few days to many months. They include sugar, salt, vinegar and various chemical compounds which must be approved by the government.

The reason for using such ADDITIVES is to maintain the quality of food or add flavour; some, such as ascorbic acid (vitamin C), which is added to fruit to prevent browning, actually increase its nutritional value.

A small number of people have an allergic reaction to some of the additives commonly used.

DANGER ZONES

- Make sure frozen food is completely thawed before cooking.
- Once frozen food has thawed, do not refreeze it.
- Be particularly careful not to undercook meat, fish or eggs.
- Do not leave food to cool and forget about it. Bacterial growth is at its most prolific between 7°C (45°F) and 60°C (140°F). Food should be left in this temperature zone for as short a time as possible.
- When reheating leftovers, you should make sure the food reaches 75°C (167°F) right through.
- Use up any refrigerated leftovers within a day or two.
- Never reheat food more than once. The repeated heating and cooling of food destroys vitamins and encourages bacterial growth.

MARKET, GREENGROCER OR SUPERMARKET?

Markets are usually the cheapest source of fruit and vegetables. However, market produce tends to be less uniform and of more variable quality than supermarket produce, so always inspect it carefully and discard any that is unduly wrinkled, dry or soft.

Greengrocers are often a good source of fresh produce, but their stocks are usually limited and reflect local demand. The inevitable deterioration of fresh fruit and vegetables, especially in hot weather, should be reflected in your greengrocer's prices.

Supermarkets have sophisticated cold storage and distribution facilities, and sell a wide range of imported produce, satisfying consumer demand for 'out of season' fruit and vegetables. Some consumer groups, however, complain that the supermarkets sacrifice flavour for cosmetic appearance. They claim ORGANIC FOODS are tastier even though they often look slightly inferior.

How to freeze and thaw foods safely

FOOD	PREPARATION	PACKAGING	TIPS	USE WITHIN (MONTHS)	THAWING (hr/0.45 kg or 1 lb)	
					IN FRIDGE	IN ROOM
Butter 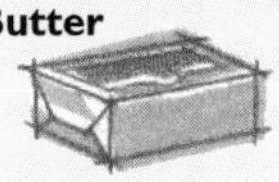	Freeze in its wrapper.	Overwrap it if it is soft.	Unsalted butter stores longer than salted.	3-8	12	1-2
Whole white and oily fish	Scale and fillet.	Wrap in polythene, freezer paper or foil.	Oily fish only stores for 3 months.	3-6	6-10	3-5
Fish steaks	Separate the portions using freezer paper.	Wrap in polythene, freezer paper or foil.	Dry fish with kitchen paper before freezing.	3-6	6-10	3-5
Apples	Wash, peel, core, slice and blanch.	Use polythene containers or freezer bags.	To pack, sprinkle sugar between layers.	9 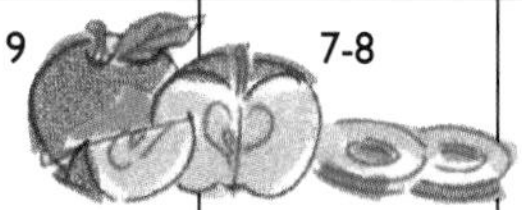	7-8	3½-4
Peaches and plums 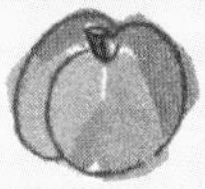	Wash, stone and peel peaches; halve plums. Pack with syrup.	Use polythene containers, or waxed cartons.	A tablespoon of lemon juice for each pint of syrup preserves colour.	9 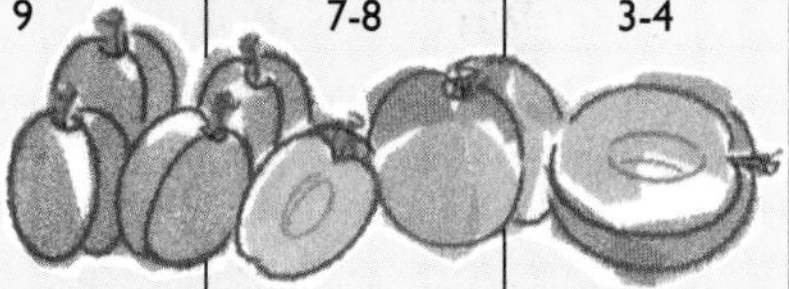	7-8	3-4
Berries	Remove hulls and pack with sugar or syrup.	Use polythene containers or waxed cartons.	Strawberries and raspberries may be frozen without sugar.	9 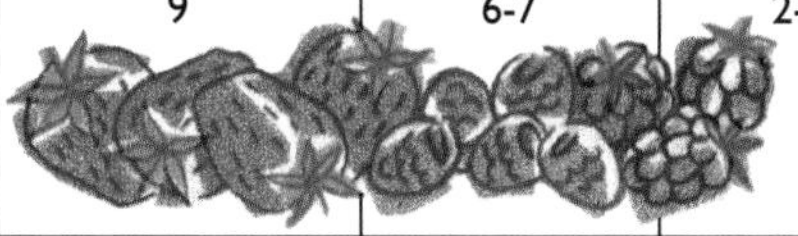	6-7	2-3
Green vegetables	Wash, trim, blanch, drain.	Use polythene bags or cartons.	Squeeze air out of the bags.	12	—	—
Beef, lamb and pork joints 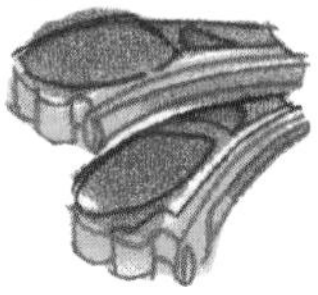	Cut joints to required size. Cover protruding bones with foil. Bone if desired, roll and tie into a neat shape.	Wrap tightly in polythene or foil. Overwrap large joints with extra layers for protection.	Boning joints before freezing saves valuable space.	4-6 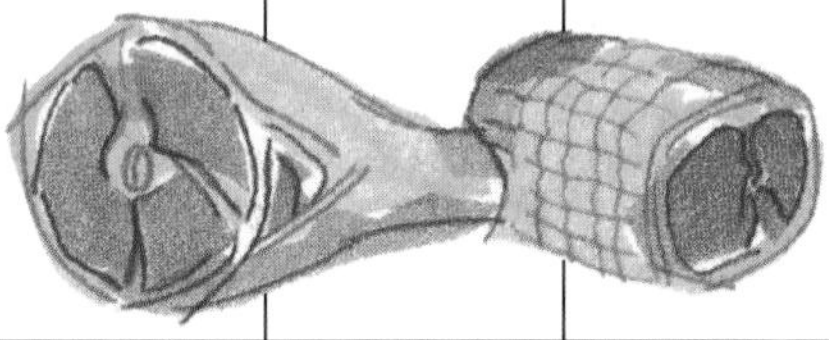	5	2
Pork and lamb chops	Separate with sheets of freezer paper.	Use polythene bags or plastic containers.	Thaw pork chops in the refrigerator.	4-6	5	2
Minced meat	Divide into portions.	Use sealed freezer bags.	Only freeze very fresh mince.	1-2	6	1-1½
Sausages (shop bought)	No preparation necessary.	Use polythene or freezer bags. Wrap tightly and seal.	Homemade sausages can be stored for up to 6 months.	3 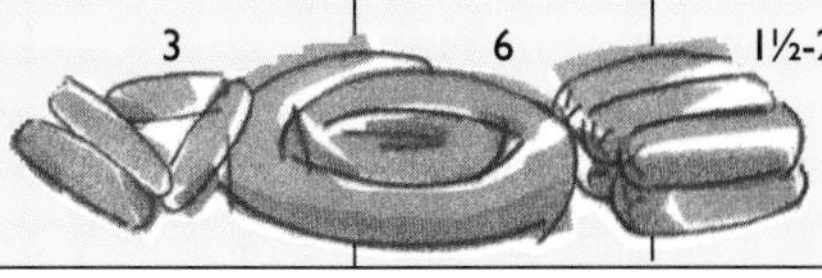	6	1½-2

PROSTATE PROBLEMS

EAT PLENTY OF
- *Zinc-rich foods such as shellfish*
- *Foods containing vitamin E, particularly wheatgerm oil, nuts, seeds and green vegetables*
- *Oily fish such as herring, mackerel and sardines*

CUT DOWN ON
- *Tea and coffee*
- *Red meat and dairy products*
- *Alcohol*

Increasing the amount of zinc in a man's diet may lead to relief of the symptoms of an enlarged prostate gland. This is because an enlarged prostate is often caused by a build-up of dihydrotestosterone (a product of the male hormone testosterone), the formation of which is retarded when adequate zinc is present. It has also been found that enlarged prostate glands contain cells with zinc levels that are lower than normal. Zinc-rich foods include whole grains, shellfish, meat, nuts and seeds (particularly pumpkin). Vitamin E and some fatty acids present in oily fish may also help due to their anti-inflammatory action.

Some medical experts advise men to drink 1.7 litres (3 pints) of fluid a day; herbalists recommend gentle diuretics such as parsley or celery seed tea. Other diuretic drinks – including alcohol, coffee and tea – are irritants and should be drunk only occasionally.

Prostate enlargement occurs most often in men over 50 years old, but especially between the ages of 60 and 70. Recent statistics show that about 4 in every 1000 men in Britain are treated for the problem each year.

The prostate is a walnut-sized gland just below the bladder that is involved in semen production. An enlarged prostate may cause frequent urination, as well as a weakening or interruption of the urinary stream. Other symptoms include pain while urinating and total stoppage of urination, which requires immediate medical help.

An enlarged prostate can also be caused by a malignant growth, so any man with any of the symptoms described above should consult a doctor as soon as possible. A US study of nearly 50000 men found a link between those who had advanced prostate cancer and also a high consumption of animal fat. Other studies suggest the risk of prostate cancer is increased by alcohol intake.

In Britain it is estimated that one in every three elderly men suffers from the early stages of prostate cancer, though it is slow-growing and seldom fatal. In its more virulent form, tumours can spread to the spine, causing back pain. Unless diagnosed and swiftly treated this form can be fatal.

Bark, berries and plants

- In Europe, extracts from the bark of *Pygeum africanum*, an African tropical evergreen tree, have been found to be effective in reducing symptoms of an enlarged prostate – including the need to urinate frequently. Unfortunately, stomach upsets are a side effect.
- An extract of saw palmetto (*Serenoa repens*) berries has been shown in studies to reduce urinary symptoms. It is claimed to be more effective than pygeum and has no side effects.
- In Germany, research has discovered the effectiveness of the roots of stinging nettles (*Urtica dioica*) in relieving some symptoms.
- An extract of flower pollen has been used to reduce urinary symptoms in several Japanese studies.

PROTEIN

BENEFIT
- *Essential for most of the body's vital functions, including the growth, maintenance and repair of cells*

DRAWBACKS
- *Too much protein can put a strain on the liver and kidneys, and may increase the excretion of some minerals such as calcium*
- *High-protein foods are often rich in calories and fats*

Every cell in the body needs protein; it is required for the growth and repair of everything from muscles and bones to hair and fingernails. Protein also helps to create enzymes that enable us to digest food, produce antibodies that fight off infection, and hormones that keep the body working efficiently.

Nutritionists recommend that you should aim to get 10-15 per cent of your calories from protein – with 35 per cent from fat and 50 per cent from carbohydrates. If your intake of fats or carbohydrates is insufficient to meet your energy needs, body proteins will be broken down and used as energy.

PROTEIN IN THE DIET

Eating too much protein is counter-productive as the body cannot store it for later use. Instead the liver converts excess protein into glucose and by-products such as urea which have to be excreted. Excess protein also leads to the production of acidic urine, which in turn leads to an increased loss of calcium from the bones – and may increase the risk of osteoporosis.

Foods that supply protein include cereals (wheat, oats, rice and bread), meat, poultry, fish, eggs, cheese, pulses (beans, peas and lentils), nuts and potatoes. The average man or teenage boy needs around 55g (2oz) of protein a day, which could be derived from a

Do athletes need more protein?

There is a myth that all athletes need extra protein, but what they really need is extra energy. The best foods for energy are carbohydrates, including bread, potatoes, rice and pasta. Excess protein is either converted into energy or transformed into fat and stored in the body. Body builders do require some extra protein to build muscle tissue, but their needs should still be met by a balanced diet because their food intake is larger than average anyway.

220g (about 8oz) portion of lean roast chicken or about 250g (9oz) steamed trout. The average woman or teenage girl requires around 45g (1½oz) of protein a day; and a child between seven and ten years of age 28g (1oz). Lactating women need extra protein because of the milk they are producing. Take care to ensure you are eating enough protein if you are on a diet, if you are ill, or recovering from a serious injury. Most Westerners, however, eat far more protein than they need – consuming around 100g (3½oz) a day.

WHAT IS PROTEIN?

The building blocks of protein are amino acids – compounds containing the four elements that are necessary for life: carbon, hydrogen, oxygen and nitrogen. Some amino acids contain sulphur as well. Although most proteins are made up of about 20 amino acids, many are present several times, so that a protein molecule may consist of 500 or more amino acid units arranged in a specific sequence.

There are many types of protein molecules in the body, and each type is specific to its function. For example, proteins such as keratin and collagen give strength and elasticity to hair, as well as to skin and tendons; haemoglobin and myoglobin are the oxygen-binding proteins of the blood and muscle, respectively; and ovalbumin, the principal protein of egg white, is responsible for the setting and foaming properties of eggs. A particularly important group of proteins, known as enzymes, directs all the body cells' chemical reactions. These reactions provide the basis of every type of cell activity, including growth, repair, the production of energy, and the excretion of waste products.

THE QUALITY OF PROTEIN

The protein we eat is broken down by digestion into amino acids, which are then absorbed and used to make other proteins. Of the 20 different amino acids commonly found in plant and animal proteins, most can be made by the human body, but eight essential amino acids can be obtained only from food. The main reason we need protein in our diet is to supply these eight essential amino acids: isoleucine, leucine, phenylalanine, valine, threonine, methionine, tryptophan and lysine. In children, histidine is also considered to be an essential amino acid since they are unable to make enough to meet their needs.

Because proteins from animal foods contain all the essential amino acids in the proportions required by the body, they used to be known as 'complete' (or first-class) proteins. Proteins from plant sources do not always contain all the essential amino acids, and were known as 'incomplete' (or second-class) proteins. However, in practice, the classification is irrelevant as human diets consist of a mixture of plant proteins, and the deficiency in one plant protein is made up by an excess in another. For example, the proteins of beans and wheat when eaten together provide similar levels of amino acids to meat. The protein intake of a vegetarian who eats a good variety of vegetable proteins will therefore be just as high as that of a person who regularly eats meat.

Nowadays proteins are simply classed as being high or low in quality. High-quality proteins include meat, poultry, fish, eggs and soya beans while low-quality proteins include nuts, pulses, bread, rice, pasta and potatoes.

PRUNES

BENEFITS

- *Rich source of potassium*
- *Useful source of fibre and iron*
- *Contain vitamin B_6*
- *Relieve constipation*

DRAWBACKS

- *High in calories*
- *May cause flatulence*

Prunes are the dried fruit of any of a number of varieties of plum tree. Like all dried fruit, they are concentrated sources of sugar, making them a useful energy-giving food. They also provide potassium, iron and vitamin B_6.

Prunes are a useful source of dietary fibre and can help to overcome constipation. Soak a cup of prunes in water overnight and then eat half of them in the morning and half in the evening. If you are not fond of whole prunes, prune juice makes an excellent substitute, and you can buy it ready bottled. Prune juice is low in fibre, yet still works as an effective laxative due to substances called hydroxyphenylisation derivatives, which stimulate the muscles of the large bowel.

You may suffer from flatulence when you first use prunes in your diet, but this symptom should disappear after about a week when your body has become accustomed to them.

Psoriasis

EAT PLENTY OF
- *Oily fish for omega-3 fatty acids*

CUT DOWN ON
- *Offal*
- *Alcohol*

Beauty is undeniably more than skin deep, and no creams or lotions will solve skin problems unless you eat to provide your skin with the nutrients it needs for repair and renewal. Psoriasis – a chronic condition which tends to run in families – affects one person in 50 in Britain and the United States. It is characterised by scaly pink patches, commonly appearing on the elbows, knees, shins and scalp; fingernails and toenails are also often affected.

Although there is as yet no cure for the disease, a combination of a healthy diet and prescribed skin ointments enables most sufferers to keep their symptoms under control.

Many people with psoriasis find that their symptoms improve after they have been in the sun. Moderately severe psoriasis may be treated with PUVA (the combination of a light-sensitive psoralen drug and exposure to longwave ultraviolet light). Recent research has found that sufferers have a faulty metabolism of vitamin D, and a patient may be prescribed the vitamin in the form of an ointment.

Psoriasis can be either helped or exacerbated by food choices. Oily fish – such as mackerel and trout – have been shown to relieve some symptoms of psoriasis and should form a regular part of the diet. They contain omega-3 fatty acids (see FATS), which have an anti-inflammatory effect, as well as large amounts of vitamin D.

Many people find that simply cutting out certain foods from their diet results in a marked improvement. Examples of foods which may be worth excluding are dairy produce, animal fats, meat and spices. Cut out offal because this contains an essential fatty acid called arachidonic acid, which the body converts to pro-inflammatory prostaglandins, which will irritate the condition. However, it is advisable to consult a nutritionist before eliminating too many foods from the diet.

Reducing alcohol intake may also be beneficial, since it is a vasodilator – it widens blood vessels and increases the blood flow to the skin – which causes the skin to become reddened and warm, exacerbating the itching and flaking of psoriasis.

Pulses

BENEFITS
- *Good source of protein and fibre*
- *Low in fat*
- *Source of minerals and B vitamins*
- *Help to control blood sugar levels, and so can be useful to diabetics*
- *Help to lower blood cholesterol levels*

DRAWBACKS
- *Can cause flatulence*
- *Soya beans are a common food allergen*

From beans on toast to dhal with rice, pulses are a nutritious and cheap alternative to meat. Dried peas, beans and lentils all contain protein, although unlike meat, fish and eggs they do not contain ideal amounts of all the essential amino acids necessary for growth and for maintaining healthy muscle tissue and organs. For this reason, most pulses should be served together with plant foods and whole grains such as rice or bread – a solution adopted by vegetarians the world over. Soya beans are the exception to this rule. Unlike the majority of pulses, they are classed as a source of high-quality protein because of their healthy balance of amino acids. Also, unlike other pulses, they contain a significant amount of fat, but most of it is unsaturated.

Pulses contain insoluble and soluble fibre: the former promotes regular bowel movements, so helping to guard against constipation, as well as possibly lessening the risk of cancers of the colon and rectum; the latter has been connected with lowering blood cholesterol levels, thereby reducing the risk of heart disease and stroke. Because the starches in pulses are digested and absorbed slowly, they allow a steady release of glucose into the blood – this is particularly useful for diabetics as it helps them to control their blood sugar levels.

Researchers are also examining the possible role of soya beans, as well as soya products such as TOFU, soya sauce, miso and soya milk, in protecting against cancer, particularly breast

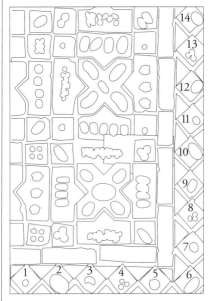

BEAN FEAST *Pulses are the cheapest protein source of all, with no waste. Aduki beans (1), broad beans (2), black-eyed peas (3), red lentils (4), chickpeas (5), cannellini beans (6), soya beans (7), mung beans (8), flageolet beans (9), borlotti beans (10), green lentils (11), red kidney beans (12), puy lentils (13), pinto beans (14).*

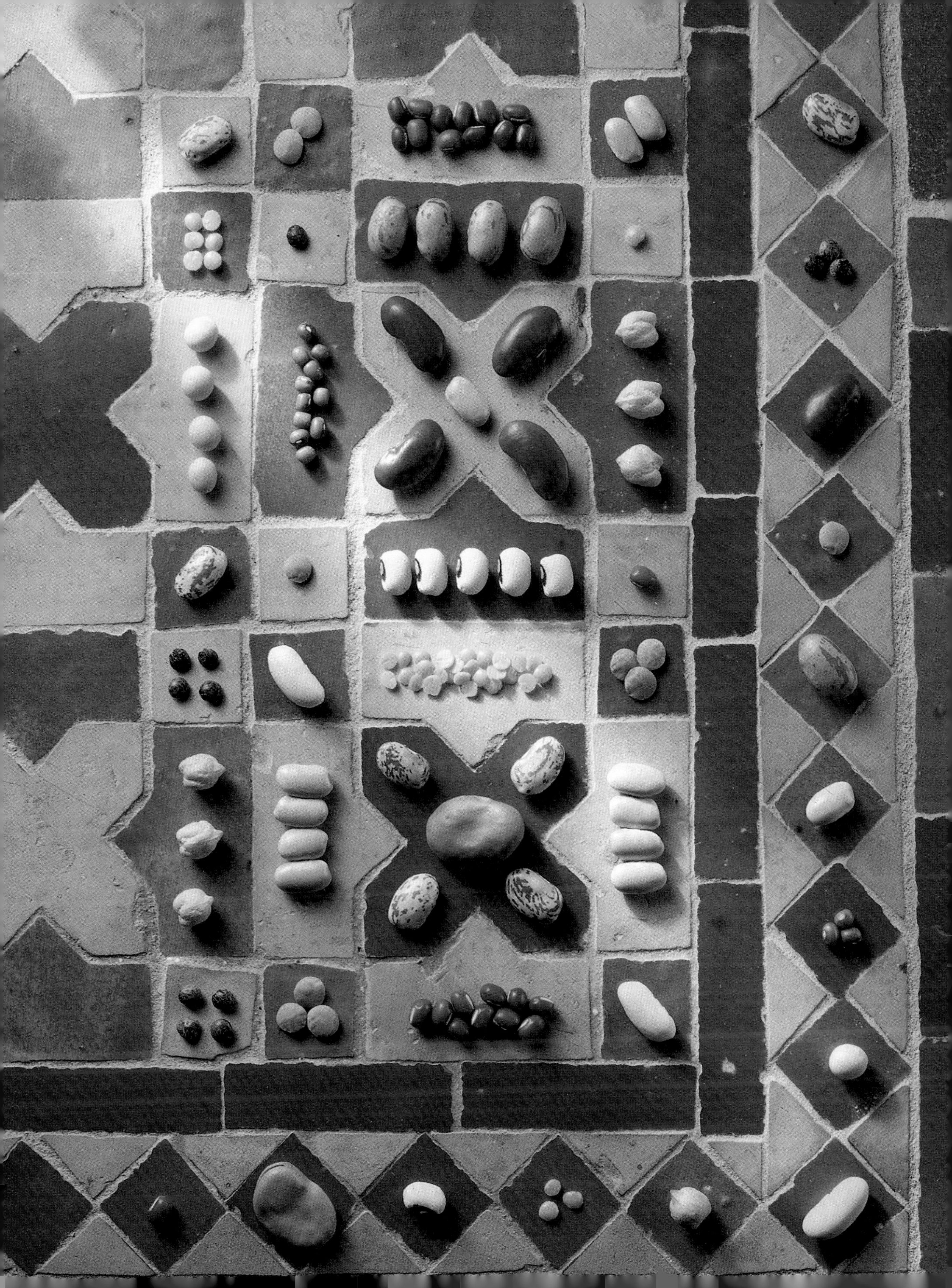

cancer, as well as osteoporosis and menopausal symptoms, because of the phytoestrogens they contain. Most cooked pulses contain iron, potassium, phosphorus, manganese, magnesium and the B vitamins (except for B_{12}); some of them also contain vitamin E. Although convenient, tinned pulses may be high in added salt.

When using dried KIDNEY BEANS it is essential to boil them rapidly for 15 minutes and then to simmer them until they are thoroughly cooked. Raw or undercooked kidney beans contain a substance that cannot be digested in the stomach and can result in severe food poisoning. Other beans contain a similar substance, but normally this is digested whether or not the beans are cooked and does not cause problems, except in people with poor digestion.

Soya beans, and any products containing them, however, are a common allergen, and can cause headaches and indigestion in susceptible people. Pulses are also moderately high in purines so should be avoided by people who suffer from gout.

Except for lentils and split peas, dried pulses need to be soaked in water for several hours or overnight before cooking. This will shorten the cooking time and reduce the levels of indigestible sugars responsible for causing wind. Discard any beans that float and then cook the drained and rinsed beans in plenty of fresh water. Adding herbs such as thyme, rosemary, sage, summer savory, lemon balm, fennel or caraway, may help to prevent flatulence.

Common pulses

Aduki bean Small, sweet-flavoured bean. Used in Oriental cuisine.

Black bean Earthy-flavoured, pea-sized bean used in Latin American, Chinese and Japanese cuisines.

Black-eyed pea Creamy, kidney-shaped bean with the characteristic black spot. A staple of southern US cooking, it is an excellent source of folate, supplies useful amounts of phosphorus and manganese, and contains zinc, iron, magnesium and thiamin.

Borlotti bean Speckled light brown bean that is popular in Italy.

Broad bean Strongly flavoured bean that can be eaten raw. A useful source of phosphorus and manganese, it also contains iron, zinc, folate, niacin, magnesium and vitamin E.

Cannellini bean Large white kidney bean commonly used in Italian cooking.

Chickpea Round with a nutty flavour, it is used in central Asian and Middle Eastern cuisines; also available as flour. A good source of manganese, it has useful amounts of iron, folate and vitamin E. Chickpeas are the main ingredient of hummous.

Flageolet bean Pale green, immature kidney bean, popular in France.

Kidney bean Large bean with a meaty flavour; usually dark red but can be black or white (see KIDNEY BEANS).

Lentils Staple of south Asian cuisine, available in various colours. Green and brown varieties are a good source of selenium, offer useful amounts of iron and manganese, and also contain phosphorus, zinc, thiamin, B_6 and folate.

Lima bean Also called the butter bean, it contains phosphorus and iron.

Mung bean Small green bean, often sold in the form of beansprouts. A source of manganese, iron, folate, magnesium and phosphorus.

Pinto bean Long, mottled bean. Among the highest in fibre of the pulses; popular in the United States and Latin America.

Soya bean Used for protein, oil, milk, tofu, flour and soya sauce. It is rich in potassium and is a useful source of magnesium, phosphorus, iron, folate and vitamin E. It contains manganese, vitamin B_6 and thiamin.

Split pea Yellow or green dried pea; excellent in purées and soups.

Pumpkin

BENEFITS

- *Good source of beta carotene*
- *Useful source of vitamin E*

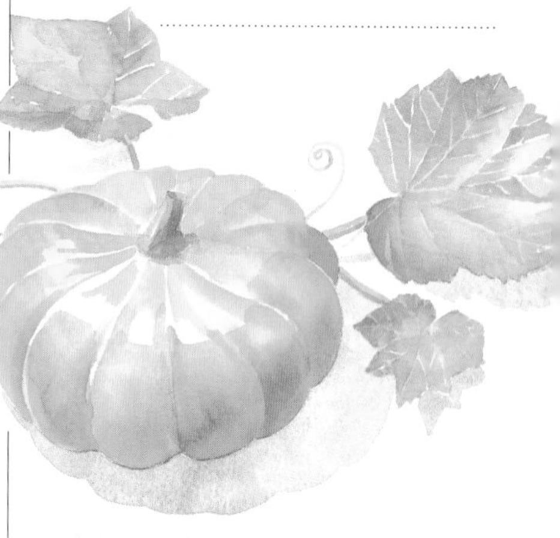

Widely used in Europe, the USA, Australia, Africa and the Caribbean, but less valued in Britain, pumpkins and other winter squash are a good source of beta carotene, which the body converts into vitamin A.

Pumpkins and the many varieties of winter squash, such as acorn and butternut, can play a particularly important role in a vegetarian diet where animal products are not available to provide vitamin A.

Beta carotene is also an ANTIOXIDANT, helping to prevent free-radical damage that might lead to certain types of cancer. Another antioxidant found in useful amounts in pumpkins is vitamin E.

Pumpkins are easily digested and rarely cause allergies, which makes them an excellent weaning food. Their SEEDS should also be saved as they are an excellent source of iron and phosphorus, and are rich in potassium, magnesium and zinc.

In natural medicine, pumpkin seeds are prescribed as a treatment for intestinal WORMS, when they must be taken in conjunction with a purgative such as castor oil. They can also be used for prostate and urinary problems.

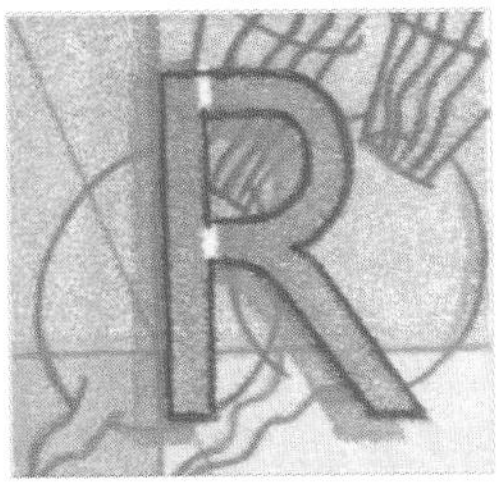

RADISHES

BENEFITS
- *Low in fat and calories*
- *Useful source of vitamin C*

Members of the cruciferous family of vegetables – which include radishes, broccoli, Brussels sprouts, cabbages and cauliflowers – contain sulphurous compounds which may help to protect against some forms of cancer. Radishes are a useful source of vitamin C, required for the manufacture of collagen which is needed for healthy skin, bones, cartilage, teeth and gums and for healing wounds and burns.

As radishes are low in calories and fat, they tend to be popular as a snack with slimmers – but they should be eaten in moderation. There are many varieties, differing in their pungency, size, shape and colour; they can be red, red and white, black or white.

In Ancient Egypt, radishes are known to have been cultivated extensively by the Pharaohs. They are used as a diuretic in herbal medicine.

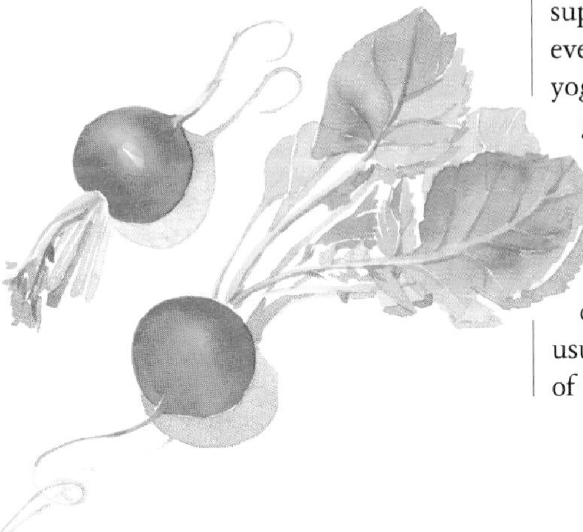

RAISINS

BENEFITS
- *Good source of potassium*
- *Contain iron*

DRAWBACK
- *High sugar content can encourage dental caries if consumed too frequently*

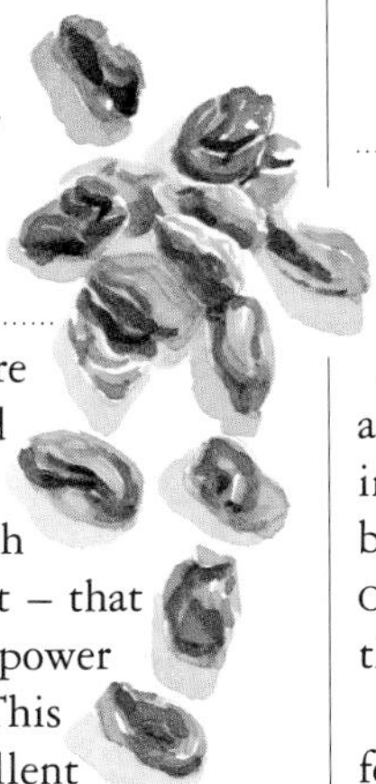

These dried grapes are such a concentrated source of calories – on account of their high natural sugar content – that they are like little power packs of energy. This makes them an excellent snack for endurance athletes and indeed anyone else who has to undergo prolonged physical exertion.

Raisins are a good source of potassium – a handful weighing 25 g (1 oz) will provide about 7 per cent of the recommended daily adult requirement – and they also contain iron.

Although high in calories, raisins are low in fat and so can be eaten by slimmers in moderation. Plain dried raisins contain around 70 Calories in 25 g (1 oz). However, dieters should be wary of eating raisins that have been dipped or coated in some sort of confectionery in the mistaken belief that they are a healthy treat. The same 25 g (1 oz) serving of chocolate-covered raisins is higher in saturated fat and supplies some 103 Calories. Perhaps even more surprising is the fact that yoghurt-covered raisins contain a greater amount of saturated fat, and provide as much as 115 Calories.

It is a good idea to brush your teeth after eating raisins, as they tend to stick to the teeth and can cause tooth decay. Diabetics are usually advised to avoid them because of their high natural sugar content.

RASPBERRIES

BENEFITS
- *Rich source of vitamin C*
- *Raspberry-leaf tea can be used to treat mild digestive problems. If drunk late in pregnancy, it may help to reduce the length of labour pains*

As a rich source of vitamin C, raspberries are both delicious and nutritious. Vitamin C is needed to maintain the health of skin, bones and teeth, to help the body to absorb iron from food, and to speed up the body's healing processes. As an ANTIOXIDANT, vitamin C may even reduce the risk of developing certain cancers.

Raspberries also contain vitamin E, folate and fibre. However, once canned in syrup their nutritional benefits are considerably diminished.

In naturopathic medicine, the juice of raspberries is widely believed to cleanse and detoxify the digestive system, to soothe childhood illnesses and cystitis, and is used as a cooling remedy for fevers. Raspberries are also thought to be useful in the treatment of diarrhoea, indigestion and rheumatism. Raspberry vinegar is used as a gargle for sore throats and may be added to cough mixtures. To make it, steep 500 g (1 lb 2 oz) of raspberries in 1 litre (1¾ pints) of wine vinegar for two weeks before straining the juice.

RASPBERRY-LEAF TEA

For centuries, raspberry-leaf tea has been used as a general tonic for the female reproductive system. It has a reputation for strengthening and toning the muscles of the womb, and of assisting contractions during labour. If drunk regularly during the last three months of pregnancy, it may lessen the risk of severe haemorrhage at birth, reduce the length of labour pains and even make delivery easier. But do not take large amounts in the early stages of pregnancy when it could initiate contractions in some women, perhaps causing a miscarriage.

Raspberry-leaf tea may have a mild relieving effect on period pains if taken for several days before the onset of menstruation. It is also suitable for treating mild digestive symptoms, including dyspepsia, diarrhoea and constipation, and is ideal for babies and children. Because of its mild astringent action, it may also be used as a mouthwash.

RAW FOOD DIET

There is little doubt that fruit and vegetables are at their nutritional best in their raw state but, for most people, the idea of maintaining a constant diet of uncooked food would be less than appealing. Yet there are many people who are happy to follow a raw food diet, often claiming that it makes them feel more energetic and 'alive'. They believe that cooking and processing not only damage the nutritional quality of food, but also reduce its health-giving properties. It is true that the nutritional content of fruit and vegetables is reduced through exposure to heat and water, especially in terms of water-soluble vitamins.

Fruit and vegetables make up the bulk of the raw food diet, but it may contain a little dairy produce and oil, both of which are likely to have undergone some form of processing. Beans, pulses, rice and other grains, pasta and potatoes are excluded as they cannot be eaten unless they are cooked – whether boiled or baked into bread.

As the raw food diet is based on fruit and vegetables, it provides plenty of B vitamins, vitamin C, beta carotene and potassium. The diet is high in insoluble FIBRE, which means that constipation is unlikely. However, an excessive intake of raw food can lead to irritable bowel syndrome. The diet is also high in soluble fibre, which is associated with a reduced risk of HEART DISEASE. Furthermore, a high consumption of fruit and vegetables is believed to help the body to fight infection, and to protect against some forms of cancer.

The raw food diet tends to be low in fat – and thus low in calories – so it is likely to promote weight loss in most people. This makes the diet unsuitable for children and those who do not need to lose weight, such as pregnant women and people with cancer. The diet is likely to be deficient in iron. If dairy products are excluded, it may

NATURALLY NUTRITIOUS *With a little imagination, uncooked food can be made into a wide range of appetising, nutrient-rich dishes.*

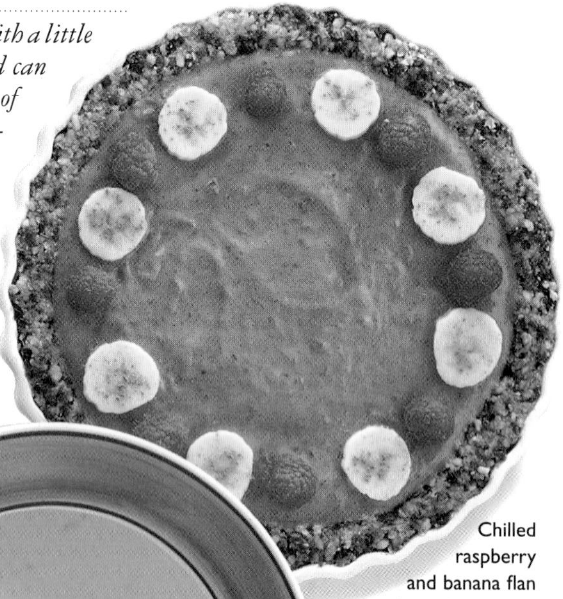

Chilled raspberry and banana flan in an almond, hazelnut, date and honey base.

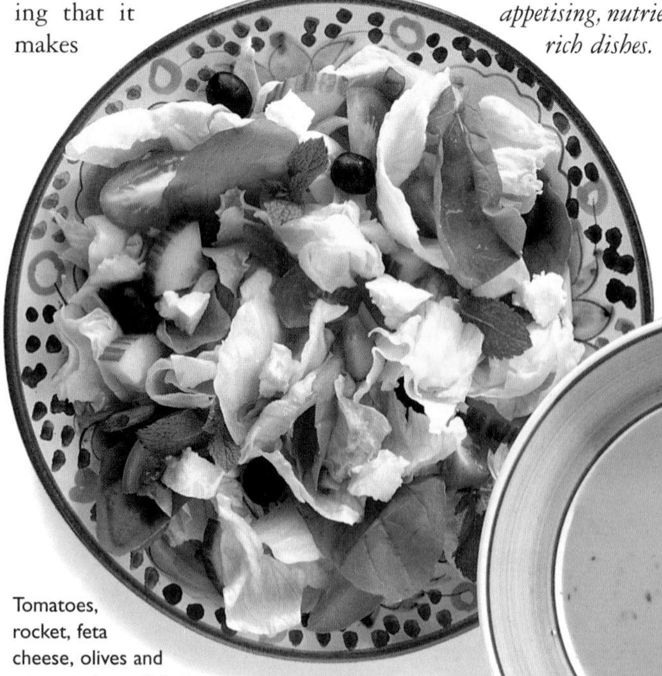

Tomatoes, rocket, feta cheese, olives and mint mix beautifully in a traditional Turkish salad.

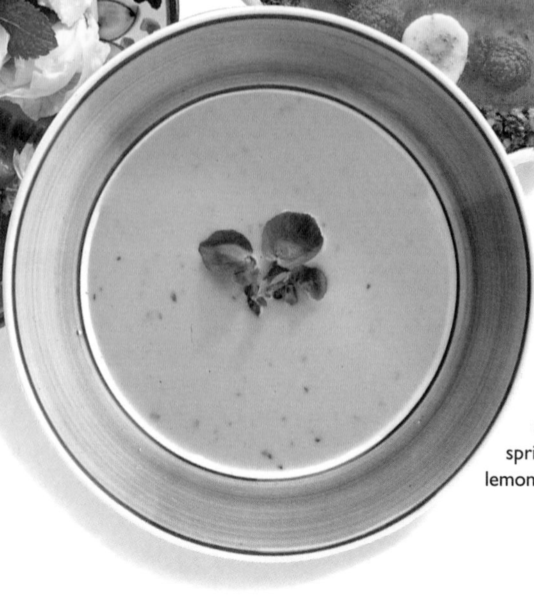

This chilled soup combines avocado, celery, spring onion, a little lemon juice and wine.

also be lacking in adequate supplies of other vital nutrients, such as calcium, vitamin B_{12} and protein.

Eaten for a week or so, the raw food diet is said by some to detoxify the system, improve vitality and may indeed help people to lose a few pounds. Others dispute this claim, and argue that the body's capacity to detoxify chemicals is reduced, and that much of the weight lost will be water, not fat. If you are considering adopting a raw food diet for any longer than a week or two, it would be wise to consult a qualified dietician first.

NUTS FOR PROTEIN

Including plenty of nuts in a raw food diet ensures an adequate supply of PROTEIN. Although the quality of protein from individual plant foods is lower than that from foods of animal origin, the overall protein quality will be just as high if a good variety of plant proteins is consumed.

Nuts also contribute vitamin E, thiamin and niacin, but their high fat content does make them calorific – most contain more than 225 Calories per 55g (2oz) serving.

RAYNAUD'S DISEASE

EAT PLENTY OF

- *Oily fish such as salmon, mackerel and sardines*
- *Foods rich in vitamin E, such as seed oils and avocados*

AVOID

- *Smoking*

Although no cure has yet been found, diet and other self-help measures are an essential part of the fight against the symptoms of Raynaud's disease. The illness is a CIRCULATION PROBLEM in which the flow of blood (and therefore of oxygen) to the body's extremities is interrupted – usually as a response to cold, a change in temperature, or stress.

As a result, the fingers and toes, and sometimes the nose and ears, turn white and dead-looking, then blue as the tissues use up oxygen. Finally, they turn red as the arteries relax and fresh blood rushes in. Other symptoms are a burning sensation as well as pain or numbness, though not every sufferer experiences all of these.

Severe cases of Raynaud's disease may need drug treatment to dilate the blood vessels. All patients should avoid vibrating tools such as hair dryers and electric drills, which can trigger the spasms. They should also try to keep their extremities as warm as possible – by wearing gloves, hats and thick socks in cool environments. If possible, they should avoid exposure to extreme cold, and try to maintain a healthy circulation through diet and regular aerobic exercise.

Frequent hot drinks and regular small meals – make sure that at least one of them is hot – help to provide fuel to keep the body warm throughout the day. Some people find it helpful to start the morning with a bowl of hot porridge or cereal with warm milk.

Case studies indicate that vitamin E is helpful in the treatment of Raynaud's disease. Rich sources include seed oils, wheatgerm and avocados. Eating plenty of oily fish, such as salmon, herring, mackerel, tuna and canned sardines, may be useful, too. These contain the omega-3 fatty acids, which may help to prevent the blood vessels from going into spasm. Adding one clove of garlic to the daily diet may also help by lowering blood pressure.

Smoking should be avoided because it has the effect of constricting the blood vessels. Alcohol, on the other hand, has the opposite effect and may therefore be helpful in small amounts. One or two units daily is a good guide, as long as patients avoid mixing it with any medication. Larger amounts of alcohol may cause the body to lose heat, thus adding to the problems associated with Raynaud's disease.

Raynaud's disease affects nine times more women than men. It is more common after the menopause, when it is believed to be caused by fluctuations in oestrogen levels.

The symptoms of Raynaud's disease can also accompany a more serious underlying disorder such as rheumatoid ARTHRITIS, LUPUS, or scleroderma (systemic sclerosis) – a condition affecting connective-tissue that causes toughening of the skin, usually of the hands and feet.

Scleroderma can also affect the internal tissues of the body, leading to loss of weight, aching muscles, joints and bones, shortness of breath and kidney problems. These symptoms collectively make up 'Raynaud's syndrome'.

REDCURRANTS

BENEFITS

- *Excellent source of vitamin C and a good source of potassium*

Although redcurrants belong to the same family as blackcurrants, their nutritional benefits are quite different. A 100g (3½oz) serving of raw redcurrants contains the full adult daily requirement of vitamin C, whereas the same quantity of blackcurrants boasts at least three times as much.

Cooking this tart-tasting fruit reduces some of its vitamin levels, but redcurrants still remain a good source of vitamin C and potassium. They also contain iron and fibre in quite useful quantities.

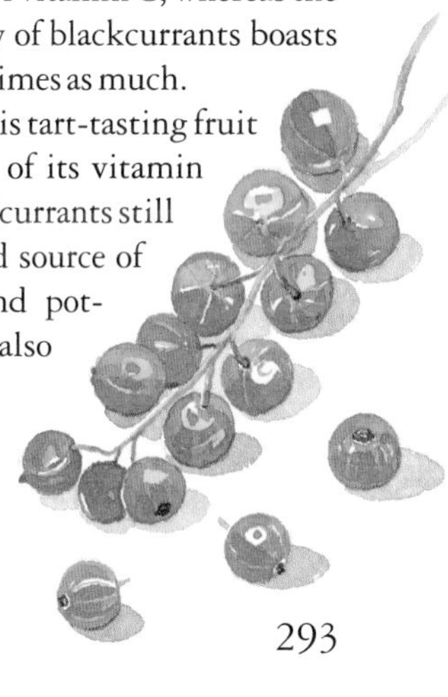

Restaurants and Eating Out

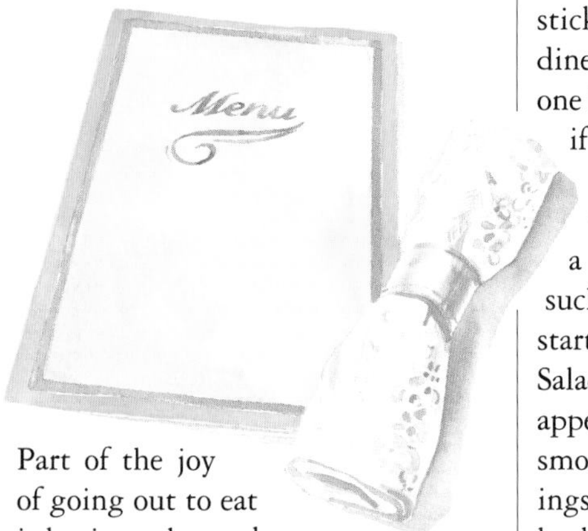

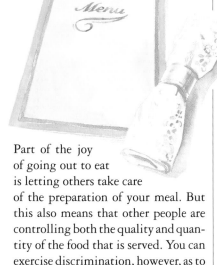

Part of the joy of going out to eat is letting others take care of the preparation of your meal. But this also means that other people are controlling both the quality and quantity of the food that is served. You can exercise discrimination, however, as to where you eat, and what you choose from the menu.

The trend towards healthier eating is reflected in many restaurants, with menus offering nutritious, low-fat dishes. Although there is always the temptation to overindulge in rich sauces and sugary desserts, it is perfectly possible to eat, and enjoy, a healthy meal in virtually any restaurant, although the type of cuisine can make a big difference.

It would not be difficult to choose a low-fat meal in a seafood restaurant or from a Japanese menu, for example. It may be a little harder in a French restaurant, where many dishes are traditionally served with heavy sauces, incorporating rich ingredients such as cream, butter and cheese.

Alcohol, too, is a source of hidden calories. A glass of wine can contain around 100 Calories. Try mixing white wine with mineral water to make a spritzer, or drink light beer. If you prefer red wine, order a bottle of mineral water as well and alternate glasses of wine with water. This is a good way of helping to prevent dehydration – and a hangover.

Bread and butter or *grissini* (breadsticks) can be irresistible to hungry diners. Limit yourself to two *grissini* or one bread roll, and do not have butter if you are watching your weight.

Try to choose dishes which add up to a balanced meal. If you select a high-carbohydrate main course, such as pasta, opt for a high-protein starter, such as oysters or poached fish. Salads make excellent low-calorie appetisers, as long as they are not smothered in mayonnaise-style dressings. A little oil and vinegar is a healthier choice. Other good starters for people who are watching their weight include tomato or vegetable soups, raw vegetables and melon or other fresh fruits.

Grilled or poached fish, poultry without its skin and any lean cut of meat – such as a trimmed rump steak – are all relatively low-fat main courses. However, cream or egg-based sauces, breadcrumb-style coatings, sautéed potatoes or vegetables *au gratin* (topped with grated cheese and breadcrumbs and grilled) will pile on the calories. In pasta restaurants, choose tomato, seafood or vegetable sauces in preference to cream and cheese-based sauces such as Alfredo or carbonara.

For many people, the dessert course is the highlight of the meal. By ending your meal with fresh fruit, fruit salad, a compôte or a sorbet, rather than a rich dessert, you will be able to leave the table without feeling bloated.

Taking a chance?

Despite strict laws governing the way that food is handled in restaurants, there are still health risks associated with eating out. Many outbreaks of FOOD POISONING can be traced back to restaurants. Short of inspecting an establishment's kitchens, people have no way of assessing hygiene standards. A lot can be judged, however, by a restaurant's general appearance, and by its reputation. Good indicators are a clean dining area and, if you can see it, a clean, well-organised kitchen.

On the other hand, chipped or discoloured crockery, dirty cutlery, smeared glasses and stained table linen probably indicate poor standards of hygiene behind the scenes. Food that is tepid and stale-tasting, or looks as though it has been kept warm, are all common warning signs. Skin on sauces or dried-out vegetables, for example, are a good indication that your chosen dish has been kept warm for far too long. If food and plates that are meant to be hot arrive only lukewarm, they could have provided an environment in which bacteria may well have had a chance to breed.

In restaurants serving buffet meals, where dishes of food might stand around for a long time, there is a risk of

High-risk foods on restaurant menus

If you are especially worried about the risks of food poisoning, you may wish to avoid those foods on restaurant menus most frequently reported to cause outbreaks. These include all dishes or sauces incorporating raw or lightly cooked egg, such as omelette, quiche, steak tartare (raw steak with raw egg yolk); the sauces hollandaise, béarnaise and mayonnaise; and desserts such as tiramisu, lemon meringue pie and chocolate mousse. Shellfish is another culprit (especially on Mondays when it may not be fresh from the market). Undercooked chicken, whether in a hot or cold dish, is believed to be one of the most common causes of food poisoning.

food poisoning because cold dishes may not be kept thoroughly chilled, and hot dishes not kept adequately hot.

Never be afraid to send something back if you think it is undercooked or off. In a busy restaurant mistakes can happen and most restaurant owners would be happier if you spoke up so that the problem can be solved instead of enduring a miserable meal and vowing never to return.

Restless legs

EAT PLENTY OF

- *Wheatgerm, nuts, pulses, parsley and green leafy vegetables for folate*
- *Liver, as a source of iron, vitamin B_{12} and folate*
- *Safflower oil, unsalted peanut butter and avocados for vitamin E*
- *Bananas for potassium*

CUT DOWN ON

- *Caffeine in coffee, tea and cola*
- *Salt*

AVOID

- *Smoking*

The condition of restless legs is fairly common. Symptoms such as pins and needles, burning sensations, pain and frequent involuntary jerking movements of the legs are normally felt soon after sitting down or going to bed. Apart from the obvious annoyance, this can interfere with sleep.

The most likely cause, especially in women, is iron deficiency. Eat plenty of iron-rich foods, such as liver (but not during pregnancy), kidneys and dried apricots. Vitamin B_{12}, found in meat, may help too. Make sure that your daily diet also includes wheatgerm, nuts, pulses, parsley and green leafy vegetables to provide ample amounts of folate, which is used by the body in the formation of red blood cells. The condition may be due to a circulatory disorder, so safflower oil, unsalted peanut butter and avocados should be included in the diet to provide vitamin E – which helps to ensure the healthy functioning of the peripheral circulatory system. Bananas are a good source of potassium, which aids the control of blood pressure and is needed for the proper functioning of muscles. Reduce your salt intake to keep your blood pressure down.

Caffeine and nicotine constrict the blood vessels, impairing the circulation. Restrict coffee and tea intake to no more than two or three cups a day. Try to avoid nicotine altogether. Very rarely, these spasms are the result of epilepsy, spinal-cord injury or neurological disease. Always consult your doctor if symptoms are severe.

Rheumatism

The term 'rheumatism' is used to describe a multitude of ailments where pain occurs with or without signs of inflammation in joints, muscles, tendons and connective tissues. It is not an illness in itself, though it is often regarded as such. People who complain of having rheumatism may in fact be suffering from conditions ranging from rheumatoid ARTHRITIS to fibrositis or lumbago.

Many people believe that if they feel a twinge after they have been caught out in the rain, they must be suffering from rheumatism. In fact, in this instance they are likely to be suffering from fibrositis. This is where the connective tissue of the muscles becomes inflamed causing considerable pain. Little is known about this common ailment, although it does tend to be brought on by damp, cold conditions. It is most commonly felt in the lower back, shoulders and neck. There is some suggestion that a low intake of the antioxidants selenium and vitamins A, C and E may increase the risk of rheumatic illnesses. So make sure that your diet includes plenty of fresh fruit and vegetables for vitamin C and beta carotene (which

Case study

Robin, a landscape gardener, was finding it difficult to use his hands. During a round of golf a friend noticed that he could not grip his clubs properly and looked unwell. He advised Robin to see a doctor. Thinking it was just a bit of 'rheumatism', Robin was surprised when the doctor diagnosed rheumatoid arthritis. The condition was eased with anti-inflammatory drugs and diet (eating oily fish and plenty of fresh fruit and vegetables). After a few weeks his hands felt less stiff and before too long he had even managed to reduce his golf handicap.

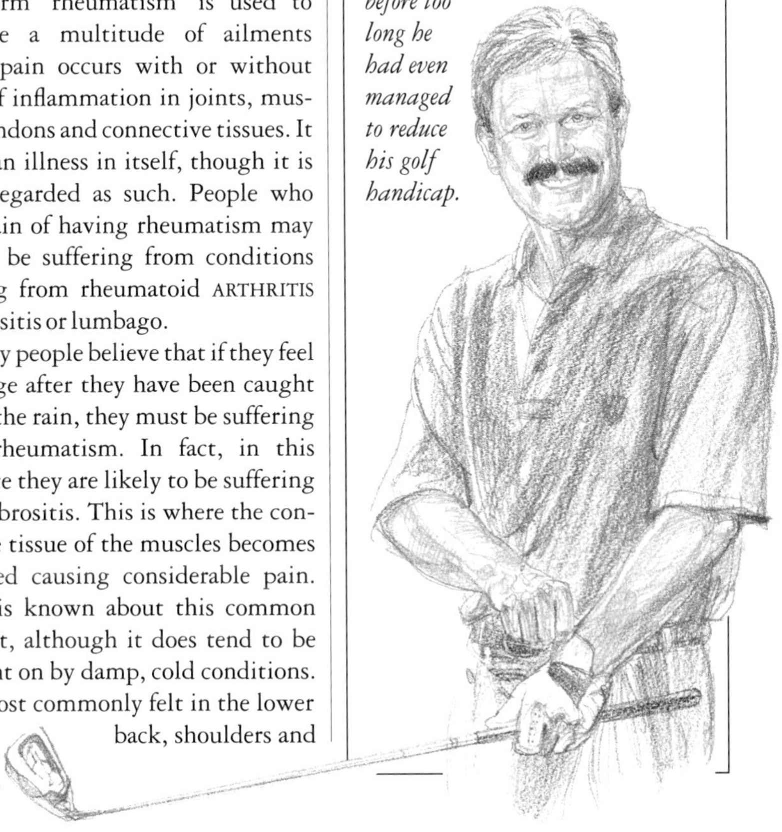

the body converts to vitamin A). Avocados, fresh nuts and olive oil will provide vitamin E and fish oils, cereals, eggs and brewer's yeast will supply selenium. Fish oils also contain omega-3 fatty acids which have an anti-inflammatory effect in the body.

Conditions where pain is felt in the muscles may be helped by taking supplements of selenium with vitamin E. A study in the USA showed that these supplements could help to reduce disabling muscular pain, stiffness and aching. Other studies have found that supplements of fish oil or evening primrose oil can reduce the need to take painkilling drugs.

An immediate and effective treatment is to place a hot-water bottle or hot flannel on the painful area. In any case of severe muscular pain it is sensible to take plenty of rest. Since the symptoms of 'rheumatism' cover a variety of illnesses you should consult your doctor in the first instance.

Did you know?

The following painful ailments all come under the umbrella term of soft-tissue rheumatic conditions: frozen shoulder, tennis elbow, golfer's elbow, carpal tunnel syndrome, repetitive strain injury, plantar fasciitis (inflammation of the sole of the foot, and policeman's heel), Achilles tendonitis, and trigger finger. All can involve considerable pain, though none is regarded as medically serious.

Usually, patients are offered analgesics, anti-inflammatories, physiotherapy and, if all else fails, steroid injections. Sometimes an injection of corticosteroids is combined with a local anaesthetic to relieve acute pain. Many sufferers can benefit from manipulative therapies such as osteopathy.

Rhubarb

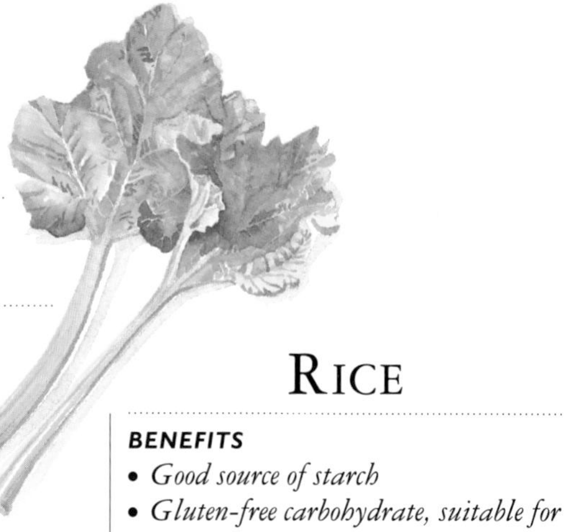

BENEFIT
- *Good source of potassium*

DRAWBACKS
- *Oxalic acid content inhibits calcium and iron absorption*
- *May aggravate joint problems in those with arthritis or gout*
- *May promote development of kidney stones in some people*
- *Leaves are highly poisonous*

Although it is thought of as a fruit, rhubarb is in fact a vegetable. Its characteristic sourness means that it is usually cooked with sugar to make it more palatable. While this considerably increases its calories, it does not alter its vitamin and mineral content significantly. Rhubarb contains vitamin C and manganese, and is also a good source of potassium.

Unfortunately, rhubarb also contains oxalic acid. This inhibits calcium and iron absorption, and can exacerbate the painful joint problems of people with gout or arthritis. It may also promote kidney stone formation in susceptible people.

In traditional Chinese medicine, rhubarb was often used as a purgative. According to Mrs Grieve's *A Modern Herbal* (1931), English rhubarb is a mild treatment for diarrhoea.

Rhubarb watchpoints

Rhubarb leaves are highly poisonous and should never be eaten. When cooking rhubarb, avoid using an aluminium saucepan. The metal of the pan reacts with the acids and other constituents of the juice. A shiny pan after cooking is a sign that the outer layer of oxidised aluminium has gone into the stewed fruit. Consuming excessive amounts of the MINERAL may well be harmful.

Rice

BENEFITS
- *Good source of starch*
- *Gluten-free carbohydrate, suitable for people with coeliac disease*
- *Helps to steady blood sugar levels*
- *Rice bran may reduce the risk of bowel cancer*

DRAWBACKS
- *Diets high in white rice may be deficient in thiamin*
- *Diets high in brown rice can contribute to iron and calcium deficiencies*

Rice is the staple food for over half the world's population, for whom it not only provides energy but is also an important source of protein. With any grain, the more refined the product,

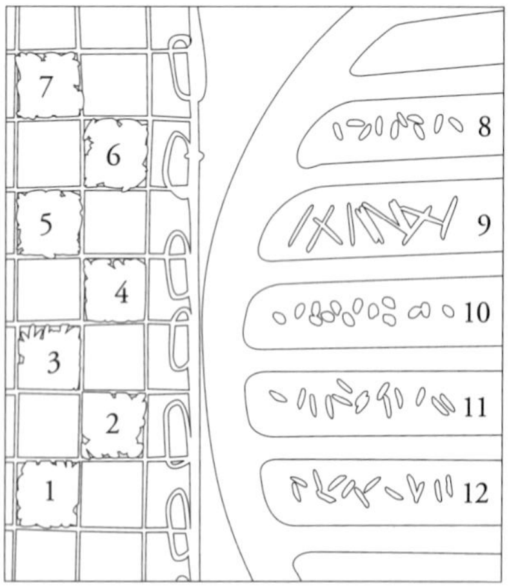

THE LONG AND THE SHORT OF IT *Varieties of rice include: risotto (1), glutinous (2), easy-cook basmati (3), easy-cook long-grain brown (4), long-grain brown (5), long-grain white (6, 8), easy-cook long-grain white (7), wild (9), pudding (10), brown basmati (11) and basmati (12).*

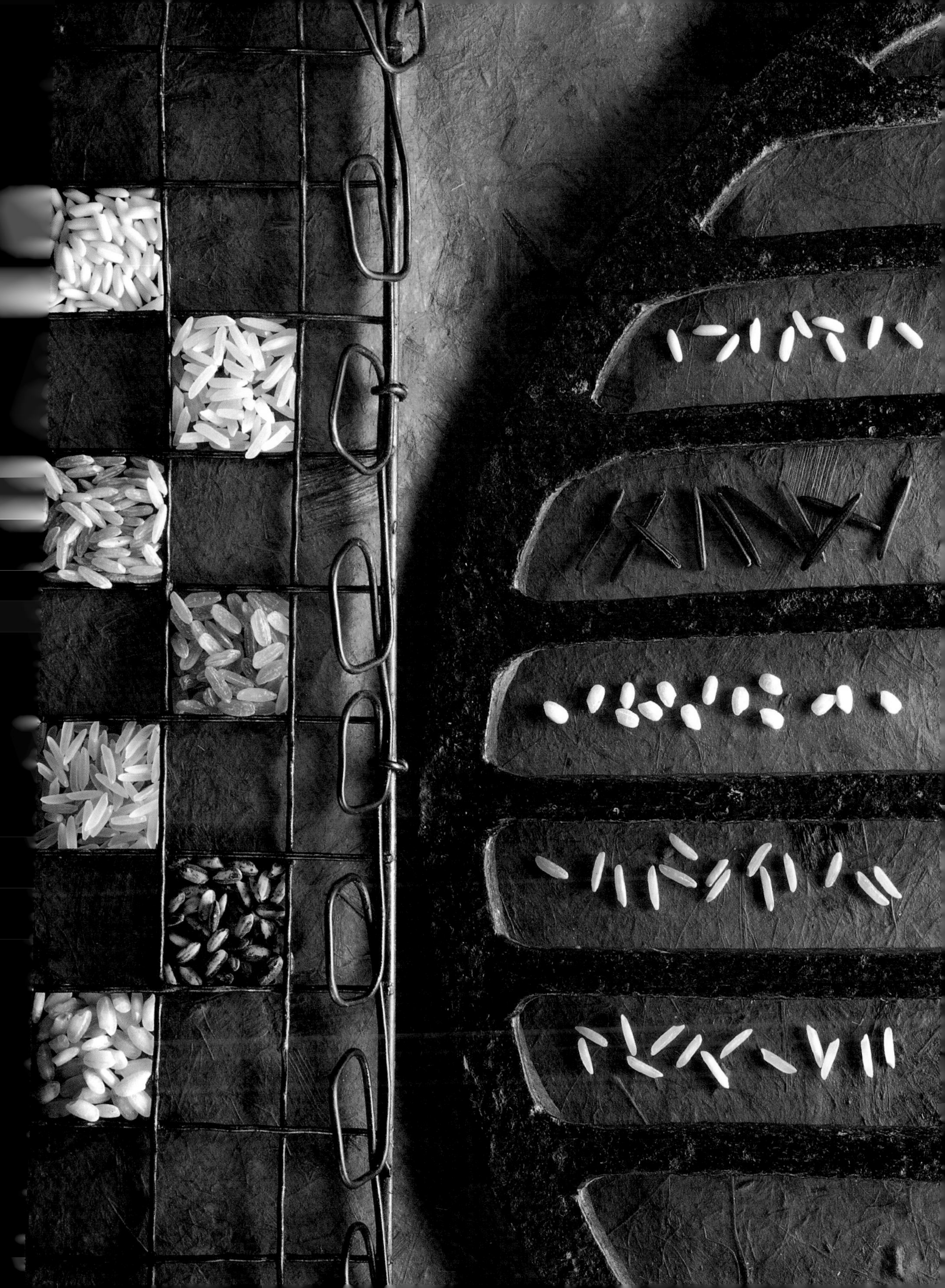

Did you know?

Rice is believed to have originated in southern Asia – it is known to have been cultivated in India and China for more than 6500 years. Yet it did not make an appearance in Europe until around AD1000. It reached England's shores during Elizabethan times, when it was imported from Spain.

Rice cannot be grown in the cold British climate and a large proportion of the rice now eaten in Britain comes from Carolina in North America. On a world scale, however, 90 per cent of all rice is still grown and consumed in Asia.

In some oriental cultures, rice is the symbol of life and fertility. Perhaps that is the origin of the widespread custom of throwing rice at newly married couples.

the fewer vitamins and minerals it contains. Rice is no exception to the rule. Many of its nutrients are contained in the bran and germ. In populations who subsist on white rice, thiamin deficiency is common. However, the bran, present in brown rice, also contains anti-nutritional factors such as phytic acid, which inhibits the absorption of iron and calcium.

Removing the bran makes rice cook more quickly, and many of the vitamins in rice can be retained if it is parboiled before milling. In Britain, parboiled rice is known as 'easy cook'. 'Enriched' white rice has vitamins and minerals added after it has been milled. Although white rice is low in fibre, some of the starch is resistant to digestion and acts like dietary FIBRE.

The starch in rice, particularly brown rice, is digested and absorbed slowly, thereby providing a steady release of glucose into the blood, which is helpful for controlling blood sugar levels in people with DIABETES. Rice is gluten-free, so it is useful for anyone with a wheat intolerance or COELIAC DISEASE and it also makes a safe weaning food.

Macrobiotic diets based on brown rice became very popular in the 1960s. Several deaths occurred when people tried to live on brown rice alone. Because diets high in brown rice can cause mineral deficiencies, they are particularly unsuitable for children.

MEDICAL BENEFITS

Rice has long been used in natural medicine to treat digestive disorders, from indigestion to diverticular disease. It is also believed to relieve mild cases of diarrhoea and constipation. Furthermore, research now suggests that eating rice bran, which can be bought in health-food shops, may reduce the risk of bowel cancer.

POPULAR TYPES OF RICE

Rice is classified according to its size. There are long-grain varieties and short-grain; wholegrain and easy cook. Long-grain white rice is still one of the most popular varieties. It has a delicate flavour and is milled to remove the outer layers of the husk and bran. Brown long-grain rice is more flavoursome and retains the bran layer after minimal milling. This means that brown rice contains more vitamins, minerals and fibre than white rice and is therefore more nutritious.

Arborio A medium-grain, absorbent rice, cooking to a creamy mass. It is used in the Italian dish risotto.

Basmati A long-grain, aromatic rice typically used in Indian dishes. It has been described as the prince of rice.

Glutinous A sticky rice popular in the Far East. Almost round in shape, it has a slightly sweet flavour.

Jasmine A fragrant rice, similar to basmati, but with a stickier texture. It is widely used in Chinese cooking.

Pudding rice A short-grain rice that, as its name suggests, is ideal for use in puddings and sweets. The grains are starchy and tend to clump together as they are being cooked.

Wild rice This is not a true rice at all, but the seeds of a North American wild aquatic grass. The 'grains' are long, slim and black. They are rich in the B vitamins (with the exception of vitamin B_{12}). Wild rice is often used in salads – mixed in with basmati rice.

RUNNER BEANS

BENEFITS

- *Useful source of vitamin C*
- *Contain folate*
- *Contain iron*

Containing a reasonable amount of nutrients and fibre, runner beans are coarse-textured, succulent green pods encasing immature, pink kidney-shaped beans. A 100g (3½oz) helping of cooked runner beans provides a quarter of an adult's daily vitamin C requirements and about a fifth of the recommended intake of folate, as well as a small amount of iron.

Most people tend to boil runner beans, but young, tender beans are delicious raw – thinly sliced into salads. (Make sure you wash them thoroughly to remove all traces of chemical pesticides that may have been applied to the growing crop.) Raw runner beans contain the greater amount of nutrients – about a third of their vitamin content is lost once runner beans have been boiled.

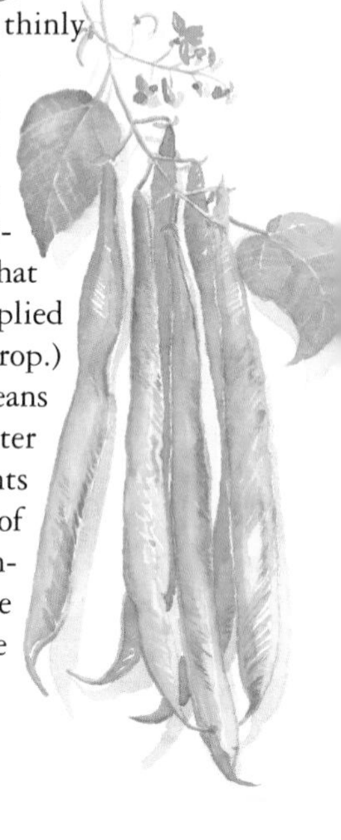

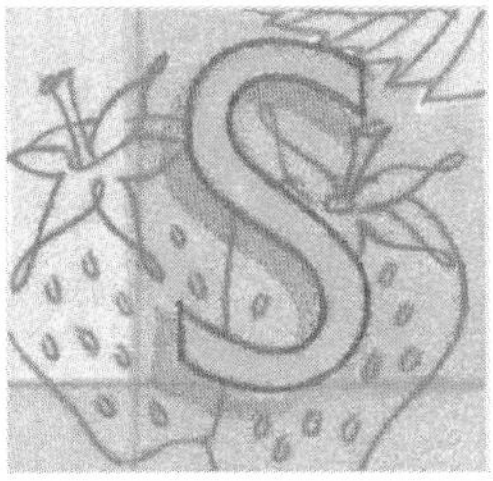

SAD (SEASONAL AFFECTIVE DISORDER)

TAKE PLENTY OF
- *Complex carbohydrates, such as wholemeal bread, pasta, pulses, vegetables and brown rice*

AVOID
- *Alcohol, which can worsen depression*
- *Excessive intakes of sweets, biscuits and cakes*

People who always feel abnormally depressed and lethargic during the gloomy winter months – and whose symptoms subside in spring – may well be suffering from Seasonal Affective Disorder, or SAD. This depressive condition is due to the chemical effects of light deprivation on the brain. It afflicts mainly women living in northern climates, such as Scandinavia, where there is a high incidence of depression and suicide during the long, dark winters. SAD was not officially designated an illness until 1987, although back in the 1920s it was common for doctors to send depressed patients off to have a holiday in the sun during the winter months.

LIGHT THERAPY

The majority of SAD sufferers feel better after one or two weeks of light therapy. This involves extra exposure to natural sunlight or high-intensity bright white light (between 5 and 20 times brighter than ordinary room lighting) for periods of half-an-hour to several hours each day. This treatment tends to be more effective than the antidepressant drugs that are sometimes prescribed for SAD.

FOOD CRAVINGS, especially for sugary carbohydrates, are often associated with the disorder – a starchy 'fix' makes SAD victims feel better for a while. Scientists in Switzerland have suggested that eating sweet things might trigger the release of the same mood-altering chemicals as sunlight or bright white light. Once light therapy is initiated, the craving for sugary foods may drop.

If you have SAD, try to satisfy any carbohydrate cravings by eating pasta with light sauces, beans and pulses, fresh vegetables and bread instead of high-fat, high-sugar sweets, biscuits and cakes, and try to avoid alcohol, as it can worsen depression. Aim to undertake more outdoor activities, and if you work in an office, ask if your desk can be moved near to a window. If possible, escape the winter blues by taking a winter holiday in a sunny place.

SALAD DRESSINGS

BENEFITS
- *The vegetable oils used in salad dressings are low in saturated fat and a good source of vitamin E*

DRAWBACK
- *High in calories*

A classic vinaigrette, or French dressing, adds interest to the plainest salad, but at a heavy cost in terms of fat and calories. However, the vegetable oils used in salad dressings contain mostly the healthier monounsaturated and polyunsaturated FATS rather than the less healthy saturated fats, an excess of which can lead to heart disease. We need relatively small quantities of fats to stay healthy and to maintain normal body function. Our intake of calories from fats should not exceed 35 per cent of total calorie consumption, and can be safely reduced to about 25 per cent (of which only 10 per cent should be saturated fat). It is, therefore, best to use oily salad dressings in moderation.

When making a vinaigrette, choose a cholesterol-free, cold-pressed oil, such as extra-virgin olive oil. Salad oils generally have a high vitamin E content. Olive, peanut and rapeseed oils contain a high proportion of monounsaturated fats, while soya bean, corn, sunflower, walnut and safflower oils are rich in polyunsaturated fats.

Commercial vinaigrettes and other salad dressings usually contain a range of additives and egg or soya derivatives which can cause allergic reactions in some people: check the label if you are in any doubt. Low-calorie versions of

Healthy homemade dressings

Homemade salad dressings can be healthy and fresh, as you have complete control over what is in them. Try whisking the following ingredients together for a tasty dressing to use with a fresh green salad: 150ml (¼ pint) crème fraîche, 1 tablespoon of white wine vinegar, 1 tablespoon of lemon juice, ¾ teaspoon of Dijon mustard and a little black pepper.

Alternatively, peel and crush one clove of garlic and mix with 3 tablespoons of virgin olive oil and 1 tablespoon of balsamic vinegar. Season to taste. For a dressing to serve with a tuna and bean salad, mix the juice of half a lemon with 3 tablespoons of virgin olive oil and season to taste.

dressings are available – and are a useful alternative if you are trying to control your calorie intake – but they are not to everyone's taste.

Although Thousand Island and Caesar salad dressings are made with the addition of raw egg to the basic salad-dressing recipe, manufacturers always use pasteurised egg yolk to avoid the risk of salmonella. When making your own dressing, be sure to use eggs from a trustworthy supplier.

Roquefort and similar blue-cheese dressings are increasingly popular – but even if you keep the cheese content as low as tastiness will allow it will still boost the dressing's calorie count and saturated fat content.

SALT AND SODIUM

BENEFITS

- *Maintain fluid balance and blood pressure*
- *Improve the flavour of many foods*
- *Useful food preservatives*

DRAWBACKS

- *Excessive intakes can cause a rise in blood pressure, and an increased risk of stroke, heart disease and kidney failure*
- *High intakes promote an increase in calcium excretion and may exacerbate osteoporosis*

Most people eat more salt than they need. In Britain, the average adult eats 9g (about 2 level teaspoons) of salt per day, as opposed to the World Health Organisation's recommended figure of 6g. Doctors and nutritionists associate excessive salt consumption with an increased risk of high BLOOD PRESSURE, which can eventually result in strokes, heart disease and kidney failure.

Every cell in the body needs sodium in order to function properly. It helps to regulate the body's fluid balance and to maintain healthy blood pressure levels. It is also needed for the healthy functioning of the nerves and muscles – including those in the heart – and the absorption of certain nutrients in the small intestine and kidneys.

Sodium requirements vary according to age, and how much is lost in sweat – either through physical exertion, or just from living in a hot, humid climate. Some people naturally perspire more than others – this is not necessarily a sign of being unhealthy. Although any salt that the body loses through sweating will need to be replaced, too much salt can be just as damaging to your health as too little.

Sodium in everyday foods

A level teaspoon of salt supplies 2g, or 2000mg, of sodium. The level in some foods is surprisingly high. For example, a bowl of cornflakes contains as much as a bag of crisps.

Bacon, lean, grilled: 2240mg per 100g; 800mg per average rasher.

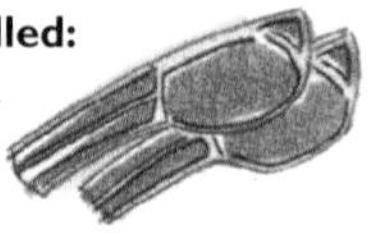

Bread, all types: 550mg per 100g; 200mg per slice from a large loaf.

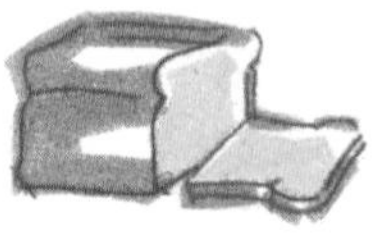

Blue cheese: 1095mg per 100g; 430mg per helping.

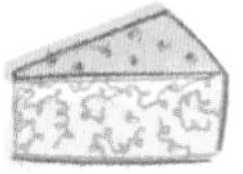

Cornflakes: 1110mg per 100g; 360mg per bowl.

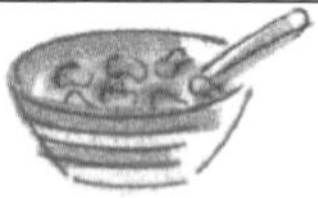

Crisps, various: 1070mg per 100g; 270mg per packet.

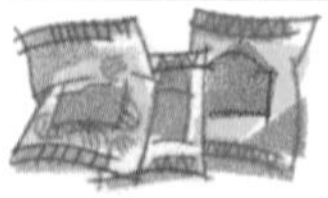

Peanuts, roasted and salted: 400mg per 100g; 100mg per small bag.

Tinned tomato soup: 450mg per 100g; 1125mg per bowl.

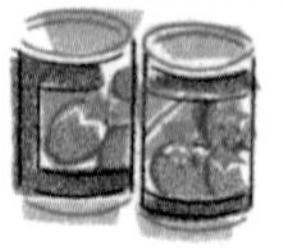

HOW MUCH SALT?

The salt (sodium chloride) that we add to food when cooking, or at the table, accounts for only one-fifth of our total sodium intake. Another fifth comes from naturally occurring sodium in unprocessed foods – there are low levels of sodium in all fruits, vegetables, meat, fish, grains and pulses. But more than half of the sodium in our diet – at least 60 per cent – comes from manufactured foods, which contain salt or sodium compounds, such as the preservative sodium nitrate, the flavour enhancer monosodium glutamate, or sodium bicarbonate, which is a raising agent.

The minimum daily amount of sodium needed by the adult body is 1.6g, contained in about 4g of salt. A level teaspoon of salt weighs 5g; a heaped teaspoon weighs about 8g. Salt is made up of 40 per cent sodium and 60 per cent chloride, by weight. This means that one gram of salt contains 0.4g of sodium, and conversely one gram of sodium is the equivalent of 2.5g of salt.

EATING LESS SALT

Many foods, such as bread, breakfast cereals and biscuits, contain 'hidden' salt, but it is not always practical to cut these foods out of the diet. The most obvious way to cut down on salt is to use less in cooking and at the table. Salt does not need to be added to vegetable water, for example; in fact, salt detracts from the natural sweetness of many vegetables.

If you are in the habit of adding salt at the table, try omitting it from cooking altogether. Use fresh or dried herbs and spices to add extra flavour to cooked dishes and salad dressings. Avoid foods which are high in salt. By weight, these include stock cubes (on average around 60 per cent) and gravy mixes (15 per cent), smoked salmon (5 per cent), cooked bacon (4 per cent), ham (4 per cent), potato crisps (1 per cent), olives (2 per cent) and sauerkraut (2 per cent).

CHILDREN AND ADULTS

Babies and children are less efficient than adults at excreting sodium, so they are much more vulnerable to excessive sodium intake – which can cause severe dehydration. This is why babies and young children should not have salt added to their foods. Packaged baby foods have to meet strict health regulations, and do not have any salt or sodium compounds added to them at all.

Adults need salt, but only in small quantities. Large intakes of salt cannot be tolerated by our bodies – which is why you should never drink sea water. Excessive amounts of salt can increase calcium excretion and so increase the risk of developing osteoporosis.

ALTERNATIVES TO SALT

Miso, tamari or soya, used in oriental dishes, are concentrated sources of sodium, but only small amounts of them are used. Lemon juice, garlic or pepper are healthier alternatives.

Low-sodium salt – half sodium and half potassium – is now widely available. Avoid using low-salt substitutes, however, if you are diabetic or suffer from kidney disease. Diabetics often retain potassium so must guard against accumulating dangerously high levels; people with kidney disease may also have difficulty excreting potassium, and they too should watch their intake.

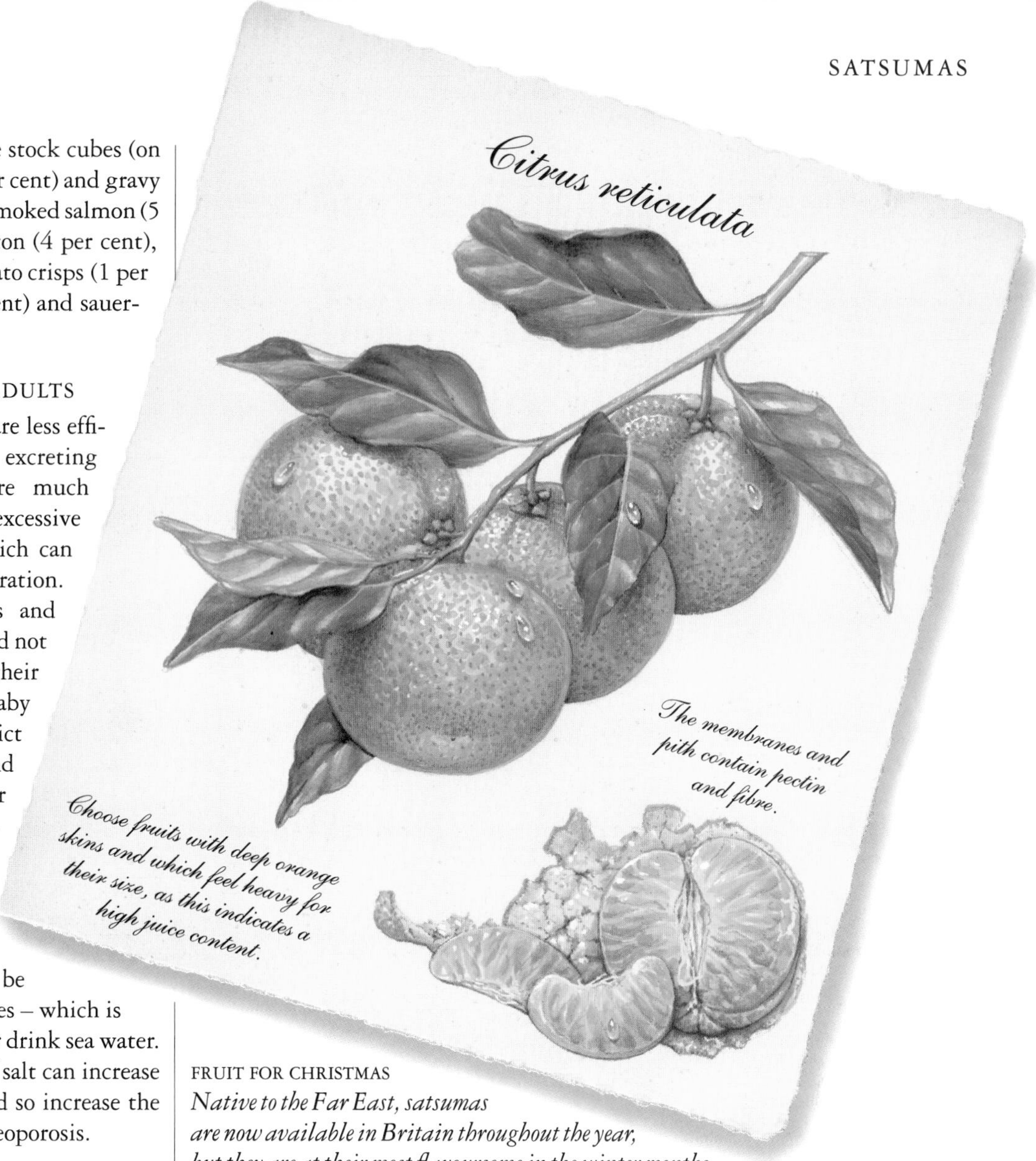
Citrus reticulata
The membranes and pith contain pectin and fibre.
Choose fruits with deep orange skins and which feel heavy for their size, as this indicates a high juice content.

FRUIT FOR CHRISTMAS
Native to the Far East, satsumas are now available in Britain throughout the year, but they are at their most flavoursome in the winter months.

SATSUMAS

BENEFITS
- *Good source of vitamin C*
- *Contain pectin, a form of soluble fibre which may help to lower blood cholesterol levels*

Along with tangerines, mandarins and clementines, satsumas belong to a group of bright-orange citrus fruits with thin, easily peeled skins. Like the other varieties, satsumas are a good source of vitamin C. Low levels of the vitamin increase our susceptibility to infection. Vitamin C is also an antioxidant, which may help to prevent the damage caused by FREE RADICALS and so offer protection against various forms of cancer.

Make sure you eat the membranes between the segments as well as some of the pith which clings to them. These contain pectin – fibre which may be helpful in lowering blood cholesterol levels. The membranes and pith also contain bioflavonoids, which act in much the same way as antioxidants.

Sauces

BENEFITS

- *Enhance the flavour, texture and appearance of many foods*
- *Hot, spicy sauces can help to clear blocked nasal passages*

DRAWBACKS

- *May be high in salt and sugar*
- *May be high in fat*

Some sauces are eaten in such small amounts as to offer only minimal nutritional benefits. Unfortunately, the majority of the sauces that are usually eaten in larger quantities, such as cream and egg-based sauces, contain a lot of fat and calories.

Many sauces also have high levels of sugar and salt – tomato ketchup and brown sauce are both examples. Commercially prepared 'cook-in' sauces can contain a wide variety of ADDITIVES, from thickeners, emulsifiers and stabilisers to preservatives and colourings. Check labels carefully if you know that you have an allergy to any of these additives.

Creamy sauces

Béarnaise and hollandaise are classic French sauces made from egg yolks and butter, sharpened with lemon juice or vinegar. They are a source of vitamin A, but are extremely high in calories and saturated fats. Therefore, as with all cream-based sauces, they are best avoided if you have high blood cholesterol levels.

Béchamel or white sauce, traditionally made from butter, flour and milk, is usually not quite so high in calories and fat. If it is made with semi-skimmed milk and not too much butter, it can be enjoyed, at least occasionally, by almost anyone.

Further calories and saturated fats are added when béchamel is flavoured with cheese, turning it into a Mornay sauce. Another milk-based sauce is traditional bread sauce. These sauces all supply vitamins B_2, B_{12} and niacin, as well as calcium and phosphorus.

Gravy made with meat dripping can be very high in fat. A healthier version can be made by skimming the fat from the meat juices first. Gravy made from granules may be a lower-fat alternative, but is usually high in salt.

Pasta sauces

A commercially prepared tomato-based pasta sauce is a rich source of potassium and a useful source of vitamin B_2. It is usually low in fat and calories, but remember to check the label as some brands may be high in SALT, or sodium. A cheaper, easy and nutritious alternative can be made using fresh or tinned tomatoes, onions, olive oil and garlic. Pesto, made from fresh basil, Parmesan cheese, pine nuts and olive oil, is higher in fat, but is eaten in relatively small quantities. Cream and cheese sauces, such as those used in spaghetti carbonara and fettucini Alfredo, contain substantial amounts of fat and are high in calories.

Far Eastern cuisine

Soya sauce, used extensively in Far Eastern cooking and made from fermented soya beans, is an extremely concentrated source of sodium – it contains almost six times as much sodium as brown sauce. It also contains wheat and should therefore be avoided by anyone with a gluten or wheat intolerance. Japanese and Chinese sauces often contain monosodium glutamate (MSG), which was thought to cause headaches in susceptible people (part of the so-called Chinese Restaurant Syndrome), but recent research suggests that other foods commonly used in oriental cuisine are to blame.

Researchers are currently examining the possible role of soya beans and related products such as tofu and soya bean paste in protecting against breast cancer, cardiovascular disease, osteoporosis and menopausal symptoms.

Oyster sauce is another salty condiment widely used in Chinese cuisine. It may produce allergic reactions in people sensitive to shellfish. The Thai version is made from salted dried fish.

Black and yellow bean sauces are also frequently used in Chinese cooking. Both are made from soya beans, either salted or fermented, and are high in salt. Bottled bean sauces may be thickened with wheat flour and should therefore be avoided by anyone with a gluten intolerance.

Hoisin sauce is a salty-sweet condiment made from soya beans and red rice (tinted by red beans). It is used to flavour Peking duck, which is traditionally accompanied by a sauce made from tart, pickled plums and sugar.

The Malaysian and Indonesian dish satay, which consists of meat kebabs, is usually served with a spicy peanut sauce. Although it is high in fat, the sauce also offers some vitamins and minerals, especially vitamin E, thiamin and manganese.

All oriental sauces that are high in sodium should be avoided by people on a low-salt diet.

Hot and spicy sauces

Spicy sauces, such as Tabasco, a hot and tangy seasoning made from Mexican chilli peppers, vinegar and salt, and Worcestershire sauce can be helpful in clearing blocked nasal passages. Although they are used too sparingly to offer any nutritional benefits, they should still be avoided by anyone suffering from indigestion or an ulcer.

Bottled sauces

Most brands of tomato ketchup and brown sauce are high in salt and sugar. However, unless they are eaten in large quantities their contribution to sugar intake is not significant.

SAUSAGES, SALAMIS AND FRANKFURTERS

BENEFITS
- *Good sources of energy*
- *Good sources of protein*

DRAWBACKS
- *Fat typically accounts for more than 70 per cent of a sausage's calories*
- *High in salt*
- *Usually high in additives including preservatives, colourings, flavourings and 'fillers'*
- *Contain nitrosamines*
- *Contain cholesterol*

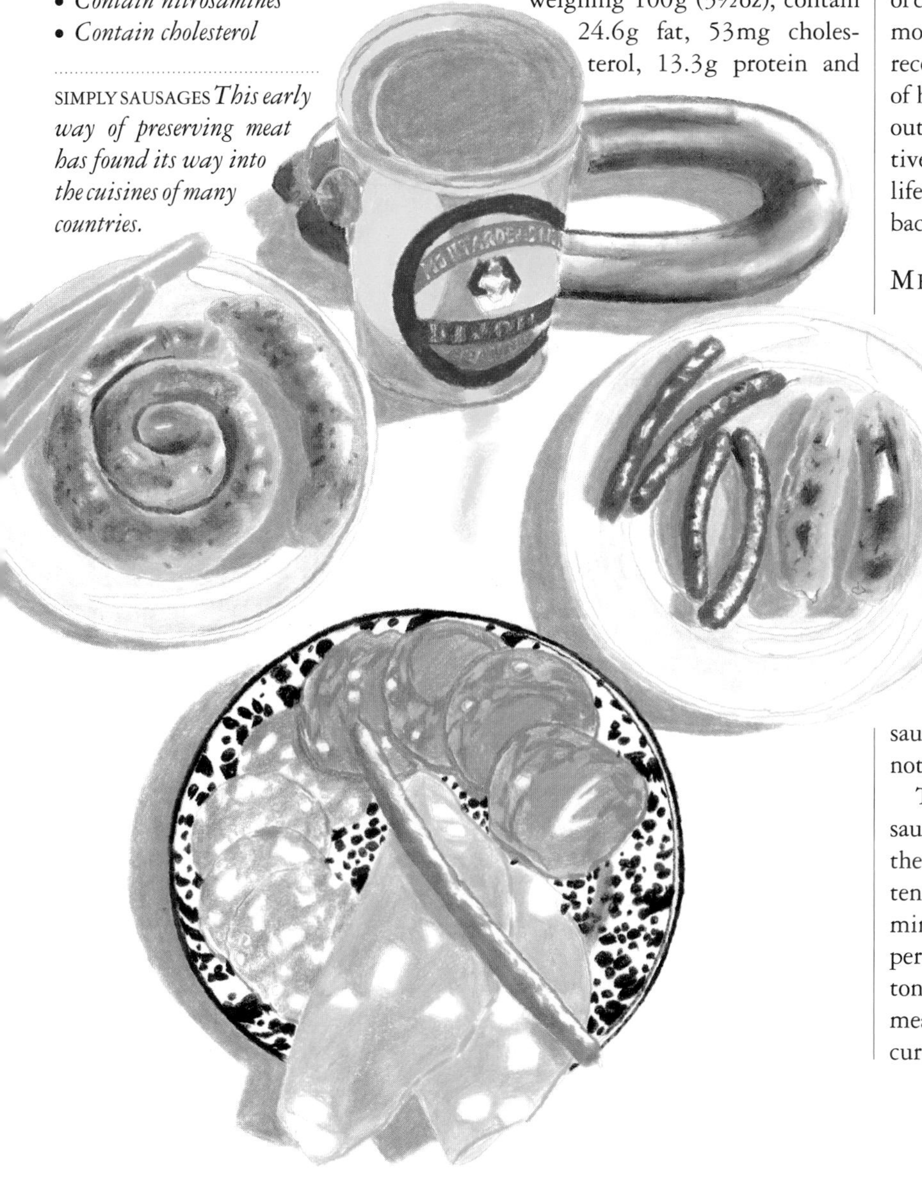

SIMPLY SAUSAGES *This early way of preserving meat has found its way into the cuisines of many countries.*

In all their many guises, sausages are processed forms of meat. They are usually high in fat and salt, although they do provide protein. As far back as Greek and Roman times sausages have been used as a way of preserving meat – the name sausage derives from the Latin *salsus* meaning 'salted' – and there is a limit to how far the salt and fat content can be reduced if the sausage is to have much flavour and retain its shape.

Sausages are generally of less nutritional value than fresh meat, although they contain the same range of nutrients. Three grilled pork sausages, weighing 100g (3½oz), contain 24.6g fat, 53mg cholesterol, 13.3g protein and 2.5g salt. Sausages also tend to contain many ADDITIVES. Although there is now stricter legislation controlling the use of colours, preservatives and flavourings, one group of additives – the nitrates and nitrites – has caused particular concern.

Nitrites (and nitrates which readily convert to nitrites) can react with substances in the meat and in the stomach to form nitrosamines. In very large doses, these additives have been linked with cancer in laboratory animals, but research indicates that the amounts in which these chemicals are used in processed foods pose a minimal threat of cancer to humans. They are carefully monitored and permitted only at recognised 'safe' levels. The possibility of harmful effects is thought to be far outweighed by the ability of the additives to inhibit the proliferation of life-threatening bacteria such as the bacterium that causes botulism.

MEAT CONTENT

As well as additives to preserve the meat, sausages may contain herbs and spices to add flavour, and they nearly always contain 'fillers', such as oatmeal, breadcrumbs or a special type of biscuit, to make the meat go further. The European Union regulations for meat and fish products do not actually stipulate what fillers are permitted in sausage manufacture, but they must not pose any hazards to the consumer.

The regulations state that if a sausage is qualified by the name pork, the minimum permissible meat content is 65 per cent; if it is called beef the minimum meat content must be 50 per cent; and if it is called liver or tongue, then at least 30 per cent of the meat must be liver or tongue. For cured meat and other sausages where the name of the meat is stated, the sausages must comprise at least 80 per cent of the named meat. If the sausage is not linked to any type of meat in its name, then all the consumer knows is that at least 50 per cent of the sausage is meat, but this could be made up of any mixture of meats.

The regulations do not state which part of the animal the meat must come from, so that meat which has been mechanically recovered can find its way into sausages. This meat can take two forms: muscular tissue taken from the surface of bones (and which is permitted in sausages made for cooking), and the paste-like bone marrow which may be used in sausages with pâté-like fillings, such as liver sausage spreads.

A HEALTHY SAUSAGE?

There are some manufacturers who take pride in producing top-quality 'traditional' sausages, which many people consider to be much more wholesome than the typical product. These companies adhere to a rigid code. No fat or mechanically recovered meat is allowed; the meat is organically farmed – which means that it comes from animals which have not been given growth hormones – and the meat content of the sausage is maintained at a minimum of 80 per cent. No artificial colourings, preservatives or flavourings are added.

SALT AND SALAMI

The famous Italian salami is a particularly unhealthy sausage because it contains dramatically high levels of both sodium and fat, compared with other sausages. Although salami is not usually eaten in such large quantities as other sausages, only 50g (1¾oz) provides nearly half the 6g daily intake of salt recommended by the World Health Organisation.

Salamis, as well as frankfurters and other smoked sausages, usually contain a substance called tyramine which has been known to cause an allergic reaction in susceptible people. Anyone with a medical condition that demands a low-fat, low-salt diet should try to avoid salami and only occasionally eat most other sausages.

VEGETARIAN SAUSAGES

Vegetarian sausages tend to have fewer calories than meat sausages but they usually contain only slightly less fat. Unlike meat sausages, however, most of their fat content does not come from saturated fats and they generally contain a lot less sodium.

Vegetarian sausages usually contain vegetable proteins, vegetable oil and grains with spices and flavourings. They also provide much more fibre than their meat equivalents, but they generally do not supply iron, zinc and vitamin B_{12} in the same amounts as meat sausages. The vegetable proteins which are used in vegetarian sausages can include soya beans or peanuts and so they should be avoided by people who have allergies to these foods.

The nourishment found in sausages (100g, 3½oz)

SAUSAGE	CALORIES	PROTEIN (g)	FAT (g)	CARBOHYDRATE (g)	FIBRE (g)	VITAMINS	SODIUM (mg)
Frankfurter	274	9.5	25.0	3.0	0.1	3.0mg niacin 1.0mcg vit B_{12}	980
Salami	491	19.3	45.2	1.9	0.1	8.2mg niacin 1mcg vit B_{12}	1850
Beef sausages (fried)	269	12.9	18.0	14.9	0.7	9.7mg niacin 1mcg vit B_{12}	1090
Pork sausages (fried)	317	13.8	24.5	11.0	0.7	7.3mg niacin 1mcg vit B_{12}	1050
Low-fat pork sausages (fried)	211	14.9	13.0	9.1	1.4	5.0mg niacin 1mcg vit B_{12}	950
Vegetarian sausages	219	17.0	15.0	4.0	5.0	1.2mg vit B_1 285mcg vit A	700
Ready-made, textured vegetable protein sausages	219	14.1	13.8	9.2	1.7	1.6mg vit E 90mcg folate	700

Schizophrenia

EAT PLENTY OF
- *Fresh fruit and vegetables*
- *Dark green leafy vegetables, dried fruits and nuts*

CUT DOWN ON
- *Caffeine in tea, coffee and colas*

AVOID
- *Alcohol, which often reacts dangerously with medication*
- *Foods to which you may be allergic*

Half a million people suffer from schizophrenia in Britain. Personality changes, delusions, hallucinations and paranoia are classic symptoms of the illness, a susceptibility to which may be genetically inherited. People with this debilitating psychiatric illness may also suffer from eating and sleep disorders as well as deep depression.

The onset of schizophrenia most commonly occurs in adolescence or early adulthood; and while correct medication is of vital importance, careful attention to diet can also help.

Schizophrenics often suffer from low BLOOD SUGAR LEVELS or HYPOGLYCAEMIA. To combat this, the diet should contain plenty of fresh fruit and vegetables and regular snacks of foods containing carbohydrates. Depending on the type of medication, drug treatment may necessitate the use of vitamin and mineral supplements.

Some people who develop schizophrenia are found to have had learning difficulties or to have been hyperactive as children and it is possible that some of their problems may be caused by allergies. Certainly, both gluten-free and milk-free diets have been claimed to improve the symptoms of some chronic schizophrenics. Cutting out milk, however, can reduce calcium intake. When adopting a milk-free diet it is important to compensate by eating plenty of calcium-rich foods, such as dark green vegetables, dried fruit and nuts and tinned sardines – complete with bones. Also, cut down on caffeine (found in coffee, tea, colas and chocolate) which increases excretion of calcium through the kidneys. Wheat and other foods which contain gluten can be replaced with potato products and grains such as corn, millet and rice. Avoid alcohol as it often reacts dangerously with medication.

Schizophrenics rarely exhibit symptoms continuously and most have periods of apparent normality. This has led some researchers to suspect that the psychiatric symptoms might be produced by the abnormal metabolism of some commonly eaten foods, which affects the body chemistry of the whole body, including the brain.

Although it must be stressed that schizophrenia cannot be controlled by diet alone, a healthy diet which supplies all the essential nutrients and cuts out any known or possible allergens, combined with an appropriate drug regime, should offer real relief.

Seaweed

BENEFITS
- *Most types of seaweed are an excellent source of iodine*
- *Provides a wide range of minerals including calcium, copper, iron, magnesium, potassium and zinc*
- *Contains varying amounts of B vitamins and beta carotene*

DRAWBACK
- *Some seaweeds are high in sodium*

The Japanese have been harvesting vegetables from the ocean for centuries. They eat seaweed in sufficiently large amounts to benefit from its concentrated mineral content; as much as a quarter of all food in the Japanese diet contains some variety of seaweed, used to enhance the flavour of salads, soups and savoury dishes.

Sea vegetables are also an important ingredient in the MACROBIOTIC DIET. Some seaweed, such as laver, can be gathered from British shores, though do check that the area is not polluted (see COUNTRYSIDE FOODS).

Many seaweeds are an excellent source of iodine, a mineral which is vital for normal functioning of the thyroid gland. The THYROID gland produces hormones that regulate the body's metabolism, and therefore its growth and development. A characteristic sign of iodine deficiency is the swelling of the thyroid gland in the front of the neck, known as goitre.

Other minerals normally found in seaweed include copper and iron for healthy blood; magnesium for the proper functioning of muscles and nerves; calcium for healthy bones; potassium for the maintenance of the

SEASIDE BREAKFAST *The Welsh and Irish make mineral-rich seaweed called laver into flat cakes. They are then fried and traditionally served up with tomatoes and bacon.*

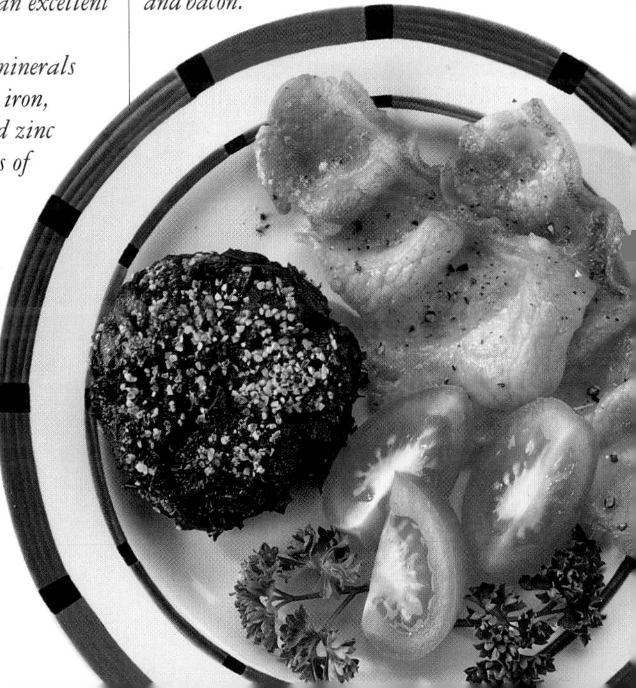

Seaweed seasoning

Dried sheets or strips of seaweed are sold in Japanese grocers and health food stores. They have a naturally salty flavour due to their high mineral content.

The seaweed strips are often crumbled and used as a seasoning to give soups and noodle dishes a fresh sea-water flavour. Dried strips of *nori* are used as edible wrappers for sushi and rice cakes.

body's cells and balance of fluids; and zinc for the body's immune system. Most seaweed contains some B vitamins, and beta carotene – the plant form of vitamin A, but the amount varies according to the type of seaweed and how it is served. Beta carotene is an ANTIOXIDANT and may help to prevent degenerative diseases such as cancer.

Unusually for a plant, seaweed also contains vitamin B_{12}. However, there is some debate as to whether the B_{12} in seaweed is 'biologically active' – in other words, whether it can actually be used by the body.

Seaweeds only seem to have one drawback – their high sodium content; many of them are unsuitable for anyone on a low sodium diet.

In traditional medicine, seaweed has long been used to treat a wide variety of ailments, including constipation, colds, arthritis and rheumatism.

ALGAE SUPPLEMENTS

Kelp tablets are a convenient way to include some seaweed in the diet. Because of their high iodine content, some herbalists prescribe them for mild thyroid disorders.

The freshwater algae supplements spirulina and chlorella are increasingly popular. They contain all the nutrients that you would expect to find in green vegetables, including beta carotene, vitamin C, calcium and iron. They also contain protein and vitamin B_{12}. It is claimed that spirulina is a good source of the essential fatty acid, gamma linolenic acid (GLA). However, claims that these algae can boost the immune system, detoxify the body, promote energy and increase longevity, have not been substantiated.

These algae are either gathered from lakes or cultivated in man-made ponds, then harvested, dried and sold either in powder or tablet form.

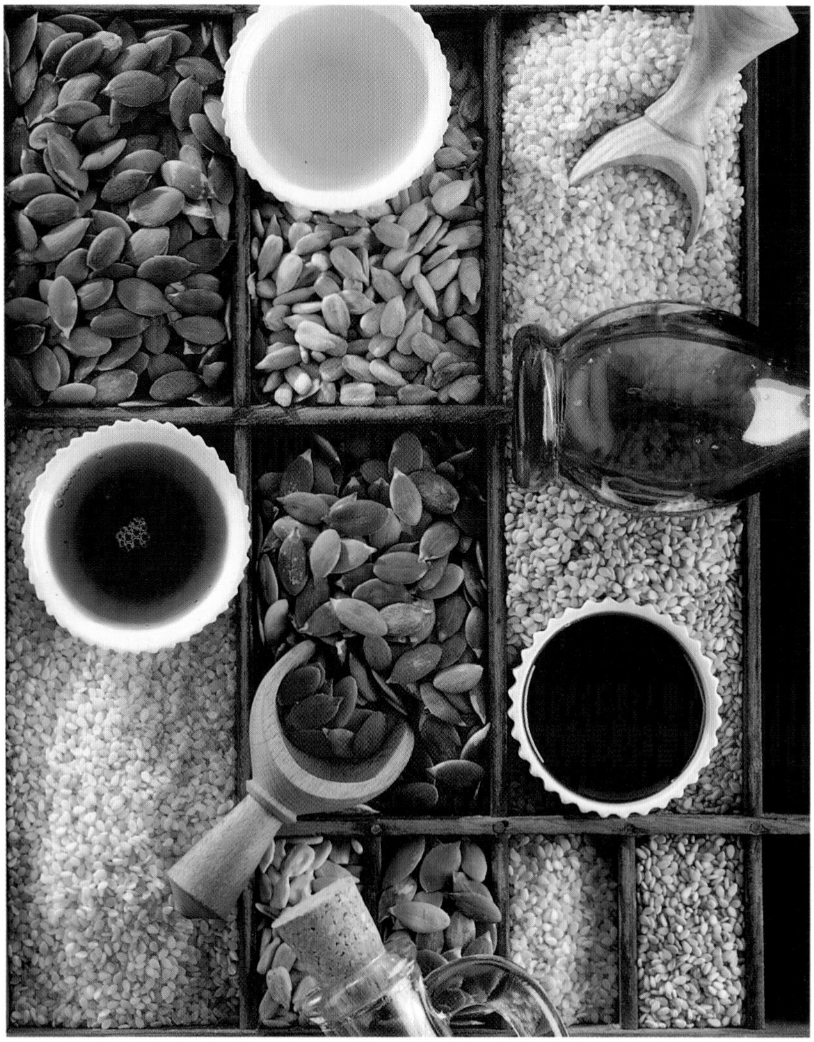

THE SEEDS OF HEALTH *Sprinkled into soups and salads, seeds impart a nutty flavour. Try (clockwise) pumpkin, sunflower, hulled sesame (white) and unhulled sesame seeds.*

SEEDS

BENEFITS
- *Excellent source of protein*
- *Usually a good source of vitamin E and the B vitamins, except for vitamin B_{12}*
- *Good source of fibre*
- *High in unsaturated fats*

DRAWBACK
- *Salted seeds are high in sodium*

Along with nuts, cereals and pulses, seeds contain protein. They are also a good source of vitamin E and the B vitamins, as well as dietary fibre – which is essential for regulating the bowels.

Seeds are high in calories – a tablespoon can contain about 100 Calories. They may help to lower blood cholesterol levels because the fat content (58per cent in sesame seeds and 48per cent in sunflower seeds) is largely unsaturated. However, salted seeds should be eaten in moderation, because they are high in sodium.

Seeds should be roasted or cooked to destroy any unwanted substances that may be present. Cooking destroys protein toxins, such as trypsin inhibitors, which reduce protein digestibility and haemagglutinins which, if they survive the digestive process, can cause diarrhoea and vomiting. Most seeds are bought already cooked and raw seeds are not normally eaten in sufficient quantities to have a harmful effect.

SEEDS FOR SNACKS

Seeds make especially nutritious additions to soups, salads, casseroles and baked foods. The following seeds make healthy snacks.

Pumpkin seeds Contain iron for healthy blood, magnesium for maintaining healthy body cells and zinc for normal growth and development.

Sesame seeds An essential cooking ingredient in the Middle East, where sesame seeds are used to make a sweetmeat called halva and the spread tahini, which is blended with chickpeas to make the dip hummous. Sesame oil adds a nutty flavour to many exotic dishes. Sesame seeds contain vitamin E and calcium.

Sunflower seeds These seeds are a useful source of vitamin E and they are high in linoleic acid (needed for the maintenance of cell membranes). The seeds are used to make sunflower oil and polyunsaturated margarines.

SEMOLINA AND CORNMEAL

BENEFITS
- *Good sources of starch*
- *Cornmeal is suitable for gluten-free diets and is a good source of potassium and a useful source of iron*

DRAWBACK
- *Low in fibre*

The CEREAL products semolina and cornmeal are widely used in Europe, the Americas and Africa, but less so in Britain. Both are good sources of starch and they also provide protein. They can be used as an alternative to potatoes, rice, pasta and bread to add a bit of variety to the diet. For vegetarians, they provide complete protein when they are combined with pulses, vegetables or milk.

SEMOLINA

Produced by milling wheat flour and mainly obtained from durum wheat, semolina is a hard wheat used in baking as well as to make PASTA. The outer coating is removed from the wheat grain, then the largest particles of the remaining portion of the grain are sifted and separated. The resulting grains form coarse semolina which is a useful source of manganese and contains phosphorus, but has little dietary fibre.

In Britain this coarse semolina is mainly used in desserts. In the United States, it is popular as a hot breakfast cereal, but in Italy it is used in savoury and sweet cooking. Coarse semolina, mixed with water and flour, is used in the North African dish known as couscous.

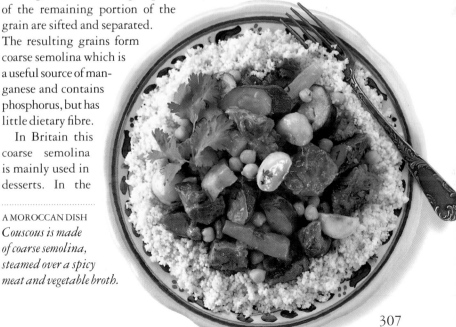

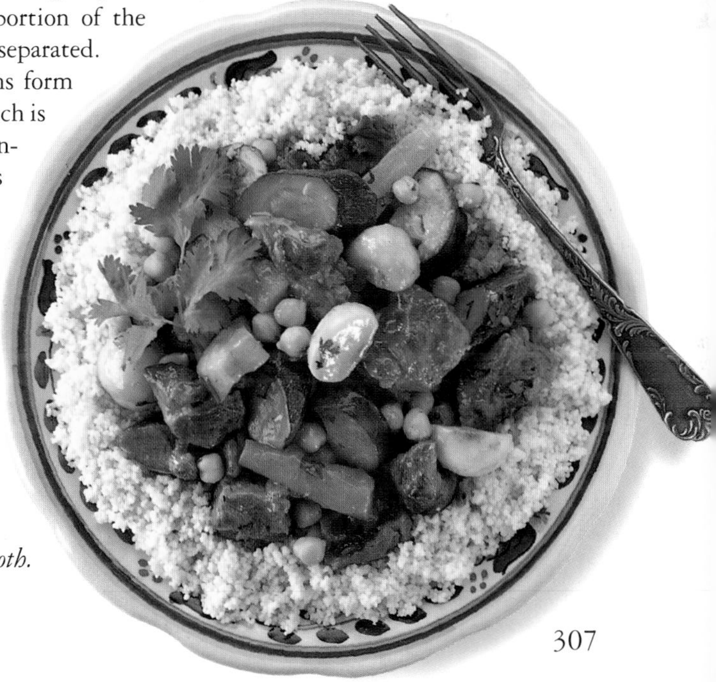

A MOROCCAN DISH
Couscous is made of coarse semolina, steamed over a spicy meat and vegetable broth.

CORNMEAL

When corn (maize) is dried and ground it is known as cornmeal. It is low in fibre, but it is a good source of potassium and a useful source of phosphorus, iron and thiamin. It is also gluten-free so it is suitable for people with COELIAC DISEASE.

Cornmeal can be white or yellow. Coarsely ground cornmeal is used to make porridge-like dishes such as polenta in Italy, hominy grits, breads and muffins in the southern states of America, tortillas and other dishes in Latin America, and mealie meal in Africa. Much of the cornmeal produced is used to make corn syrup and invert sugar, which is widely used in the food industry as a sweetener.

Since cornflour is made from finely ground and pulverised grain, it is useful for thickening sauces and as an ingredient in baking, when it gives biscuits and pastries a light texture.

SHELLFISH: FRUITS OF THE SEA

Shellfish are low in fat but high in protein and many types are excellent sources of other vital nutrients, especially zinc. They may even help to protect against heart disease.

High in protein, vitamins and minerals and low in calories, shellfish make a highly nutritious treat. They can be divided into two groups: molluscs and crustaceans. Most molluscs – clams, oysters, mussels and scallops – have two shells, although some, such as abalone, have a single shell with a soft underside. Crustaceans – shrimps, prawns, crabs, lobsters and crayfish – have segmented bodies armoured with sections of shell.

Shellfish are compact storehouses of vital nutrients. Most supply abundant vitamin B_{12}, necessary for the formation of red blood cells and maintaining a healthy nervous system, and zinc, which is important for the production of proteins, wound healing and the development of reproductive organs.

Various shellfish contain a host of other vitamins and minerals to a greater or lesser degree, including vitamins B_1, B_2 and niacin, selenium, calcium, magnesium and iodine. (See the nutrient chart on page 311.)

COLCHESTER OYSTERS

Colchester has been famous for its oysters ever since Roman times. The discovery of the distinctive River Colne oyster shells among Roman ruins suggests that the ancient invaders must have been so fond of them that they shipped them home. And it is claimed that the Roman historian Pliny once said 'The only good thing about England is its oysters'.

The town holds a yearly oyster feast every October. Some claim the feast dates from 1845 when the mayor, Henry Wolton, invited 200 guests to a luncheon where oysters were served. But others believe the feast to be a revival of celebrations dating from the 11th century that occurred around the same time of year.

SELENIUM IN SHELLFISH

Shellfish are good sources of the trace mineral selenium. This essential mineral, present in the body in minute amounts, works with vitamin E in the promotion of normal body growth and fertility. As an ANTIOXIDANT it is believed to play a role in the fight against cancer and helps to offset the effects of oxidised fats which can contribute to the growth of tumours.

Research has shown that selenium is protective against toxic metals such as mercury and cadmium: it is able to bind with their compounds which are then excreted from the system. Of all the shellfish, lobster is the richest in selenium; cockles, mussels, scallops and shrimps are also good sources.

CHOLESTEROL CONTENT

Until recently, seafood was thought to aggravate the problem of high cholesterol levels in the blood – increasing the risk of coronary heart disease. It is true that shrimps, prawns and crayfish are high in dietary cholesterol, as is squid (although curiously octopus is not), but they are very low in fat, and the cholesterol is poorly absorbed from these foods. Moreover, several studies have shown that eating shellfish tends to lower, not raise, blood cholesterol levels. In a three-week experiment at Washington University, a group of men were asked to substitute shellfish for their usual protein foods. Oyster, clam, crab and mussel diets were seen to reduce the blood levels of one particularly dangerous type of blood fat, and also appeared to lower total blood cholesterol levels. In this study, the squid and shrimp diets did not reduce blood fats in the same way.

Shellfish, in common with oily fish, contain small amounts of essential fatty acids (EFAs), which may help to protect against heart and circulation

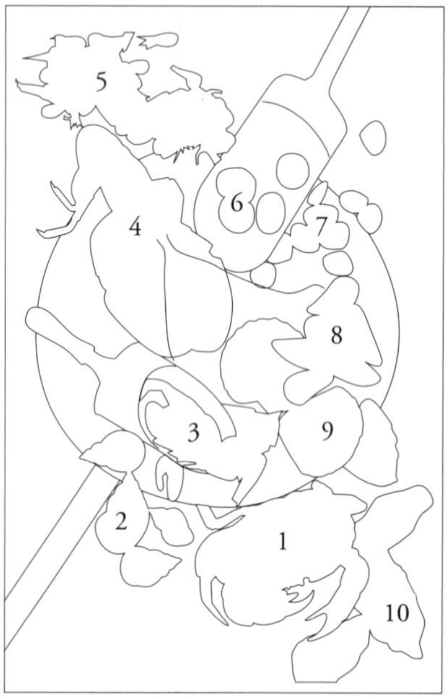

SEAFOOD PLATTER *Choose from a tasty selection of nutritious, low-calorie shellfish including: crab (1), whelks (2), prawns (3), lobster (4), shrimps (5), Amande clams (6), Venus clams (7), mussels (8), scallops (9) and oysters (10).*

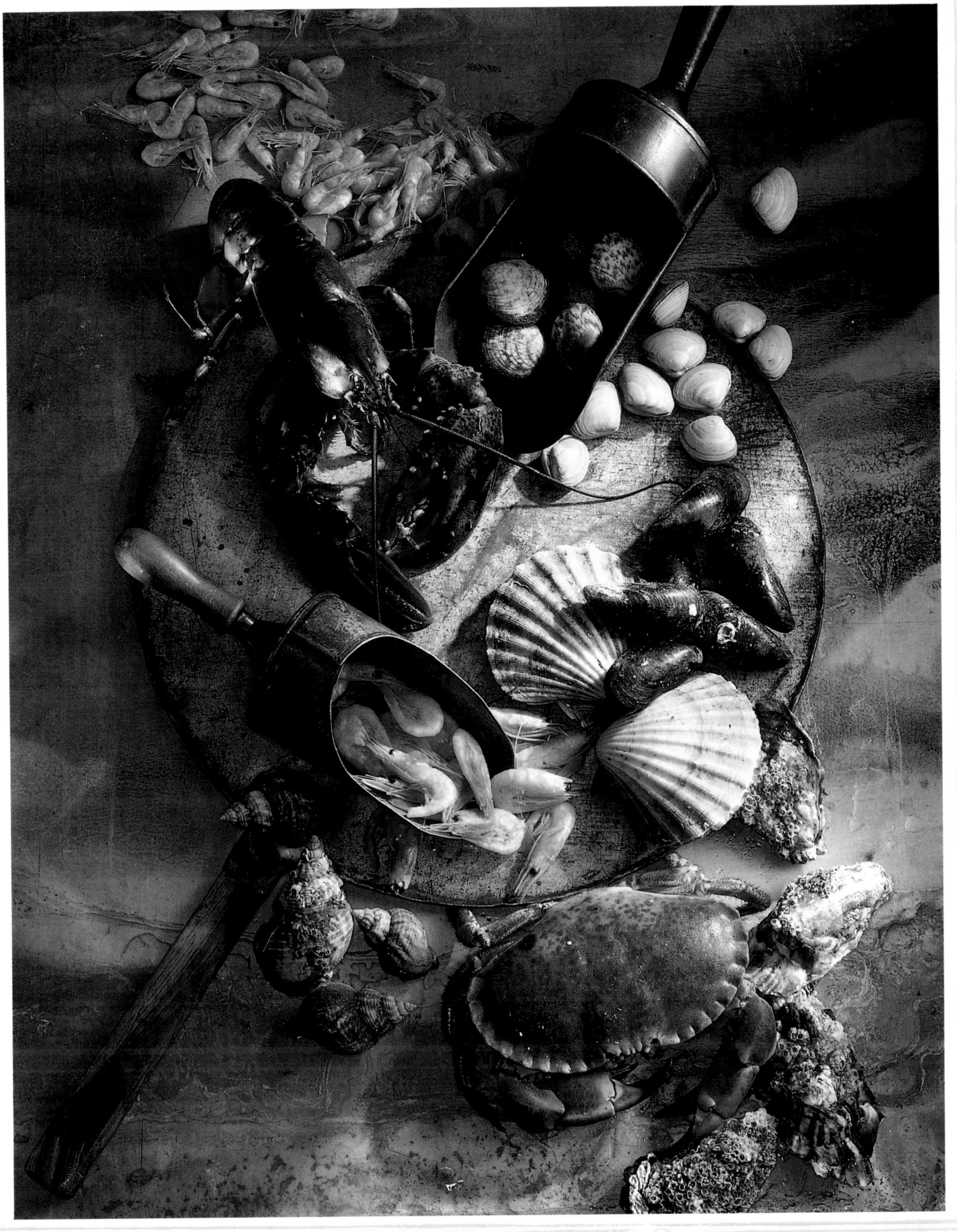

DOS AND DON'TS TO PREVENT FOOD POISONING

• Do buy shellfish from a reliable source. Scrub shells thoroughly in clean water before use.

• Do try to eat shellfish on the day of purchase.

• Do check that mussels, clams, oysters and cockles are closed tightly before cooking. Tap any open shells with a knife and if they do not close discard them. After cooking all shells should be open: discard any that remain closed.

• Do check that scallops have firm, creamy white, slightly translucent flesh with no brown markings, when you buy them. They should also have a bright orange 'coral' and a pleasant sea smell.

• Do shake a crab before purchase – it should not contain water.

• Do touch the flesh of abalone when buying it fresh – it should still move.

• Don't collect and eat your own mussels from the beach – unless you are sure that they are free from sewage pollution. Harvested mussels should be soaked in salted water to purge them of sand and grit. Use two teaspoons of salt to 4.5 litres (1 gallon) of water for about an hour – no longer. Just one or two bad mussels could infect the whole batch if left soaking together in water for too long.

• Don't buy cooked lobster if it smells 'fishy'. It should smell clean and the tail should spring back when opened out if it is fresh.

• Don't eat the green 'tomally' in lobsters or the yellow 'mustard' in crabs. They may be considered by some to be delicacies, but these organs (the livers) filter toxins and, rarely, could contain poisons.

problems. EFAs are also important for the upkeep of healthy cell membranes in the brain and the retina of the eye.

BACTERIAL HAZARD

All shellfish are highly perishable and prone to bacterial contamination. They are best eaten on the day of capture, but if this is not possible they should be kept alive until they are about to be cooked. If you have to store them, keep them at 0-5°C (32-41°F) and eat within a day or two. If you home-freeze shellfish at the peak of freshness in a domestic freezer (not the icebox of a fridge), they can be stored for up to two months.

Molluscs, such as clams and oysters, are filter feeders and will each filter as many as 90 litres (20 gallons) of water a day. So if there is any pollution in the water, it is likely to be in the shellfish too – and in a concentrated form, for they are 'biomagnifiers', concentrating heavy metals and bacteria from the water in their tissues as it passes through. If possible, check where your shellfish have come from: the safest are shellfish that have been commercially farmed in clean waters. Never take home shellfish such as mussels from the beach unless you are absolutely sure that they are safe to collect.

SHELLFISH SETBACKS

Shellfish are more likely than other types of fish or meat to trigger allergic reactions, and can produce a variety of responses in susceptible people. They may, for instance, provoke the skin condition urticaria (nettle rash or hives) in some people.

Anyone who suffers from gout should refrain from eating large quantities of shellfish because they contain chemicals called purines which can raise the level of uric acid in the bloodstream and hence aggravate the condition. Shellfish are often boiled in salted water and so tend to be high in sodium. They should, therefore, be eaten only in moderation by people with high blood pressure or by those who are following a low-sodium diet.

THE FOOD OF LOVE?

Aphrodisiac powers have long been attributed to oysters. Their reputation is probably founded on their zinc content. Oysters are the richest source of zinc there is – just one serving (six raw or steamed oysters) provides over five times the recommended daily amount. Zinc is needed for sperm production and is reputed to enhance the libido: Casanova is said to have consumed an average of 40 oysters a day. Certainly, a lack of zinc is known to cause infertility and impotence. Too much zinc, however, can produce a toxic effect.

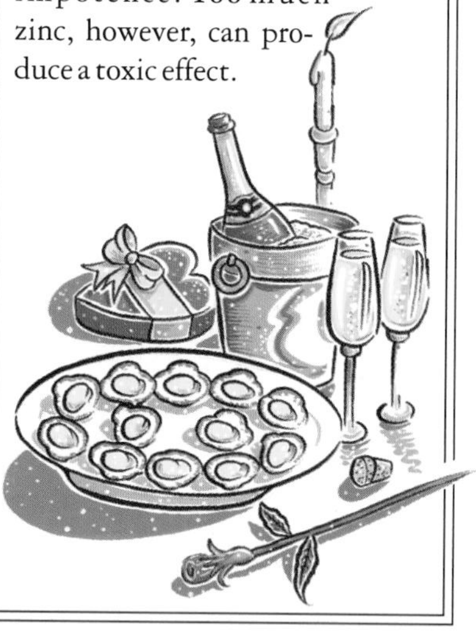

WHEN TO EAT OYSTERS

In Britain, it is illegal to harvest native oysters during the summer when they are spawning – hence the traditional saying that you should only eat them when there is an R in the month. These days, however, it is the Pacific oyster which is commercially farmed in the UK, which is unable to spawn in cold British waters. Consequently, oysters can now be enjoyed all the year round.

The important nutrients found in different shellfish

Low in saturated fat and high in protein, shellfish have many of the qualities health-conscious people are looking for; they are rich in B vitamins and are useful sources of trace minerals. However, they are prone to bacterial contamination and so extra care should be taken when buying, preparing and cooking shellfish. All values are for 100g (3½oz) of shellfish.

SHELLFISH	PROTEIN(g)	FAT(g)	SODIUM(mg)	VITAMINS	MINERALS
Oysters (raw)	10.8	1.3	510	Excellent source of vitamin B_{12}. Useful source of vitamin E and niacin. Contain thiamin and riboflavin.	Excellent source of zinc and copper. Good source of iron and potassium. Useful source of selenium and iodine.
Mussels (boiled)	16.7	2.7	360	Excellent source of vitamin B_{12}. Useful source of vitamin E and riboflavin. Contain folate.	Rich source of iron and iodine. Good source of selenium.
Scallops (steamed)	23.2	1.4	180	Excellent source of vitamin B_{12}, useful source of niacin.	Rich source of selenium. Good source of potassium. Useful source of zinc.
Clams (canned)	16.0	0.6	1200	Excellent source of vitamin B_{12}.	Excellent source of iron. Useful source of zinc.
Shrimps (boiled)	23.8	2.4	3840	Excellent source of vitamin B_{12}, useful source of niacin.	Rich source of iodine. Good source of selenium. Useful source of calcium.
Prawns (boiled)	22.6	0.9	1590	Excellent source of vitamin B_{12}.	Useful source of selenium. Contain iodine.
Lobsters (boiled)	22.1	1.6	330	Excellent source of vitamin B_{12}, useful source of niacin.	Excellent source of selenium. Useful source of zinc.
Crayfish (raw)	14.9	0.8	150	Excellent source of vitamin B_{12}. Contain folate and niacin.	Excellent source of selenium. Rich source of iodine.
Abalone (canned)	24.8	2.0	990	Useful source of niacin.	Excellent source of iron.
Crabs (boiled)	19.5	5.5	420	Good source of riboflavin. Useful source of pantothenic acid. Contain vitamin B_6.	Good source of potassium and zinc. Contain magnesium.
Cockles (boiled)	12.0	0.6	490	Excellent source of vitamin B_{12}.	Excellent source of iron and iodine. Rich source of selenium.
Whelks (boiled)	19.5	1.2	280	Excellent source of vitamin B_{12}. Contain vitamin E.	Excellent source of zinc and copper. Useful source of iron.
Cuttlefish (raw)	16.1	0.7	370	Excellent source of vitamin B_{12}. Useful source of vitamin B_6 and niacin.	Rich source of selenium. Useful source of iron.
Octopus (raw)	17.9	1.3	120	Useful source of vitamin B_6 and niacin.	Excellent source of selenium.
Squid (raw)	15.4	1.7	110	Excellent source of vitamin B_{12}. Good source of vitamin B_6. Useful source of vitamin E.	Excellent source of selenium. Contain iodine.

SEX DRIVE

EAT PLENTY OF
- *Oysters and other zinc-rich foods*

CUT DOWN ON
- *Caffeine and nicotine*
- *Alcohol*

There is a wide variation in the sex drive of individuals. People who are concerned about having a low sex drive should take steps to reduce stress, take some form of regular exercise and ensure that their diet is well balanced and provides all the vitamins, minerals and nutrients that they need (see BALANCING YOUR DIET).

Some nutrients may be particularly important. For example, zinc is needed for sperm production and is also essential for the development of the reproductive organs. A lack of zinc can cause infertility and impotence. Weight for weight, oysters contain more zinc than any other food – so perhaps their reputation in folklore as an aphrodisiac is based on truth. Crab, offal and pumpkin seeds are other good sources.

DRINKING AND SMOKING

Alcohol and nicotine are known to suppress the sex drive of people who smoke or drink heavily. The hops in beer may also play a part in reducing the libido of excessive beer drinkers. Constituents in hops are used in herbal medicine to lower the sex drive of men, but they can accentuate depression too.

Smoking also increases the risk of atherosclerosis (hardening of the arteries), and atherosclerosis of the penile artery is a common cause of IMPOTENCE in older men. The risk can be reduced if you stop smoking and include plenty of ANTIOXIDANTS in your diet.

Caffeine, found in coffee, tea and chocolate, can also reduce sex drive, though its effect depends very much on the individual. High cholesterol levels, high blood pressure and various drugs can also play a part in suppressing people's libidos.

APHRODISIAC MYTHS?

There is no scientific evidence that aphrodisiacs, such as powdered rhino horn and Spanish fly, increase sex drive. Both substances irritate the urethra, and the resulting burning sensation may be behind the myth. The claims made about Siberian ginseng restoring sex drive are much more credible.

Many people believe that a menu of eggs, broccoli and wheatgerm – all rich in vitamin E – will help to maintain a healthy sex drive, but there is no scientific evidence for this.

SEXUALLY TRANSMITTED DISEASES

TAKE PLENTY OF
- *Whole grains, fresh fruit and vegetables*
- *Lean meat, nuts and pulses*
- *Water and fruit juices*

CUT DOWN ON
- *Caffeine in tea, coffee and colas*

Anybody who has been at risk of contracting a sexually transmitted disease (STD) and shows any symptoms should seek the advice of a genito-urinary clinic as a matter of urgency and abstain from sexual activity until given a clean bill of health. Venereal diseases are usually treated with antibiotics. But as well as having the appropriate medical treatment, an infected person should adopt a balanced and nutritious diet, with plenty of whole grains, fresh fruit and vegetables, moderate amounts of lean meat, fish, poultry, nuts and pulses, and a little unsaturated fat. Try to cut down on caffeine (found in tea, coffee and cola drinks), to drink plenty of water and fruit juice, and to get plenty of rest. All these measures will help the immune system to fight the infection.

Since the discovery of antibiotics, most STDs – including gonorrhoea, chlamydia and NSU (non-specific urethritis) – have been treatable, and syphilis is no longer the killer it once was. Genital HERPES cannot be cured, but locally applied creams, along with the general advice regarding diet and rest given here, can help to lessen the severity and frequency of attacks.

It must be remembered that any symptoms – such as sores (painless or otherwise), rashes, unusual discharges, a burning sensation or bleeding upon urination – should never be ignored and may not respond to home remedies. Always seek medical advice as soon as possible. (See also AIDS.)

SHELLFISH

See page 308

SHINGLES

TAKE PLENTY OF
- *Citrus fruits, apricots, cherries, tomatoes and papaya, for vitamin C and bioflavonoids*
- *Safflower oil, olive oil, nuts, unsalted peanut butter and avocados, for vitamin E*

The virus that causes CHICKENPOX is also responsible for a painful condition known as shingles – the medical term for which is HERPES zoster. Following an attack of CHICKENPOX, some of the virus particles survive and lie dormant for many years in nerve tissue. Then, if the immune system is suppressed – perhaps after a long period of stress or medication with steroid drugs – the virus replicates and migrates along the nerve where it causes a sharp burning sensation and blisters on the skin. Shingles can occur in childhood, but is more common in later life – elderly people are the most susceptible.

An attack typically starts with extreme sensitivity and a burning sensation in the area of skin about to be affected. It most commonly strikes around the shoulder and waist, on one side of the face and one eye, and sometimes down the arm and across the front of the chest. If the virus affects an eye it can cause permanent damage by scarring the cornea.

The severity of an attack may be greatly diminished if an appropriate drug, such as acyclovir or famcyclovir, is taken at the onset of symptoms. In addition, eating a nutritious diet at the earliest signs of shingles can help to reduce the risk of post-herpetic neuralgia, a long-term side effect (where the patient continues to experience pains). Recently, doctors have begun to prescribe a cream made with extract of chilli seeds to minimise it.

Eat plenty of citrus fruit, apricots, cherries, tomatoes and papaya for vitamin C and bioflavonoids, as well as safflower oil, nuts, olive oil and avocados for vitamin E. All these foods contain ANTIOXIDANTS, which may help to prevent inflammation.

SINUSITIS

EAT PLENTY OF

- *Fresh fruit and vegetables for vitamin C and bioflavonoids*
- *Shellfish and nuts for zinc*
- *Whole grains and pulses for B vitamins*
- *Sunflower seeds, seed oils and avocados for vitamin E*
- *Garlic and onions*
- *Decongestant herbs and spices such as elderflower, thyme and ginger*

Case study

Maria was an excellent secretary, but at her annual performance review her manager told her that her habit of constantly blowing her nose and sounding as if she had a cold was distracting other staff. For some years she had suffered from persistent congestion of her nose and a watery discharge. She consulted her doctor, but there was no obvious cause for her chronic sinusitis. The doctor suggested that dairy products may be the cause. At first Maria was sure that there was no connection, but over the next few days she experimented by excluding cheese, butter, yoghurt and milk from her diet. To her surprise, her symptoms began to disappear.

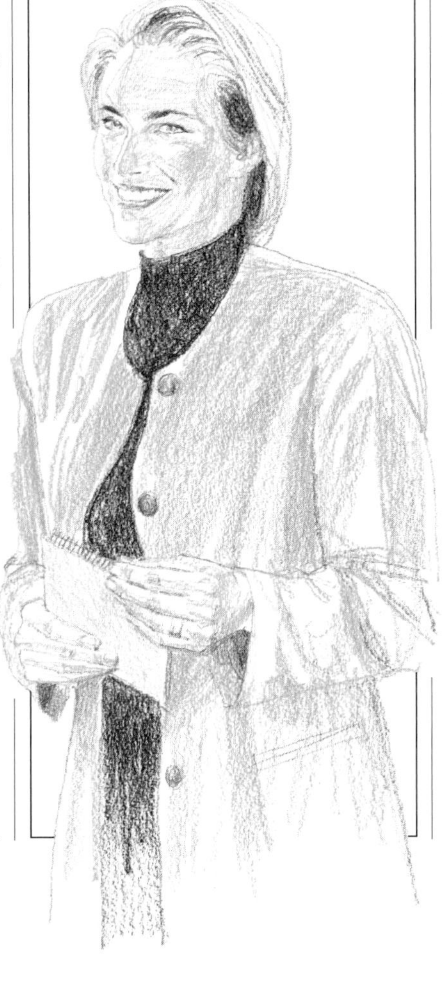

Sinuses are air-filled cavities in the bones surrounding the eyes and nose. Normally, mucus produced by the membrane that lines the nasal sinuses drains into the nasal cavity along narrow passages. However, when you are suffering from a cold or have an abscess in an upper tooth, the infection is able to travel down the passages and spread to the sinuses. The membrane lining the sinuses swells and blocks the passages which then prevent the mucus from draining. The mucus becomes infected, resulting in a stuffed up feeling and an aching face.

Because acute sinusitis is usually the result of an infection such as tonsillitis, a diet that supplies plenty of vitamins and minerals to reinforce your body's defence system can aid recovery and help to prevent further attacks. Chronic sinusitis may be the result of infection or an allergy to particular foods, such as dairy products, cereals or even soya products, causing the mucous membranes to swell. Hay fever, exposure to fumes, smoking and nasal injury can also lead to sinus problems. Always get a proper diagnosis from your doctor.

Eat plenty of whole grains, pulses and nuts for B vitamins which help to maintain a healthy immune system, and fresh fruit and vegetables to ensure a good intake of vitamin C. Citrus fruits (rather than just the juice), grapes and blackberries are particularly useful because they also contain bioflavonoids, which act with vitamin C to keep the blood capillaries healthy. Bioflavonoids also have anti-inflammatory properties.

Vitamin E, which is found in nuts, sunflower seeds, seed oils and avocados, also supports the immune system.

Eating natural decongestants may be helpful. They include raw or cooked onions and garlic, and herbs and spices such as ginger, thyme, elderflower, horseradish, cloves and cinnamon.

SLEEP AND YOUR DIET

In a world full of pressures, sleep is an antidote to daytime cares. Diet can play an important role in getting a good night's sleep, providing a chance to rest the mind and repair the body.

Most people put up with the occasional bad night's sleep without noticing any ill-effects, but if poor sleep goes on for several weeks you may start to worry about whether it is having an adverse effect on your health. The anxiety over being unable to sleep can make you even more prone to insomnia, so you become caught up in a vicious circle.

Scientists still do not fully understand what makes us sleep, but certain 'sleep centres' have been found in the brain which are thought to act as a sort of 'body clock' controlling the timing of rest and wakefulness. Some natural chemicals in the body promote sleep, and diet also plays a part. Consuming large quantities of coffee, tea and cola drinks, or a bar of plain chocolate after supper, supplies the brain with CAFFEINE which can keep you awake. However, some people who drink a lot of coffee develop a tolerance to caffeine and have no problems going to sleep.

CAUSES OF INSOMNIA

Insomnia is one of the many symptoms of ANXIETY, DEPRESSION and STRESS. Overcoming the root cause of anxiety is obviously essential to improving sleeping habits, but proper nutrition can help as well. OBESITY can interfere with sleep because it adversely affects breathing, increases the likelihood of disruptive snoring and may lead to a disorder called sleep apnoea, in which someone stops breathing when asleep – sometimes for as long as 90 seconds. Losing weight can often put an end to obstructive sleep apnoea (see DIETS AND SLIMMING).

Another condition that can interfere with sleep is RESTLESS LEGS, when there are intermittent involuntary leg movements, particularly when lying in bed. Many naturopaths consider that the most common cause of this is iron deficiency, and recommend iron-rich foods such as pulses, dried apricots, dark green leafy vegetables and nuts (especially almonds).

FOOD AND DRINK FOR SLEEP

Never go to bed hungry, and never go to bed on an over-full stomach. Too little food – and that gnawing pang in the pit of your stomach will make sure that you have a restless night; too much – and you may find yourself

TAKE PLENTY OF
- *Sweetened milky malted bedtime drinks, camomile tea or other hot drinks with honey*
- *Starchy foods such as pasta, rice and potatoes in the evening meal*

CUT DOWN ON
- *Caffeine, found in coffee, tea, cola drinks and chocolate*

AVOID
- *Late-night meals that are greasy, spicy, rich or heavy*

Dos and don'ts of insomnia

Do keep your worries and problems out of your bedroom. Entering it should not make you think of the bills you have not paid or the work you need to do the next day.

Do make the hours before going to bed as relaxing as possible to keep your mind off the day's problems. Take a warm bath, listen to some soothing music or read a book.

Do make a list of your worries if they are keeping you awake, so you can deal with them at another time. But don't leave the list by your bedside.

Do relax in bed. For example, imagine doing something peaceful, such as sunbathing on a deserted beach. Try to relax all the muscles in your body; start with your forehead and jaw, and work down to your feet.

Do get up at your normal time.

Don't nap during the day.

Don't smoke or drink excessive amounts of alcohol or stimulants such as tea and coffee too soon before going to bed.

Don't eat a rich or heavy meal less than 3 hours before bedtime.

Don't over-stimulate your mind near bedtime, for example, by doing a difficult crossword or having an intense discussion.

Don't exercise late at night. Evening workouts can keep you awake.

Don't keep looking at the clock at the side of your bed.

Don't lie awake for hours worrying; get up and do something useful but relaxing for 20 minutes or so, until you feel tired again. A snack, such as an oatmeal biscuit or a piece of bread, may help you to get to sleep.

lying awake all night because you are suffering from INDIGESTION, heartburn or FLATULENCE. Rich or spicy meals can also cause these symptoms.

Milk A sweetened milk drink at bedtime helps to encourage better sleep because the sugars in the drink enable the brain cells to absorb more tryptophan (provided by the milk protein) from the blood stream. The brain then converts the tryptophan into a soothing chemical called serotonin.

Starchy foods While a meal that is rich in starch can improve physical endurance, it can also act like a sedative on the brain. This could be due to the effect of starch on blood glucose levels, or possibly because it can also encourage the release of serotonin.

Honey This is a folk remedy that can act as a mild sedative. Stir a little honey in warm milk or camomile tea.

Herbal teas Many herbal teas are claimed to ensure a good night's sleep; camomile, lime blossom and valerian are said to be the most effective.

DO YOU NEED EIGHT HOURS?

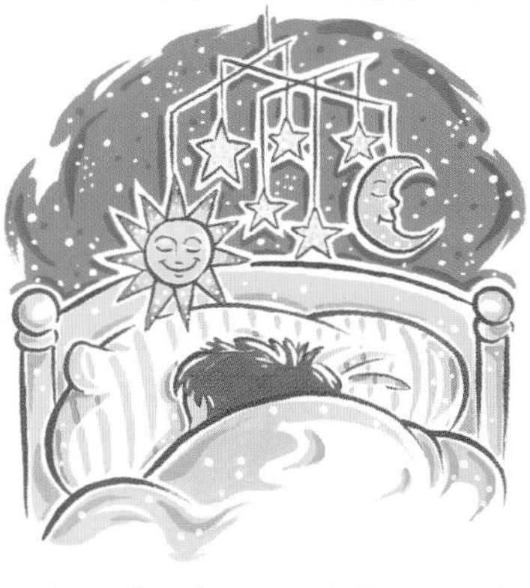

It has often been said that people should get at least eight hours' sleep at night, but individuals tend to need different amounts. Throughout our lives, as well as from day to day, each person's needs are constantly changing. As you age, it becomes normal to sleep less, to take longer to get to sleep, and to wake more during the night. If you get eight hours, but still feel tired, experiment by going to bed earlier for ten days, noting how refreshed you feel during the day, and how you cope with difficult tasks. A little extra sleep may be all you need to feel revitalised.

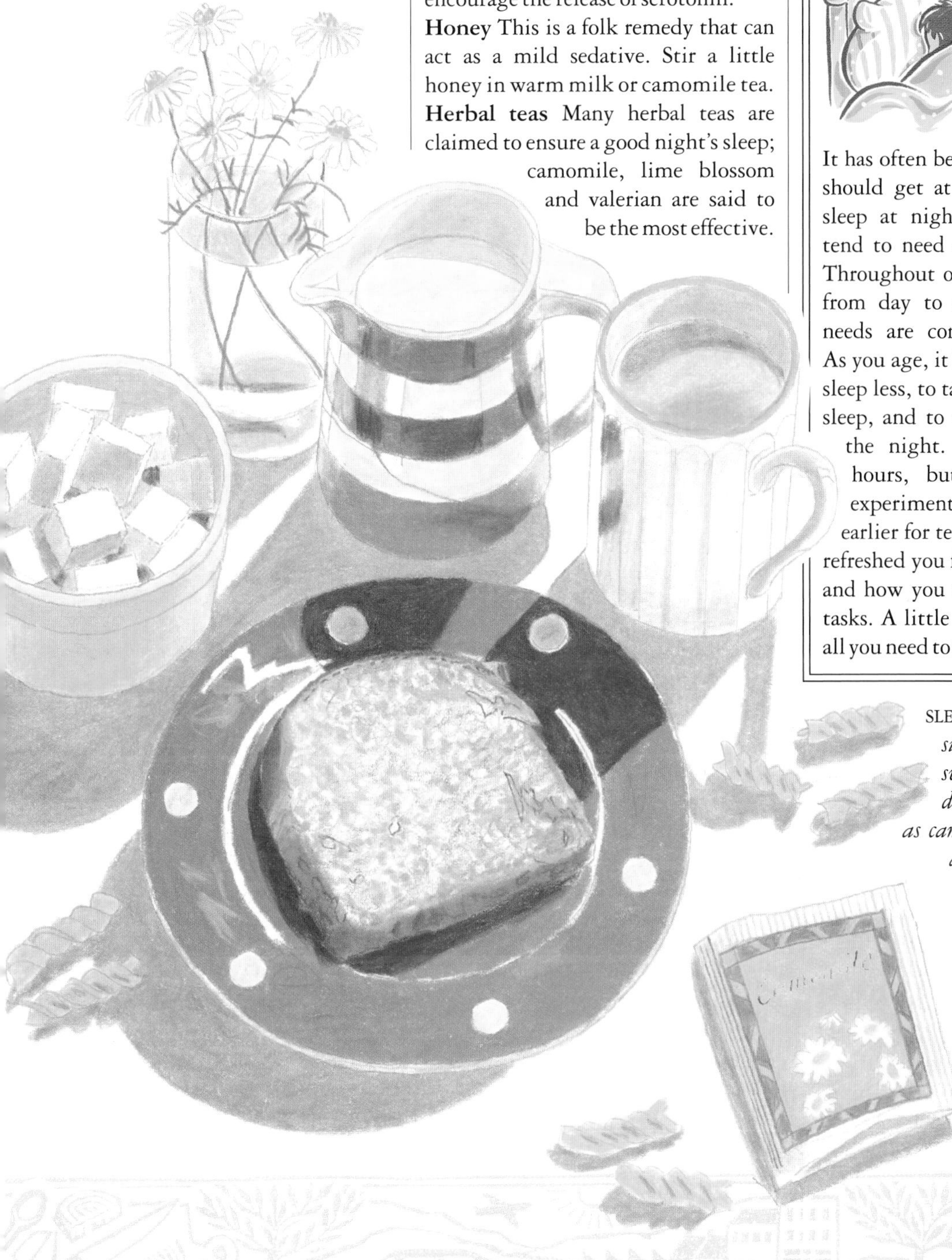

SLEEP WELL *Starchy foods such as bread and pasta, sweetened milky malted drinks, herbal teas such as camomile, and honey can all help to promote sleep.*

SMOKED, CURED AND PICKLED FOOD

For thousands of years food has been smoked, cured and pickled as a means of preserving it. Modern technology has made most of the traditional preserving methods redundant, but they survive because people still enjoy the strong flavours they create.

SMOKING

The distinctive flavour of smoked food comes from chemicals found in the smoke, combined with the effects of slow, very low-temperature 'cooking' and drying. Many foods are smoked, including fish, meat and cheese. The smoky taste is so popular that it is sometimes added artificially to crisps.

Smoke is made up of hundreds of chemicals, its composition depending on the substance being burned and the extent of combustion. It contains aldehydes, ketones, carboxyl acids and phenols. Some of these compounds are toxic to bacteria, some slow down fat oxidation and prevent rancidity, while others impart the flavour of burning wood to the food. Different woods, such as hickory, juniper, apple or oak, produce distinctive flavours.

Some of the substances in smoke are known to be harmful: carcinogenic agents are often present, including tars from a group of complex molecules known as polycyclic aromatic hydrocarbons (PAHs). However, unless large amounts are eaten regularly, the risks associated with eating smoked or barbecued foods are much lower than those associated with being exposed to tobacco smoke.

CURING

Smoking is often carried out in combination with salt curing – another effective method of food preservation – but the vast majority of foods that have been cured are high in sodium. Bacon is a typical example: 100g (3½oz) of back bacon contains 2g of sodium (the equivalent of 5g, or one teaspoon, of salt). Since most nutritionists agree that a high level of salt in the diet is detrimental to health, it is best not to eat bacon or similar cured and smoked products every day.

Smoking salmon

First salmon is cured by soaking it in a strong brine solution for up to 24 hours; the fillets are then rubbed all over with salt, stacked in boxes and pressed. After another short soaking in brine, the fillets are cold smoked, traditionally using smoke from oak chippings, and then finished off with a slightly warmer smoke to bring the natural oils to the surface.

The salts used in curing are sodium chloride (table salt), which dries out bacteria through dehydration, plus nitrates and nitrites. Nitrates and nitrites react with the pigment present in meats to produce an attractive pink colour when the meats are cooked. They also dramatically reduce the risk of food poisoning by inhibiting the growth of *Clostridium botulinum*, the bacterium responsible for botulism, which is sometimes lethal. Although the toxins produced by these bacteria can be destroyed by cooking, they are a major hazard if they are produced in meats that have been cooked and are then eaten without further heating (cold, boiled ham being an example). The addition of nitrates or nitrites can therefore be of vital importance.

There are strict government guidelines to control the levels of nitrates and nitrites added to food. This is necessary because nitrites can react with foods to form substances known as nitrosamines, which have been shown in tests with laboratory animals to have carcinogenic properties. However, there is no evidence to suggest that, at the levels which are allowed in foods, nitrites are harmful to humans.

THE EFFECTS OF DYEING

Many fish products are dyed before they are smoked. These include cod's roe (dyed pink), cod fillets, haddock and whiting (dyed yellow) and kippers (dyed brown). Azo dyes are often used and some of these, notably tartrazine and sunset yellow, may provoke an allergic response in some people; they are also believed to promote hyperactivity in some children. The addition of dyes is monitored and controlled by law. Tartrazine and sunset yellow may only be added up to a maximum of 100mg per kilogram of fish, although even this is enough to spark asthma in susceptible people.

It is better to buy undyed smoked fish. Natural smoked haddock is a creamy golden hue, as opposed to bright yellow and kippers are a delicate creamy beige before colouring is added. Undyed taramasalata is pale beige rather than pink.

PICKLING

The process of pickling began as a way of preserving fruit and vegetables through the winter months. The food to be pickled is usually placed in sterile containers and immersed in hot or cold vinegar then the containers are sealed. Vinegar discourages the growth of harmful microbes and gives the food a tangy flavour. PICKLES often improve with age and, as long as the container stays sealed, can be stored for years.

Many nutrients are lost in the pickling process, although some vitamin C is retained. Common pickled foods include onions, gherkins, walnuts and beetroot. People who are sensitive to moulds or yeasts should avoid pickles.

SMOKING AND DIET

EAT PLENTY OF

- *Fresh fruit and vegetables for vitamin C and beta carotene*
- *Nuts, seeds and vegetable oils for vitamin E*
- *Whole grains, lean meat and offal for B vitamins*
- *Starchy foods, such as bread, pasta and potatoes*

CUT DOWN ON

- *Saturated fats*
- *Salt*
- *Alcohol*

Cigarette smokers face a greatly increased risk of heart and respiratory disease, of cancer of the lungs, mouth, throat, stomach, pancreas, bladder and rectum as well as a form of leukaemia. About half of all smokers die as a direct result of the habit, while many suffer minor symptoms such as indigestion. The best advice is to give up smoking completely. But for those who still smoke, a change in diet may help to mitigate some of its harmful effects.

LIMITING THE DAMAGE

Stressful living, poor nutrition, high consumption of saturated fats, salt and alcohol all increase a smoker's risks of developing a serious disease. Even with a healthy diet, the most a smoker can do is limit the damage.

There is evidence that smokers have an increased need for vitamin C. One theory is that it is used by the body when fighting the free radicals in smoke and to prevent the formation of nitrosamines – cancer-forming agents made from nitrogen compounds in food. Tests have shown that smokers can have up to 30 per cent less vitamin C in their blood than non-smokers. Since smokers use up vitamin C at a faster rate, they should eat plenty of fresh fruit and vegetables to ensure an adequate intake of the vitamin. The Department of Health recommends that smokers have a daily intake of 40-80mg more vitamin C than the 40mg recommended for non-smokers.

ANTIOXIDANT ANTIDOTES

Vitamins C and E and beta carotene are used by the body as ANTIOXIDANTS to destroy FREE RADICALS found in cigarette smoke. Vitamin E is found in wheatgerm, avocados, vegetable oils, nuts and seeds. Beta carotene is abundant in most fresh fruit and vegetables.

Some studies have found lower levels of beta carotene in the blood of smokers compared with non-smokers. And those smokers with the lowest levels of beta carotene were found to have an increased risk of lung cancer.

Bioflavonoids, found in fruit and vegetables, including grapes, citrus fruits, peppers, tomatoes and broccoli, also have antioxidant properties and so help to neutralise free radicals.

B VITAMIN DEPLETION

Smoking depletes the body of B vitamins due to the increased load it puts on the liver's function of filtering toxins out of the blood. Vitamin B_{12} is used for the detoxification of cyanide which is present in cigarette smoke. The B vitamins can be found in offal, whole grains, lean meat and fish.

Recent research also suggests that a diet high in omega-3 fatty acids, found in oily fish and shellfish, may reduce the risk of lung disease in smokers.

BECOMING A NON-SMOKER

It is almost never too late to give up tobacco, and there is always a health gain. Irritation of the lungs and nasal passages will reduce almost immediately and 10-15 years after giving up smoking an ex-smoker will have the same risk of heart disease as a lifelong non-smoker. However, some damage does tend to persist, such as a predisposition to strokes.

Many smokers worry that they will put on weight if they stop smoking. Nicotine suppresses the appetite and dulls the tastebuds. It also increases the metabolic rate, and when they give up smoking some people find that they put on weight as a result of a decreased metabolic rate. Try to reduce your intake of fatty foods when you first give up smoking and replace them with starchy foods such as pasta and potatoes. Do not allow your smoking habit to be replaced by another addiction. If you crave sugar, it is better to eat fruit rather than sweets.

The weight gain that ex-smokers often suffer can also be caused by the need to keep the mouth and hands busy. Sweets, soft drinks and snacks often take the place of cigarettes. Try to resist fattening foods, try chewing sugar-free gum instead.

A DIET FOR GIVING UP?

The cravings associated with the withdrawal of nicotine might be reduced if the rate of excretion of nicotine through the kidneys is decreased. This can be achieved by increasing the alkalinity of the urine. To do this you need to increase the levels of alkaline foods in your diet while decreasing the amounts of acidic foods.

For a few days, reduce all sources of protein in your diet (especially that from meat, fish, eggs and most cereals), though milk and milk-based products can be taken in moderation because of their high calcium content (calcium has an alkaline effect). At the same time, substantially increase your intake of foods high in potassium and magnesium, which are alkaline (including fruits and vegetables). There is no guarantee that this diet will work for everyone, although some people have found it helpful.

Snacks, Crisps and Dips

Though some manufactured snacks come loaded with fat, there are healthy alternatives. Balanced, nutritious snacks take the guilt out of eating between meals and boost your energy, too.

Most people eat snacks between meals and, in moderation, this should do no harm provided the right kind of snacks are chosen. Unfortunately, the majority of the manufactured snacks on offer do not supply much in the way of nutrients. Though chocolate bars contain calcium and protein, and crisps are an excellent source of potassium and supply vitamin C, both are usually high in fat.

As long as the food is nutritious, however, the 'little and often' way of eating has its advantages. Some people say that it makes them feel more energetic. After a long period without food, blood sugar levels drop, leaving you feeling tired and depressed. Small, regular quantities of nutritious food can keep energy levels high without overloading the digestive system.

Small appetites

With their smaller stomachs, young children often cannot eat enough of a meal at one sitting to gain all the nutrients they need. It makes sense, therefore, to divide the food into small portions or snacks which the child can eat at regular intervals through the day. Growing children have high nutritional demands and by feeding them mini meals instead of trying to force them to eat adult portions, you can ensure that they receive all the nutrients their energetic and rapidly growing bodies need.

Look at the label

It is a good idea to check the number of calories in commercial snack foods. For example, a 50g (1¾oz) packet of nuts can provide around 300 Calories – as much as a small meal. Look on the packet to see exactly what each manufactured snack contains. High-calorie

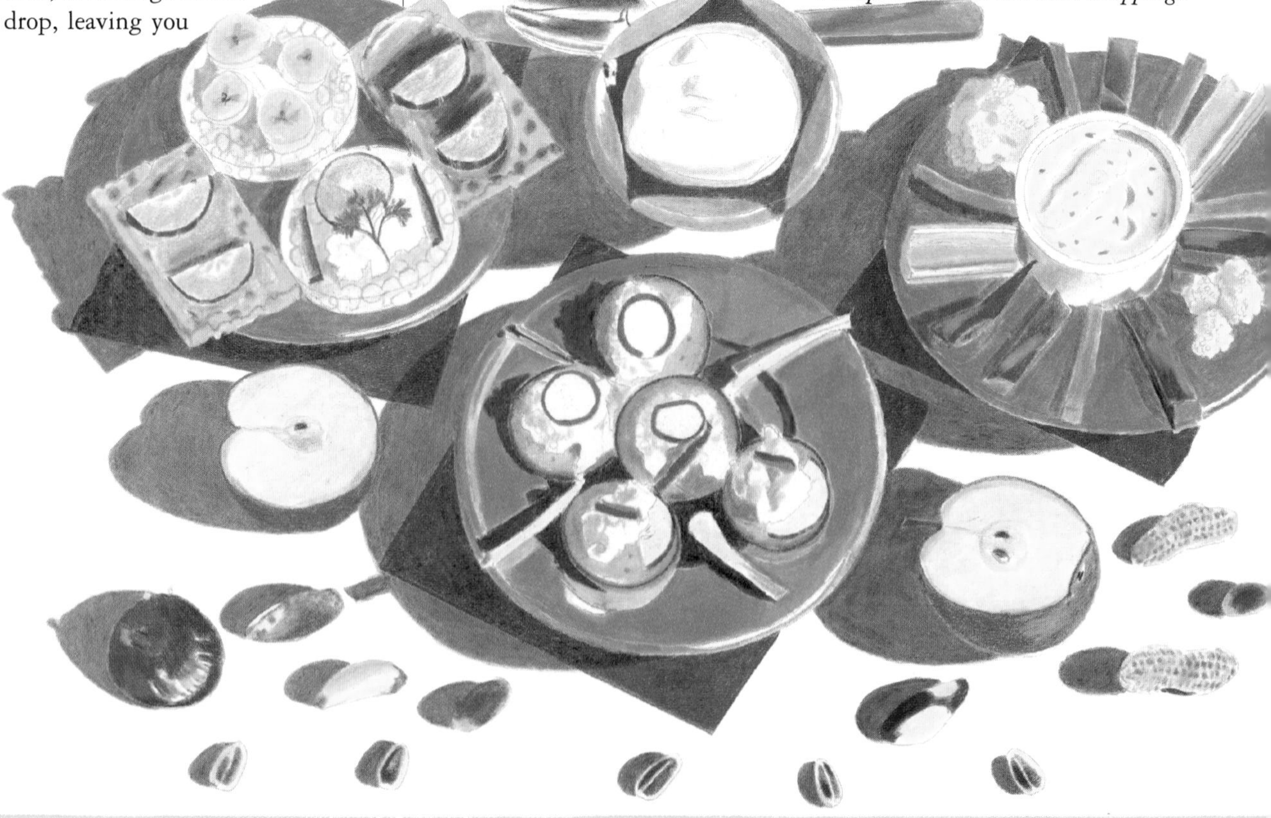

NUTRITIOUS SNACKS *Prepare your own snacks of fruit, nuts, dips and rice cakes or crispbreads with low-calorie toppings.*

snacks are not necessarily bad for you, however, as long as your calorie intake matches your body's energy demands.

Should you wish to check the salt content of a packaged snack, bear in mind that some declare added salt, others sodium, and that 1g of sodium is equivalent to about 2.5g of salt. It is better to choose crisps cooked in vegetable oils rather than hydrogenated vegetable oils. The label will reveal this and also how much fat a packet provides. A small packet of crisps provides about 9g of fat, of which a third may be saturated. Crisps can form part of a balanced diet if eaten in moderation.

Snack attack

Another school of thought questions why people eat snacks at all, arguing that if meals supply sufficient nutrients to meet their bodies' needs, they should not need to eat any extra food. The modern fashion for eating between meals hints at something other than pure physical hunger, such as boredom or discontent. We are constantly bombarded with advertising for confectionery and encouraged to overindulge. Children are the major consumers of snack foods and manufacturers target them using cartoon characters, television personalities and clever packaging.

If you decide to abandon the conventional three meals a day in favour of more frequent snacks, make sure these mini meals fit in with your daily requirement of nutrients. Prepare your own snacks in advance and keep them on hand, so you will not have to buy less healthy packaged snacks.

Healthy alternatives

Everyone will occasionally feel a real and urgent hunger between meals, but this can be satisfied with a number of healthy options. Fresh fruit, such as apples, pears, bananas and oranges, is nutritious and comes in convenient portions. A handful of dried fruit or unsalted nuts provides instant energy and can be added to a small carton of yoghurt and sprinkled with a teaspoon of wheatgerm for a highly nutritious between-meal filler. But remember that nuts are high in calories.

Raw vegetables, such as carrots, celery, cauliflower florets or sliced red, yellow and green peppers, can be eaten alone or with dips. Bear in mind, however, that dips can be high in fat and calories (although you can reduce the fat and calories by making them with yoghurt or fromage frais instead of cream or mayonnaise). Rather than eating a sticky bun, try oatcakes, crispbreads or rice cakes with a topping of cottage cheese, low-fat soft cheese, low-sugar fruit jam, yeast extract or peanut butter. A banana is often all it takes to ease the hunger pangs. If you plan your snacks carefully, you will be able to boost your energy levels, while keeping to a healthy diet.

If you are in the habit of eating snacks do not forget dental hygiene, as the frequent presence of food in the mouth and around the teeth encourages the build-up of the bacteria which cause plaque. Try to brush and floss your teeth regularly.

What is in your favourite dip? (100g, 3½oz)

Guacamole Made from avocado, lemon juice, tomatoes and salt, this dip is a good source of vitamin E, contains pantothenic acid and is a useful source of vitamin C. It contains no cholesterol, 1.4g protein, 12.7g fat and 2.2g carbohydrate.

Hummous Consisting of chickpeas, garlic, olive oil, lemon juice, salt and pepper, hummous contains iron and thiamin. The chickpeas provide plenty of protein, 7.6g, and it contains 12.6g fat, 11.6g carbohydrate but no cholesterol.

Taramasalata Made of white breadcrumbs, smoked cod's roe, olive oil, pepper and lemon juice, taramasalata is high in fat, 46.4g (although 22.6g of this is monounsaturated). It is an excellent source of vitamin B_{12}, but it contains 37mg cholesterol. It has 3.2g protein and 4.1g carbohydrate and contains 446 Calories.

Blue cheese A typical mix of Stilton, sour cream and mayonnaise produces a dip that is high in calories and fat, about 34g (15g of which is saturated). For a lower-fat version substitute crème fraîche for the sour cream and mayonnaise.

Salsa Made of tomatoes, onion, lemon juice, olive oil, chilli peppers, garlic and spices, this dip supplies just 1g of protein. It also provides only 64 Calories, containing 3.5g fat and 7.2g carbohydrate.

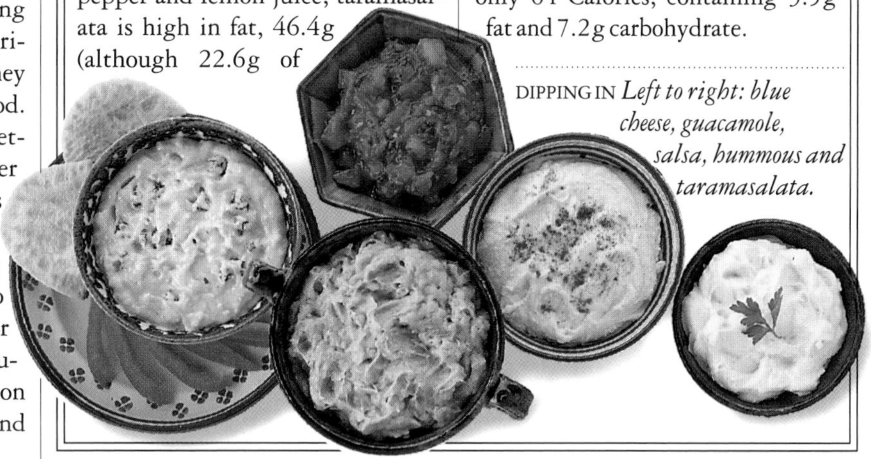

DIPPING IN *Left to right: blue cheese, guacamole, salsa, hummous and taramasalata.*

SOFT DRINKS

BENEFITS

- *Isotonic drinks help to replace lost fluid and energy very quickly after vigorous activity*

DRAWBACKS

- *Can be high in sugar, which may contribute towards tooth decay*
- *Acidic drinks can erode the enamel on your teeth*
- *It is possible to consume excessive amounts of caffeine if you drink too many cola drinks, as well as coffee*

Most sweetened soft drinks provide 'empty calories'; they supply plenty of energy, but no other useful nutrients. Typically, a 330ml (10½fl oz) can of a regular, non-diet cola drink contains just over seven teaspoons of SUGAR. Too many sweet drinks can therefore contribute to weight problems as well as to TOOTH AND GUM DISORDERS.

There are, however, an increasing number of low-calorie, sugar-free soft drinks now available. Some of them claim to be good for you. Isotonic drinks, which are specifically produced for sports enthusiasts, are designed to boost energy – and to replace the electrolytes (mineral salts such as sodium, potassium, magnesium and chloride) that are lost through sweating. The isotonic drinks usually contain 5 per cent sugar, which allows the water in the drink to be absorbed much more quickly by the body than from a glass of pure water.

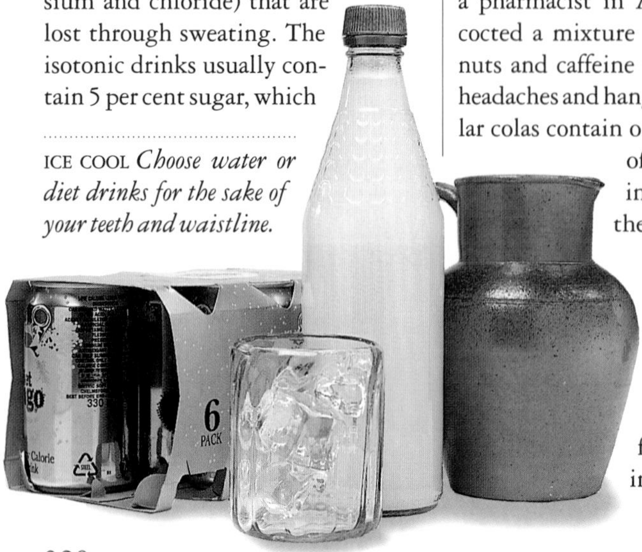

ICE COOL *Choose water or diet drinks for the sake of your teeth and waistline.*

Hidden sugar in drinks

PER 200ml (7fl oz)	CALORIES	SUGAR (g) (5g=1 tsp)
Coca-Cola	86	21
Diet Coca-Cola	0.9	No sugar
Lemonade	42	11
Diet orange drink	3	1
Lucozade	152	37
Lime juice cordial	58	10
Ribena	98	24
Rosehip syrup	77	21
Tonic water	50	11
Orange squash	36	10

FIZZY DRINKS AND SQUASHES

The original cola drink was invented in 1886 when John Styth Pemberton, a pharmacist in Atlanta, USA, concocted a mixture of coca leaves, cola nuts and caffeine to sell as a cure for headaches and hangovers. Today, regular colas contain only about one-third of the caffeine found in a cup of coffee, and there are also decaffeinated versions. The sugar contained in diluted squashes ranges from a single teaspoon per glass to four or even more in the case of some blackcurrant drinks, but these may also provide useful amounts of vitamin C. The sugar in soft drinks is broken down by bacteria growing on teeth – to produce acid. If you sip sugary drinks over long periods, this increases the risk of tooth decay by prolonging the time that enamel-destroying acids are in the mouth. Acidic fruit-juice cordials can also erode your teeth. Try to drink soft drinks at mealtimes, and clean your teeth regularly.

In a recent survey, researchers at Southampton University found that some children are gaining almost half their daily energy intake from sugary drinks, and that these empty calories are leading to irritability, loss of appetite, poor weight gain and diarrhoea. And doctors who treated eight toddlers referred to Southampton General Hospital with eating or behavioural problems found that the children's symptoms disappeared when their consumption of sweetened soft drinks was reduced.

LOW-CALORIE DRINKS

Made with artificial sweeteners, low-calorie drinks are suitable for almost everyone, including diabetics. They do not contribute to tooth decay by promoting the formation of plaque, or to weight problems. Sparkling waters with added herbs, minerals and ginseng claim to act as a natural pick-me up, but tend to be more expensive than other soft drinks. They are usually sweetened with fruit juice.

ALLERGIES

Some ADDITIVES used in soft drinks, such as the azo dyes sunset yellow (E110) and tartrazine (E102), found in some orange, lemon and lime squashes, have been alleged to cause allergic reactions in susceptible individuals. The symptoms can range from skin rashes and upset stomachs to irritability and hyperactivity.

Did you know?

- In the UK, we consume about 8.25 billion litres of soft drinks every year, comprising fruit juice, waters and carbonates.
- The British began to bottle lemonade during the early 1700s, using sulphur as a preservative. By 1789, Nicholas Paul of Geneva, in Switzerland, had developed a method of manufacturing carbonated waters in bulk.
- By 1891, sole ownership of the Coca-Cola formula had been acquired by Asa Candler for just $2300. Less than 30 years later, the Candler family sold on the Coca-Cola company to banker Ernest Woodruff for $25 million.
- Coca-Cola's stimulating effect now comes from caffeine; the leaves of the South American coca tree are no longer used. Once the main ingredient of many soft drinks, the dried leaves are nowadays probably best known as a source of the drug cocaine.
- Pepsi-Cola was created by Caleb D. Bradham in 1898. The drink was intended as a remedy for dyspepsia – hence its name.

SORE THROAT

TAKE PLENTY OF

- *Fruit and vegetables for vitamin C*
- *Foods rich in vitamin A and beta carotene such as liver (unless you are pregnant), carrots and spinach*
- *Oily fish for vitamin D*
- *Olive oil and avocados for vitamin E*
- *Live or bio-yoghurt to protect against the effects of antibiotics*

CUT DOWN ON

- *Tobacco and alcohol*

A raw, stinging throat can often be the first sign of a cold, influenza or tonsillitis. The cause is usually a virus, although the *Streptococcus* bacterium can also produce a sore throat and fever known as 'strep throat'. One factor that can lead to tonsillitis and other infections is an unhealthy diet – high in refined carbohydrates such as cakes, biscuits and table sugar, and low in the micronutrients important for the efficiency of the body's natural defences. tiredness, stress, smoking and drinking too much alcohol may also lower the body's resistance to infection.

To ward off sore throats, make sure that your diet is providing you with a good intake of vitamin D – found in oily fish – and vitamin E, in olive oil, nuts, seeds and avocados. These vitamins, along with the essential fatty acids found in vegetable and fish oils, are very important for maintaining a healthy immune system.

Deficiency in vitamin C can increase people's susceptibility to infections. Excellent sources of the vitamin include blackcurrants, oranges, strawberries, red peppers and watercress. Dietary iron in the form of liver, sesame seeds and bread may also help because it too is necessary for the formation of antibodies.

If you do develop a sore throat, it may be helpful to eat yellow or orange fruit and vegetables such as apricots or carrots, and dark green leafy vegetables such as spinach. As well as containing vitamin C, they provide beta carotene, which the body converts to vitamin A. This vitamin is important for the health of mucous membranes, including the lining of the throat. Other sources include liver, as well as polyunsaturated margarines and low-fat spreads, which the law requires to be fortified with vitamin A.

Anyone who has been taking antibiotics may benefit from eating live or bio-yoghurt once the course has finished. This can help to replace the intestinal bacteria – an important source of some of the B vitamins – that are destroyed by the medication.

Naturopaths recommend adding the juice of half a lemon and a teaspoon of honey to a glass of hot water to make a soothing drink for a sore throat. The lemon juice contains vitamin C which stimulates the production of saliva – soothing irritated membranes, and the honey also soothes your sore throat.

Another natural approach to curing a sore throat is to gargle with sage tea. It is made by pouring a cup of boiling water onto a teaspoon of dried sage or a dessertspoon of chopped fresh leaves. Red sage is preferable to garden sage, but both are claimed to work.

A sore throat usually lasts three to four days; if symptoms continue for any longer, consult a doctor as they may be an early sign of an illness such as glandular fever or mumps.

OLD SOCKS AND DEAD FROGS

An old English remedy for a sore throat was to tie an old sock around the patient's throat. A bizarre cure for infants was to wrap a dead frog in a pure-white linen cloth and let the unfortunate baby suck on it. An old-fashioned remedy that is still in use is to drink a glass of hot milk laced with a teaspoon of honey.

Allergy alert

A common cause of sore throats is tonsillitis. The tonsils protect the throat from invading germs, but when the germs become too much for them, the tonsils themselves become infected and inflamed. Some naturopaths believe that recurrent attacks of tonsillitis may be caused by an allergic reaction to cow's milk, in which case dairy products should be eliminated.

Soup

Various forms of cooking inevitably rob vegetables of many of their vitamins and minerals, but soup makes a filling and nourishing meal. It has the added advantage of retaining most of the nutrients of its ingredients.

Homemade soups

Soup can be made with almost any ingredient, so you can create a number of dishes that meet your family's particular nutritional needs; a list of healthy soups is suggested on the next page. A number of easily digestible meals can be produced by using a good homemade stock that is made with various combinations of pulses, grains, meat, fish and vegetables. Most good supermarkets now sell fresh stock, and this is a much healthier convenience choice than stock cubes, which are high in sodium and usually contain additives.

Homemade stock is made by boiling up meat, poultry bones, gristle, or vegetables with herbs and spices. The long, slow cooking process concentrates the flavours. A good fish stock can be made with almost any clean trimmings – but will start to smell strongly and take on a bitter taste if overcooked (20 minutes is usually long enough). If you chill meat stock thoroughly before using it in soup, it sets as a soft jelly and you can easily lift off the solid layer of fat that rises to the surface. Even poultry fat will set enough to be lifted off the stock.

If you have a freezer, you can make stock in large quantities, and freeze it for up to six months. But make sure that the stock is labelled and dated.

The milk added to some soups enriches them by increasing their protein and calcium content. However, if you use whole milk, it will also add significantly to the fat content.

STOCK IDEAS *Suitable for any occasion; soups can be as humble or as extravagant as you want to make them.*

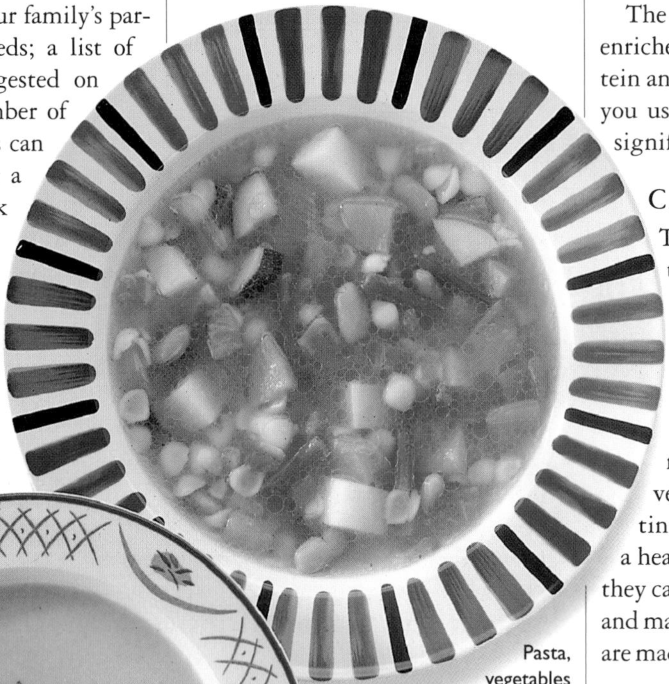

Pasta, vegetables and beans combine to make minestrone.

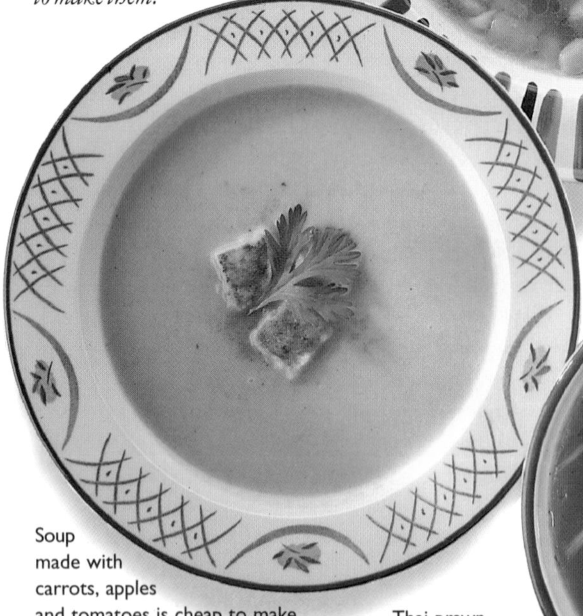

Soup made with carrots, apples and tomatoes is cheap to make but very nourishing.

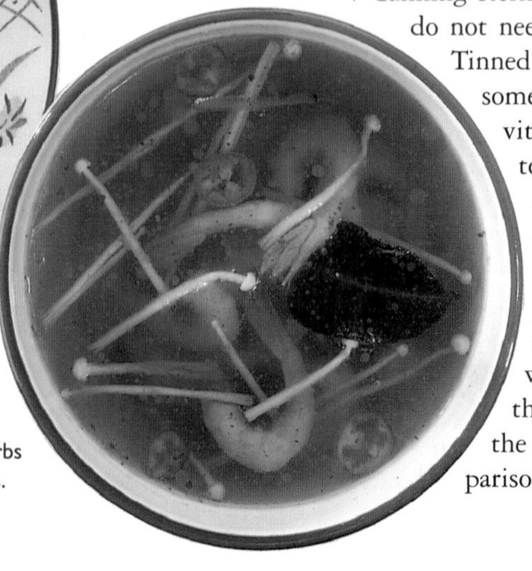

Thai prawn soup is made with chillies, herbs and lemon grass.

Carton soups

These soups are the next best thing to homemade because they use fresh ingredients which retain most of their nutrients. This is due to the way that carton soups are prepared; they are pasteurised, rather than being heated to a very high temperature like a tinned soup. Cartons are therefore a healthier choice than tinned – but they can contain large amounts of salt, and may be very high in calories if they are made with milk or cream.

Tinned soups

Canning sterilises soups so that they do not need added preservatives. Tinned tomato soup contains some beta carotene, but the vitamin C content tends to be low as the soup is subjected to prolonged cooking before it is canned. Most tinned or packaged soup contains salt, the quantity of which has to be stated on the label. The chart on the next page gives comparisons of sodium contents.

The contents of a tomato soup

The nutritional content of a soup can vary significantly, according to the way it is made. Taking tomato soup as an example, this chart shows the differences. You can see that while the protein content remains more or less the same, homemade creamed tomato soup contains the most fat and calories; condensed has the most sugar; tinned has the most salt; while homemade is low in sugar and salt. Dried soup is the lowest in calories – but it is also the lowest in nutrients.

NUTRITIONAL VALUE (per 220 g)	TOMATO & BASIL (CARTON)	CREAM OF TOMATO (HOMEMADE)	CREAM OF TOMATO (TINNED)	CREAM OF TOMATO (CONDENSED)	TOMATO SOUP (DRIED)
CALORIES	88	179.1	121	136	68
PROTEIN	1.76g	2.5g	1.76g	1.98g	1.32g
FAT	4.2g	14.9g	7.26g	7.48g	1.1g
SUGAR	7.5g	4.9g	5.72g	12.32g	7.7g
SODIUM	900mg	213.5mg	1012mg	902mg	858mg

Dried packet soups

Packet soups generally contain fewer nutrients and more additives than their tinned or homemade equivalents. In addition to dried foods, they contain thickening agents, salt, colourings and flavourings.

Consumer pressure has resulted in levels of monosodium glutamate – a flavour enhancer that was thought to cause headaches in some people – being reduced in many brands. Packet soups may contain lower levels of vitamins than other types of soup because of the losses that can occur during the drying of the food ingredients.

The thickeners found in many commercial soups and stock cubes may be derived from wheat, so people with a gluten intolerance should always check the labels.

Soups and joint pain

People who suffer from GOUT should choose soups made with vegetable stocks if possible. This is because meat stocks may contain high levels of purines which raise the amount of uric acid in the body – and uric acid crystals cause the painful joints experienced by people with gout. Asparagus soup, especially if the tips are used, also contains some purines, and is therefore best eaten in limited amounts.

Popular, healthy soups

Bouillabaisse A thick fish soup based on a famous recipe from Marseilles, which can be made with any mixture of fish. It provides vitamin C from tomatoes, calcium from vegetables, and iron and protein from the fish.

Chicken In folk medicine, chicken soup is said to clear a blocked nose. It contains protein and most B vitamins. Try a curried mulligatawny soup.

French onion A warming soup, long regarded in folk medicine as an antidote to fatigue, chills, head colds and even hangovers.

Gazpacho A cold, summer soup that originated in southern Spain, made with breadcrumbs, tomatoes and salad vegetables such as spring onions and cucumber. It provides vitamin C.

Lentil A good soup for vegetarians as lentils are an excellent source of protein, as well as fibre and iron.

Minestrone This wholesome Italian soup is made with fresh vegetables, dried beans and pasta or rice. It provides protein, fibre and vitamin C.

Tomato A homemade tomato soup is much more nutritious than tinned varieties. If you want a sweet flavour, make it in the summer and use tomatoes that are almost overripe. It provides fibre and vitamin C.

What is in a stock cube?

Commercial stock cubes are made with highly concentrated extracts of beef, chicken, mushroom or mixed vegetables. They can also include many other ingredients such as monosodium glutamate (a flavour enhancer that is contained in hydrolysed vegetable protein), salt, sugar, yeast extract, herbs, spices and thickeners. Although monosodium glutamate has now been removed from many tinned soups, it is no longer blamed for Chinese Restaurant Syndrome (CRS) and is still widely used in stock cubes.

If you have been told that you should be following a low-salt diet, you should avoid using stock cubes, as one cube can contain up to one level teaspoon of salt.

Spices: A Taste of the East

The fragrant aromas of exotic spices have been prized since the dawn of civilisation. Today, spices and seeds are still valued for their culinary and medicinal properties.

With their distinctive colours and flavours, spices stimulate the appetite and enhance our enjoyment of food. Used in small amounts, spices are of little nutritional value. However, with their intense and distinctive flavours, spices can be a healthy alternative to salt in the diet.

Spices, such as juniper, cloves and pepper, have long been used to improve the flavour of preserved food as well as to make bland, staple foods more appetising. However, a few contain compounds that can cause adverse reactions in susceptible people.

Spicy remedies

Practitioners of alternative medicine have ascribed specific health benefits to certain spices. Although the majority of their claims have not been substantiated by scientific studies, many of the remedies have been used for hundreds of years.

Allspice Thought to aid digestion.

Black pepper Stimulates digestion, eases flatulence, relieves constipation and improves circulation.

Caraway seeds Said to relieve flatulence, colic and bronchitis. They also stimulate the appetite, can be used to relieve menstrual pain and increase milk flow in nursing mothers.

Cardamom Relieves indigestion and sweetens the breath when chewed. It also helps to stop vomiting, belching and acid regurgitation. It can be used in the treatment of colds and coughs as well as bronchitis.

Cayenne pepper A spice claimed to act as a tonic to the digestive and circulatory systems. It can be used to treat indigestion and has been found to be helpful in the treatment of chilblains.

Chillies Have been found to be useful in clearing the mucus from airways, so relieving congestion.

Cinnamon Used for indigestion, flatulence and diarrhoea. It also acts as a nasal decongestant.

Cloves The oil has long been used to ease toothache.

Coriander seeds Help to stimulate the digestive system. Coriander has also been prescribed in the treatment of diarrhoea and cystitis, as well as infections of the urinary tract.

Cumin seeds The strong aroma and slightly bitter taste of this spice makes it a popular component of curries. In the past cumin has been used to cure flatulence and colic, though today its medicinal use is usually confined to veterinary practice.

Ginger Aids digestion, is a popular remedy for nausea, notably for travel and morning sickness, and improves circulation. In natural medicine it is also used to protect against respiratory and digestive infections and to ease flatulence and griping pains. Ginger can be chewed to relieve toothache.

Taken at the first signs of a cold or flu, hot ginger tea makes a comforting drink and may help to clear a blocked nose and stimulate the liver to remove toxins from the bloodstream. It is made with a teaspoon of freshly grated ginger, the juice of half a lemon and a teaspoon of honey, topped up with boiling water.

Juniper berries Since they have antiseptic properties, juniper berries have been used to treat infections of the urinary tract, such as cystitis. They are a kidney irritant so should not be used if the kidneys are infected or otherwise diseased. Do not take juniper berries during pregnancy since they can cause the uterus to contract, which may lead to a spontaneous abortion.

Mustard seeds The black seeds are hotter than the white. Hot water poured onto crushed mustard seeds and used as a foot bath is said to ward off flu and relieve headaches.

Nutmeg and mace Two spices from the same plant (mace is the lacy covering around the seed). Both contain myristicin, a substance which can cause hallucinations and drowsiness. Although toxic in large quantities, nutmeg and mace may alleviate nausea and vomiting, flatulence and diarrhoea when taken in moderation.

Saffron One of the most expensive spices, saffron is used for the treatment of a variety of ailments. It is said to ease menstrual pain and menopausal problems, depression, chronic diarrhoea and neuralgic pain.

Star anise Relieves flatulence. In the East the fruit is believed to cure colic.

Turmeric In alternative medicine, this spice is said to be a tonic for the liver, to help calm inflammation and to relieve digestive problems. Turmeric improves circulation and also has an antibacterial action.

SOOTHING SPICES *It is a common misbelief that peptic ulcers are caused by a spicy diet. In fact, recent research suggests that a bacterium is the usual culprit. In herbal medicine, spices such as cardamom and ginger are actually used to aid digestion.*

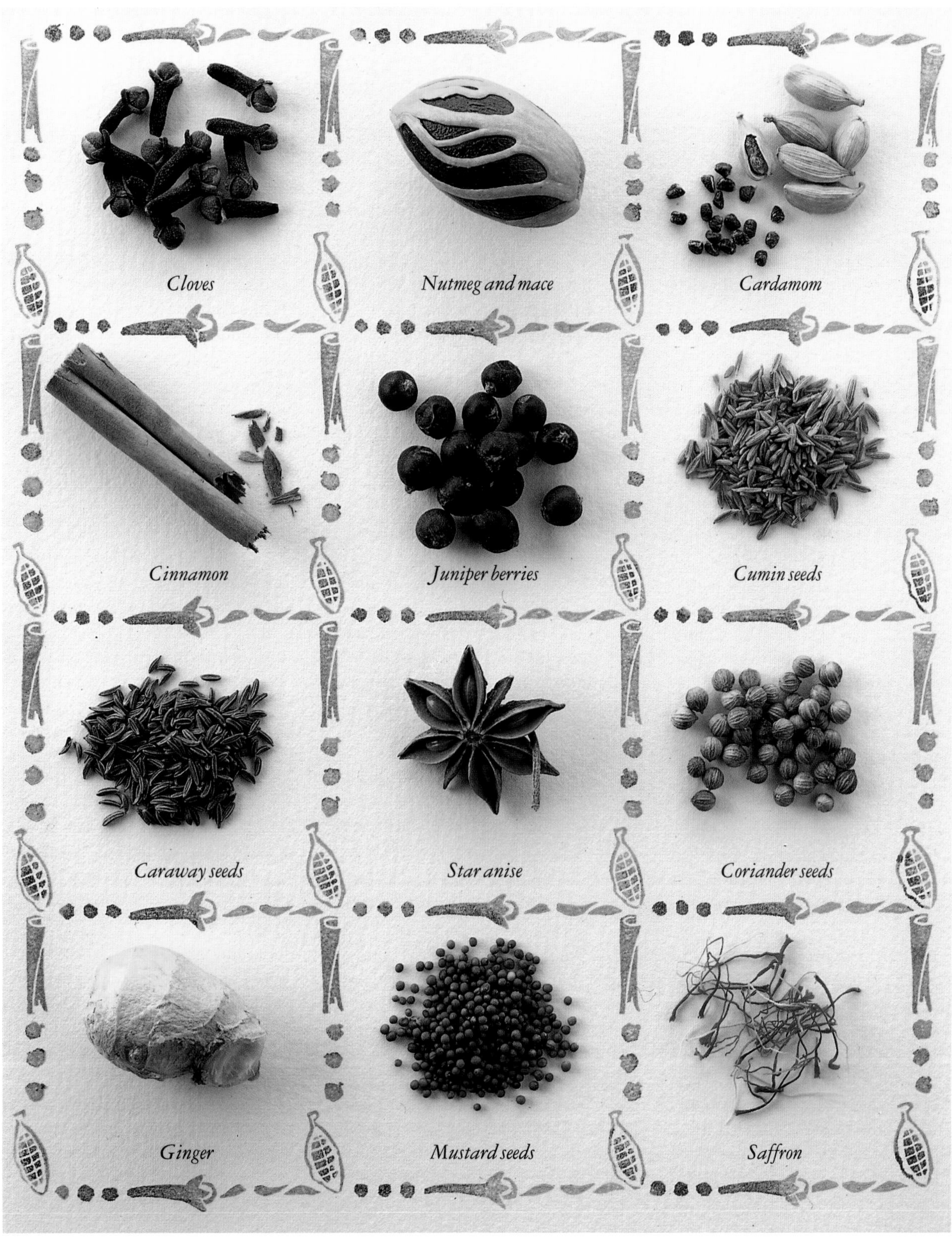
Cloves
Nutmeg and mace
Cardamom
Cinnamon
Juniper berries
Cumin seeds
Caraway seeds
Star anise
Coriander seeds
Ginger
Mustard seeds
Saffron

Spina bifida

Before conception and during the first three months of pregnancy, women should

EAT PLENTY OF

- *Brussels sprouts and broccoli*
- *Yeast extract*
- *Pulses (beans, peas and lentils)*
- *Breakfast cereals and bread which are fortified with folic acid*
- *Brown rice, wheatgerm and barley*
- *Nuts and seeds*

AVOID

- *Liver*

Women can reduce the likelihood of their children developing spina bifida (a condition that develops in the womb and is present at birth) by taking a daily supplement of folic acid, as well as eating foods that contain folate. (Folate and folic acid are both names for an important B vitamin which, together with vitamin B_{12}, is needed to form blood cells.)

The critical period for women to make sure that they are getting enough folate in their diet is actually before conception – and then during the first three months of pregnancy. So if you are trying to conceive, you should start taking a daily folic acid supplement immediately.

The literal meaning of spina bifida is 'split spine'. This condition occurs when the developing baby's spine fails to form correctly, and leaves a gap or a split somewhere along the spinal column. The spinal cord and spine are part of the neural tube, which begins to develop two or three weeks after conception. The reasons why it sometimes develops incorrectly are not fully understood, but dietary, genetic and environmental factors are all involved. Many babies born with spina bifida also have hydrocephalus – water on the brain – due to abnormalities in the physical structure of the brain which prevent proper drainage of cerebrospinal fluid. Thirty years ago many babies born with neural tube defects died, but today medical and surgical treatment have greatly improved their chances of survival.

Women who have given birth to one baby with a neural tube defect have a 1 in 35 chance of having another. Trials carried out by the Medical Research Council over a seven-year period found that the risk was reduced by 75 per cent through the inclusion of folic acid supplements for at least one month (preferably two or three) before conception, and throughout the first 12 weeks of pregnancy.

The Medical Research Council has recommended a daily intake of 4 mg – available on prescription only – for women who have already had a child with spina bifida. Women who are not in a high-risk group should take a daily 0.4mg supplement, available from chemists and health food shops.

Good sources of folate include Brussels sprouts, broccoli, green leafy vegetables, yeast extract, chickpeas, cauliflower, lentils, peas, brown rice, soya beans, wheatgerm, wheat bran, nuts, endives and seeds, as well as breakfast cereals and bread that have been fortified with folic acid.

Don't eat liver

In the past, liver was regarded as an essential part of the expectant mother's diet. Although liver contains plenty of valuable nutrients such as folate and iron, the modern advice is that pregnant women should not eat liver, liver pâté or liver sausage. Liver has high concentrations of vitamin A which, when added to the vitamin A present in a properly balanced diet, could result in an overdose which might harm the developing foetus. An excess of vitamin A can build up because it is a fat-soluble vitamin, and cannot be excreted through the urine.

Spinach

BENEFITS

- *Excellent source of carotene and a good source of vitamin C, which may help to prevent cancer*
- *Good source of potassium*
- *Useful source of folate*

DRAWBACKS

- *Oxalic acid may interfere with calcium and iron absorption*
- *Can aggravate kidney and bladder stone formation in susceptible people*

Contrary to popular belief, spinach is not an especially good source of iron although its dark green leaves do contain a lot of other valuable nutrients. Indeed, some research suggests that it is one of the most potent of all vegetables in helping to prevent cancer.

Spinach contains a high concentration of carotenoids, including beta carotene which is the plant form of vitamin A. It is also a rich source of lutein, a carotenoid pigment that has ANTIOXIDANT effects. Several studies have now suggested that eating dark green vegetables regularly might protect against many types of cancer.

A study carried out at Harvard Medical School in 1994 showed that a diet rich in carotenes reduced the risk of age-related macular degeneration –

Spinach for soldiers

During the First World War, according to Mrs Grieve writing in *A Modern Herbal* (1931), spinach juice was mixed with wine and given to French soldiers who were weakened by heavy blood loss, to help try to restore their strength. Since spinach contains folate – which is important for blood formation – as well as some iron, the remedy may actually have helped.

a common cause of blindness among the elderly. This problem, caused by a deterioration of the area at the centre of the retina, was less likely to develop in people who consumed plenty of green leafy vegetables.

Spinach is also a useful source of folate, the consumption of which is highly recommended for pregnant women to help to prevent spina bifida.

The wisdom of traditional medicine is shown by some long-standing uses for spinach. It has been prescribed for high blood pressure as well as anaemia and constipation; and spinach is a good source of potassium, now recognised by doctors to be an important element in regulating blood pressure.

THE POPEYE MYTH

Spinach has long been thought of as a particularly rich source of iron; back in the 1950s, many children were forced to eat it by their parents – who thought that it would make them fit and strong. A big influence on this super-healthy spinach image was the cartoon character, Popeye, who gulped down tins of the vegetable to give his muscles an instant boost.

This popular misconception arose from a simple mathematical error by a food analyst when calculating the iron content of spinach; a decimal point in the wrong place led many people to believe that spinach contained ten times as much iron as it really did.

Your body will absorb more of the iron that is in spinach if you eat the vegetable with foods that contain vitamin C, such as fruit or tomatoes.

RAW SPINACH

Many people dislike the strong taste and soggy texture of cooked spinach. Why not try experimenting with raw spinach instead, as it is among the most nutritious of salad greens? You can make a wide variety of salads by substituting young spinach leaves for lettuce; a warm salad made with raw spinach, grilled bacon, avocado and sliced mushrooms is just one example.

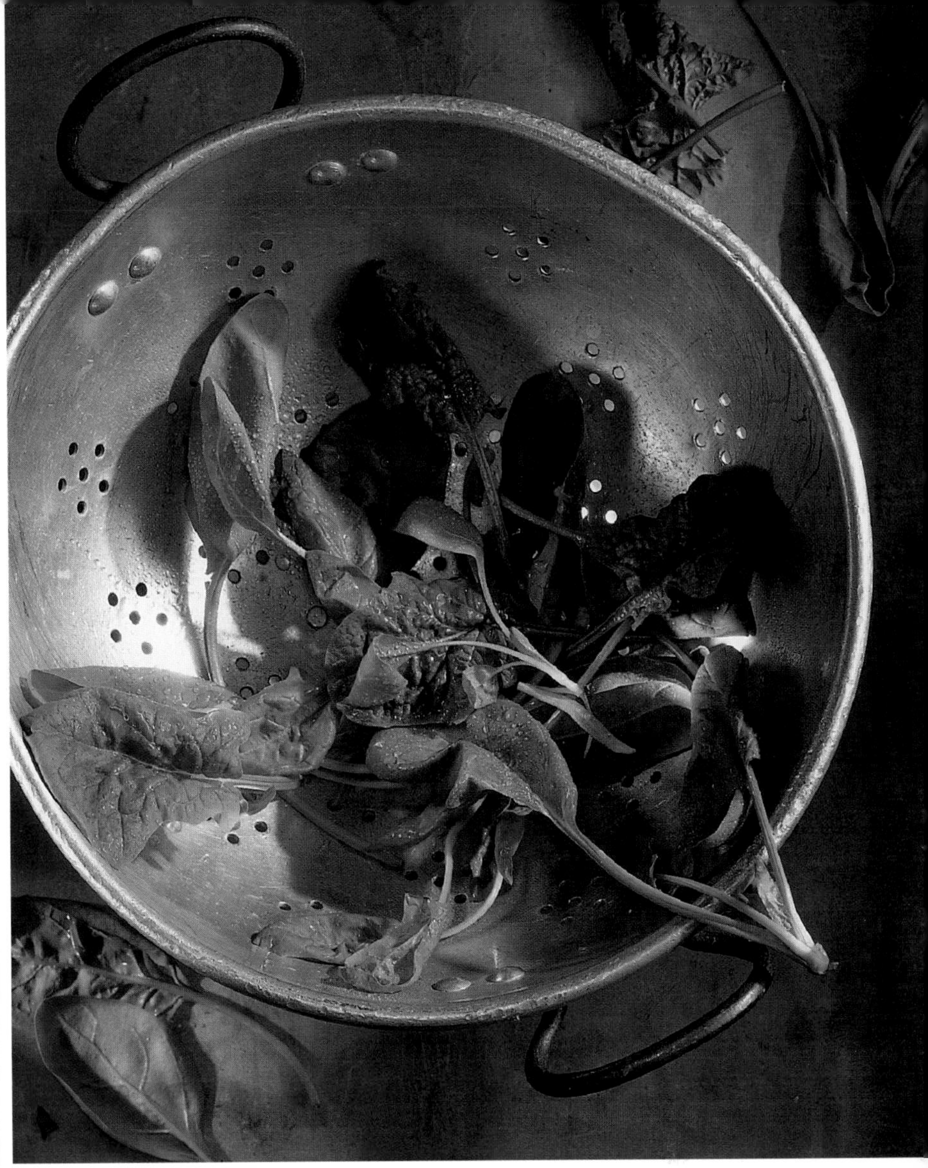

VERSATILE VEGETABLE *Young spinach leaves can be eaten raw or lightly cooked. Always wash spinach thoroughly to remove grit, and discard damaged leaves and tough stalks.*

DRAWBACKS

The nutritional benefits of spinach are tempered by its high concentration of oxalic acid. This combines with the iron and calcium in spinach, limiting their absorption – the amount of iron that can be absorbed is considerably reduced and only a fraction of the calcium the spinach contains can be used by the body. This has led to claims that eating spinach affects the absorption of calcium generally – but studies have shown that massive amounts would have to be eaten before interference of oxalic acid became a serious problem. Eating spinach (and other foods that contain significant amounts of oxalic acid, such as rhubarb), while also taking vitamin C supplements, can aggravate the formation of oxalate kidney and bladder stones. These arise from a build-up of oxalate deposits, in susceptible people. Spinach can also contain high levels of nitrate, recently the subject of much discussion within the European Union (see CELERY).

Sports nutrition to beat the competition

For the modern athlete, nutrition is taken as seriously as the training programme. There are no shortcuts or false starts to a winning diet – the answer lies in balancing intake with output.

The physical and psychological benefits of exercise are undeniable but, when strenuous physical exercise is part of your daily life, you must make sure that you are eating the right diet for long-term health. Athletes have similar nutritional requirements to those of the average person but, because of physical exertion, they may have increased carbohydrate needs. An endurance athlete's diet may consist of up to 67 per cent carbohydrate.

Athletes should be wary of manipulating their diet to achieve short-term performance at the expense of lifelong health. No single food can magically enhance performance; only a good range of foods can enable an athlete to compete in peak condition. When a sports activity demands a high energy expenditure, an adequate intake of calories, macronutrients (carbohydrates, proteins, fats and fibre), and micronutrients (vitamins, most minerals and trace elements) is essential to maintain energy and fluid balance.

Athletes should follow a balanced diet which is 'scaled up' to meet increased energy needs. Contrary to popular opinion, there is no need to eat a high-protein diet when undergoing training; in most cases it is better to obtain extra calories from carbohydrates, although athletes with very high energy demands, such as oarsmen, need a greater than average intake of fat so that the diet is not too bulky. However, some less energetic sports – snooker for example – do not require any increase in calories.

The fluid factor

During physical exercise, breathing out and sweating deplete the body's reserves of fluids. Excessive perspiration can lead to a reduced flow of blood to the extremities, a reduction in blood volume and, in extreme cases, to dehydration, heatstroke and collapse. Therefore it is vital to drink water before, during and after exercise.

Commercial 'isotonic' sports drinks contain low levels of salts (to induce thirst and to replace minerals lost through sweating) and sugars for energy. Since these drinks are designed to prevent dehydration, they are not retained in the stomach and pass quickly into the small intestine for absorption. A cheap substitute is to dilute fruit juice 1:1 with water.

More minerals

The mineral content and requirements of tissues and cells differ. Bone contains a lot of calcium, muscle cells large amounts of potassium and magnesium, while blood carries high levels of sodium and chloride. A shortage of MINERALS will normally be compensated for by reduced excretion or by the release of some of the minerals stored in the body's tissues.

If you run a marathon and are temporarily depleted of minerals, these will probably be restored without you making any changes to your diet, but prolonged mineral deficiency can be serious. Some authorities advise the use of multi-mineral supplements, although there is no scientific proof that these significantly improve the performance of athletes.

The potassium in muscles is gradually lost as they work repeatedly during exercise. The body needs this mineral for the release of energy, a regular heartbeat and movement of digested food. Replenish stores by including plenty of potassium-rich foods in your diet; good sources are lean meats, vegetables, nuts, pulses and fruit – especially bananas.

Low magnesium levels have often been found in athletes engaged in endurance exercise. When too little magnesium is available for use it can interfere with the release of energy, causing fatigue and possibly muscle cramps leading to poor muscle tone. Foods rich in magnesium include seafood, dark green leafy vegetables, whole grains, nuts and pulses.

Much of the zinc in our bodies is stored in bone and muscle; only a small amount is readily available, mainly in the blood. Zinc is lost primarily through urine and sweat, so athletes need to watch their daily intake. Good sources include seafood, offal, eggs, wheatgerm and pulses.

Anaemia in female athletes

Although the exact reasons are not fully understood, female athletes are known to be at risk from anaemia. It is important, then, that they should have an adequate intake of iron, folate and vitamin B_{12} to support normal blood formation. Good dietary sources of iron include red meat, offal, egg yolks and dark green vegetables. Folate can

GLYCOGEN: THE MUSCLE FUEL

Glycogen is the main fuel the muscles use when they move. It is produced from the glucose provided when carbohydrates are digested, and is stored in muscles and in the liver. Unfortunately, the body can store only a relatively small amount of glycogen, so athletes need a high-carbohydrate diet to make sure glycogen stores are always full before any activity.

be obtained from liver, wheatgerm, cabbage, pulses, broccoli and yeast extract, while sources of vitamin B_{12} include offal, poultry, fish, eggs and dairy produce.

LOOK AFTER YOUR BONES

Almost all the body's calcium is in the bones: 1 per cent is available elsewhere in the body, and may be lost through sweating. Bones, despite their deceptive hardness, constantly need to absorb and release calcium and, when calcium intake is low, bones become weaker. Ensure that the diet contains adequate calcium by taking plenty of milk and other dairy produce, as well as green leafy vegetables.

THE RISK OF OSTEOPOROSIS

Young women athletes, especially long-distance runners, are particularly susceptible to reduced bone density, or OSTEOPOROSIS, when exercise, stress and weight loss leads to depressed oestrogen levels, resulting in irregular or missed periods and inefficient calcium metabolism. This is probably a consequence of the very low levels of body fat that the runners strive to maintain. Tennis players and swimmers are less likely to have problems because they usually have more body fat. Women who take regular, medium-impact exercise – such as walking or jogging in good sports shoes – can take heart, as this type of exercise actually lowers the risk of osteoporosis.

BEAT THE FATIGUE 'WALL'

When glycogen stores are exhausted, for instance during a marathon, an athlete hits the 'wall' of fatigue and feels too exhausted to continue the event. Gradually increasing training in the run-up to an event, while maintaining a diet high in complex carbohydrates, such as potatoes and rice, can increase the period of efficient performance.

Some athletes used to prepare for major events by 'carbo loading', that is: cutting down on carbohydrate-rich foods for several days, and then overloading with foods such as bread and pasta for two or three days immediately before an event. These days most athletes keep to a diet high in complex carbohydrates all the time.

WHY FATS ARE NEEDED

Because the emphasis in an athlete's diet is on a high carbohydrate intake, fat intake need only make up about 30 per cent of calorie intake. Muscle uses fat as its preferred fuel during light exercise, but carbohydrate is used up faster at higher levels of activity. A high carbohydrate intake can improve endurance, but it makes for a very bulky diet. Adding fat to food can double its energy value without adding too much bulk. When adding fat to the diet, unsaturated fats (found in vegetable oils and oily fish) are healthier than saturates (the hard fats in cheese, butter and meat) and the trans fatty acids (present in most margarines). However, you should not attempt to exclude all saturated fats from the diet. For current guidelines, see FATS.

Case history

Olympic champion sprinter Linford Christie believes in a good breakfast whenever he is competing or training. This includes fried plantain, eggs and bacon or an omelette followed by Earl Grey tea. If there is time in his training schedule for lunch he will generally eat some fruit. His evening meal is often fish or chicken served with rice and peas. Extra energy during the day comes from snacks of fruit. Linford, who won the 100m gold medal in Barcelona at the age of 32 in 1992, does not vary this diet, which he has eaten since his early days as an athlete, but he does alter the amount he eats depending on the level of training. On the morning of a competition he eats a good breakfast and then nothing until after the event.

He recommends that newcomers to athletics should aim to eat plenty of fruit, fish and chicken, but try to cut down on red meat consumption.

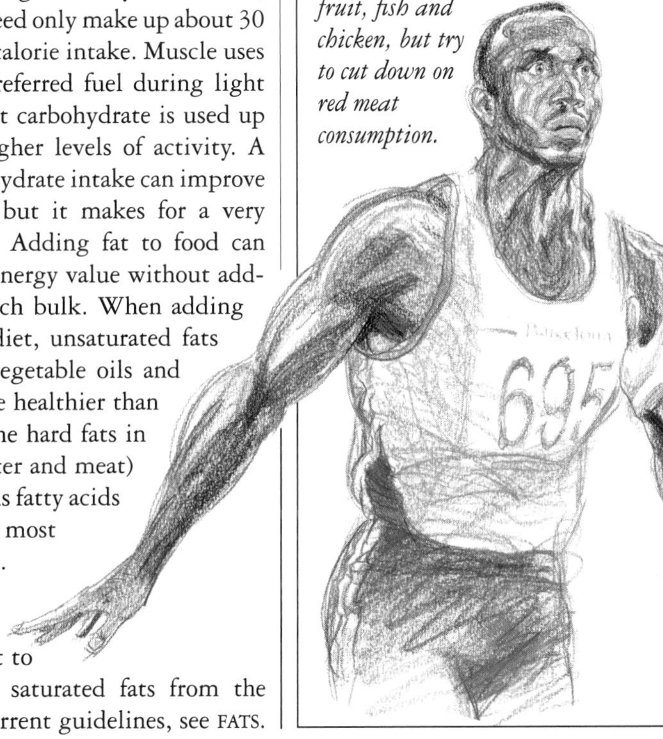

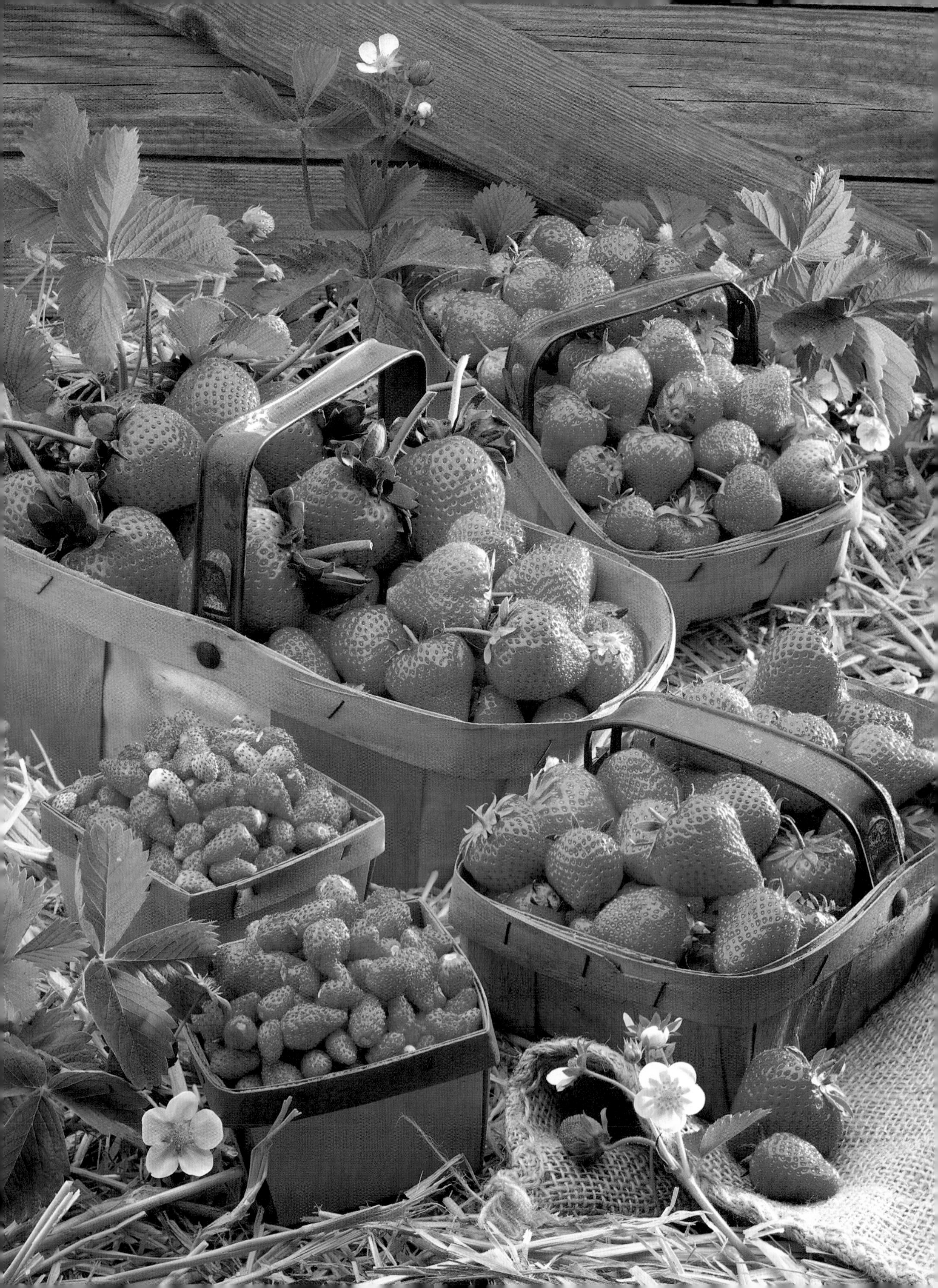

STRAWBERRIES

BENEFIT

- *Excellent source of vitamin C*

DRAWBACKS

- *Can cause allergic reactions*
- *Seeds may be an irritant to people with bowel disorders*

One of the favourite foods of high summer, strawberries contain higher levels of vitamin C than any other berry and a serving of 100g (3½oz) contains only 27 Calories.

Eating strawberries, or any other food high in vitamin C, after eating iron-rich vegetables will help to improve the body's absorption of iron. This is especially useful for people whose diets do not contain much meat.

In traditional medicine, strawberries have long been used to cleanse and purify the digestive system; they are said to act as a mild tonic for the liver and to have antibacterial properties.

ALLERGIC REACTIONS

Some people have an allergic reaction to strawberries, and develop an itchy rash known as hives. This rash is the result of an excess production of histamine by the body, which appears to be triggered by a substance in the fruit. It has been suggested that an allergic reaction is more likely when the fruit has not ripened on the vine.

Strawberries are high in compounds known as salicylates and should be avoided by people with an intolerance to aspirin – which is made of a similar substance called salicylic acid. People with bowel disorders such as colitis should also avoid the fruit because the seeds may be a source of irritation.

BERRY BASKETS *No one knows for sure, but one reason for the strawberry's name is that for centuries straw has been used to keep the berries clean and away from the soil.*

Herbal folklore

Over the years strawberries have been credited with many curative properties – they were believed to eliminate kidney stones and also to relieve arthritis, gout and rheumatism. In 1653, Culpeper's *English Physician and Herbal* claimed that the berries made 'an excellent water for inflamed eyes and to take away a film or skin that beginneth to grow over them'.

In Mrs Grieve's *A Modern Herbal*, published in 1931, the cosmetic benefits of strawberries are discussed. The book says that 'the juice left on the teeth for 5 minutes removes discoloration', and that a cut strawberry 'rubbed over the face immediately after washing will whiten the skin and remove slight sunburn'.

STRESS

See page 334

SUGAR AND ARTIFICIAL SWEETENERS

BENEFITS

- *Enhance the taste of some foods*
- *Almost immediate source of energy*
- *Sugar alcohols used in some sweets actually help to prevent dental caries*
- *Some artificial sweeteners provide very few calories*

DRAWBACKS

- *Too much sugar causes tooth decay*
- *Some people are intolerant of the milk sugar, lactose*
- *Sugary snacks can displace more nutritious foods from the diet*

To most people, sugar means table sugar (sucrose). In fact, there are many types of sugars imparting varying degrees of sweetness. The sweetest form is fructose (in fruit and honey), then sucrose (the main component of sugar cane and sugar beet), glucose (in honey, fruit and vegetables), maltose (in sprouting grains) and lactose (in milk).

Nutritionists distinguish between two types of sugars: intrinsic sugars, which are contained in the cell walls of plants, and extrinsic sugars, which are not. Intrinsic sugars occur in fruit and sweet-tasting vegetables such as carrots and beetroot. As well as providing vitamins and minerals, these foods contain fibre, which helps to make you feel full.

Extrinsic sugars include table sugar, glucose, honey, syrup, molasses and the sugar in milk. The sugar in fruit juice is also extrinsic as the fruit cells have been broken down in the juicing process. Because extrinsic sugars are damaging to teeth, the Department of Health recommends that they should make up only 10 per cent of your total calorie intake.

A SOURCE OF ENERGY

Together with starch, sugars are one of the main types of energy-providing CARBOHYDRATES. During digestion sugars are broken down into glucose, which is then released into the bloodstream and carried around the body as fuel for muscles, organs and cells.

Levels of glucose in the blood are controlled by the hormones insulin (which reduces blood glucose) and glucagon (which increases it). If the body cannot regulate its BLOOD SUGAR LEVELS, as happens with DIABETES, this can cause either hyperglycaemia, when levels become too high, or HYPOGLYCAEMIA, when levels fall too low.

Most sugars are digested quickly and so provide an almost immediate source of energy. However, the faster your blood sugar rises, the faster it falls, which is why the boost you get from a sugary drink or snack does not last and can leave you feeling rather lethargic afterwards. Eating small, regular meals and plenty of complex carbohydrates makes it easier for your body to control blood sugar levels.

IS SUGAR BAD FOR YOU?

Although links have been investigated between high intakes of sugar and increased risks of heart disease, diabetes and kidney disease, none has been scientifically proven. There is even doubt that eating a lot of sugar leads to obesity, since some studies have found that thin people eat more sugar than those who are fat.

Sugar itself does not provide any vitamins, minerals or fibre, and even though honey and brown sugar have a healthier image, they contain only very small amounts of vitamins and minerals. It is therefore important to ensure that snacks and drinks that are high in sugar do not displace more nutritious foods from the diet.

Sugar also has a suppressant effect on the appetite. This can be worrying if children fill themselves up before mealtimes with 'empty calories' from sugary drinks or CHOCOLATES AND SWEETS and therefore reduce their appetite for more nutritious foods.

Apart from the link with tooth decay, sugar itself is not thought to be harmful. Provided the overall diet is well-balanced – with adequate intakes of vitamins, minerals and fibre, and suitable proportions of fat, protein and carbohydrate – moderate amounts of sugar are nutritionally acceptable. And for most people it adds to the enjoyment of food.

One controversial theory links a diet high in refined sugar with HYPERACTIVITY. Chromium is needed for the metabolism of sugar, but it is removed from sugar during the refining process. Without it, insulin is less effective in controlling blood sugar levels, and it has been suggested that this may lead to or exacerbate hyperactivity and behavioural problems such as AGGRESSION AND DELINQUENCY. But there is insufficient scientific evidence for this theory to be accepted by the medical establishment.

The sugar in milk – or lactose – is a problem for anyone with lactose intolerance. Due to a deficiency of the enzyme lactase, they are unable to digest milk, although yoghurt and some cheeses may be tolerated. (See ALLERGIES AND FOOD INTOLERANCES.)

SUGAR AND TOOTH DECAY

Sweets and SOFT DRINKS are major causes of tooth decay, although all starches can contribute to TOOTH AND GUM DISORDERS because bacteria on the teeth can break them down to form an acid that destroys tooth enamel. Eating between meals and sipping sugary drinks and fruit juices over long periods is particularly bad for teeth because it prolongs the time they are in contact with sugar. Babies should never be given dummies that contain syrup or fruit juice to suck.

Sticky sweets and dried fruit are both high in concentrated sugar and cling to the teeth, allowing more time for acid to form. Chewing sugar-free gum after a meal can help to prevent tooth decay by stimulating the production of saliva, which washes a lot of the harmful acid away.

READING FOOD LABELS

Because sucrose (table sugar) is a preservative, and gives bulk as well as sweetness to certain foods, it is widely used in food processing. However, the food industry uses many different sorts. Sucrose, glucose, dextrose, maltose, molasses, lactose, fructose, honey, corn syrup and invert syrup are all commonly used types of sugar.

Artificial sweeteners

Artificial sweeteners fall into two categories. Although the bulk sweeteners (such as mannitol, sorbitol, xylitol and hydrogenated glucose syrup) have about the same calorific value as sugar and replace it in many processed foods, they are not so readily absorbed. The sugar alcohols, hydrogenated glucose syrup and xylitol, actually help to prevent dental caries and are used in tooth-friendly sweets and chewing gums. However, any of these bulk sweeteners can cause diarrhoea if consumed in excess of 25 g (1 oz) daily.

Intense sweeteners, such as acesulfame K, aspartame (widely sold as NutraSweet) and saccharin, provide virtually no calories and are used mainly in diet drinks and desserts and table-top sweeteners. Amazingly they are as much as 200-400 times sweeter than sugar.

Aspartame has a similar taste to sugar and unlike saccharin it does not leave a bitter aftertaste. Various claims that aspartame causes adverse reactions such as headaches, blurred vision and hyperactivity have been countered by numerous studies that have found no link. Manufacturers point out that saccharin has been used safely for more than 50 years. Equally, claims that artificial sweeteners may sometimes stimulate the appetite are dismissed by most experts.

Low-calorie drinks made with artificial sweeteners are suitable for almost everyone, including people with diabetes. However, although they do not cause tooth decay, acidic varieties, such as sugar-free fruit cordials, can harm teeth by eroding tooth enamel.

Sunburn

TAKE PLENTY OF

- *Water*
- *Orange-coloured fruits and vegetables and dark green leafy vegetables for beta carotene and vitamin C*
- *Nuts and wheatgerm for vitamin E and zinc*
- *Whole grains, fish and pulses for their B vitamins*

The painful redness of sunburn is thought to be the result of ultraviolet light penetrating the top layer of skin and forming FREE RADICALS, which then attack cell membranes and DNA. The immune system responds to this 'attack' by releasing more free radicals, which then destroy the tissues surrounding the damaged cells. Sunburn victims should drink plenty of water to combat dehydration.

Vitamin A, found in dairy produce and liver, helps in the growth and repair of body tissues and plays a role in maintaining healthy skin. Apricots, carrots and spinach are other good sources, as they contain beta carotene, which the body converts to vitamin A. The possibility that beta carotene may provide protection against sunburn by neutralising free radicals is being investigated; it may also reduce the risk of developing skin cancer caused by excessive exposure to sun. In any event always use a sun screen when exposing yourself to strong sunlight.

B vitamins are also essential for healthy skin and are found in fish and poultry, whole grains, pulses and seeds. Vitamin C, found in fruit, helps to heal burns and is essential for the formation of collagen, the protein that gives skin its elasticity. Zinc also helps to heal burns and is found in wheatgerm and nuts. Vitamin E, provided by seed oils, wheatgerm and avocados, is an ANTIOXIDANT and may help to protect against free radical damage.

Supplements

Each week, nearly a third of all adult Britons take some form of supplement in the hope that they will feel healthier. Some take a general vitamin and mineral supplement to ensure against possible deficiency; others take extracts and concentrates of specific plants to treat a particular condition. While a few supplements offer some genuine benefits, nutritionists stress that random supplementation with large amounts of individual VITAMINS and MINERALS can be harmful.

Who needs supplements?

Where requirements for specific nutrients cannot be met by the diet alone, vitamin or mineral supplements are often recommended, particularly for young children, pregnant women, vegans and elderly people.

In Britain, the government advises that until the age of two – preferably until the age of five – children should be given supplements of vitamins A, C and D. Children particularly in need of these vitamins include those from traditional Asian communities; those on diets, such as the macrobiotic diet, that exclude certain foods; and poor eaters whose source of foods is limited.

Folic acid supplements provide higher levels of intake than a normal diet can offer; they are recommended both before and during the early stages of pregnancy to reduce the risk of giving birth to a child with a neural tube defect such as spina bifida.

Some experts argue that, taken with vitamin B_{12}, folic acid supplements can also benefit middle-aged men and the elderly, since a deficiency may raise blood levels of an amino acid linked to increased risk of heart disease.

Because vegans exclude all foods of animal origin from their diet, they need to eat fortified foods, such as breakfast cereals, or take supplements of vitamin B_{12} and possibly also of vitamin D and riboflavin, and the minerals zinc, calcium, iodine and iron.

Among the elderly, normal diets seldom meet all the body's needs for vitamin D so that supplements are useful, especially for the housebound. For those with a poor appetite or a restricted diet, a multivitamin supplement may be useful to help prevent infections, boost the immune system, and reduce the risk of degenerative diseases such as cancer. Iron and vitamin C supplements are the most effective treatment for advanced iron-deficiency ANAEMIA.

Proceed with caution

There is growing evidence that more than the recommended daily amounts (RDAs) of some nutrients can reduce certain health risks – extra vitamin E, for example, may counter the threat of cardiovascular disease. But excessive quantities of some vitamins and minerals can be extremely dangerous. Vitamins A and D, for example, are fat-soluble and cannot be excreted from the body if excess amounts are taken in. Too much vitamin A can cause damage to the liver and bones, as well as birth defects. Pregnant women should therefore always avoid eating liver or taking supplements containing more than the RDA of vitamin A. Too much vitamin D can cause a build-up of calcium deposits in soft tissues such as the heart and kidneys and cause irreversible damage.

The Department of Health has put limits on levels of some vitamins, such as vitamin A, that can be sold over the counter. Any decision to take supplements in large amounts should be based on the advice of a doctor or qualified nutritionist. If you have children, always buy supplements in child-resistant containers. Iron supplements are among the most common causes of fatal poisoning among children.

STRESS: A DISEASE OF MODERN LIVING

We live in a stressful world, with little time to release the tension. If stress is not to rule our lives and ruin our health, we must take steps to relieve it – using diet, exercise and relaxation.

Good nutrition is a powerful ally when it comes to dealing with stress. Research shows that prolonged periods of day-to-day pressure can weaken the immune system and cause a high incidence of minor illnesses such as colds, coughs and flu.

Certain nutrients are used up more quickly when you are under stress: your body needs extra B vitamins for a healthy central nervous system, and vitamin C and zinc for resistance to infection. These extra requirements can easily be met by eating plenty of the foods listed in the 'anti-stress larder' (on page 336). You can boost your energy levels and reduce fatigue caused by stress by eating small, frequent meals (at least every 3 hours) based around complex carbohydrates such as wholemeal bread, pasta, rice and potatoes. Set aside a peaceful time for eating – so that you can eat slowly, relax and enjoy your meal – no matter how busy and rushed you may be during the rest of the day. Remember that excessive amounts of tea and coffee are far more likely to stimulate feelings of anxiety, rather than to calm them. Some people turn to smoking and alcohol during times of stress, but both of these rob the body of valuable nutrients. While the short-term effect of alcohol is to induce a sense of well-being, long-term use can lead to depression.

FIGHT OR FLIGHT

The body reacts to stress with a 'fight or flight' response, which harks back to our primitive beginnings, when a quick reaction was needed for survival. But this long-held instinct to react instantly to a threat or challenge is inappropriate for the present day, as the codes

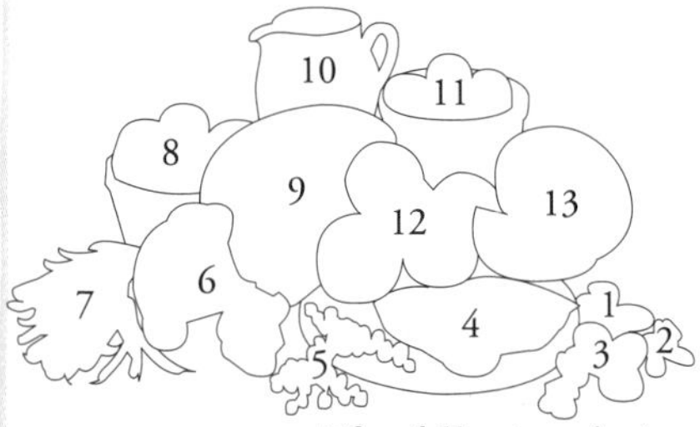

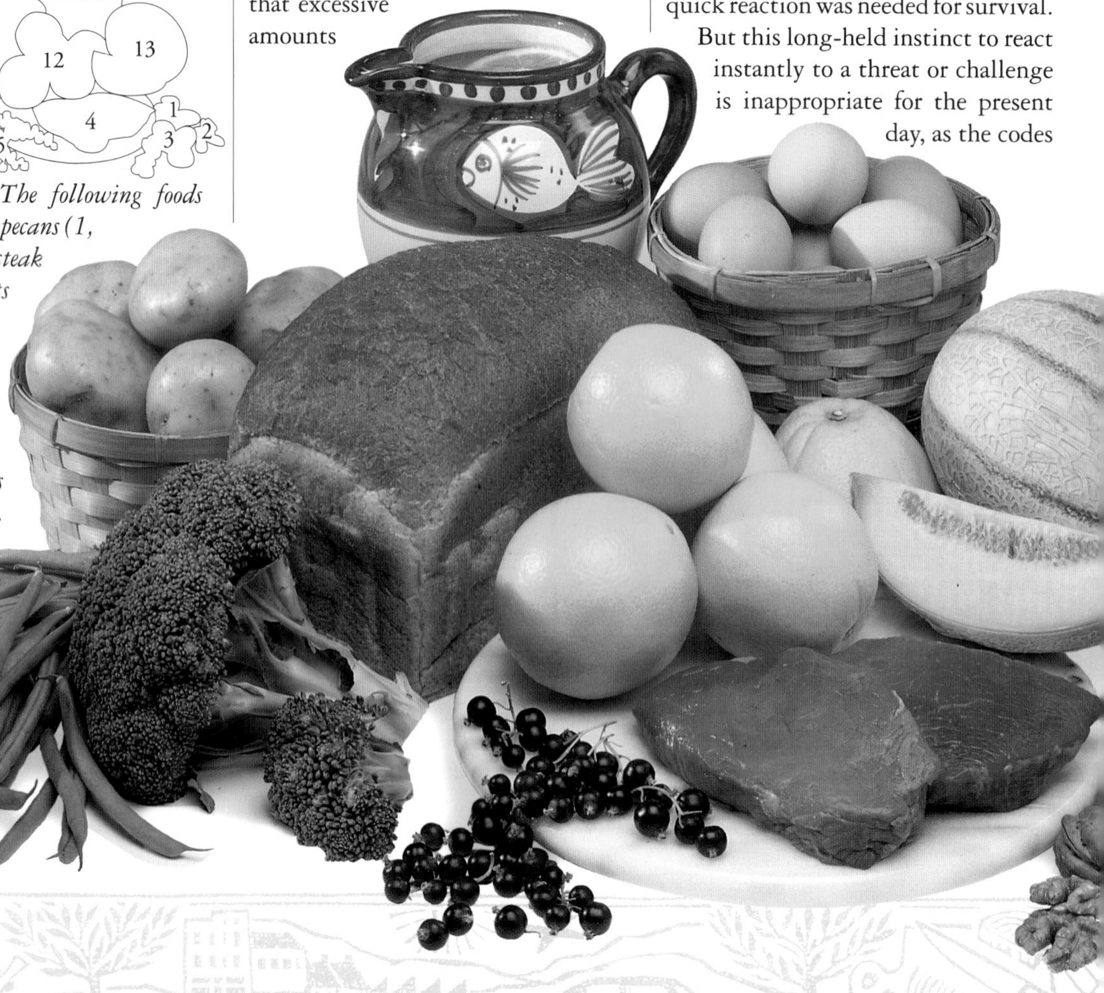

CALMING FOODS *The following foods help to beat stress: pecans (1, 2), walnuts (3), steak (4), blackcurrants (5), broccoli (6), green beans (7), potatoes (8), wholemeal bread (9), water (10), eggs (11), oranges (12), melon (13).*

STRESS RELIEVERS

- Take regular holidays.
- Eat regular and healthy meals.
- Avoid excessive amounts of caffeine, alcohol and tobacco.
- Take regular exercise.
- Practise some form of relaxation technique such as yoga, meditation and deep breathing exercises.
- Face up to work or relationship problems and do something to resolve them.
- Learn to recognise your own threshold for stress, and do not push yourself past it.
- Consider having a pet; stroking an animal can help you to relax.
- Talk about your problems. A professional counsellor will be able to help you to take an objective view of yourself, and put your problems into perspective.

of acceptable social behaviour make it impossible to choose either 'fight' or 'flight'. People often have to grin and bear it. If you can, it is better to let off some steam immediately. You could take a brisk walk or talk your problems over with a friend.

During the 'fight or flight' response, the stress hormone adrenaline causes your blood pressure to rise, giving you that familiar heart-pounding sensation. At the same time, the blood flow to the digestive system is reduced so that a greater supply can be directed towards the muscles, producing the feeling of butterflies in the stomach. Adrenaline also stimulates the release of fatty acids and glucose into the bloodstream ready to fuel the muscles.

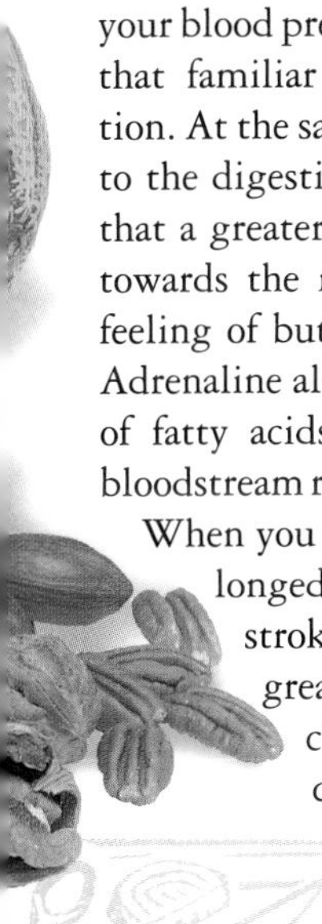

When you are under stress for prolonged periods, the risk of strokes and heart disease is greater, because the levels of circulating fats and blood cholesterol are increased, and blood platelets participate in clot formation more readily (because their 'stickiness' has increased). Physical exercise will help to clear the fat from your bloodstream.

THE MANY SIGNS OF STRESS

Stress affects the whole person – body, mind, feelings and behaviour – and can cause a wide range of symptoms. Among the most common are neck pain, headaches, pain in the lower back, teeth-grinding, feeling a 'lump in the throat', high-pitched or nervous laughter, trembling, shaking, excessive blinking and other nervous tics. Stress can also lead to more serious symptoms and disorders such as high blood pressure, migraine and digestive problems, including irritable bowel syndrome.

Other symptoms include a fast pulse, a thumping heart, hyperventilation, sweating, dryness of the throat and mouth, and difficulty in swallowing. Insomnia is common, and there

Case study

Martin, a 40-year-old GP, serves 2400 patients. In recent years he had been in the habit of starting earlier in the morning and working later into the evening, keeping himself going with cups of strong black coffee. His wife was increasingly unhappy with this arrangement; when he came home he was always irritable and tired and their three young boys hardly saw him at all. As if this were not enough, he also worked voluntarily for a local hospice, spending much of his free time there.

Although Martin was spending longer and longer at the surgery, he found that he was not actually getting through more work. The more tired he became, the longer it took to do even the most routine tasks, leaving him frustrated and even more tense. Fortunately, he recognised the symptoms of stress and took the advice that he had been giving to his patients for years. He acknowledged that he needed to take regular exercise and joined a local fitness club. Playing basketball, five-a-side football and other team sports for an hour, three times each week, left him physically exhausted but feeling mentally refreshed.

The next step was to give up coffee. The caffeine in coffee was keeping Martin wide awake, even when he wanted to get off to sleep. He found himself in the vicious circle of drinking too much coffee, not resting, feeling tired, and reaching for the coffee again. Once the cycle had been broken, Martin was able to sleep soundly when he needed to, giving him energy to face the next day. Martin has moderated the time he spends at the surgery, finding that his renewed vigour means he is more efficient. He still helps at the hospice, and has a lot more energy. But perhaps the greatest benefit is that he is able to spend more time with his family.

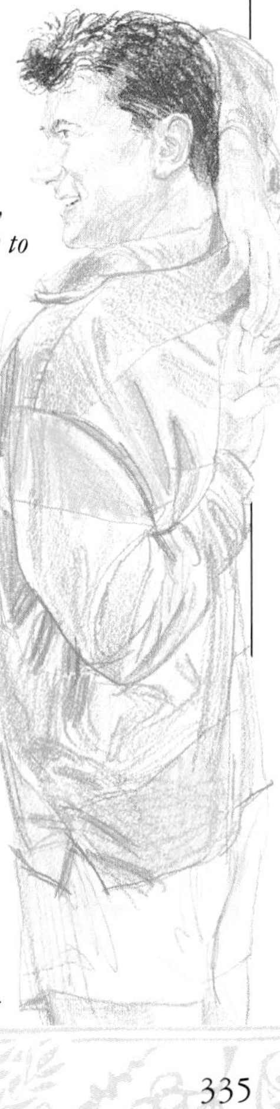

may also be dizziness, weakness and a lack of energy. In addition stress may cause increased stomach acid secretion which can lead to ulcers.

The manifestations of stress are not limited to physical symptoms: you can also end up with poor concentration, vague anxiety or fear for no apparent reason, and periods of irritability followed by depression and lethargy.

A POSITIVE VIEW ON STRESS

You cannot spend your life avoiding stress, and you should not try to. Stress is a normal and natural element in life, and many people find it enjoyable to use their stress to overcome physical, intellectual and social challenges. Extending yourself in this way helps to keep you healthy, active and young – as long as you also know how to relax.

TIME TO RELAX

It is important to balance times of stress with periods of relaxation. Do something that takes your mind off your problems, such as gardening, walking, playing a sport, meditating or listening to soothing music.

By learning to face each new challenge as it arises, and by knowing how to switch off before fatigue and frustration set in, you can use your stress to motivate you and make life more interesting and fulfilling.

ANTI-STRESS LARDER

Take care to include some of the following foods in your diet when you are under stress, because vital nutrients are being used up more quickly.

B vitamins, to release energy and to maintain a healthy nervous system. Found in green vegetables, potatoes, fresh fruit, wheatgerm, wholegrain cereals (such as brown rice), eggs, dairy products, yeast extract, seafood, lean meat, liver, kidney, poultry, pulses (peas, beans and lentils), nuts, seeds and dried fruit.

Vitamin C, to help the body to resist infection and for wound healing. Found in fresh fruits, especially citrus fruits and blackcurrants, fruit juices and fresh vegetables.

Zinc, for resistance to infection and for wound healing. Found in liver and red meat, egg yolks, dairy produce, wholegrain cereals and seafood – particularly oysters and other shellfish.

Complex carbohydrates, to boost energy and calm the mind. Found in bread, rice, pulses, oats, pasta and potatoes. These foods supply a steady stream of energy to the body, and also have a calming effect on the brain.

ARE YOU STRESSED?

It is often difficult to take an objective view of yourself to see how stressed you really are. However, some common signs of stress are easy to spot. Do you:

- Often feel close to tears?
- Easily snap and shout at those around you at home and work?
- Have a reduced sex drive?
- Sleep badly?
- Fidget, bite your nails or fiddle with your hair?
- Find it hard to concentrate, and impossible to make decisions?
- Find it increasingly hard just to talk to people?
- Eat when you are not hungry or skip meals altogether?
- Feel tired most of the time?
- Think that your sense of humour has gone for good?
- Feel suspicious of others?
- Drink or smoke more to help you through the most difficult days?
- Feel that you just cannot cope?

If you answer yes to more than four of these questions, then you are stressed and need to incorporate some 'stress relievers' (see page 335) into your routine.

THE STRESS HIT LIST

Stress can be set off by important changes in life – even pleasant ones. Individual responses vary, but some events and changes are much more likely to cause stress than others. They are rated here according to the amount of stress they are likely to cause.

Highest stress rating
Death of partner
Divorce or separation
Prison sentence
Death of a close relative
Personal injury or illness
Marriage
Loss of job
Moving house

High stress rating
Reconciliation with partner
Retirement
Serious ill health in the family
Pregnancy
Sexual problems
New baby/family member
Change of job
Money problems
Death of a close friend

Moderate stress rating
Family arguments
Taking on a large mortgage
Legal action over a debt
New responsibilities at work
Child starting/finishing school
Son/daughter leaving home
Difficulties with in-laws
Change in living conditions
Problems with boss

Lower stress rating
Change in working conditions
Change of schools
Holidays
Change in contact with relatives
Minor violations of the law
Joining/leaving a social group
Christmas
Small mortgage or loan

The many sources of stress

People have always experienced stress, right from the earliest times, although in prehistoric days people were probably better at working it out of their systems. But with our increasingly ordered and controlled lifestyles, stress can build up to intolerable levels, causing all manner of illnesses. It is not just the bad things in life which cause stress, but happy occasions, too. We are creatures of habit and fear the unknown, so that stress occurs whenever there is a major change in our lives, be it a death, a divorce, a wedding or a birth. However, if you can cultivate a positive attitude towards stress you can make it work for you instead of letting it ruin your life.

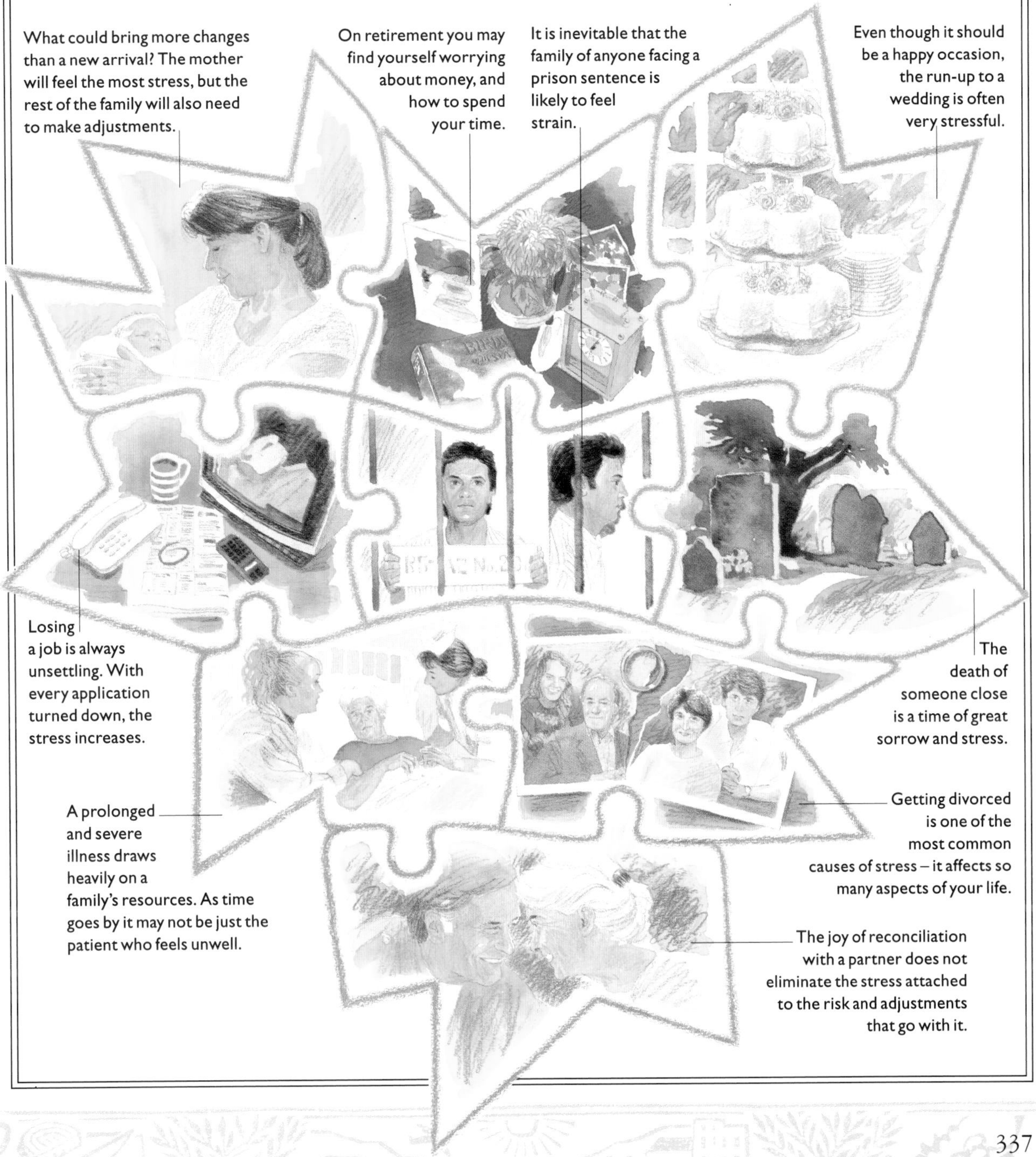

What could bring more changes than a new arrival? The mother will feel the most stress, but the rest of the family will also need to make adjustments.

On retirement you may find yourself worrying about money, and how to spend your time.

It is inevitable that the family of anyone facing a prison sentence is likely to feel strain.

Even though it should be a happy occasion, the run-up to a wedding is often very stressful.

Losing a job is always unsettling. With every application turned down, the stress increases.

The death of someone close is a time of great sorrow and stress.

A prolonged and severe illness draws heavily on a family's resources. As time goes by it may not be just the patient who feels unwell.

Getting divorced is one of the most common causes of stress – it affects so many aspects of your life.

The joy of reconciliation with a partner does not eliminate the stress attached to the risk and adjustments that go with it.

SWEATING TO EXCESS

TAKE PLENTY OF

- *Fluids – at least 1.7 litres (3 pints) per day to replace lost fluids*

Loss of moisture through the skin is a normal, vital function that helps the body to regulate its temperature. Although it can be troublesome, it seldom indicates a medical problem. Moderately active adults are advised to make up the lost fluid by drinking at least 1.7 litres (3 pints) of water a day. Athletes and very active people need to drink more – an extra litre (1¾ pints) per hour of activity – while patients with fever should drink as much as they can, within reason, even if they do not feel thirsty.

Very heavy sweating can lead to excessive salt loss, which is usually accompanied by dehydration. Because consuming salty foods can exacerbate dehydration, it is best to rehydrate by drinking water together with food, or by taking a rehydration solution made by mixing eight teaspoons of sugar and one teaspoon of salt with 1 litre (1¾ pints) of water.

Doctors do not know why some people sweat more than others, but they believe that the condition can be inherited. Excessive sweating can occasionally be a sign of illness. It is one of the symptoms of an overactive thyroid gland, which increases the body's metabolic rate – the speed at which food and oxygen are burned to provide energy. Other symptoms include a rapid pulse, weight loss, irritability and an increased appetite. Sweating is also obviously exacerbated by heat, but ANXIETY and OBESITY can also accentuate the problem.

Some herbalists believe that the unpleasant body odour that accompanies heavy sweating may be due to a deficiency of zinc, which can lead to kidney complaints and excess urea being excreted through the skin. Once the deficiency is corrected, the odour may disappear. Lean meat, nuts and shellfish are all good sources of zinc. Many practitioners of natural medicine also believe that sweating helps in the removal of toxins from the body, and that while attention to personal hygiene is desirable, it should not involve the complete suppression of sweating with antiperspirants.

SWEDES

BENEFITS

- *May help to protect against cancer*
- *Useful source of vitamin C*

DRAWBACK

- *High intakes increase the requirement for iodine*

Cruciferous vegetables, which include swedes and turnips, as well as members of the cabbage family, contain chemical compounds that many scientists believe may help to prevent some cancers. The two most widely studied of these chemicals are indoles and isothiocyanates. Experiments indicate that indoles may protect against breast cancer by stimulating enzymes that reduce the effects of the hormone oestrogen, which is thought to encourage this type of cancerous growth. Isothiocyanates are thought to trigger the formation of enzymes that protect DNA (the genetic material that is found in all cells) against damage by carcinogens.

One disadvantage of these compounds is that they rob the thyroid gland of iodine and can cause an iodine deficiency if you do not get much of this mineral from your diet. Iodine is found in seafood and seaweed, and is needed for the thyroid gland to be able to produce the hormones that control the body's metabolism and therefore its healthy growth and development.

Cooking swedes makes it easier for the body to absorb indoles and isothiocyanates, but as with other vegetables, it reduces the vitamin C content. Nevertheless, a 100g (3½oz) portion of boiled swede is still a useful source of this vitamin. They are also an excellent food for anyone who is trying to lose weight: a typical 100g (3½oz) cooked serving contains only 11 Calories.

Although swedes originated in Bohemia, they came to England via Sweden – hence their name, shortened from Swedish turnips. In Scotland, they are still called turnips or 'neeps'.

SWEET POTATO

BENEFITS

- *Excellent source of beta carotene*
- *Good source of potassium and a useful source of vitamin C*

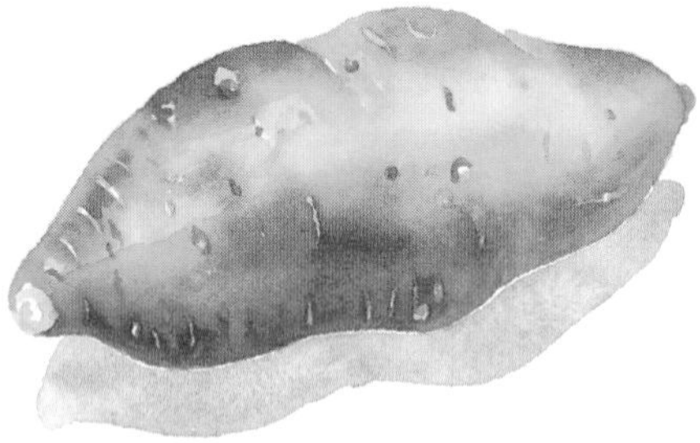

Despite their sweetness, sweet potatoes are a starchy vegetable. They supply about the same amount of calories as new potatoes – 84 Calories per 100g (3½oz) portion compared with the 77 Calories provided by white potatoes. There are two sorts of sweet potato: the moist, orange-fleshed variety and the dry, creamy-fleshed type. Both contribute potassium, vitamin C and fibre to the diet, but the orange-fleshed sweet potato is also an excellent source of beta carotene, which may help to prevent certain types of cancer.

TEA

See page 344

THROMBOSIS

EAT PLENTY OF

- *Oily fish, for omega-3 fatty acids*
- *Oat bran and pulses for fibre*
- *Onions and garlic which may help to prevent blood clots*

CUT DOWN ON

- *Animal and dairy products which are high in saturated fats and cholesterol*
- *Salt, which raises blood pressure*
- *Smoking*

A diet that is low in saturated fats, high in fibre and contains plenty of fruit and vegetables helps to reduce the risk of atherosclerosis, a form of HEART DISEASE, in which fatty deposits build up in the linings of the blood vessels. This can lead to thrombosis, which occurs when one of the fatty plaques narrows a blood vessel and a blood clot, or thrombus, forms, blocking the flow of blood. Cut down on foods high in saturated fat, such as dairy products, as well as foods that have a high salt content (which can raise blood pressure), such as yeast extract, bacon or sausages.

HELPFUL FOODS

Not all fats are bad for you, however. Some polyunsaturated fats contain omega-3 fatty acids which make blood

REDUCING THE RISKS *The key to avoiding thrombosis is a diet low in saturated fat and high in fibre and omega-3 fatty acids found in some oils and oily fish.*

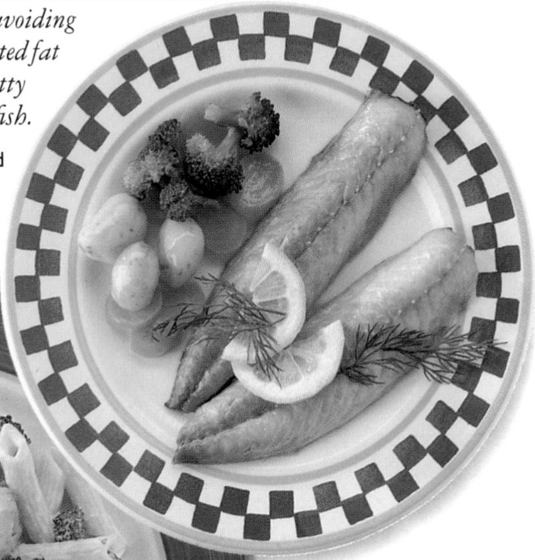

Grilled mackerel served with vegetables provides essential omega-3 fatty acids and plenty of fibre.

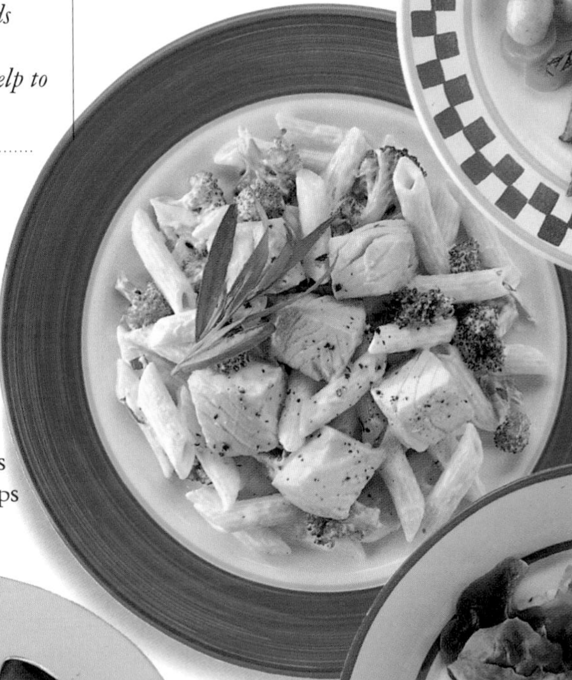

Broccoli and salmon pasta is high in fibre and vitamin C, but low in saturated fat.

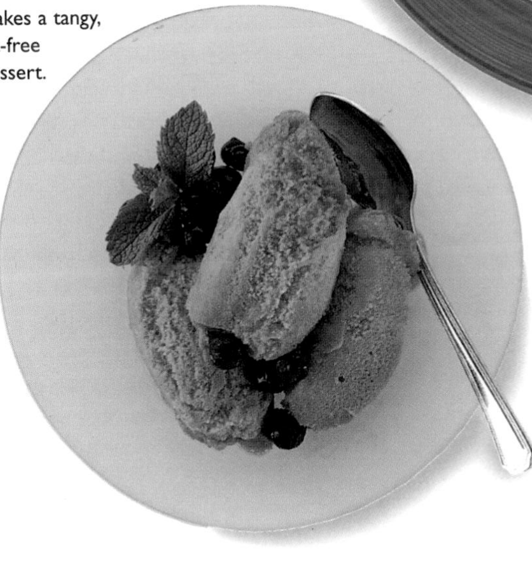

Blackcurrant sorbet makes a tangy, fat-free dessert.

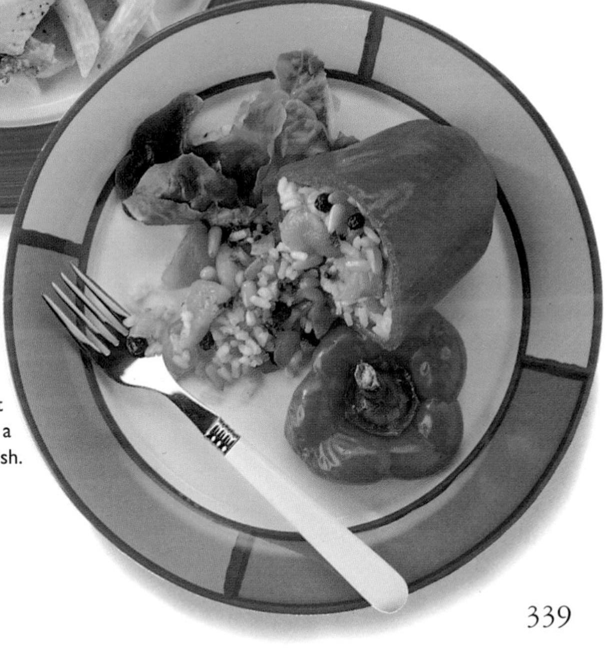

Peppers with moist pine nut and apricot stuffing is a high-fibre dish.

platelets less 'sticky' – so helping to prevent blood clots. They are found in oily FISH such as mackerel, herring and trout. Try to eat a meal including one of these fish two or three times a week.

Raw ONION is thought to guard against the harmful effects of fatty foods by increasing the rate at which blood clots are broken down. Fresh GARLIC is also thought to reduce the risk of blood clots. However, you would have to eat ten or more cloves a day for a significant effect.

The risk of thrombosis increases with age, while other factors known to make it more likely include obesity, smoking and physical inactivity. Although you cannot stop the years passing, you can help to reduce your risk of thrombosis by cutting down on smoking, keeping to a healthy weight and taking regular exercise. Moderate ALCOHOL consumption (two glasses of wine a day) is acceptable and may also lower the risk of thrombosis by causing the dilation of small blood vessels.

Types of thrombosis

If a thrombus blocks an artery, the part of the body beyond it is deprived of blood and therefore of oxygen and nutrients. If a limb is affected, the deprived area soon becomes pale, swollen and painful. If a coronary artery is blocked, the heart muscle is deprived of blood, which can then trigger a heart attack. A clot in the blood vessels supplying the brain may cause a stroke.

A thrombus in the veins can be just as serious. Deep-vein thrombosis usually occurs in the legs. It can sometimes follow surgery, but is less likely to occur if patients get up and about as soon as possible. Other contributory factors are obesity, some contraceptive pills and immobility.

If a clot from a deep-vein thrombus becomes dislodged, it can cause an embolism. If it moves to the lungs (a pulmonary embolism) it can be fatal. Thrombophlebitis is an inflammation of the veins closest to the skin. It usually affects the legs and may be associated with varicose veins.

THRUSH

Also known as candidiasis, thrush is a fungal infection caused by the yeast organism *Candida albicans*. Oral and vaginal thrush are the most common forms, followed by skin infections in areas where surface damage is caused by a combination of damp and friction – under the breasts, for example. Young babies can develop thrush in the mouth, and the fungus can exacerbate the problems of nappy rash.

Severe candida infections usually arise when the immune system is compromised in some way. For example, when the body is already fighting off another illness or infection such as flu. Anyone taking antibiotics, hormonal or steroidal drugs such as those prescribed for asthma, or people suffering from stress are also susceptible.

UNFRIENDLY INVASION

Candida albicans is one of many micro-organisms which live naturally in the mouth and gut and on the skin. These micro-organisms cause problems only when they multiply out of control and the benign yeast form changes into its invasive fungal form.

Normally *Candida albicans* is kept in check by the body's 'friendly' bacteria. But if the protective bacteria are destroyed or the immune system is weakened, for example by taking a broad-spectrum antibiotic over a long period of time, the candida cells can multiply and cause infections. All babies are born without protection and receive their first dose of 'friendly' bacteria from their mother's birth canal, skin and breast milk, which helps their gut to establish immunity to all sorts of infections. Formula and cow's milk contain as little as 20 per cent of the friendly bacteria found in breast milk. However, the mother will also pass *Candida albicans* on to her baby.

Yoghurt cure for thrush

The most common form of this condition is vaginal thrush, which results in a white discharge and irritation and soreness in and around the vagina. For years some doctors have advised women to insert live yoghurt into the vagina to produce a more acid environment in order to encourage the growth of protective natural bacteria to help fight the infection.

In a letter to *The Lancet* from the Department of Microbiology at the University of Western Ontario in Canada, researchers describe the treatment of one patient using a more sophisticated technique. In 30 months a 33-year-old woman had suffered 20 episodes of vaginal infection, many of them thrush. She was given one pessary, which contained freeze-dried lactobacillus bacteria (similar to the friendly bacteria found in live yoghurt) to insert into her vagina. Within two days she was free of her symptoms and remained so for seven weeks. In the following six months she used two more pessaries and stayed free from thrush.

THE YEAST FACTOR

Although it is refuted by orthodox medicine, some alternative practitioners claim that people who suffer from recurrent thrush should avoid all foods that contain sugar, which yeasts feed on, and foods containing any form of yeast, mould or fungi, such as bread, mushrooms, grapes, wine, yeast extracts and 'mouldy' cheeses. They claim that if a person is already sensitive to one type of yeast, they should avoid all other forms as well. This sensitivity to yeasts is blamed for a host of problems: fatigue, bloating in the stomach, depression, anxiety, aches in the muscles and joints, other fungal infections and skin rashes.

The alternative practitioners go on to say that in its invasive form, *Candida albicans* can eventually penetrate the mucous membrane of the gut, allowing toxins to leak into the bloodstream and infect the whole body.

However, many doctors argue that there is little scientific proof that a yeast exclusion diet is of any more benefit than a healthy, balanced diet.

THYROID DISORDERS

EAT PLENTY OF

- *Foods rich in B vitamins, such as fish, whole grains, pulses and seeds, to counter the weight loss associated with an overactive thyroid gland*

CUT DOWN ON

- *Raw cabbage, turnips, swedes, peanuts and mustard, which can inhibit the body's ability to use iodine*
- *Smoking, alcohol and caffeine, if the problem is an overactive thyroid gland*

The thyroid gland, which sits in front of the windpipe just below the Adam's apple, produces iodine-containing hormones that control the body's metabolic rate – the speed at which food and oxygen are burnt to produce energy for growth, exercise and times of stress. Iodine is needed in the diet for the normal functioning of the thyroid gland. Iodine-deficiency is one of the world's most common nutritional diseases and results in a condition called endemic goitre. The term goitre is used to describe the enlargement of the thyroid gland which is associated with the condition.

Iodine deficiency is, however, quite rare in the developed world, usually occurring in areas where dietary iodine intake is low because of low levels of the mineral in soil and water. In such areas, the amount of iodine in the diet should be increased. The richest food sources are saltwater fish and seaweed. Eggs, yoghurt, milk, hard cheese and iodised salt are also useful sources.

FOODS TO WATCH

Some foods, such as raw cabbage, turnips, swedes, peanuts and mustard, can interfere with the body's ability to use iodine in the production of the thyroid hormones. These foods are called goitrogens, but are not of any nutritional significance unless their intake

Case study

Dorothy went to see her doctor because she had been experiencing pain in her left hand for the past few weeks. The doctor soon realised that she had carpal tunnel syndrome, a painful condition where a nerve in the wrist becomes squeezed by swelling in the tissues. He also noticed that Dorothy had dry, rough skin and coarse hair and her face was puffy and pale. These symptoms indicated that she might have a form of hypothyroidism. He asked her some questions and found that Dorothy always felt the cold, tended to be constipated and had been gradually putting on weight. Blood tests were arranged and the results showed that she had too little thyroid hormone in her blood.

To his surprise the doctor discovered that because of previous cases of thyroid disease in her family Dorothy had a fear of thyroid disease and had been eating foods with a high iodine content, such as seafood, seaweed and watercress, in addition to regularly taking iodine supplements. She had been making the condition worse. Although her thyroid gland was producing thyroid hormone in the correct quantities, the excess iodine was preventing its release into the bloodstream.

Dorothy was persuaded not to take the iodine supplements and was given dietary advice to reduce the amount of iodine-rich foods she ate. When she returned to her doctor a few months later most of her symptoms had improved: she was pleased to report that she had regained her old energy and that her hand was no longer painful at night.

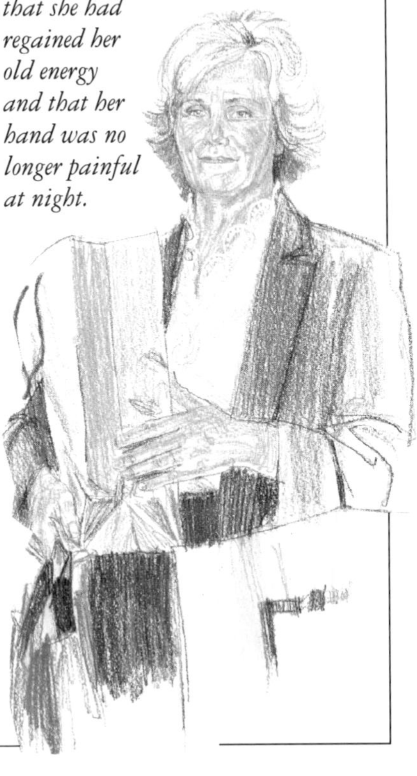

is excessive. They precipitate goitre only when iodine intake is marginal. Groups most at risk include vegans.

In developed countries, goitre is more likely to be the result of an auto-immune disease, which impairs the functioning of the thyroid gland, leading to underactivity.

AN UNDERACTIVE THYROID

Hypothyroidism, the term used to describe an underactive thyroid gland, causes the body's metabolism to slow down. The illness develops slowly; apart from goitre, early symptoms include tiredness, forgetfulness, weight gain, sensitivity to cold, constipation and dry skin and hair. If the condition is due to an auto-immune disease, hypothyroidism arises because the body develops antibodies against its own thyroid gland, which leads to a reduction in hormone production. Hypothyroidism is prevalent in the elderly, but can affect people of all ages. If it occurs in childhood, it may cause retarded growth, inhibit normal brain development and delay sexual maturity. As a precaution, babies are now screened for it at birth.

An underactive thyroid gland is a common cause of raised blood cholesterol levels in women. It is usually treated by giving the thyroid hormone thyroxine. Patients with thyroid disease have a reduced capacity to convert beta carotene – found in some orange-coloured fruit and vegetables and dark green leafy vegetables – to vitamin A. This results in the build up of carotene in the blood and tissues, giving a yellow tinge to the skin.

AN OVERACTIVE THYROID

Hyperthyroidism (overactivity of the thyroid gland) is where the gland is producing excessive amounts of the two main thyroid hormones, with the result that many of the body's processes, such as the heart rate, speed up. Other symptoms of an overactive thyroid gland include weight loss, fatigue, increased appetite, irritability, goitre, sweating, sensitivity to heat and bulging eyes.

Because of the increase in their metabolic rate, people with an overactive thyroid burn calories and use vital nutrients much faster than normal. A diet rich in all nutrients should therefore complement medical treatment.

If weight loss is a serious problem, additional protein, in the form of fish and eggs for example, may be necessary to replace muscle tissue that has been lost. Adequate intake of the B vitamins, which can be found in whole grains, potatoes and dairy products, is essential for the metabolism of the extra carbohydrates and protein.

The cause of thyroid overactivity is usually the presence of antibodies that stimulate thyroid cells, but what causes these antibodies to be produced by the body is still unknown. Hyperthyroidism tends to run in families and the condition is more common in women than in men.

If you suffer from hyperthyroidism, limiting nicotine, alcohol and caffeine (found in tea, coffee, colas and plain chocolate) may reduce the symptoms as they can all raise the metabolic rate.

Goitre

A swollen neck due to an enlargement of the thyroid gland is known as a goitre. The swelling is usually soft, although it may be hard and lumpy. In some cases goitres can grow to be quite large, causing a considerable increase in collar size, and can even compress the windpipe.

When an overactive thyroid gland produces a goitre, it will probably be accompanied by various other symptoms, such as sweating, racing pulse, slightly bulging eyes and weight loss.

Alternatively, when an underactive thyroid leads to the formation of a goitre, it may be accompanied by symptoms such as dry and coarse hair, sensitivity to cold, weight gain and fatigue.

A goitre may also result from a lack of dietary iodine. In this case it is not accompanied by any other symptoms. Iodine-rich foods such as seaweed may help, but avoid foods such as raw cabbage, turnips and swedes, which inhibit the body's ability to use iodine in the production of thyroid hormones.

TINNED OR CANNED FOODS

BENEFITS

- *Long shelf-life*
- *Retain many nutrients, including protein, and vitamins A, D and riboflavin*
- *Sterile and safe*

DRAWBACKS

- *Many tinned foods are high in salt*
- *Colour, texture and taste of foods are altered*
- *Some nutrients are lost*

The process of canning preserves food by sealing it in airtight containers and cooking it to a sufficiently high temperature to ensure that it is sterile. Because any micro-organisms inside the container are killed and air is excluded, tinned foods will keep for a long time without deteriorating.

Most tinned foods will keep for at least a year; others, such as corned beef, salmon and fish in oil are perfectly safe after four or five years. A 'best-before' date is usually found stamped or indented on one end of the tin. After that date it does not necessarily mean that the food is dangerous, but it may no longer be at its best. Even tinned foods start to deteriorate eventually.

The canning process has virtually no effect on protein, carbohydrates, fats, or the vitamins A, D and riboflavin that the food may contain. But, the high temperatures involved in the process tend to destroy thiamin (vitamin B_1) and vitamin C in vegetables and savoury foods. Tinned fruit and fruit juices, however, retain most of their vitamins. The extent of the vitamin loss largely depends upon the acidity of the product; most acid foods retain their vitamin C well.

As with any other form of cooking, the canning process will usually produce changes to the colour, texture and flavour of foods. Furthermore, tinned foods often contain relatively high levels of salt, so it is always worth checking the label.

If you open a tin and use only part of its contents, do not store the remainder in the tin in case the metal taints the food once it is exposed to the air. Instead, transfer leftovers into a covered container, store in a refrigerator, and use within two days.

AVOID DAMAGED TINS

Tins should not be used if they are dented or rusty, particularly along the seam. If the tin looks distorted, and the ends appear swollen, it means that gas-producing micro-organisms are likely to be inside. Throw away the tin, and do not attempt to open it, because it may contain poisonous bacteria.

There used to be widespread concern over the dangers of fatal FOOD POISONING from botulism. This is caused by the toxin produced by the bacterium *Clostridium botulinum*, the spores of which are very heat resistant, and may survive inadequate heat sterilisation of tinned foods. Technology is now so advanced that botulism from this source is extremely rare.

TOFU (SOYA BEAN CURD)

BENEFITS
- *High in protein*
- *Low in saturated fats*
- *Good source of calcium and a useful source of vitamin E*
- *May help to protect against some forms of cancer and heart disease*

DRAWBACK
- *Soya is a common food allergen*

Known as the 'cheese of Asia', soft creamy coloured tofu is made by grinding cooked soya beans to produce a milk that is then solidified with a mineral coagulant (calcium sulphate). Tofu is high in protein, very low in saturated fats, and cholesterol-free. A 100g (3½oz) serving of steamed tofu contains about 73 Calories.

Tofu is naturally bland and can therefore be used in both sweet and savoury dishes. There are two basic types: silken tofu, which is soft and suitable for making dressings, sauces and dairy-free products such as ice cream or cheesecake, and firm tofu, which is more solid and can be marinated to give it some flavour. Firm tofu can be stir-fried, grilled, scrambled, pickled, smoked, baked and even barbecued.

Steamed tofu is a good source of calcium (from the calcium sulphate used to make it) and a useful source of manganese and vitamin E. It also contains phosphorus and iron, and is therefore a particularly useful part of a balanced vegetarian diet. Tofu can be substituted for meat in many recipes, from traditional English shepherd's pie to oriental dishes such as teriyaki.

Soya beans and soya-bean products such as tofu and soya sauce are also being examined for their possible role in protecting against cancer (particularly breast cancer), osteoporosis and menopausal symptoms. Their protective qualities are attributed to the hormonal activity of phytoestrogens present in these foods. Soya beans and their products may also help to lower blood cholesterol, thereby protecting against cardiovascular disease.

Because the soya bean's fibre is removed during the manufacturing process, tofu is extremely easy to digest. However, it will absorb about 15 per cent of the fat used for frying. Soya is also known to be one of the more common food allergens.

When buying fresh tofu, smell it first to make sure that it is not sour. Packaged tofu will have a freshness date stamped on the wrapping. Rinse the tofu and store it in the refrigerator in fresh cold water. Change the water daily and use within three to four days.

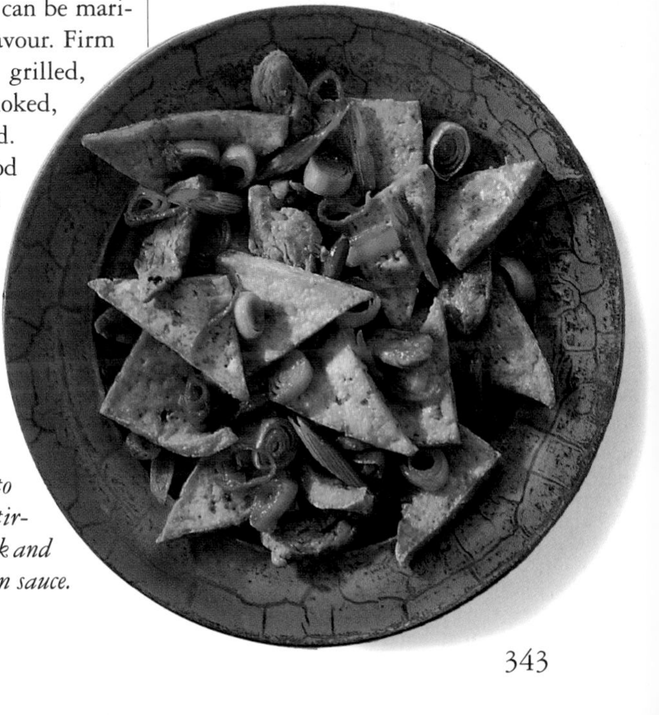

FOOD FROM THE ORIENT
In this dish, tofu is cut into triangles, deep fried then stir-fried with thin slices of pork and vegetables in a yellow-bean sauce.

TEA: A GENTLE STIMULANT

The British have been drinking tea for more than 300 years; today, it accounts for nearly half the fluid intake of a British adult. But can you have too much of a good thing?

There is sometimes nothing more reviving than a cup of tea, but in fact it has little nutritional value – although the milk or sugar added may supply around 40 calories. However, the stimulants such as caffeine that tea contains can accelerate the heart rate, increase alertness, and help respiration by dilating the airways of the lungs. A single cup of tea provides about 40mg of caffeine, which is almost twice the amount present in most cola drinks and about two-thirds the level found in a cup of instant coffee.

The tannins in tea are not as useful however. They give it body but can interfere with iron absorption, especially if tea is drunk with iron-rich foods. Toddlers should not be given tea because their digestive systems are less able to cope with its chemical stimulants and there is the possibility of developing iron-deficiency anaemia.

Tannins can also stain teeth, particularly dental work. Mouthwashes which contain chlorhexidine should not be used immediately prior to drinking tea because the chemical can accentuate the staining effect.

Tea also contains considerable levels of quercetin, one of the many naturally occurring chemical compounds that are known as bioflavonoids. Although preliminary research indicated that quercetin might be involved in causing cancer, more recent work suggests that high intakes of bioflavonoids, which are strong antioxidants, are associated with a decreased risk of cancer and heart disease. In particular, green tea and Oolong tea are thought to have specific anti-cancer properties. However, there is still conflicting evidence and the encouraging results of laboratory experiments have not yet been replicated in population studies.

Other constituents of tea, besides added flavourings such as bergamot, include fluoride (0.25 mg in a cup) and manganese (0.5 mg per cup).

People suffering from peptic ulcers should avoid strong black tea because, like coffee, it stimulates acidic gastric secretion and may cause irritation; instead, they should drink weak tea with milk. Tea has also been known to precipitate MIGRAINE in sensitive individuals; it is not known, however, whether this is due to its bioflavonoid or its caffeine content.

BENEFITS

- *Mild stimulant*
- *Supplies quercetin – an antioxidant that may lower the risk of heart disease and cancer*

DRAWBACKS

- *Decreases the absorption of iron from food when consumed at mealtimes*
- *Tannins in tea can stain teeth*
- *May trigger migraine in susceptible individuals*
- *May cause gastric irritation*

HERBAL TEAS

These teas, tisanes or infusions made from the leaves, blossoms and fruits of many plants, have become increasingly popular. Many are credited with medical benefits although there is as yet little scientific evidence to justify the claims. There is now an enormous range of herbal teas available in health food shops and supermarkets, but the herbal remedies (overleaf) – which have all been recommended by the National Institute of Medical Herbalists – can be safely and easily prepared at home. Allow one teaspoon of the dried herb (or two of the fresh) per cup. Pour boiling water over the herb, cover and infuse for about 5 minutes, then strain before drinking. Use honey or sugar to sweeten the tea, if desired.

ICED TEA – A SUMMER TREAT

An English merchant, Richard Blechynden was visiting the United States in 1904 in order to promote Indian tea. Finding few takers on a scorching day at the St Louis World Fair, he decided to pour tea over ice cubes – and iced tea was born.

Tea experts recommend the following method of preparation: Steep 60g (2oz) of tea in 1.2 litres (2 pints) of freshly drawn cold water for at least three hours, or overnight. Strain the cold tea into a large jug and keep refrigerated. Pour into a glass over ice cubes; an added slice of lemon is optional.

Many people sweeten their iced tea with a little sugar, while adding fresh mint leaves makes a refreshing summer variant.

HEALING TEAS *Leaves, seeds and flowers are all used by herbalists in their quest for the most effective natural remedies.*

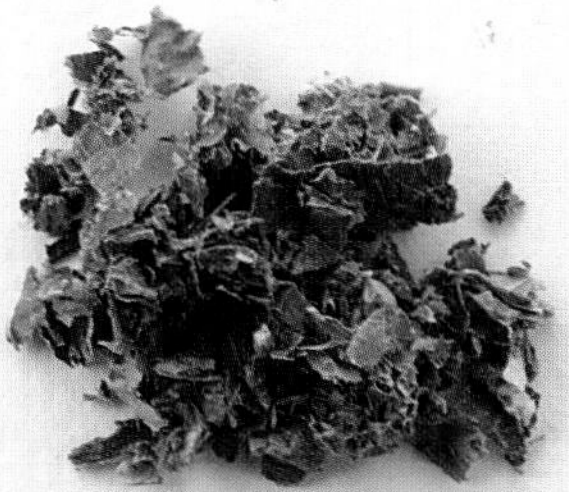

Raspberry leaf

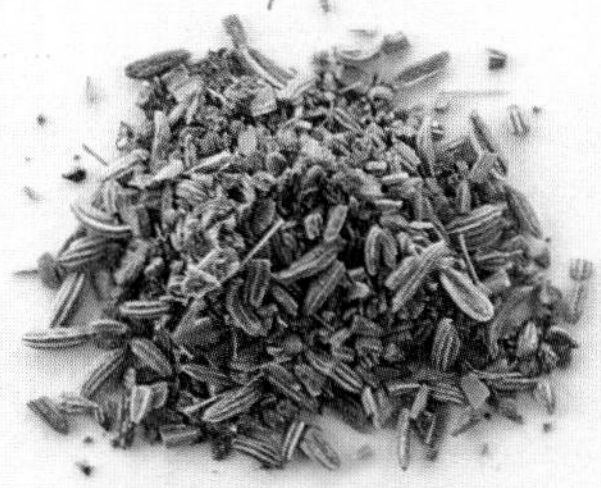

Fennel seed

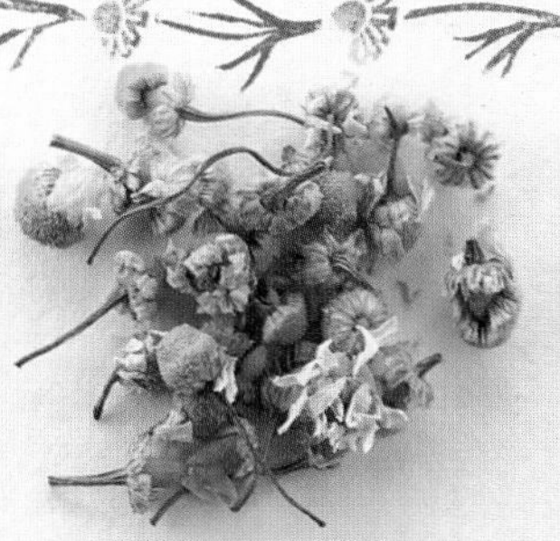

Camomile

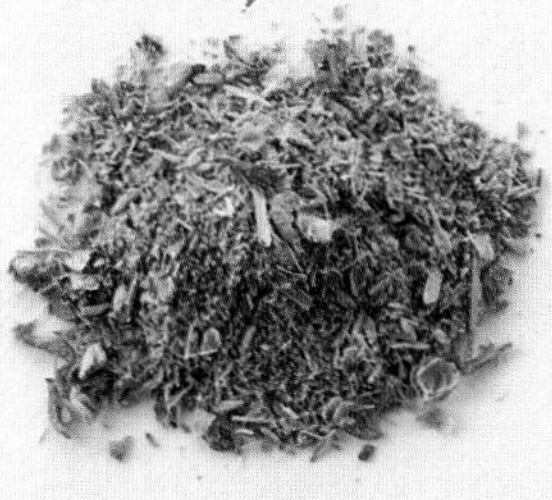

Thyme

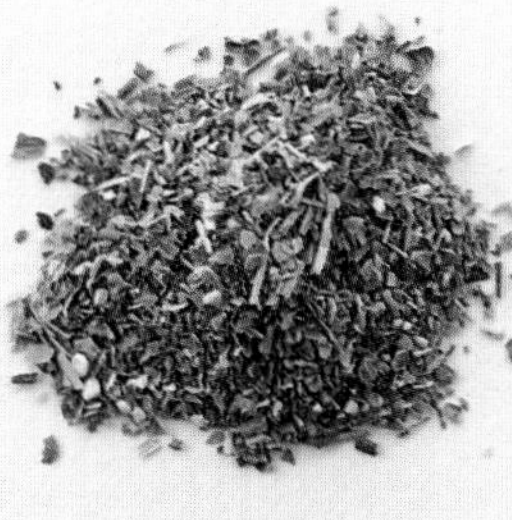

Dandelion

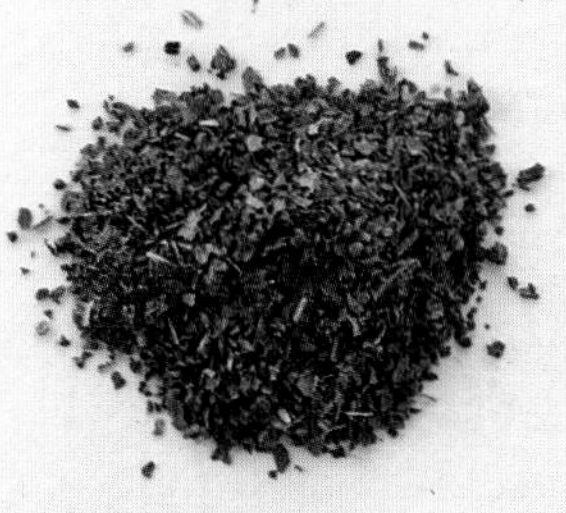

Nettle leaf

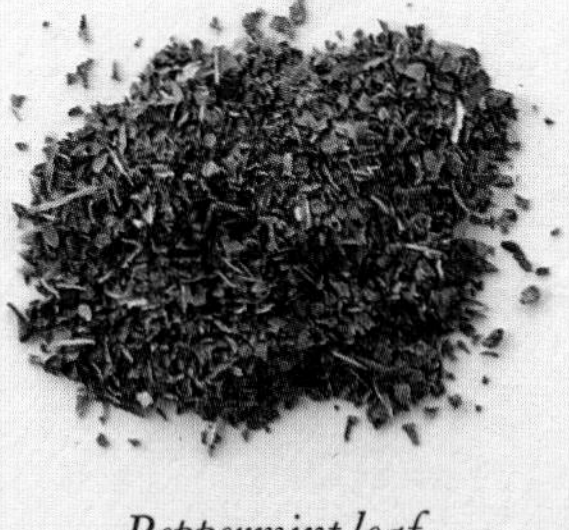

Peppermint leaf

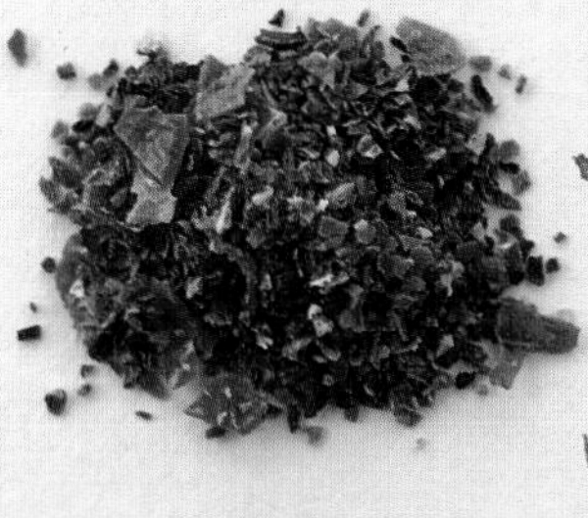

Rosehip

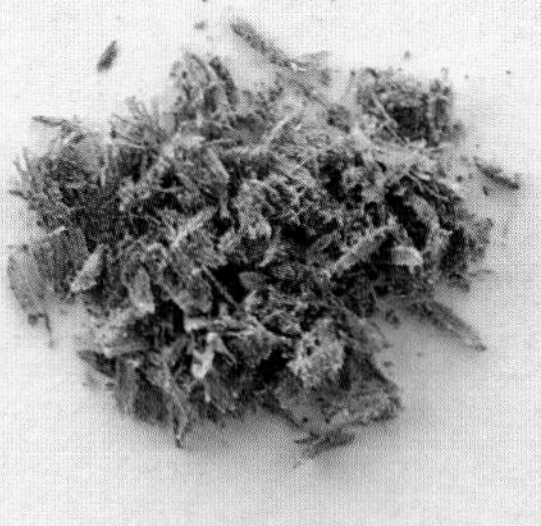

Lavender flower

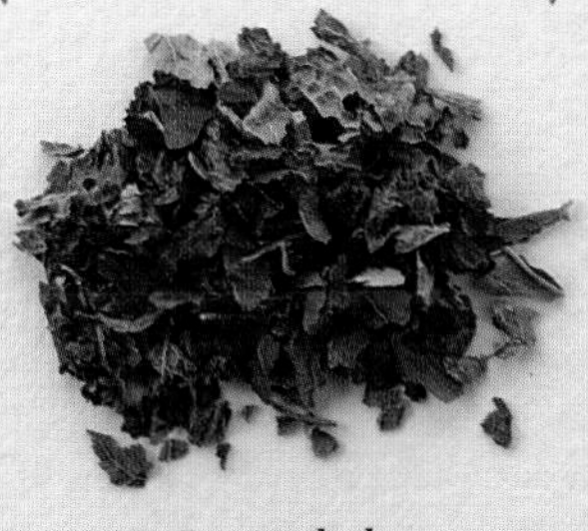

Lemon balm

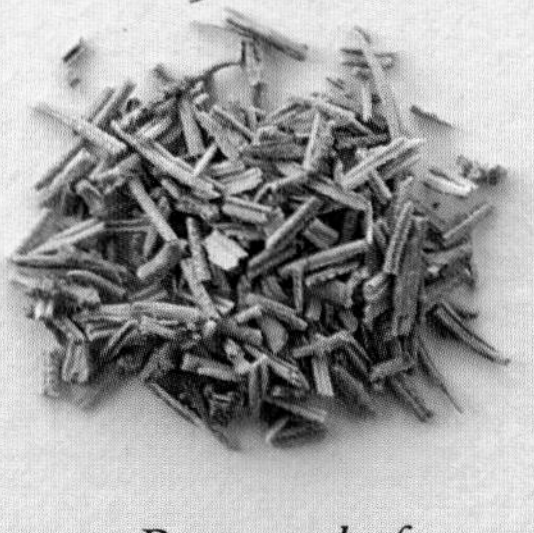

Rosemary leaf

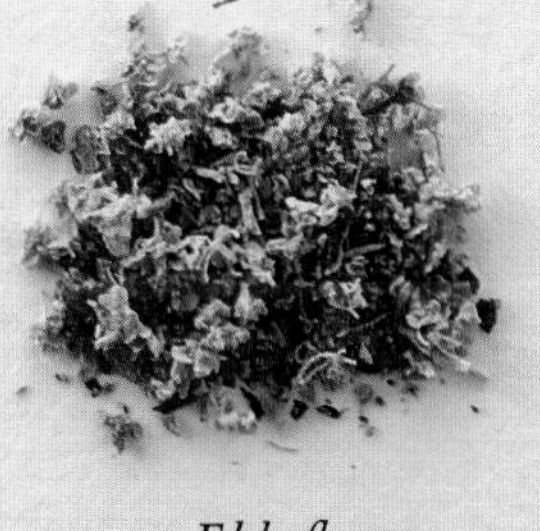

Elderflower

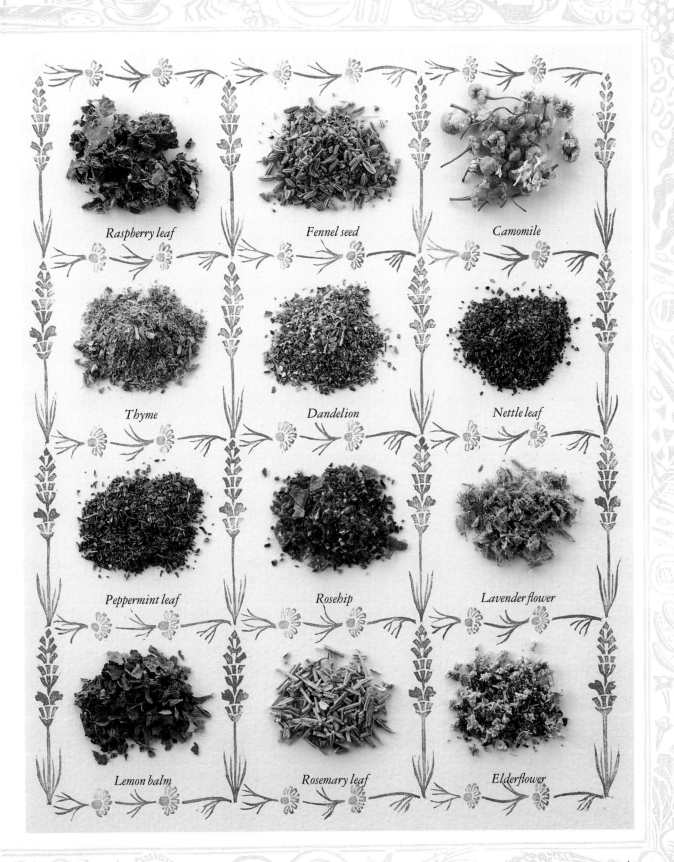

Camomile has long been used to ease indigestion, calm the nerves and reduce anxiety. It is said to aid sleep, and used tea bags (soaked in boiling water and cooled) can be applied to soothe inflamed, itching or tired eyes.

Dandelion leaf tea can be an effective diuretic – helping the excretion of excess fluid from the body.

Elderflower is a comforting tea to drink if suffering from flu, catarrh or painful sinuses; it is said to be anti-inflammatory and makes you perspire. It is also useful for chesty conditions and may help to ease hay fever.

Fennel seed tea helps digestion: it can relieve nausea and a stomach which is bloated because of wind. If taken by a breastfeeding mother, it is said to increase milk flow and at the same time relieve colic or wind in the baby. However, fennel seeds are also thought to encourage menstruation so should be avoided by pregnant women.

Lavender flower tea is a relaxing brew and should be taken at bedtime to help to induce sleep.

Lemon balm, a tea best made with fresh leaves, eases tension without

WARNING

Some herbal infusions used in alternative medicine may contain potentially harmful substances; pregnant women should not take such preparations. Pyrrolizidine alkaloids, for example, found in over 300 plant species, including comfrey, have been linked to liver damage. As a result, comfrey tea should strictly be used for medicinal purposes only.

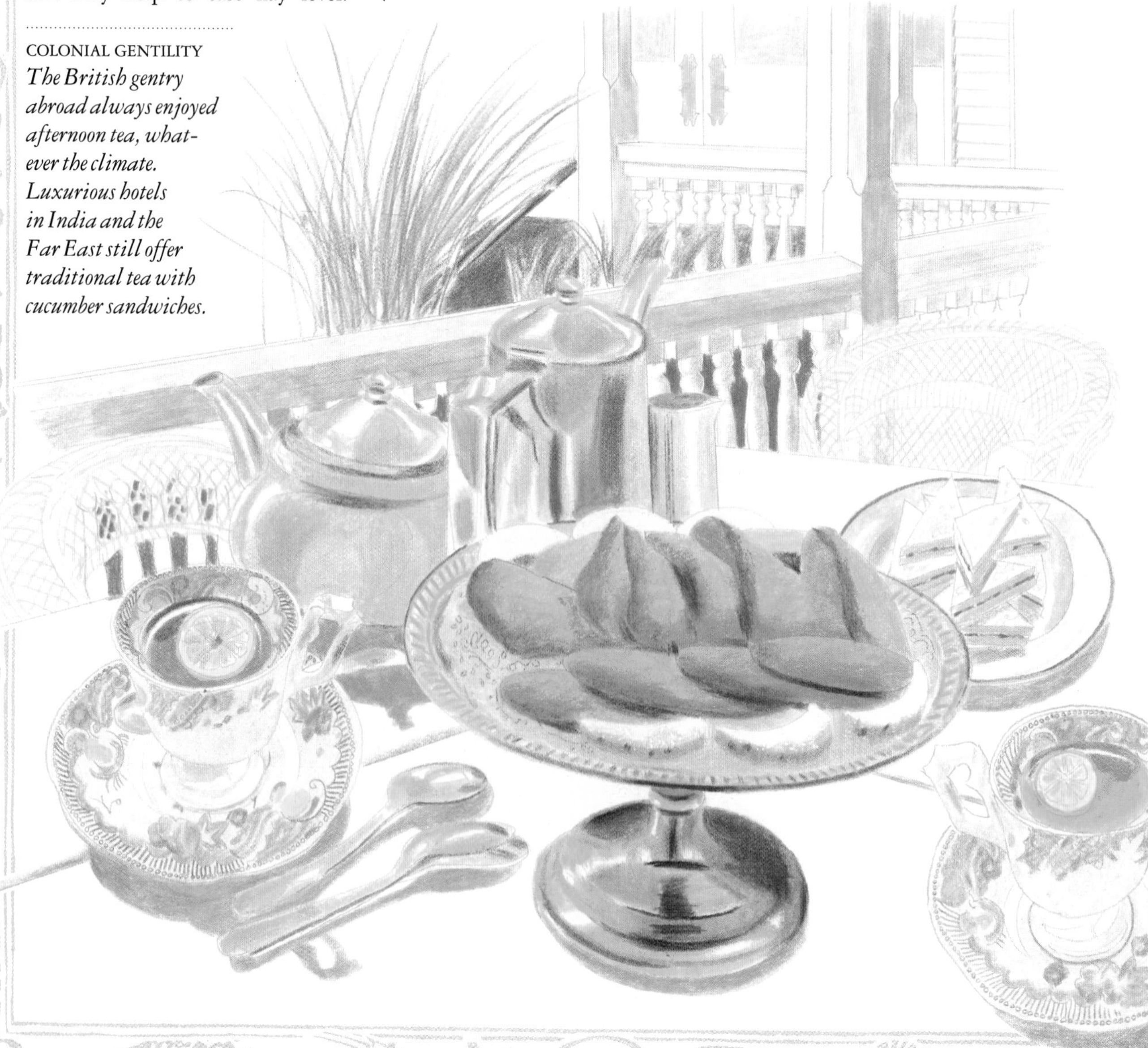

COLONIAL GENTILITY
The British gentry abroad always enjoyed afternoon tea, whatever the climate. Luxurious hotels in India and the Far East still offer traditional tea with cucumber sandwiches.

causing drowsiness. It can also aid digestion and soothe frayed nerves and may help to alleviate feverish conditions such as influenza.

Limeflower tea is soothing and especially popular in France, where it is known as *tilleul*. It is said to ease stress headaches, calm a busy mind, reduce nervous tension and aid sleep. It was used by doctors during the Second World War as a mild tranquilliser. Limeflower tea may also reduce the fever caused by colds and flu.

Nettleleaf tea is a tonic. It contains vitamins and minerals, including iron. It may also relieve allergic reactions, such as hayfever and nettle rash.

Peppermint leaves make an excellent tea to drink after a rich meal to aid digestion and to relieve flatulence. It can also help to control nausea and is useful in the treatment of colds and flu, especially in a traditional combination with elderflowers.

Raspberry leaf tea is mildly astringent and can be used as a mouthwash or gargle for throat infections. If drunk regularly during the last few weeks of pregnancy, it is also said to reduce the length of labour pains and make delivery easier. However, it should not be taken in early pregnancy because it may cause a miscarriage.

Rosemary tea is taken as a pick-me-up to increase alertness at the start of the day, or when energy is fading. It may ease headaches and can be taken for indigestion. It is even claimed to improve the memory and morale.

Rosehip tea, made with crushed, chopped rosehips, is rich in vitamin C and can be taken to help ward off colds and infections. Its mild flavour may be enhanced by adding a little lemon juice or a twist of lemon peel.

Thyme tea is recommended for all types of infections, including colds, flu, bronchitis, earache and sinusitis. It is also said to relieve the pain of indigestion and to lift the spirits.

Tea tales and tips

- Tea is said to have been discovered more than 5000 years ago by the Chinese emperor Shen Nung.
- Tea arrived in Britain during the 17th century, when sailors with the East India Company brought back packets of the leaf from China for their relatives and friends.
- By 1700 there were more than 500 coffee houses in London selling tea, and sales of alcohol declined.
- In the early 1800s, Anna, wife of the 7th Duke of Bedford, began the tradition of afternoon tea to ward off hunger pangs between lunch and dinner. The concept was developed in the same era when the 4th Earl of Sandwich, unwilling to leave the gaming table for a meal, put a filling between two slices of bread.
- Since tea was introduced into Britain, it has been credited with healing powers. This is reflected in a few current brand names – P.G. is said to stand for pre-gestive and Typhoo is Chinese for doctor.
- Superstitions surrounding tea abound: tea leaves strewn on the doorstep, for example, are said to keep evil spirits and poverty at bay.
- Professional tea tasters smell, taste, and some also listen to the leaves while rubbing them together, to determine how dry they are.
- A New York merchant, Thomas Sullivan, inadvertently invented the first tea bag in 1904 when he sent out samples enclosed in silk.
- Drinking tea with or without milk is a question of taste. In Britain most people prefer to take black teas with milk for a less astringent taste. Milk poured in first blends more readily with tea; if milk is added, it precipitates the release of tannins, which then stain the cup.
- Adding lemon to tea was a Russian habit, introduced by the eldest daughter of Queen Victoria, the Princess Royal, who was married to the Emperor of Prussia.
- Teapots should be made of glazed earthenware, porcelain or glass, which hold the heat better than silver or stainless steel. Aluminium or cast-iron pots taint the flavour.
- The pot should be warmed to ensure that the water poured onto the tea stays around boiling point for as long as possible.
- To remove stubborn tea stains from the pot, soak for an hour in a mixture of hot water and a tablespoon of bicarbonate of soda, or wash the pot in a dishwasher.
- Tea is an evergreen plant, and a member of the camellia family. It has smooth, glossy, oval leaves.
- India produces some 30 per cent of the world's tea. The main tea-growing area is Assam, which stretches from the Himalayas down towards the Bay of Bengal.
- Darjeeling, a light delicate tea grown more than 2000m (7000ft) above sea level in the foothills of the Himalayas, is widely regarded as the 'champagne' of teas.
- Earl Grey is treated with oil of bergamot, which gives it its characteristic scented flavour.
- In Britain, tea is the most popular beverage, accounting for 43 per cent of everything we drink.
- As a nation, the British drink a staggering 175 million cups of tea daily, which is the equivalent of 3½ cups for every man, woman and child over the age of ten.
- A cooling cocktail called Planter's Punch is made with iced tea, apple juice, lemon juice and brandy.

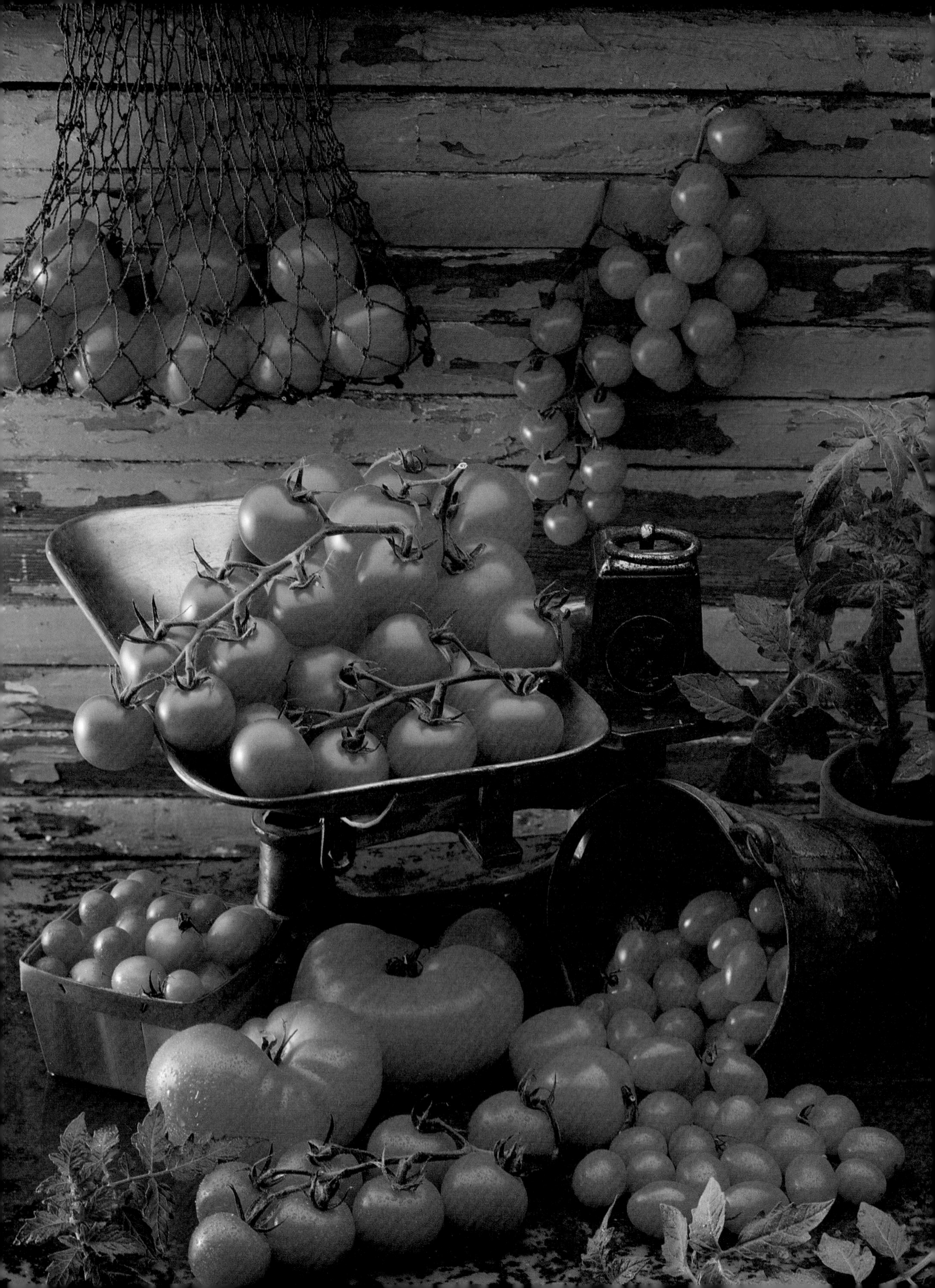

TOMATOES

BENEFITS
- *Good source of carotenoids and potassium*
- *Useful source of vitamins C and E*

DRAWBACKS
- *Common trigger of allergies, especially eczema*
- *Green tomatoes may cause migraine in susceptible people*

As well as being delicious in salads, tomatoes are extremely good for you. For instance, recent research carried out in Britain suggests that lycopene, the carotenoid pigment that turns tomatoes red, may help to prevent some forms of cancer by lessening the damage caused by FREE RADICALS.

Tomatoes are a good source of both potassium and beta carotene and they are a useful source of vitamins C and E, while containing very few calories. Two medium-sized tomatoes contain only around 22 Calories between them – a fact that makes them a useful element in any weight-reducing diet. Common varieties include the small, sweet cherry tomatoes, Italian plum tomatoes, and the round, slicing tomatoes. Yellow varieties are sweeter with a higher sugar content.

Some people have adverse reactions to tomatoes. Recurrent mouth ulcers and eczema can be signs that tomatoes do not agree with you. The solanine in green tomatoes can trigger migraine.

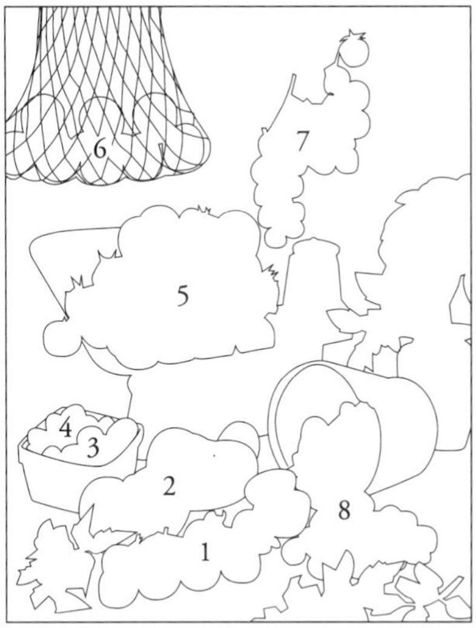

BETTER ON THE VINE? *A tomato's flavour depends more on the variety and how ripe it is than on where it has ripened. Choose from vine (1, 5), beefsteak (2), yellow cherry (3), baby cherry (4), plum (6), vine cherry (7) or baby plum (8).*

'Apple of love'

The tomato, which botanically is a fruit rather than a vegetable, used to be called the love apple. This was nothing to do with its passionate colour or suggestive shape. In fact, the name stems from Italy, where tomatoes were called *pomi dei mori*, 'apples of the moors'. When said out loud it sounded to the French ear like *pomme d'amour* – in English, 'apple of love'.

TOOTH AND GUM DISORDERS

EAT PLENTY OF
- *Calcium-rich foods such as low-fat milk, yoghurt and cheese*
- *Fresh fruit and vegetables for vitamin C*

AVOID
- *Sweet drinks and snacks between meals*
- *Sticky foods that lodge between the teeth*
- *Regular consumption of acid drinks, such as fruit juices and cordials*

Although the need for regular brushing and flossing is well established, the importance of diet in dental health is not so widely known. Tooth decay (dental caries) and gum disease are caused by bacteria growing on teeth, particularly the colonies of bacteria that constantly form a sticky film known as plaque. If plaque is not brushed away, the bacteria break down sugars and starches in food to produce acids that dissolve tooth enamel.

Diet helps to prevent decay by providing fluoride, which makes teeth resistant to decay, and other nutrients essential for healthy teeth and gums.

A DIET FOR DENTAL HEALTH

During pregnancy, make sure you are getting plenty of the calcium necessary for forming your baby's teeth: low-fat dairy products, canned sardines and pilchards eaten with the bones, sesame seeds and dark green leafy vegetables are all good sources. Vitamin D, found in oily fish, aids calcium absorption.

Dental caries can be prevented, to a large extent, by giving your children fluoride in the first few years of life. If the water in your household is not fluoridated, you can give them fluoride drops or tablets. Because children are particularly prone to tooth decay, parents should ensure good brushing and diet, especially up to the age of three. Minerals required for the formation of tooth enamel in the early years are: calcium; fluoride, added to most brands of toothpaste; phosphorus, found in meat, fish and eggs; and magnesium, found in wholemeal bread, spinach and bananas. Vitamin A also plays a role in the growth of strong, healthy bones and teeth; good sources of beta carotene, which the body turns into vitamin A, are orange fruit and vegetables such as apricots and carrots, as well as dark green leafy vegetables.

THE SUGAR FACTOR

Sucrose, the main component of sugar cane and sugar beet, has long been blamed for causing tooth decay, but it is far from being the only culprit. Although sweets and sugary drinks are major offenders, starches can also contribute to tooth decay. This is because they are broken down by saliva into simple sugars that are converted to enamel-destroying acids by the bacteria in the mouth. Starchy foods that stick to the teeth are the most likely to cause tooth decay because the acids formed from them remain in contact with the enamel, rather than being washed off by saliva.

Dried fruit can have a similar effect to sticky sweets because it is high in concentrated sugars and clings to the teeth, allowing more time for bacteria to produce acid. Unsweetened fruit juices, such as orange and grapefruit, can often contribute to decay owing to their acidity levels and their high levels of simple sugars. Artificially sweetened drinks can also cause harm. Although they do not cause tooth decay, acidic varieties such as sugar-free fruit cordials can erode the enamel from the teeth. Fresh fruit is less problematic because chewing promotes the release of saliva, thereby lessening the amount of time that sugars and acids are in contact with tooth enamel.

Eating snacks between meals and sipping sugary drinks and fruit juices over long periods, or just before bed, increase the risk of tooth decay. Parents should not, therefore, put infants to bed with a bottle of milk (which contains the sugar lactose), fruit juice or sugar solution, nor should they give babies a dummy dipped in sugar or syrup as a comforter.

HELPFUL FOODS

Finishing a meal with foods that do not promote and may even prevent cavities can also protect your teeth. CHEESE, for example, is thought to protect dental enamel: eaten at the end of a meal, and not followed by anything else such as tea or coffee, cheese reduces levels of mouth acidity. And chewing sugar-free gum (see CHOCOLATE AND SWEETS) after a meal can be helpful in preventing decay because it stimulates the flow of saliva which washes away acid.

LIQUORICE ROOT, which is found in some toothpastes, also helps to fight decay; it is an anti-inflammatory agent, and contains a substance that may help to control plaque development. However, the use of fluoride toothpaste is almost certainly the most important factor in combating tooth decay.

Case study

Brian, a postman, was only 25 and already had a young family to support. It was not unusual for him to begin his day by preparing his morning round at 5.30am and continue to work, doing overtime in the sorting office, until 8pm. He would often skip meals, just grabbing a chocolate bar when he needed energy. After several weeks had gone by, Brian's wife noticed that he seemed unwell. He had bad breath and his gums were inflamed and bleeding. Brian admitted to feeling run down and said that he was worried about the little bruises that were appearing around his ankles. The family doctor saw that he had vitamin C deficiency, and gave Brian a course of high-dose vitamin C tablets and made him promise to eat more fresh fruit and vegetables.

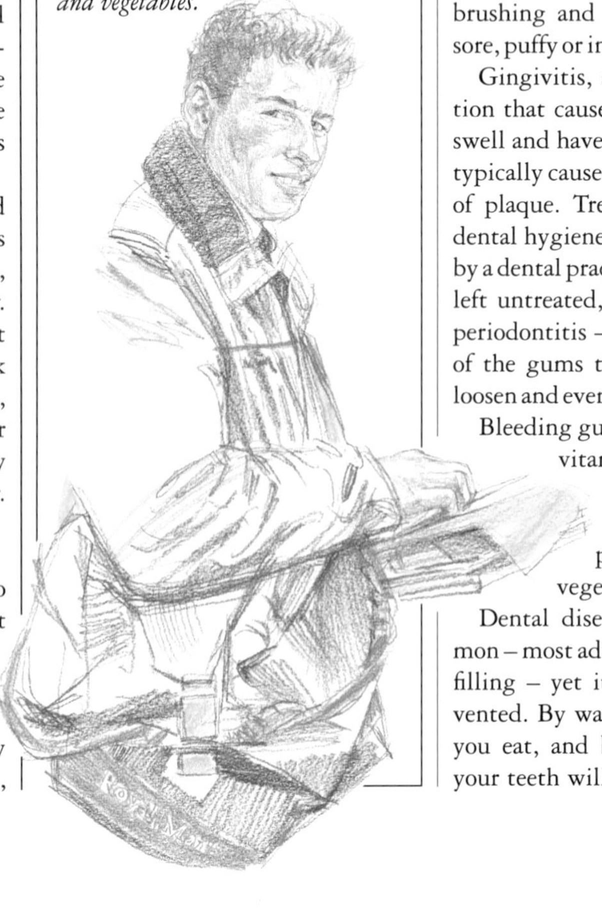

GUM DISEASE

More teeth are lost through gum disease than through tooth decay; it is likely to affect those who persistently neglect oral hygiene or fail to ensure that they have a balanced diet. Those suffering from alcoholism, malnutrition or AIDS, and people being treated with steroids or certain anti-cancer drugs, are particularly at risk. Regular brushing and flossing help to avoid sore, puffy or inflamed gums.

Gingivitis, a very common condition that causes the gums to redden, swell and have a tendency to bleed, is typically caused by a gradual build-up of plaque. Treatment involves good dental hygiene and removal of plaque by a dental practitioner or hygienist. If left untreated, gingivitis can lead to periodontitis – an advanced infection of the gums that can cause teeth to loosen and eventually fall out.

Bleeding gums can also be a sign of vitamin C deficiency. To combat this condition make sure you include plenty of fresh fruit and vegetables in your diet.

Dental disease is extremely common – most adults have more than one filling – yet it can so easily be prevented. By watching what and when you eat, and by brushing regularly, your teeth will last you a lifetime.

TRAVELLERS' HEALTH

See page 352

TUBERCULOSIS

EAT PLENTY OF
- *Fish, lean meat, grains and pulses*
- *Fresh fruit and vegetables*
- *Eggs and dairy foods*

AVOID
- *Unpasteurised milk*

Poor nutrition and poverty contribute to the incidence of tuberculosis (TB), which is responsible for more deaths globally than any other infectious disease. Although TB is most prevalent in the developing world, there is fresh cause for concern in Britain.

Thanks to vaccination programmes and better living conditions the number of cases reported in England and Wales went into decline after the 1950s. However, from 1987 to 1993, new notifications rose by 12 per cent – contributing to a total of 5961 cases.

A healthy diet plays an important role in preventing tuberculosis. In particular, eating meat and fish may be significant both for preventing the disease and in its treatment. Recently, in a study of Asian immigrants in south London, it was found that vegetarians who ate no fish and meat, and no milk or dairy products, were at least eight times more likely to develop TB than other Asians who ate either meat or dairy products every day.

Precisely why this is true is not well understood, but research suggests that a lack of vitamin B_{12} (provided almost entirely by foods from animal sources or fortified foods) increases the risk of developing TB. People with pernicious anaemia (which is caused by an inability to absorb vitamin B_{12}) are also susceptible to the disease. It is also known that vitamin D deficiency affects immunity to disease generally.

Eggs, oily fish and dairy foods are good sources of vitamins B_{12} and D. Eating plenty of these foods and also lean meat, whole grains and pulses, together with fresh fruit and vegetables, will ensure the full complement of nutrients required. This will aid recovery and help to protect against any recurrence of the disease.

WHO IS AT RISK?

In Britain during the 1960s and 1970s, TB was mainly associated with ethnic minorities – particularly from the Indian subcontinent. However, a detailed survey of new cases in Liverpool between 1985 and 1990 indicates that, as in pre-war Britain, tuberculosis is more widespread, affecting the poor and badly nourished, whatever their ethnic origin.

There is also some indication that a strain resistant to current antibiotics is surfacing in the United States where the disease has become increasingly common among people infected with the AIDS-related HIV virus.

Tuberculosis is caused by a bacterium known as *Mycobacterium tuberculosis*. The strain causing pulmonary TB is spread through coughing and sneezing. Symptoms range from fatigue, lack of appetite and weight loss to fever, rapid loss of weight and diminished strength but, in some cases, the infected person may show no symptoms at all.

TREATING TUBERCULOSIS

Young, unvaccinated children, elderly people and those who are undernourished or generally in poor health are the most susceptible to TB. Treatment involves rest and medication with antibiotics which must be taken daily for six to nine months for a complete cure. Anyone travelling to countries with a high incidence of TB should be wary of unpasteurised milk and butter, since it may have come from cows that are infected with a bovine strain of the bacterium. The bovine bacilli are slightly different, but the disease is occasionally transmitted to people.

TURNIPS

BENEFITS
- *Useful source of vitamin C*
- *Source of fibre*
- *Low in calories*
- *May help to ease bronchial problems*

The fibre contained in turnips helps to maintain bowel regularity and may help to prevent colonic or rectal cancer. Turnips are a useful source of vitamin C, which is needed for healthy skin and tissues. They consist mainly of water and are low in calories.

Some herbalists suggest that a few teaspoons of homemade turnip syrup a day may relieve respiratory ailments, such as bronchitis and asthma. The syrup, which is watery rather than thick, is made by boiling a portion of chopped turnip in a little water.

The green tops of turnips are gaining greater recognition: they are an excellent source of beta carotene, vitamin C and a good source of folate. They make a sweet-tasting green vegetable when boiled until tender.

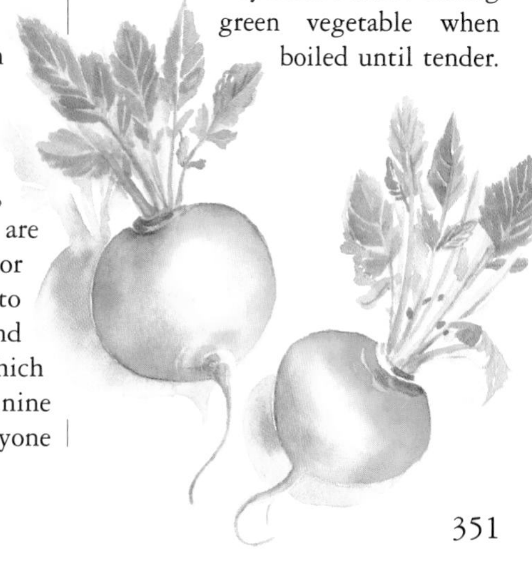

TRAVELLERS' HEALTH

The excitement of visiting faraway places is often marred by health hazards. But by taking a few simple precautions you can travel with much greater peace of mind.

Visitors to areas of the world where certain diseases are endemic should make sure that they are immunised before they travel. Ask your doctor which vaccinations you require, and what medicines you should take with you.

PROTECTING YOURSELF FROM SERIOUS DISEASE ABROAD

Cholera Although there are outbreaks of cholera in Europe – the majority occurring in Eastern Europe – it is more often found in tropical regions. Travellers to areas where cholera is rife, such as Africa, South America and South-east Asia, should be particularly careful what – and where – they eat and drink. Although there is a vaccine for cholera, it is not particularly effective so doctors rarely recommend it.

The disease is highly infectious; it is spread by bacteria which breed in food or drinking water contaminated by sewage from cholera victims. It is characterised by the sudden onset of vomiting and severe watery DIARRHOEA, commonly known as rice-water stools. In severe cases, it causes rapid dehydration accompanied by acute thirst and muscle cramps, and can be fatal within 24 hours if not treated quickly. Cholera is treated with antibiotics, and by replacing lost fluids – by mouth or intravenously.

Dysentery There are two forms of dysentery, both

DOS AND DON'TS

- Do have the necessary immunisations – visit your doctor at least two months before you travel.
- Do observe hygiene precautions and be careful what you eat and drink, as vaccines do not always confer 100 per cent immunity.
- Do peel fruit and avoid salads.
- Do drink boiled or bottled water – well-known brands of carbonated water should be safest – but always check the seal is intact. Use it for cleaning your teeth, too.
- Don't take ice in your drinks: it is probably made with tap water.
- Don't swallow swimming pool water, or swim in lakes or streams unless you know they are safe.
- Don't ignore persistent diarrhoea: dehydration can be sudden and fatal. Find a doctor.

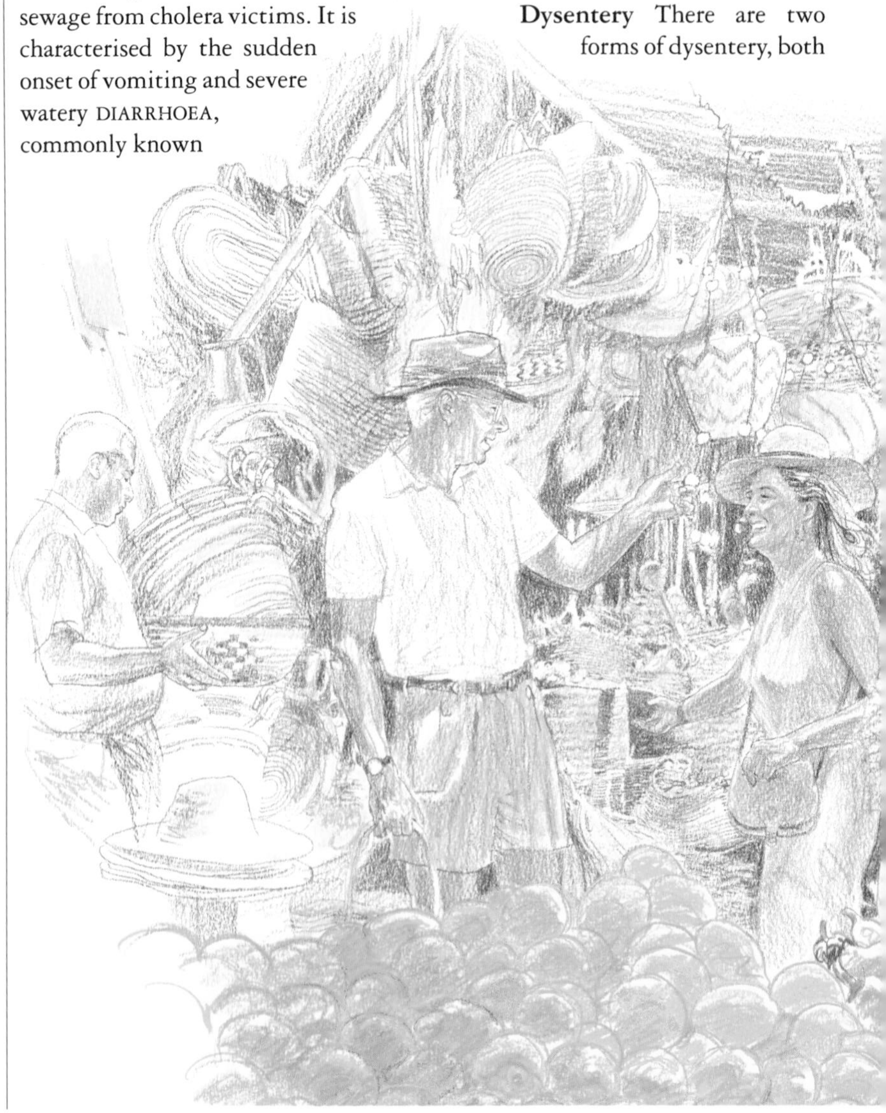

of which cause severe, often bloody diarrhoea. Amoebic dysentery is most often found in tropical countries. It is caused by a parasite spread by poor hygiene, infected food and contaminated water. Symptoms can appear days – or in rare cases, even years – after infection. It is normally treated with antibiotics and other drugs.

Bacterial dysentery is also spread through contaminated food or water. It is associated with insanitary and overcrowded conditions, and sometimes occurs in epidemics in schools. Symptoms occur within a week of infection, and include diarrhoea, vomiting and stomach cramps. Patients are prescribed antibiotics, and must take care to replace lost fluids and minerals.

If you are struck down with dysentery far away from medical help, a useful rehydration mixture is eight teaspoons of sugar and a teaspoon of salt dissolved in a litre (1¾ pints) of boiled water and half a litre (just under 1 pint) of orange or lemon juice. However, if you are so cut off from civilisation that not even boiled water is available, drinking any water is better than risking severe dehydration.

There is no vaccine for either form of dysentery so, to avoid it, you must be scrupulous in observing commonsense hygiene. Be wary not only of local tap water and ice cubes but also unbottled local beers, which may not have been pasteurised. Peel raw fruit, avoid salad and eat only vegetables which have been thoroughly cooked.

Hepatitis A People intending to visit areas where hepatitis A is endemic should be vaccinated against the virus. If you are travelling to any developing country where it is likely that hygiene and sanitation will be poor, avoid untreated water, undercooked food, raw meat or fish, raw vegetables, milk and all shellfish. Also be careful not to swim in water polluted with sewage.

Anyone who has hepatitis A is advised to eat a high-carbohydrate, low-fat diet that supplies plenty of energy and is rich in micronutrients. However, in the early stages, when sufferers feel too ill to eat much at all, they should supplement their diet with vegetable soups, meat broths, fruit juices and sugar. Spicy and barbecued foods should be avoided as these cannot be metabolised by a sick liver. Alcohol must be avoided at all costs, for anything up to a year. The damaged liver cannot metabolise it, and alcohol can destroy damaged liver cells.

Few people die of hepatitis A, but it can cause long periods of illness and severe liver damage.

Yellow fever and malaria Both yellow fever and malaria are transmitted by mosquito bites, so in countries

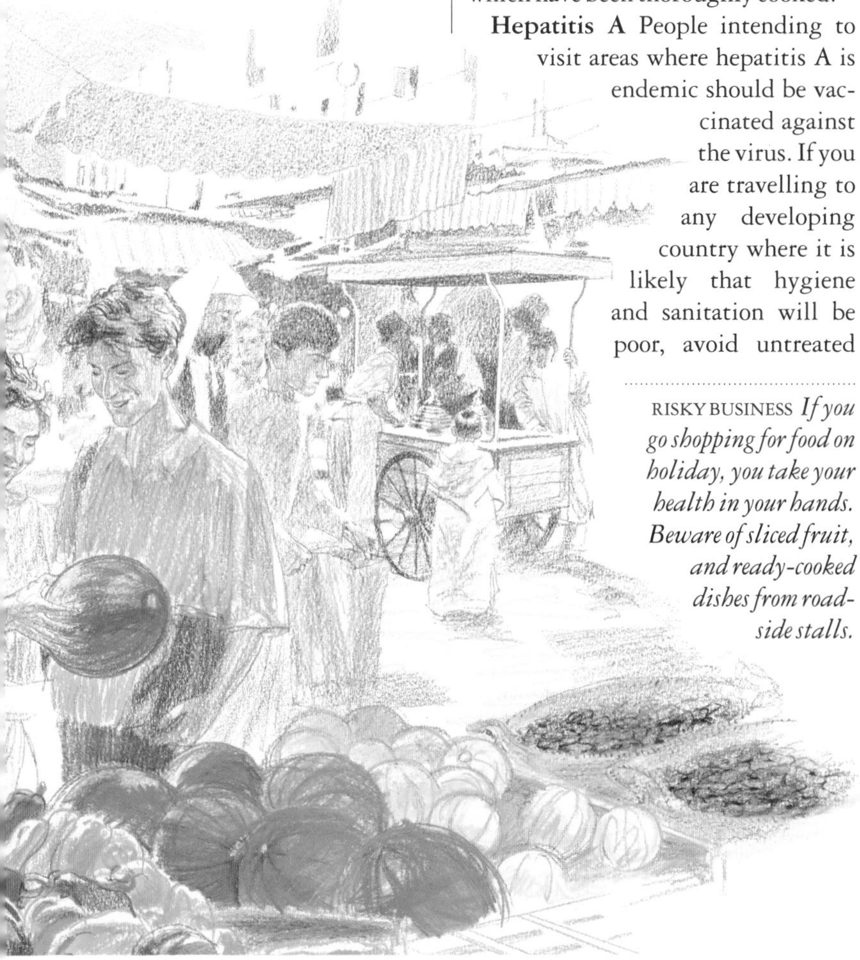

RISKY BUSINESS *If you go shopping for food on holiday, you take your health in your hands. Beware of sliced fruit, and ready-cooked dishes from roadside stalls.*

FOODS TO AVOID OR TREAT WITH CAUTION

- Shellfish and fish unless in a reputable hotel or restaurant.
- Avoid uncooked shellfish, such as oysters, altogether.
- Raw fruit unless you are able to peel it yourself.
- Undercooked food, or any food which has either been kept warm, or is served lukewarm.
- Food exposed to flies.
- Ice-cream from potentially unreliable sources, including street vendors or market stalls.
- Unpasteurised milk.
- Salad unless you can be sure that it has been washed in boiled or bottled water.
- Soft drinks which may have been diluted with tap-water, such as orange squash.

where these diseases are endemic, it is vital to take measures against being bitten. Wear long sleeves and trousers, and button shirts up to the neck (especially in the evenings). Apply mosquito repellent to all exposed skin and, at night, sleep under netting and burn mosquito coils.

Yellow fever is a potentially fatal virus-borne disease prevalent in tropical Africa and some northern parts of South America. Anyone going to these areas must be vaccinated. Symptoms include chills, headache and aching limbs – as well as JAUNDICE, hence the name 'yellow' fever. The virus is treated by replacing lost fluids.

Travellers can contract malaria in more than 100 countries worldwide. The risks vary but they are particularly high in tropical Africa, where medical services may also be remote. No vaccination exists for malaria but, if you intend to visit an infested area, you will be prescribed daily or weekly anti-malarial tablets which you must take for one week before you travel and continue taking for four weeks after you return home. Although this medication will greatly reduce the risk of contracting the disease, resistant strains of malarial parasites are on the increase and can cause serious illness.

If you are bitten by an infected mosquito, symptoms may take anything from 12 days to 10 months to appear. This means that the severe aches and pains, shivers, high fever and delirium may well occur after you have forgotten all about your holiday. Malaria can be fatal if not treated promptly so, if you think you may have the disease, consult your doctor without delay.

Typhoid Anyone planning to travel to regions where sanitation might be poor – particularly Asia, the Middle East, Africa or Central and South America – should be vaccinated against typhoid. However, an injection will not offer complete immunity if you happen to ingest large amounts of *Salmonella typhi*, the bacteria that are responsible for the disease. This means that you must be careful about what you eat and drink. Foods which should be avoided include shellfish, reheated foods, raw or unwashed fruit

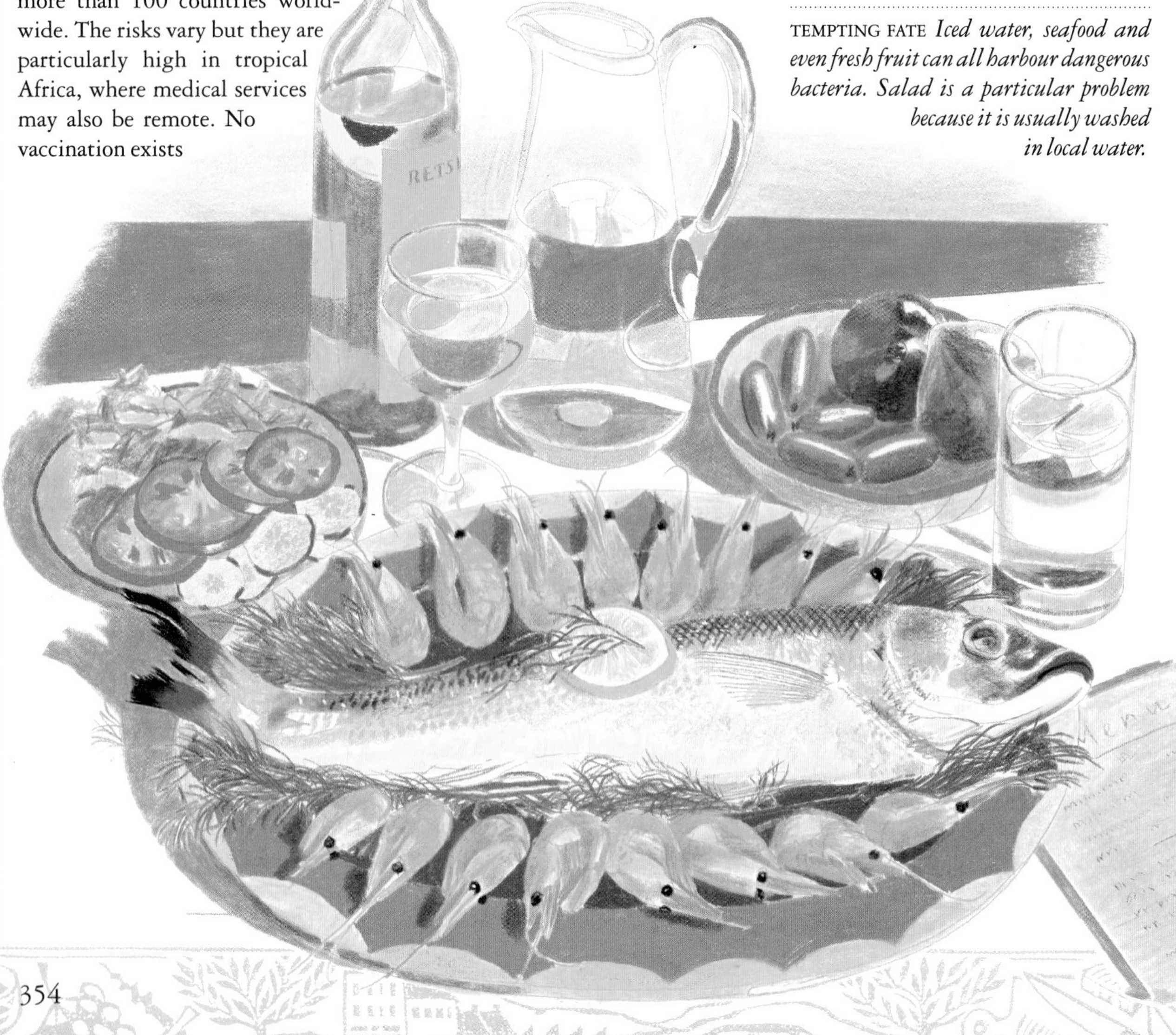

TEMPTING FATE *Iced water, seafood and even fresh fruit can all harbour dangerous bacteria. Salad is a particular problem because it is usually washed in local water.*

and vegetables, and tap water. If you contract typhoid, medical help is vital. The disease starts off with flu-like symptoms, weakness and a rash of red spots on the chest and abdomen. In serious cases, patients can suffer inflammation of the spleen and bones, delirium, and intestinal haemorrhage. Recovery occurs naturally, but is accelerated with antibiotics.

Acquiring a tan

Prolonged or unaccustomed exposure to the ultraviolet radiation in sunlight can lead to premature ageing of the skin and an increased risk of skin CANCER, and often causes SUNBURN.

Largely because of the growing problem of skin cancer, doctors now recommend extreme caution when sunbathing. They advise people to lie in the sun for no more than half an hour on the first day (redheads and blue-eyed blondes should aim for 10-20 minutes maximum exposure), increasing it a little each day. Always use a sunscreen lotion – doctors now regard anything below factor 8 as ineffective and most experts recommend factor 15 – and re-apply regularly, especially after swimming. Do not be tempted to sunbathe during the hottest part of the day – usually between 11am and 3pm, particularly if you have fair skin. So if you are set on returning home with a bronzed skin the safest way is to be patient, building up the tan gradually.

People with red hair and fair skin are particularly susceptible to burning. Babies should be kept out of direct sunlight altogether, and you should be extra vigilant with children. Try to ensure that they wear T-shirts and wide-brimmed sun-hats all the time, even when they are swimming. After bathing or showering, moisturise skin with soothing after-sun lotion.

Some people mistakenly believe that by using a sunbed for several sessions before travelling abroad, they can acclimatise their skin to the sun, and will therefore be able to tan more safely. Moreover, there are those who use sunbeds on a regular basis to maintain a year-round tan. The view held by the British Photodermatology Group is that 'the use of ultraviolet A sunbeds ... should be discouraged'. People who, despite this advice, want to use UVA sunbeds should not have more than two courses a year, neither of which should exceed ten sessions.

Increased dietary levels of beta carotene, found in carrots and other orange-coloured vegetables and fruit, and dark green leafy vegetables, may afford some protection against sunburn. This could be due to one of two reasons: either the beta carotene dissolved in the lipids of skin cells helps to filter ultraviolet radiation, or it neutralises harmful free radicals through antioxidant action.

Jet lag

Long-distance airline flights which travel from east-to-west or west-to-east, crossing the world's time zones, upset the body's natural 24-hour cycle. Travellers feel sleepy at the wrong time of day and their eating patterns are disturbed. Other symptoms of jet lag include fatigue, irritability and inability to concentrate. Most people adapt more easily to flying west than east. This is because as you fly west, the day becomes longer and conversely, as you fly east, the day becomes shorter, and the body seems to adjust more readily to a lengthening day.

Wherever possible, book daytime flights which arrive at their destination in the evening. Once on board the aircraft, set your watch to the correct time as at your destination so that you can start to get a feel for the local time straight away.

Doctors believe that the effects of jet lag can be greatly reduced by drinking plenty of non-alcoholic fluids during long-haul flights in order to avoid the dehydration caused by pressurised cabins. Alcohol will only increase dehydration, which is often the real culprit for the ill-effects normally blamed on jet lag.

During the flight, eat light meals that are easy to digest and try to get as much sleep as possible. Once at your destination, adopt the rhythm of the local time immediately – eating and sleeping to the new pattern. This will reset your 'body clock' by stimulating production of the hormone melatonin. Treatment with melatonin pills has also been reported to combat jet lag.

TRAVEL OR MOTION SICKNESS

The nausea and headaches that some people suffer when they travel by road, sea or air are all symptoms of travel sickness. The condition is caused by a conflict between what the eyes see and what the delicate organs of the inner ear feel, during movement. The eyes adjust to motion, but the inner ear does not, so the brain receives two opposing messages, and the result is nausea.

If you tend to suffer from travel sickness, do not eat a large meal before or during a journey, and avoid alcohol. Instead, take regular small amounts of water or soft drinks to avoid dehydration, and eat regular light snacks.

There are many effective over-the-counter remedies for travel sickness, most of which need to be taken before you travel. Alternatively chew a few pieces of peeled fresh root ginger before and during your journey. In clinical trials ginger has proved more effective in preventing travel sickness than a number of over-the-counter drugs, without causing drowsiness.

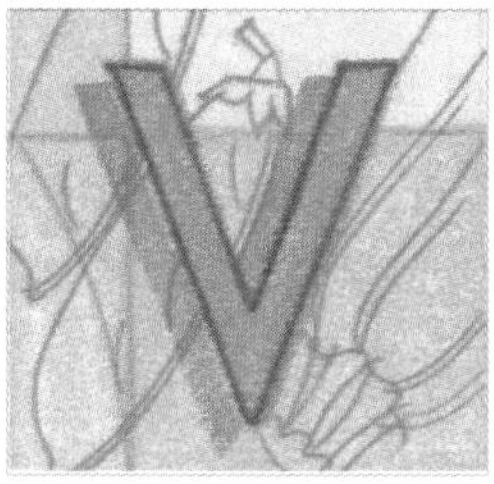

VARICOSE VEINS

TAKE PLENTY OF

- *Fibre-rich foods such as wholemeal bread, fresh fruit and vegetables*
- *Water – at least 1.7 litres (3 pints) a day*
- *Foods rich in vitamin E, such as seed oils, wheatgerm, avocados and nuts*

CUT DOWN ON

- *Refined carbohydrates, such as cakes and biscuits*

While heredity can be an important factor in determining who will develop varicose veins, dietary measures and regular exercise may help to prevent them. Although varicose veins can occur anywhere in the body, they are most commonly found in the legs. Damaged valves in the veins allow blood to collect so that the vein walls are stretched until they lose their elasticity and are unable to contract to their normal shape.

Women are more prone than men to varicose veins. They can arise during pregnancy, when the flow of blood back from the limbs is restricted. Varicose veins associated with pregnancy may cease to be a problem after childbirth; otherwise they can persist indefinitely. Jobs that involve long periods of standing still are also known to increase the risk. Obesity also increases susceptibility to varicose veins because it can impair the flow of blood back from the feet and legs. People who eat a high-fibre diet, so avoiding constipation, appear to have a reduced risk of varicose veins. You can cut down on refined carbohydrates such as cakes and biscuits, and increase your intake of soluble and insoluble fibre by eating plenty of apples, pears, green leafy vegetables, wholewheat pasta, wholemeal bread and brown rice. Bran can also be added to the diet, but do not eat more than one tablespoon daily as too much can aggravate some digestive problems, such as irritable bowel syndrome, and can inhibit the body's absorption of certain minerals, including calcium. Drinking at least 1.7 litres (3 pints) of water a day also helps to prevent constipation.

Bioflavonoids, found in the pith of citrus fruits, as well as in blackcurrants, grapes and apricots, have been claimed to help prevent or treat varicose veins. However, this theory is still controversial as it has not been tested in controlled clinical trials. It has also been claimed that vitamin E in the diet may reduce the likelihood of varicose veins. Good sources include wheatgerm, seed oils, avocados and nuts.

The best dietary advice for preventing varicose veins is to avoid obesity and eat plenty of fruit and vegetables and fibre in the form of starchy foods. Regular exercise, especially walking, can also help. Try not to stand for long periods without a break, never cross your legs, and put your feet up whenever you can.

VARICOSE ULCERS

These usually painless open sores may occur when a varicose vein is injured – perhaps by a blow to the leg – or more commonly when blood leaks out of the distended, damaged vein. Varicose ulcers can take months or even years of repeated treatment to heal. There is evidence to suggest that zinc can play a part in healing the sores; good sources include shellfish, lean meat and nuts.

VEAL

BENEFITS

- *Good source of protein*
- *Good source of vitamin B_{12}*
- *Useful source of zinc and niacin*

DRAWBACK

- *Controversy over the way in which calves are reared and transported, particularly on the Continent*

Weight for weight, raw veal contains just under half the fat and fewer calories than raw, lean beef, and has similar amounts of micronutrients. It contains protein and zinc for the growth and repair of body tissue and B vitamins for a healthy nervous system.

Traditionally, veal was produced from calves that were kept in crates to restrict their movement and fed only milk; this diet made them anaemic, resulting in white flesh. Such practice is now illegal in the UK; the more humane diet and treatment means the meat is now darker. On the Continent, the traditional method of veal production prevails and it is both the rearing process and methods of transportation that have caused public concern.

VEGETABLES

Children are repeatedly reminded that vegetables are good for them, and that they need to eat their greens to grow big and strong. This belief is upheld by nutritionists and doctors who have long recognised the value of vegetables in terms of the vital FIBRE, VITAMINS and MINERALS they provide.

In recent years, scientists have further reinforced the link between a diet containing plenty of vegetables and good health. The American Institute for Cancer Research estimates that as many as 40 per cent of all cancers in men, and 60 per cent of those in women, are linked to diet, while other authorities suggest an overall figure of 35 per cent. And several studies have confirmed that populations with diets that are rich in vegetables and fruit run a lower risk of cancer. There is much speculation as to how this protection is afforded, and several non-nutritional compounds are among the potential candidates suggested by scientists. Phytochemicals – derived from the Greek word *phyto*, meaning plant – is the term popularly used to describe these compounds.

PLANTS PROTECT THE BODY

Phytochemicals are found in all fruits and vegetables, although the cruciferous vegetables – including Brussels sprouts, cabbage, cauliflower, broccoli, kale and turnips – seem to contain more of the compounds than most.

Initially, scientists thought that some phytochemicals would actually cause cancer, and they were surprised that they had a protective effect. Most of these studies were based on animals, however, and it is possible that they may not be so relevant to cancer in humans. Now, researchers are also investigating the significance of phytochemicals in reducing the risk of other ailments including diabetes, circulation problems, heart disease, osteoporosis and hypertension.

FREE RADICAL FIGHTERS

Among the different groups of phytochemicals are the plant pigments known as carotenoids, many of which have antioxidant properties. Research has shown that ANTIOXIDANTS neutralise FREE RADICALS – potentially harmful molecules which can damage the membranes of healthy cells as well as DNA. Although free radicals are produced by the body, and play a role in the body's defence against disease, sometimes too many are made and the increase can be linked with heart disease and cancer. Factors which can lead to the overproduction of free radicals include smoking, ultraviolet light, exposure to environmental pollution and the ageing process.

ANTI-CANCER CAROTENOIDS?

Many vegetables are good sources of carotenoids. Carotenoid pigments include the red colour lycopene (found in tomatoes and red peppers) and beta carotene (the orange pigment in carrots and cantaloupe melon). Among the best vegetable sources of carotenoids are watercress, broccoli and spinach, yellow-fleshed squashes, red peppers, carrots and pumpkins. Some studies have shown that populations whose diets are high in carotenoid-rich fruit and vegetables run a lower risk of certain cancers, especially lung cancer. However, a trial in Finland contradicted these findings, and more studies are now underway.

EYESIGHT PROTECTION

In addition to helping to protect against cancer, increased intake of the carotenoid beta carotene, together with vitamin C, may possibly help to reduce the risk of cataracts.

HELPING THE BODY TO HEAL

Many phytochemicals stimulate enzymes in the liver that render some carcinogens harmless and help the body to eliminate others, thus bolstering the body's natural ability to fight off cancer. Among those under investigation are indoles, allicin compounds, isothiocyanates and bioflavonoids.

Indoles, present in cruciferous vegetables, have been found to render the female hormone oestrogen less potent which may be helpful in reducing the risk of hormone-related breast cancer. Other infection-fighting and anti-cancer phytochemicals include allicin compounds, present in garlic, onions, chives and leeks; isothiocyanates, in cruciferous vegetables such as Brussels sprouts, broccoli and cabbage; and bioflavonoids, found in virtually all fruit and vegetables.

Tomatoes, green peppers and carrots contain coumaric acid and related substances which appear to inhibit the formation of potentially carcinogenic nitrosamines in the gut. Processed tomato products, such as ketchup, also contain these protective compounds.

RAW OR COOKED?

Many people believe that raw vegetables are much better for them than cooked, and it is true that if you boil vegetables you will lose much of their vitamin C, which is water-soluble and sensitive to heat.

But cooking can also increase the availability of some other nutrients; when carrots are cooked, for example, the cell membranes are softened, thus making beta carotene more available for absorption by the body.

Breeding healthier vegetables

Scientists at the American Institute for Cancer Research are investigating all sorts of vegetables for a wide variety of possible beneficial effects. It is a major project as just one fruit or vegetable may contain dozens of different phytochemicals. By using genetic engineering and selective breeding they are hoping to create vegetables which contain higher levels of these disease-fighting substances.

So far, they have looked at garlic, soya beans, carrots, parsley and celery. The scientists will have to exercise some caution, however, because some phytochemicals that are highly beneficial when eaten in small quantities may be harmful in larger amounts.

VEGETARIAN AND VEGAN DIETS

As growing numbers of Britons cut meat from their diets and turn to fruit, vegetables and nuts as healthier – and more humane – alternatives, they must keep a wary eye on nutritional balances.

A study involving 11000 people, published in the *British Medical Journal* in 1994, found that vegetarians are 40 per cent less likely to develop cancer at an early age than meat eaters. As vegetarians and vegans tend to be slimmer than meat eaters, eat less saturated fats (found mainly in animal products) and eat more fibre, they also have lower levels of blood cholesterol and therefore heart disease.

Meat aside, vegetarians do not eat poultry or fish but they do eat eggs and dairy products. Vegans eat only foods of plant origin. This reduction or elimination of animal foods can lead to mineral and vitamin deficiencies: poor iron absorption in vegan or vegetarian women, and lack of calcium and vitamins B_{12} and D in vegans.

Vegetarians, vegans and a third group, pescatarians (who eat fish but not meat) usually eat more fibre and complex carbohydrates than meat

Important nutrients for vegetarians

Though some essential minerals and vitamins are more readily available from meat or fish than non-animal sources, a balanced diet which includes a wide variety of foods will provide vegetarians (but not vegans) with all the nutrients they need. However, care may need to be taken to ensure adequate intakes of iron, vitamin B_{12}, calcium and folate.

NUTRIENT	NON-MEAT SOURCES	WHY NEEDED	SYMPTOMS OF DEFICIENCY	HOW TO ENSURE A HEALTHY INTAKE
Iron	Beans, lentils, wholemeal flour, oatmeal, dried fruits, dark green leafy vegetables, nuts, parsley, fortified breakfast cereals and egg yolks.	Necessary for the production of haemoglobin in red blood cells; especially important for girls when menstruation starts.	Fatigue and anaemia. 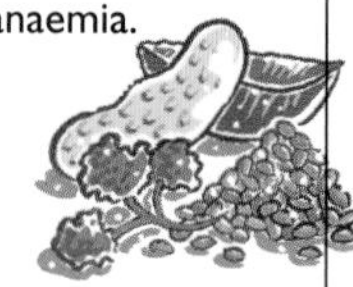	As the body needs vitamin C to convert iron from non-meat sources into a usable form, fruit, vegetables or fruit juice should be included with meals that provide iron.
Vitamin B_{12} 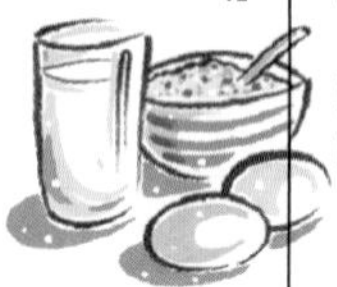	Milk, dairy products, eggs. Foods fortified with B_{12} such as soya milk, breakfast cereals and yeast extract. Vitamin supplements.	Essential for a healthy nervous system and the formation of red blood cells.	Fatigue, anaemia and irritability. Pins and needles in the hands and feet.	Many vegetarians increase their intake of dairy products in place of meat – choose the lower-fat varieties. Vegans need to eat fortified foods or take supplements.
Calcium	Milk and dairy products, fortified soya products (milk, yoghurt, cheese and tofu), nuts (especially almonds), dark green leafy vegetables, sesame or sunflower seeds.	Needed to form and maintain healthy bones and teeth. 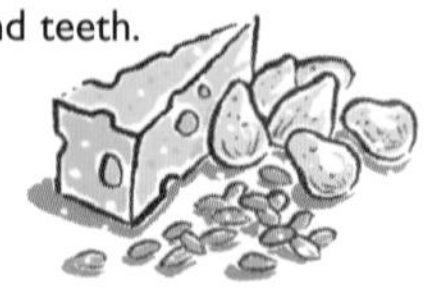	Rickets in children and osteomalacia – the equivalent of rickets – in adults. Also, osteoporosis.	Vitamin D is essential for the absorption of calcium. Most people get enough from exposure to sunlight, but it is also found in margarines, and breakfast cereals fortified with the vitamin.
Folate 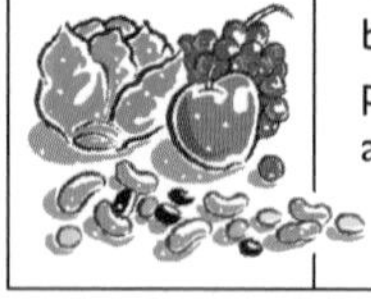	Green leafy vegetables, beans, eggs, fruit, peanuts, yeast extract and wholegrain cereals.	Necessary in forming red blood cells. Protects against spina bifida prior to and in the very early stages of pregnancy.	Anaemia, fatigue, and birth defects.	Take folic acid supplements prior to conception and up to 12 weeks into pregnancy. Eat fortified breakfast cereals and plenty of folate-rich vegetables.

eaters, in the form of wholegrain cereals, nuts and pulses (beans, peas and lentils). A high-fibre diet can protect against several diseases of the bowel, and helps food to pass more quickly through the digestive tract of vegetarians, making them far less likely to suffer from constipation. Vegetarians also have a lower risk of developing gallstones and diverticular disease.

It has been suggested that the lower incidence of cancer among vegetarians is due to eating more plant foods – such as fresh fruit and vegetables, cereals, pulses and nuts – rather than the absence of meat. However, some studies have linked high intakes of red meat with cancer of the colon.

It has also been noted that vegetarians generally live a healthier lifestyle than non-vegetarians. For example, people who give up meat are also more likely to drink moderately, be non-smokers and take regular exercise.

Not all vegetarian groups have low rates of coronary heart disease, however. A large proportion of the Asian population in Britain is vegetarian, but has a higher rate of coronary heart disease than the national average.

A well-balanced vegetarian diet should be based around nourishing staple foods such as wholemeal bread, pasta, potatoes and rice, which are eaten with a good variety of vegetables, fruits, nuts and seeds.

IS PROTEIN A PROBLEM?

Contrary to popular belief, getting enough protein is not a problem for vegetarians. Most common staple foods contain enough protein, and even those on a vegan diet can get plenty from cereals, potatoes, nuts and pulses. The protein quality of individual plant foods is lower than food of animal origin (except for soya). But when different plant sources of protein are eaten in a diet, the overall protein quality is as good as that from a mixed diet. There is no need to worry about protein quality except with young children, when it is important to combine cereals and pulses in a meal.

PREGNANCY, CHILDREN AND VEGETARIANISM

It is perfectly safe for pregnant women to follow a vegetarian diet, if they include foods that contain iron, calcium, folate and vitamin B_{12}. Vegan mothers-to-be may need to take calcium and vitamin B_{12} supplements, but they should consult their doctor first. Unless women are iron-deficient during pregnancy, their babies are born with enough iron in their bodies to last about six months; after that, it is important to include good sources of iron in the infant's diet. Prolonged breastfeeding can lead to iron-deficiency anaemia in the baby as milk is a poor source of iron. Good vegetarian iron sources include leafy green vegetables, cereals, mashed lentils and beans.

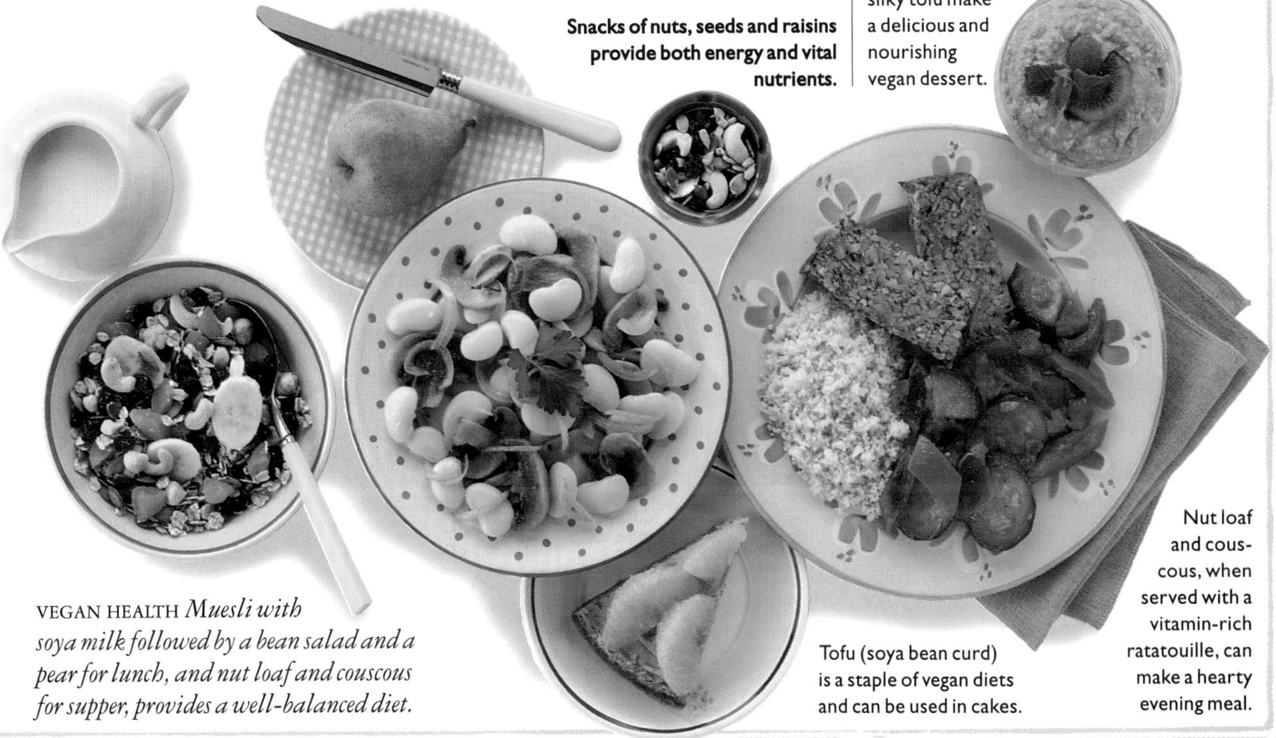

Snacks of nuts, seeds and raisins provide both energy and vital nutrients.

Fresh raspberries whipped with silky tofu make a delicious and nourishing vegan dessert.

VEGAN HEALTH *Muesli with soya milk followed by a bean salad and a pear for lunch, and nut loaf and couscous for supper, provides a well-balanced diet.*

Tofu (soya bean curd) is a staple of vegan diets and can be used in cakes.

Nut loaf and couscous, when served with a vitamin-rich ratatouille, can make a hearty evening meal.

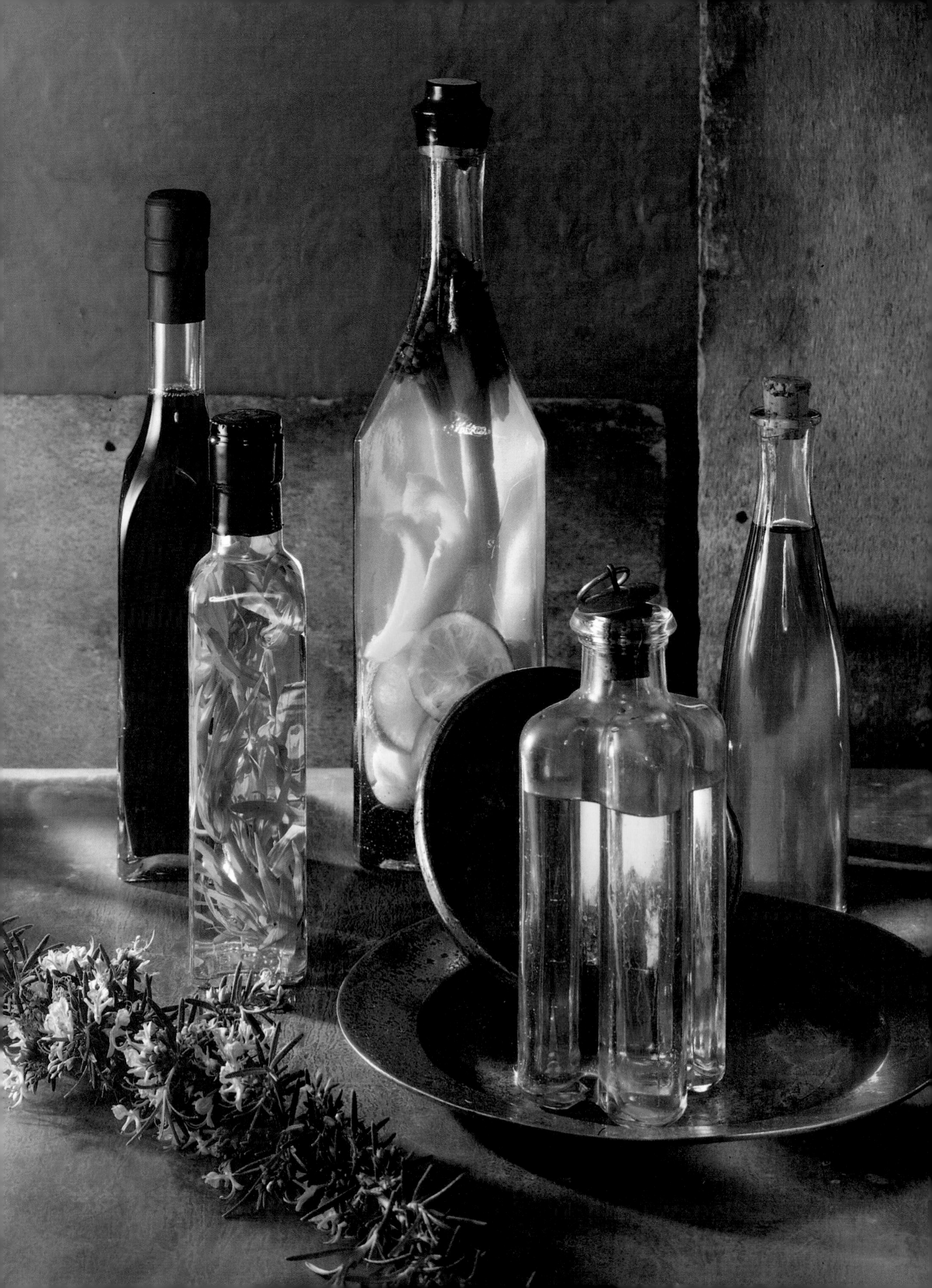

VINEGAR

BENEFIT

- *Naturopaths believe that cider vinegar may help people with arthritis*

DRAWBACK

- *May trigger an allergic reaction in people sensitive to yeasts or moulds*

With its familiar tangy flavour, vinegar may be used to make a zesty, fat-free alternative to oily salad dressings, and can spice up a low-calorie or low-sodium diet. It is mainly water, flavoured with acetic acid, although it may contain other related compounds. It is the acetic acid – typically 5g per 100ml – which gives vinegar its characteristic flavour and which makes it such an effective preservative.

Vinegar is made in two stages, under controlled conditions to ensure there is no contamination. First, yeasts turn natural sugars into alcohol and then bacteria convert the alcohol into acetic acid. In rare cases, people who have allergies to yeasts, moulds or fermented foods can develop an allergic reaction to vinegar and may experience symptoms such as headaches or hives (an itchy rash).

VINEGAR VARIETIES

Vinegars vary in colour and flavour depending on the source of alcohol; these sources include red wine, white wine, cider, malt, sherry and rice wine (in China and Japan). Speciality vinegars are made with white or red wine vinegar infused with a particular herb, spice or fruit, such as tarragon, dill, rosemary, lemon balm, garlic, green peppercorn, chilli or raspberry.

SHARP FLAVOURS *As a preserving liquid, vinegar has no equal – once sealed it can last indefinitely. Enliven salads with (from left to right) balsamic, tarragon, citrus, wine and sherry vinegars.*

Not all vinegars are what they seem. White malt vinegar, for example, is merely brown malt vinegar which has been filtered through charcoal to remove its colour, while the vinegar most often available at fish and chip shops is really non-brewed condiment (NBC). It is produced from synthetic acetic acid, artificial colour, vinegar flavourings, salt and sugar.

CIDER VINEGAR

Made from fermented apple juice, cider vinegar is believed by naturopaths to have therapeutic properties even though it contains very small amounts of minerals such as potassium and calcium. Naturopaths believe that, when taken with honey, cider vinegar can help to relieve the symptoms of arthritis and stimulate the liver to produce more bile. Cider vinegar is used in shampoos to make hair glossier, and in preparations claiming to restore hair growth.

Naturopaths also believe that cider vinegar can inhibit diarrhoea, regulate metabolism and help digestion; and that it cures gastrointestinal infections and chronic fatigue – claims that are difficult to substantiate scientifically.

In most therapies, the recommended dose is one or two teaspoons of cider vinegar in a glass of water, two or three times a day. One rather unlikely claim for combating obesity involves drinking cider vinegar, diluted in cold or hot water, first thing in the morning on an empty stomach.

STEEPED IN HISTORY

The name vinegar comes from the Latin *vinum acer* meaning 'sharp wine'. Rich, dark balsamic vinegar, produced from red wine in Modena, Italy, is the most expensive of all vinegars. It is bottled for sale at anything between 15 and 50 years old. At least ten of those years will have been spent ageing in wooden barrels.

VIRAL AND BACTERIAL INFECTIONS

The human body is vulnerable to bacteria and viruses which are capable of overwhelming the immune system and causing infection. Some foods have antibacterial or antiviral properties and can destroy or inhibit the growth of infectious micro-organisms. Other foods act indirectly, by stimulating the immune system, so helping the body to fight infection. GARLIC has well-documented infection-fighting properties, and the juice of CRANBERRIES has long been used in the prevention and treatment of urinary tract infections. Infusions of peppermint and ginger are used by herbalists to treat colds – they are thought to improve the circulation and relieve catarrh. An infusion of thyme may be used as a gargle to relieve sore throats.

Did you know?

- Eating yoghurt can combat the aftereffects of taking antibiotics. Live yoghurt restores the 'friendly' bacteria in the gut which are often destroyed by these drugs.
- Garlic can help to fight infection. It has both antibacterial and antiviral properties and may also reduce the risk of blood clots. You can help to combat 'garlic breath' by chewing fresh parsley.
- People under stress are more likely to become ill. Your immunity can be weakened considerably when you are under stress. One US experiment which looked at people's susceptibility to the common cold found that those who had higher levels of psychological stress had a significantly greater chance of catching a cold.

VITAMINS: CORNERSTONES OF HEALTH

The body is unable to manufacture most vitamins for itself, so they are an essential part of the diet. Each vitamin has several specific roles and a deficiency can lead to serious illness.

Vitamins have been one of the major nutritional discoveries of the 20th century and, in the past three decades, vitamin additives have been used to promote anything from health foods to cosmetics.

Although the effects of vitamins had been observed for more than two centuries – the use of lemons and limes to combat scurvy on sea voyages is part of nutritional folklore – their earliest identification was not until 1896, by Christiaan Eikman, a Dutch medical officer working in Java. His discovery was to revolutionise nutritional and dietary theories which, until then, had been based on the concept that proteins were the basis of a healthy diet.

As scientific knowledge and understanding expanded and, one by one, more vitamins were discovered, it became apparent that they were organic dietary compounds and that – unlike fats, carbohydrates and some proteins – they were not metabolised to provide energy. It also emerged that, by and large, vitamins could not be manufactured by the body and therefore could only be supplied by food. More recently, science has established that vitamins are required in small amounts and each performs several specific functions or is needed to prevent an associated deficiency disease.

In Britain, the Department of Health has recommended guidelines for the daily levels of nutrients which an average healthy person requires from his or her diet. Known as RNIs (reference nutrient intakes), they indicate the amount of a nutrient sufficient for up to 97 per cent of the population; in effect this means that the specified RNI level should be more than adequate for the vast majority of people.

Each individual's needs, however, will vary slightly: sometimes, men's requirements are higher than women's – or vice versa; the needs of pregnant or lactating women may differ from those of other women; babies, children and adolescents all have specific needs; and convalescents, the elderly or people who are ill may have unusually high requirements of certain nutrients.

Nutritionists usually classify vitamins according to whether they are soluble in fat or water. The fat-soluble vitamins are A, D, E and K. These vitamins are not passed out of the body in the urine, so excessive intake may be hazardous to health. The eight B vitamins and vitamin C are water-soluble, and, except for vitamin B_{12}, they cannot be stored by the body.

VITAMIN A (RETINOL)

Vitamin A plays a number of important roles in the body. It is necessary for normal cell division and growth; it is involved in maintaining the mucous membranes of the respiratory, digestive and urinary tracts; it is vital to good eyesight, playing a key role in converting light into electrical signals; and it is important for normal embryonic development. Deficiency causes a generalised drying up of mucous membranes and increases the risk of infection. It also results in an inability to see in poor light – a condition known as night blindness. A continued lack of vitamin A results in progressively worsening vision which can lead to blindness. Although rare in developed countries, vitamin A deficiency is one of the biggest causes of preventable blindness worldwide.

An adequate daily supply of vitamin A for an adult is set at about 700 micrograms (mcg) – this could be derived from the beta carotene found in about 50g (2oz) of raw carrots. Pregnant or breastfeeding women may need a slightly higher intake, and young children slightly less.

Because vitamin A has a specific function in the retina of the eye, it is known as retinol. It is found in foods of animal origin, such as full-fat dairy produce, eggs and liver. The vitamin is

WHAT'S IN A NAME?

The discovery of vitamins cannot be credited to any one person: a number of scientists working in several different countries all made important contributions.

In 1912, Dr Casimir Funk, a 28-year-old Polish biochemist who was working in London, coined the term 'vitamines' for important substances which he, and others before him, had identified in food. The name alluded to the idea that the substances were vital to life and thought to be similar to amines – previously identified nitrogen compounds. Although the chemical parallel was disproved, the name had captured the public imagination and, from 1920, the 'e' was dropped and the term vitamins was adopted.

also available, indirectly, from plant foods where it occurs as a carotenoid called beta carotene, a pigment which gives many plant foods their yellow or orange colours, and which the body converts into vitamin A.

Retinol is a pale yellow solid which dissolves easily in oils and fats. It can be produced synthetically and in this form is used to enrich margarines. The richest source of retinol is liver: just 3g

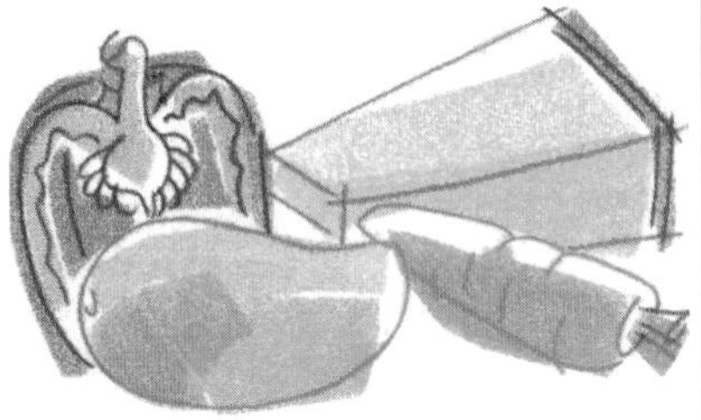

– an acorn-sized piece – of calves' liver would meet the entire adult daily requirement. Because the vitamin is fat-soluble and is not easily broken down by the body, excessive intakes of retinol are poisonous, and are associated with damage to the foetus during early pregnancy. This is the reason why women who are pregnant or trying to conceive are always advised to avoid liver. Unlike retinol, carotenoids pose no risk to health, although continued high intakes of beta carotene can lead to a condition called carotenaemia in which the skin takes on a yellow tinge, particularly on the palms of the hands and soles of the feet. This is not harmful, and the skin slowly returns to its normal colour when carotenoid intake is reduced.

Weight for weight, six times as much beta carotene is needed to provide an equivalent amount of retinol. In most Western diets, some 80 per cent of vitamin A is absorbed as retinol. Vegans, however, who not only exclude meat and fish, but also avoid dairy produce and eggs, obtain most of their vitamin A in the form of beta carotene. Carrots, red peppers, mangoes and cantaloupe melons, as well as green leafy vegetables such as spinach and kale, are all rich in this nutrient. As a rule, the more intense the colour of the fruit or vegetable the more beta carotene it contains.

As well as supplying vitamin A to the body, beta carotene has another important role as an ANTIOXIDANT. Scientists have observed that diets high in carotenoids are often associated with a reduced risk of certain cancers. However, this protection seems to be afforded only if the source of beta carotene is a food: studies where supplements have been used have not had the same positive results.

One study has claimed that two carotenoids – lutein and zeaxanthin – may be important in protecting against age-related macular degeneration (AMD), the most common cause of irreversible blindness among adults in industrialised nations, but the findings are not conclusive.

VITAMIN C

Best known as a popular, though unproven, remedy for the common cold, vitamin C (or ascorbic acid) is vital for the production of collagen, a protein needed for healthy skin, bones, cartilage, teeth and gums, and which plays an important role in healing wounds and burns. Vitamin C also helps to produce the neurotransmitters noradrenaline, which regulates blood flow, and serotonin, which helps to promote sleep.

Deficiency in vitamin C can cause fatigue, loss of appetite and increased susceptibility to infection. In severe cases it leads to scurvy – for centuries the scourge of mariners on long voyages with no access to fresh fruit or vegetables. Scurvy causes loss of teeth due to diseased gums, poor wound healing, weakened bones and mental confusion. Although vitamin C had not been identified at the time, the British Navy succeeded in staving off scurvy by issuing sailors with limes to suck – hence the term 'limey', an American slang word for a Briton.

Unlike most animals, people are unable to produce their own vitamin C from glucose and so need a regular intake from food. Vitamin C is one of the most unstable vitamins, easily destroyed by oxidation, exposure to light or high temperatures. The best sources, therefore, are fresh, raw fruits and vegetables. High levels are found in citrus fruits, strawberries, blackcurrants, guavas, kiwi fruit and peppers.

The normal adult requirement is 40mg a day, which could be provided by a small orange, a large peach or a single kiwi fruit. Smokers, whose requirements for vitamin C are at least twice as high as non-smokers, need 80mg a day or more. A medium-sized potato supplies a quarter of a non-smoking adult's daily requirement. In spite of their relatively modest vitamin C content, potatoes contribute significantly to total intakes where

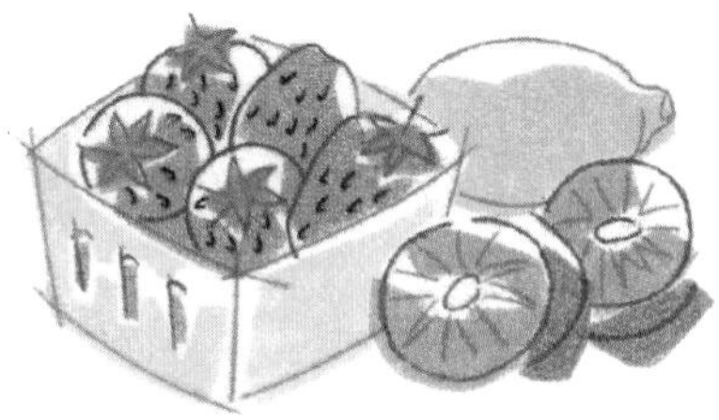

they are eaten as a staple food. In the British diet potatoes – and to a lesser extent green vegetables, fresh fruit and fruit juices – are the most important sources of vitamin C.

Vitamin C improves the iron intake of vegetarians or people who do not eat much meat because the iron present in many plant foods (known as non-haem iron) is absorbed more efficiently when these foods are accompanied by foods or fruit juices containing vitamin C.

A reduced risk of some cancers and of heart disease has been linked to diets high in fruit and vegetables, but it is still not clear how great a part vitamin C plays in this. Claims that a daily intake of 1000mg or more of vitamin C will protect against, or cure, the common cold have never been substantiated; while taking supplements may lead to a lessening of the symptoms and their duration, it cannot actually prevent people from catching a cold. Furthermore, in the long term, megadoses of vitamin C can lead to kidney stone formation in susceptible people; as well as headaches, sleep disturbances and stomach upsets.

THE B VITAMINS

Originally thought to be a single vitamin because the roles which they play in nutrition are very similar, B complex is really a combination of eight different vitamins. All except B_{12} and folate are involved in releasing energy from food. Because they are soluble in water to a greater or lesser extent – with the exception of B_{12} – the body lacks the ability to store them, and any surplus intake is therefore usually excreted in the urine.

THIAMIN (VITAMIN B_1)

The function of thiamin is to convert carbohydrates, fats and alcohol into energy. It also helps to prevent the build-up of toxic by-products of metabolism in the body, which would otherwise damage the heart as well as the nervous system.

Potatoes, pork, liver, heart, kidneys, Brazil nuts, seeds, beans and brown rice are all good sources of the vitamin. Many breakfast cereals are fortified with it and, in Britain, flours used for baking white bread are required by law to have thiamin added.

The recommended adult daily requirement for thiamin is about 1mg, which is easily supplied by the average British diet. Major sources in the UK are fortified white bread, breakfast cereals, potatoes and meat. It would take 12 slices of white bread or six and a half slices of wholemeal bread to meet an adult's daily need.

As thiamin is water-soluble, up to half the amount present in many vegetables is lost when they are boiled. Fortunately, potatoes lose less of their thiamin than most other vegetables: boiled in their skins, they lose about one-tenth, and if peeled before boiling, they lose about a quarter.

Four average portions of boiled brown rice would meet an adult's daily need. Polished white rice, however, contains hardly any thiamin and, in countries where it forms a major part of the diet, has been pinpointed as the main cause of the thiamin deficiency disease, beri-beri. In industrialised nations thiamin deficiency has been

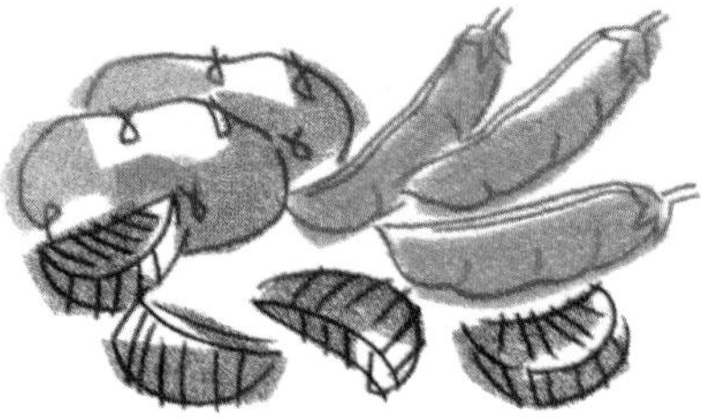

largely eliminated, but it is still found among down-and-out alcoholics who exist on alcohol alone. Symptoms of deficiency include appetite loss, confusion, swelling of the limbs, numbness and muscle weakness.

Enzymes called thiaminases can also cause deficiency symptoms. Found in some raw foods – such as blueberries, red cabbage, betel nuts and certain types of fish – thiaminases reduce thiamin activity. They are destroyed by cooking, but anyone eating large amounts of the listed raw foods may need extra dietary thiamin.

RIBOFLAVIN (VITAMIN B_2)

Riboflavin is vital for the release of energy from food; it is also needed for the proper functioning of vitamin B_6 and niacin. The body's ability to store

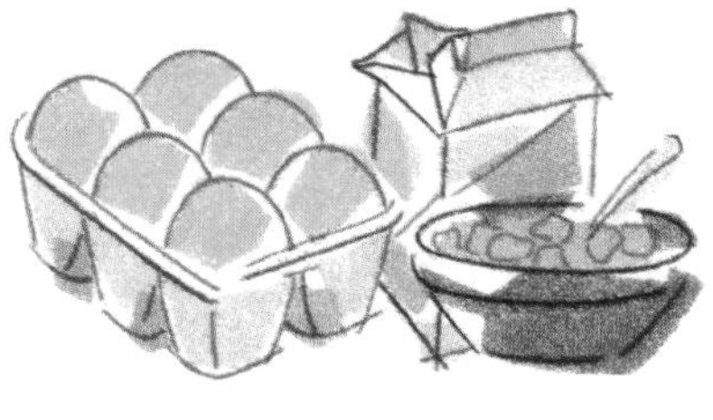

riboflavin is very limited so it is important to ensure an adequate daily intake. Riboflavin requirements are governed by the rate at which people burn energy. An adult male needs about 1.3mg a day; higher amounts are needed by pregnant or breastfeeding women, as well as by children and teenagers during growth spurts.

Milk is an excellent source of riboflavin; 750ml (just under 1½ pints) of milk will meet an adult's daily needs. However, if milk is exposed to sunlight the vitamin is rapidly lost – indeed as much as three-quarters of the riboflavin may be lost if a bottle or jug of milk is left for three and a half hours in the sun.

Riboflavin is also found in other dairy produce, as well as eggs, meat, poultry, yeast extract and fortified breakfast cereals. In fact, one bowl of fortified cereal could provide as much as half of the adult daily requirement for riboflavin. An egg will provide one-fifth, and two slices of lean roast beef a quarter of the necessary amount. Even beer contains a little riboflavin, but in such insignificant amounts that you would have to drink at least 4.5 litres (8 pints) to meet the full daily requirement.

Deficiency symptoms – common in developing countries, but rarely seen in the West apart from occasionally among the elderly or sick – include cracked lips, bloodshot eyes, dermatitis and some forms of anaemia.

NIACIN

Niacin is used in the formation of two coenzymes involved in the production of energy in cells. It is also needed to form neurotransmitters, and it helps to maintain a healthy skin and digestive system. Widely distributed in food, the best sources of niacin (nicotinic acid) are liver, lean meat, poultry, pulses, nuts and fortified breakfast cereals: niacin is manufactured commercially and is commonly used to enrich flours and fortify cereals.

Some of the body's niacin needs are met from tryptophan – an amino acid present in many proteins – which the body can convert into the vitamin. So while milk, cheese and eggs are low in niacin, they can still help to prevent a niacin deficiency because of their high tryptophan content; furthermore, the niacin they provide is in a form which is readily available to the body.

Niacin deficiency can cause fatigue, depression and a skin rash which is more likely to appear when the skin is exposed to sunlight. Pellagra, an ailment which causes diarrhoea, dermatitis and dementia, can be caused by a niacin deficiency and used to be widespread in communities whose staple foods were deficient in the vitamin. A man needs about 17 mg of niacin per day; women need slightly less – about

13mg. Three slices of lean roast beef, 150g (5½oz) of roast chicken, 300g (10½oz) Cheddar cheese, or a large salmon steak, would each provide an adequate daily intake of niacin for the majority of adults.

High-dose nicotinic acid supplements (1-2 g a day) are sometimes used to treat high blood cholesterol levels. However, these should only be taken under medical supervision because an excessive intake – maintained over several weeks – can cause side effects such as flushing of the skin and, more seriously, liver damage.

PANTOTHENIC ACID

As implied by its name, which comes from the Greek and means 'widespread', pantothenic acid is present in all foods of animal or vegetable origin. Among the most convenient sources of the vitamin are wholemeal bread, nuts – especially chestnuts – and dried

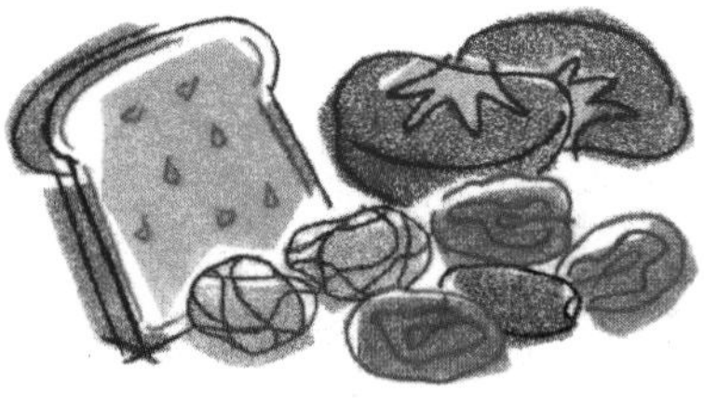

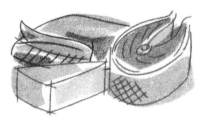

fruits such as prunes and apricots. Pantothenic acid is part of a coenzyme that enables the body to take energy from food. A deficiency – which may cause numbness in the toes – has been found only in cases of acute malnutrition such as among prisoners of war.

Indeed, pantothenic acid is so widespread in the foods we eat that no specific RNI has been recommended, although experts say that 3-7 mg daily is the minimum intake needed to maintain health. It is used as a supplement only where normal food consumption is impossible and patients are fed artificially. Problems due to an excessive intake are unknown.

VITAMIN B_6 (PYRIDOXINE)

The broad term vitamin B_6 actually describes a trio of interchangeable and related compounds (pyridoxine, pyridoxal and pyridoxamine) all of which are needed to break down and release energy from protein. It is also important for the functioning of the nervous and immune systems.

Vitamin B_6 is found in a variety of foods, particularly proteins such as offal, poultry, fish and eggs. Other important sources include potatoes and other vegetables, brown rice, nuts, soya beans, wholegrain cereals and wholemeal bread.

The more protein there is in your diet, the more vitamin B_6 you will need, but requirements vary from one individual to another. Men require slightly more of the vitamin than women; on average, an adult male requires about 1.4 mg a day, which could be provided by one large salmon steak or two servings of fortified breakfast cereal. Because vitamin B_6 is also synthesised in the gut – enabling the body to supplement dietary sources – some experts argue that our needs are higher than our dietary needs suggest.

Doctors often prescribe vitamin B_6 supplements to alleviate symptoms of premenstrual syndrome, such as mood swings or abdominal bloating, or to counteract some of the side effects of oral contraceptive pills. Do not exceed

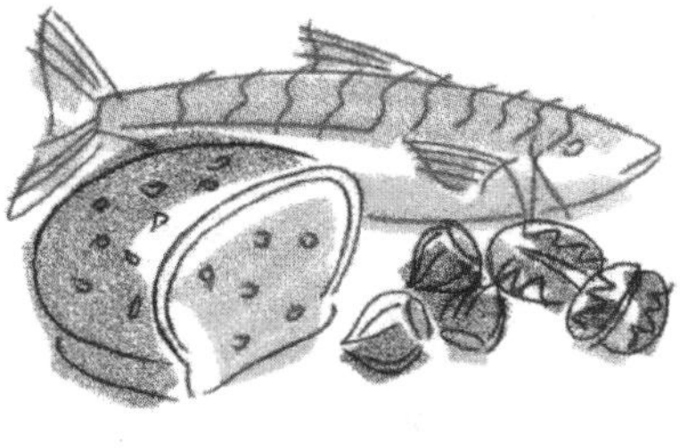

the recommended dose, however, as high doses of vitamin B_6 supplements (in amounts of 1 g or more) may cause nerve damage, reflected as weakness or numbness of the extremities.

Deficiency of vitamin B_6 is very rare. In adults, it may occur as a result of long-term medication, and can cause depression, confusion and anaemia. Symptoms may also include a scaly skin, known as seborrhoeic dermatitis, and a smooth red tongue.

BIOTIN

This coenzyme, which is widely distributed in small concentrations in all animal and plant foods, helps to make fatty acids and is needed in minute amounts in the metabolic process which frees energy from food. Liver and kidneys are both good sources of biotin and smaller amounts are found in foods such as cheese, wholemeal bread, yoghurt, peanut butter and egg yolks. However, because it is so readily available in food and so little of the vitamin is required, biotin is of little consideration when planning the diet.

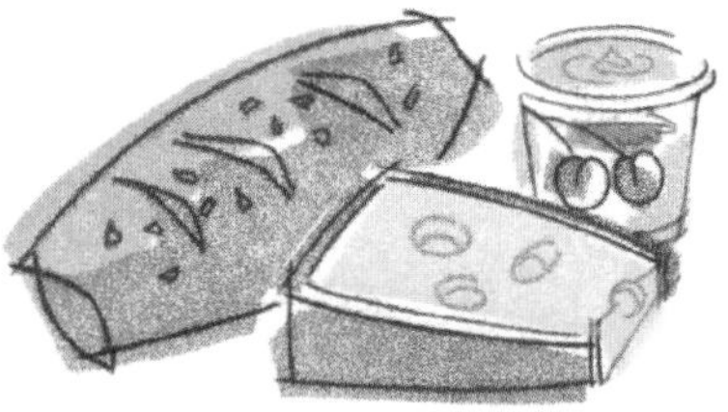

Deficiency is very rare, but is sometimes found in patients who have been fed intravenously for several weeks. If a deficiency does occur, it can lead to hair loss, scaly dermatitis, loss of appetite, nausea and muscle pains.

FOLATE

Folates are a group of compounds which are derived from folic acid. They are required for cell division and the formation of DNA (the body's genetic blueprint), RNA which transports DNA data within the cell, and for protein synthesis. Folate is also vital for reproduction and for the formation of the iron-containing protein in haemoglobin needed to make red blood cells.

The recommended daily intake is 200mcg. However, any woman trying to conceive should take higher levels of folic acid, in supplement form, for three months before conception and in the first weeks of pregnancy; there is proof that this can reduce the chances of having a baby with neural tube defects. Indeed, some nutritionists recommend an intake of 400mcg daily – double the male requirement – for all sexually active women who might, albeit inadvertently, become pregnant. In Britain, the Department of Health advises women who are, or intend to become, pregnant to take a folic acid supplement (of up to 200mcg) until at least the 12th week of their pregnancy. Liver, yeast, green vegetables such as broccoli, nuts and pulses are all good sources of the vitamin although folates are found in most foods. Pregnant women, however, should avoid liver as it may contain dangerously high levels of vitamin A.

One helping of Brussels sprouts or of a fortified breakfast cereal will provide 100mcg of folates; a large glass of fresh orange juice, 40mcg; and a slice of wholemeal bread, 15mcg. Fruit and vegetables supply about 40 per cent of folates in the average British diet.

Some experts believe that only about half of the folate in many foods is

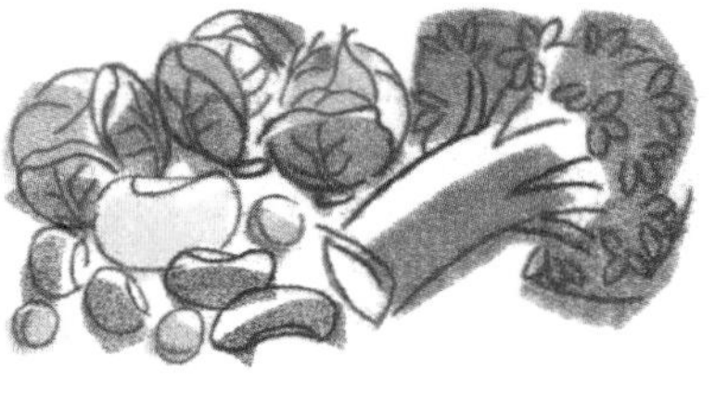

absorbed by the body, although uptake from the forms of folate used in fortified foods is known to be much higher than this. A folate deficiency, which can lead to foetal malformations and cause megaloblastic ANAEMIA, may stem from diets low in fresh foods or reduced absorption caused by diseases of the small bowel.

VITAMIN B_{12}

Found in foods from animal sources or in fortified products and supplements, vitamin B_{12} is needed for all growth and division of cells and for red blood-cell formation. It is also integral to the making of DNA, RNA and myelin – the white sheath that surrounds nerve fibres. It is required only in minute amounts – 1.5mcg fulfils the adult daily requirement – and it can only be absorbed by the body in conjunction with a glycoprotein known as intrinsic factor which is made in the stomach. Pernicious anaemia is usually the result of an inability to produce intrinsic factor, so B_{12} cannot be absorbed; it may also be caused by a dietary deficiency of the vitamin. Characterised

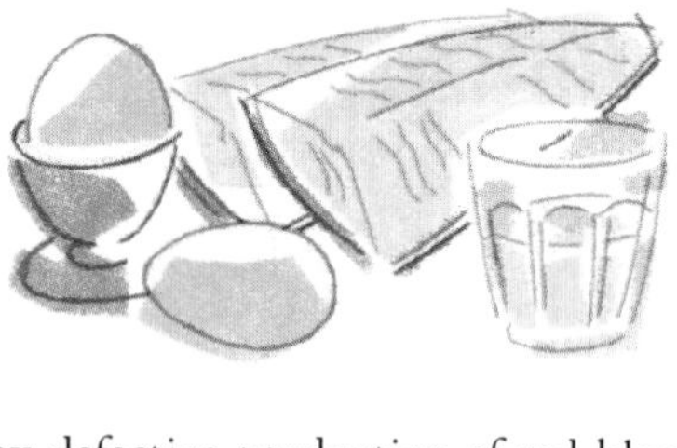

by defective production of red blood cells, and potentially fatal if left untreated, pernicious anaemia is cured by injections of vitamin B_{12}.

Any diet containing some protein from an animal source should provide adequate vitamin B_{12}. A helping of white fish or one egg, for example, will supply an adult's daily needs; a large serving of fortified breakfast cereal, or a large glass of milk, will supply about half the recommended daily intake. Furthermore, if intake is very low, B_{12} can be recycled in the body from bile.

Vegetarians usually obtain sufficient vitamin B_{12} from eggs and dairy produce, although vegans (and babies breastfed by vegan mothers) may suffer from a deficiency unless they take supplements or eat foods fortified with the vitamin. In the first instance, deficiency can cause fatigue and, in vegans, can lead to megaloblastic ANAEMIA and damage to the nervous system. Such damage may also occur without megaloblastic anaemia, because the high intakes of folate in the diets of vegans arrest the anaemia but allow the more insidious neurological symptoms to progress.

VITAMIN D

Nicknamed the 'sunshine' vitamin because it can be produced by the exposure of the skin to the sun's (and artificial) ultraviolet rays, vitamin D is needed to absorb calcium and phosphorus, and is thus vital to healthy bone structure and good teeth.

Although vitamin D is fat-soluble, not much is stored in the body. However, even in northern countries, the formation of vitamin D in the skin during summer months is sufficient to meet the body's needs for the whole year, so most adults do not have to rely on dietary sources. People most at risk of deficiency and for whom dietary vitamin D is vital are those who are compelled to stay indoors, such as babies, the sick and the elderly, or women who traditionally wear clothes which almost completely cover their bodies.

In the West, most dietary vitamin D comes from fortified foods such as

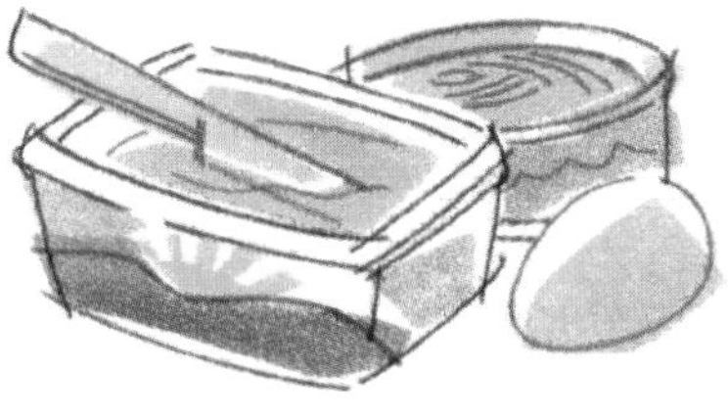

margarine – which in Britain is fortified with vitamin D by law – and breakfast cereals. Other major dietary sources include eggs and oily fish.

Vitamin D is converted into an 'active' form in the kidneys. It then acts as a hormone which controls the calcium absorbed from the intestine and regulates the levels of calcium and phosphorus in the blood and bones.

Because of its synthesis in the skin, the Department of Health sets no RNI for vitamin D, but recommends an intake of 10mcg daily (the amount found in a small can of sardines) for pregnant women and the elderly.

Deficiency causes rickets in children and OSTEOMALACIA in adults. In Britain rickets is quite rare, except among the Asian community, but osteomalacia – a softening of the bones which causes pain and makes fractures more likely – is relatively common in the elderly. However, as there is only a small margin between safe and toxic levels of the vitamin (an excess can cause kidney damage) always observe the instructions on appropriate dosage when taking vitamin D supplements.

VITAMIN E

Vitamin E is the collective name given to a group of biologically active ANTIOXIDANT compounds. It prevents damage caused by oxidation to polyunsaturated fatty acids found in cell membranes. To ensure its protective role, people with a diet which is high in polyunsaturated fatty acids should also take plenty of vitamin E.

Vegetable oils and some margarines, nuts, seeds and wheatgerm are all good sources of vitamin E. A small packet of peanuts or a small handful of almonds, or just over a teaspoon of sunflower oil would each supply about 3mg of vitamin E – an adequate daily intake of the vitamin for an adult woman.

Interestingly, some studies suggest a link between much higher intakes of vitamin E – as much as 75-100mg – and a lower risk of disorders associated with FREE RADICAL damage such as certain cancers, stroke, heart disease and atherosclerosis. Since it is not possible to obtain these levels in a balanced diet, such an intake can only normally be obtained by taking supplements. A large trial using supplements, however, failed to show that high doses of vitamin E lessened the risk of death from heart disease among smokers. There is some acceptance of its protective role in preventing atherosclerosis

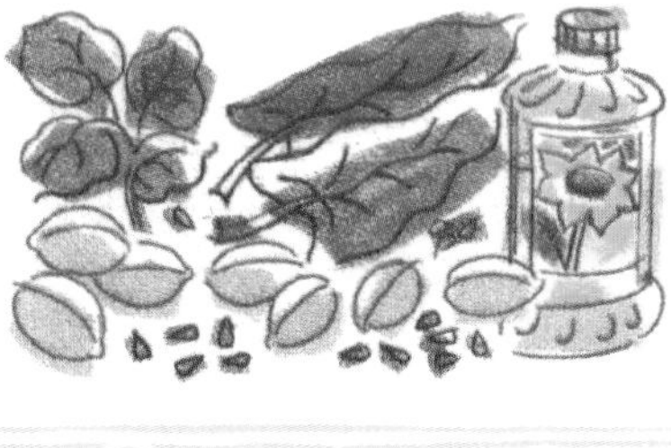

but population studies have not yet confirmed it. Vitamin E deficiency is rare, occurring only in premature babies and people who are unable to absorb fat. When it does occur, it causes haemolytic anaemia and nerve damage. High doses are not toxic but may lead to a vitamin K deficiency.

VITAMIN K

This group of compounds – found in plant foods (phylloquinones), manufactured by bacteria in the intestine (menaquinones) and created in the laboratory (menadione) – is vital in forming the glycoproteins needed for normal blood clotting. Vitamin K is also used to make other proteins needed for healthy bones and tissues.

Because the transfer of the vitamin across the placenta during pregnancy is poor and the sterile gut of the infant is unable to produce menaquinones,

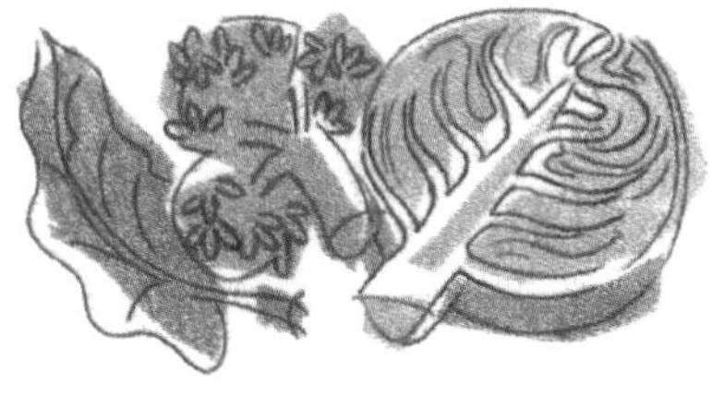

newborn babies are routinely given supplements of vitamin K either with an injection or orally. This is done not only to promote normal clotting of the blood but also to prevent any future occurrence of life-threatening haemorrhagic disease.

Dietary deficiency is rare, but can occur when the body does not absorb fat properly as in gall-bladder disease or where there is an excessive intake of vitamin E.

Reducing vitamin K is important to those undergoing anticoagulation therapy. Major sources in the diet are green vegetables including cauliflower, spinach, broccoli and cabbage – particularly in the form of sauerkraut.

VITAMIN	SOME IMPORTANT SOURCES	ROLE IN HEALTH
A (from retinol in animal foods; or from beta carotene in plant foods)	Retinol: liver, oily fish, egg yolk, butter, cheese. Beta carotene: carrots, squash, apricots, cantaloupe melon and green leafy vegetables. (6mcg beta carotene are needed to make 1mcg of vitamin A.)	Essential for growth and cell development, vision and immune function. Maintains the health of the skin and mucous membranes such as the lining of the respiratory and urinary tracts. Carotenes may act as important antioxidants in the body.
C (ascorbic acid)	Fruits and vegetables, particularly citrus fruit, strawberries, kiwi fruit, peppers, blackcurrants and potatoes.	Needed to make collagen (a protein essential for healthy gums, teeth, bones, cartilage and skin) and neurotransmitters such as noradrenaline and serotonin. Important as an antioxidant in the body; aids absorption of iron from plant food.
Thiamin (B_1)	Pork, liver, heart, kidneys, fortified white bread, fortified breakfast cereals, potatoes, nuts and pulses.	Needed to obtain energy from carbohydrates, fats and alcohol; prevents the build-up of toxic substances in the body which may damage the heart and nervous system.
Riboflavin (B_2)	Milk, yoghurt, eggs, meat, poultry, fish and fortified breakfast cereals.	Needed to release energy from food and for the functioning of vitamin B_6 and niacin.
B_6 (pyridoxine)	Lean meat, poultry, fish, eggs, wholewheat bread and cereals, nuts, bananas, yeast extract and soya beans.	Helps to release energy from proteins; important for immune function, the nervous system and the formation of red blood cells.
Niacin (nicotinic acid)	Lean meat, poultry, pulses, potatoes, fortified breakfast cereals and nuts.	Needed to produce energy in cells and to form neurotransmitters. Helps to maintain healthy skin and an efficient digestive system.
Pantothenic acid	Contained in all meat and vegetable foods, particularly liver, dried fruit and nuts.	Helps to release energy from food. Essential to the synthesis of cholesterol, fat and red blood cells.
Biotin	Present in almost all foods, particularly liver, peanut butter, egg yolk and fortified foods such as yeast extracts.	Needed to release energy from food. Important in the synthesis of fat and cholesterol.
Folate (folic acid)	Green leafy vegetables, liver, Brussels sprouts, broccoli, pulses, wheatgerm, fortified breakfast cereals and bread.	Required for cell division and the formation of DNA, RNA and proteins in the body. Extra needed before conception and in pregnancy to protect against neural tube defects.
B_{12} (cyanocobalamin)	Foods of animal origin such as meat, poultry, fish, eggs and dairy products, as well as certain fortified breakfast cereals.	Vital for making DNA, RNA and myelin – the white sheath that surrounds nerve fibres. Also needed for cell division and the transportation of folate into cells.
D (calciferols)	Fish liver oils, eggs, fortified margarines, tuna, salmon and sardines.	Needed to absorb calcium and phosphorus for normal formation of bones and teeth.
E (tocopherols)	Vegetable oils, wheatgerm, nuts, seeds and margarine.	Helps to prevent oxidation by free radicals of polyunsaturated fatty acids in cell membranes and other tissues.
K (phylloquinone, menaquinone)	Green leafy vegetables such as cabbage, broccoli, Brussels sprouts and cauliflower.	Essential in forming certain proteins and needed for normal blood clotting.

DAILY REQUIREMENT			
MALE	FEMALE	SYMPTOMS OF DEFICIENCY	SYMPTOMS OF EXCESS
700 mcg (of vitamin A)	600 mcg (950 mcg in lactation)	Poor night vision, increased risk of infection, respiratory disorders; eye damage which in extreme cases can lead to blindness.	Drowsiness, hair loss, headaches and vomiting, liver and bone damage. Increased risk of abortion and defects in newborn babies. Excess carotenes may cause the skin to become yellow.
40 mg (smokers: at least 80 mg)	40 mg (smokers: at least 80 mg)	Fatigue, appetite loss, aching joints, sore gums, scaly skin. Slow healing of wounds and consequent increased susceptibility to infection. Severe deficiency can cause mental disorders and internal haemorrhages which may lead to anaemia.	Surplus vitamin C is safely excreted in the urine. Megadoses may, however, lead to kidney stones in susceptible people. Megadoses may also cause headaches and sleep disturbance, and should not be taken by pregnant women.
1 mg	0.8 mg	Appetite loss, mental confusion, swelling of the limbs, loss of sensation, nervous disorders, muscle weakness and an enlarged heart. Common among alcoholics.	No known symptoms, as any excess thiamin is cleared by the kidneys.
1.3 mg	1.1 mg	Dry, cracked lips, inflamed, bloodshot eyes, dermatitis, mild anaemia.	No known toxicity; excess is normally excreted as bright yellow urine.
1.4 mg	1.2 mg	Deficiency in adults is rare but may be induced by antifungal and antitubercular drugs. Symptoms include anaemia, depression and confusion.	Nerve damage. High doses over a long period lead to loss of sensation and function in the hands and feet.
17 mg	13 mg	Fatigue, depression, pigmented skin rash (more likely when exposed to sunlight), dermatitis, diarrhoea and, in advanced cases, dementia.	High doses of nicotinic acid supplements may result in 'flushing' of the skin and liver damage.
3-7 mg	3-7 mg	Deficiency is extremely rare and may lead to numbness and tingling in the toes.	No reported symptoms.
10-200 mcg	10-200 mcg	Deficiency is unknown on a normal diet but can be induced if raw egg whites are eaten regularly. Symptoms include dermatitis and hair loss.	No reported symptoms.
200 mcg	200 mcg (400 mcg in pregnancy)	Megaloblastic anaemia, wasting of the gut leading to malabsorption of nutrients. Linked with neural tube defects in foetus.	Excess folate is not toxic, but it may mask vitamin B_{12} deficiency and trigger convulsions in epileptics.
1.5 mcg	1.5 mcg	Fatigue, megaloblastic anaemia, pins and needles and loss of sensation in limbs; degeneration of the nervous system.	No reported symptoms.
Enough vitamin D is made when the skin is exposed to sunlight. People who are confined indoors require about 10mcg from the diet.		Muscle weakness and tenseness; softening of the bones causing bone pain and fractures (osteomalacia). In children, leads to deformation of the skeleton (rickets).	High levels of calcium in the blood lead to calcium deposits and irreversible damage in soft tissues such as the heart, lungs and kidneys.
At least 4 mg	At least 3 mg	Occurs only in people who cannot absorb fat and in premature babies. Symptoms include haemolytic anaemia and nerve damage.	Vitamin E is not highly toxic but high doses may cause vitamin K deficiency.
70 mcg	65 mcg	In extreme cases a deficiency reduces prothrombin (a coagulation agent) so impairing clotting of the blood. In adults deficiency is usually the result of disease or drug therapy.	There may be a link between new-born babies who have been injected with vitamin K and a raised incidence of leukaemia in childhood.

WATER

See page 372

WATERCRESS

BENEFITS
- *Excellent source of vitamin C*
- *Excellent source of beta carotene*

DRAWBACK
- *Risk of bacterial contamination*

Peppery, dark green watercress leaves are among the healthiest of fresh salad vegetables. They are rich in vitamins and minerals while containing only 22 Calories per 100g (3½oz).

AN ANTI-CANCER CRUCIFER

Watercress is also a member of the cancer-fighting crucifer family (which includes broccoli, Brussels sprouts, cabbage, cauliflower and kale). It is an excellent source of the ANTIOXIDANTS beta carotene and vitamin C which 'mop up' FREE RADICALS and so protect against cancer. Watercress also contains vitamin E, another antioxidant.

Some years ago, doctors at the Roswell Park Memorial Institute, New York, USA, found that regular inclusion of cruciferous vegetables in the daily diet significantly cut their patients' risk of contracting cancer of the colon. They also found that the more frequently these vegetables were eaten, the lower the risk became. A number of other studies have also indicated that eating plenty of cruciferous vegetables may help to reduce the risk of cancers of the rectum and bladder.

POTENTIAL HAZARDS

Never gather watercress from the wild. It often grows in streams inhabited by water snails, which are carriers of the liver fluke. Droplets of water or tiny snails adhering to the leaves can pass on the parasite, which attacks the liver. Wild watercress may also carry bacteria that cause listeriosis. Even cultivated watercress, grown in controlled conditions, should be washed thoroughly before consumption.

RESTORATIVE POWERS

In traditional medicine, watercress has long been used to treat kidney disorders and liver malfunctions. *Culpeper's Herbal* (1653), suggested applying watercress juice to the skin to clear up spots. It is a natural antibiotic, and has been used in complementary medicine to speed up the body's detoxification processes. It has also been claimed to relieve stomach upsets, respiratory problems and urinary tract infections.

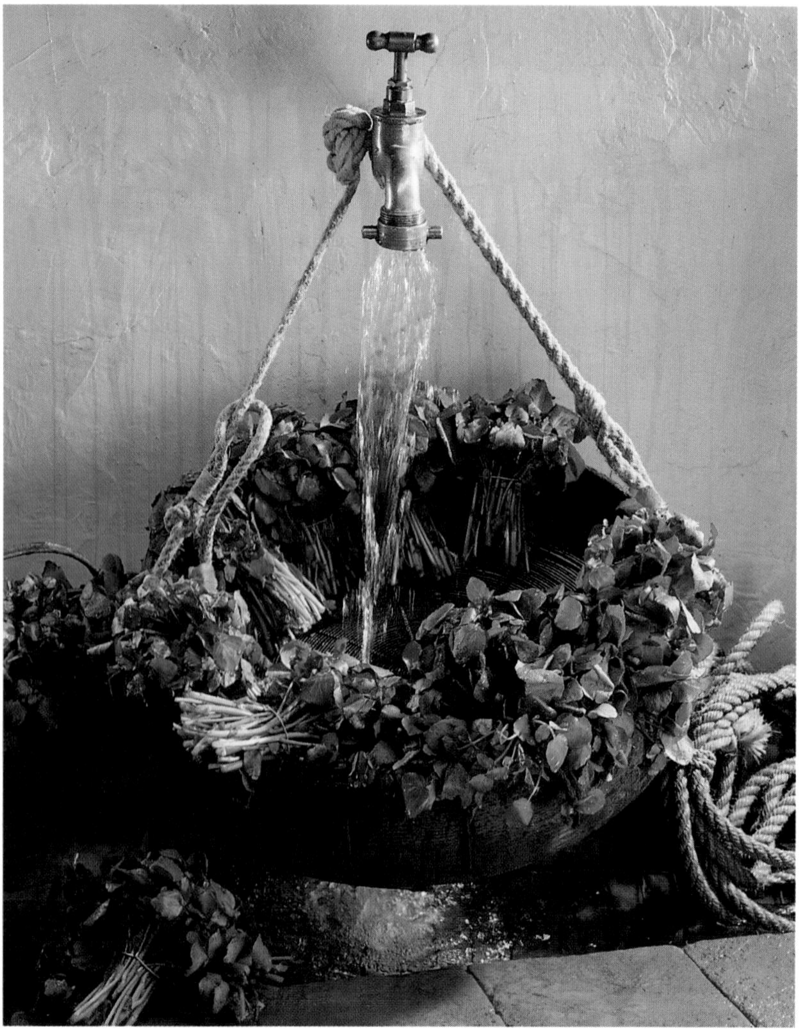

COOL AND FRESH *Watercress, which is grown in running water, is at its best in the summer months. It should be well washed to remove any harmful bacteria.*

WINE

ADVANTAGES
- *In moderation, wine may decrease the risk of heart disease, especially in middle-aged and elderly men*
- *Wine consumed with food enhances the body's absorption of iron*

DRAWBACKS
- *Red wine may induce migraines*
- *Sulphur dioxide and histamine in wines can induce asthma attacks and other allergic reactions*
- *Drunk to excess, wine can lead to hangovers, alcoholism and cirrhosis*

Medical opinion is divided as to whether wine is beneficial or harmful to health, though there is growing support for the argument that moderate consumption – particularly of red wine – may reduce the risk of heart disease later in life. On the other hand, some substances in wine are suspected of causing cancer.

Wine has little nutritional value except for its alcohol content. A glass of red wine (125 ml) supplies about 85 Calories and white about 90 Calories.

Red wines typically contain about 12 per cent ALCOHOL (ethanol) by volume, or 9.5 per cent by weight, and minimal amounts of sugar. White wines contain more variable amounts of alcohol and sugar. Wine also contains some iron but, more importantly, it helps the body to absorb iron in food when it is drunk at mealtimes.

There are elements in wine that can trigger asthma attacks in susceptible people. One of them is sulphur dioxide – used to inhibit the activities of some yeasts and bacteria – which is released when the wine is first uncorked. The other is histamine, which is found predominantly in red wine.

It is often claimed that, in spite of the high fat intake in French diets, coronary heart disease rates are low in France because of the high level of red wine consumed there. However, many other wine-drinking countries, such as Bulgaria and Hungary, have high rates of heart disease. Moreover, a recent World Health Organisation study found that the French rates of heart disease were somewhat higher than had previously been claimed. Mouth and throat cancers are common in France and this has been linked to the high wine consumption. Anyone who drinks a lot of wine and also smokes is particularly at risk from these forms of oral cancer. Numerous studies have confirmed that moderate quantities of alcohol (about two glasses a day) offer some protection against heart disease regardless of the source of alcohol. Some recent studies also suggest that a substance in red wine may offer additional health benefits by decreasing the tendency for blood to clot, as well as acting as an antioxidant.

However, some individuals find that red wine triggers migraine. It is thought that this may be due to the polyphenols it contains. Studies also show that for some people wine can spark allergic reactions which include nausea, rashes and wind.

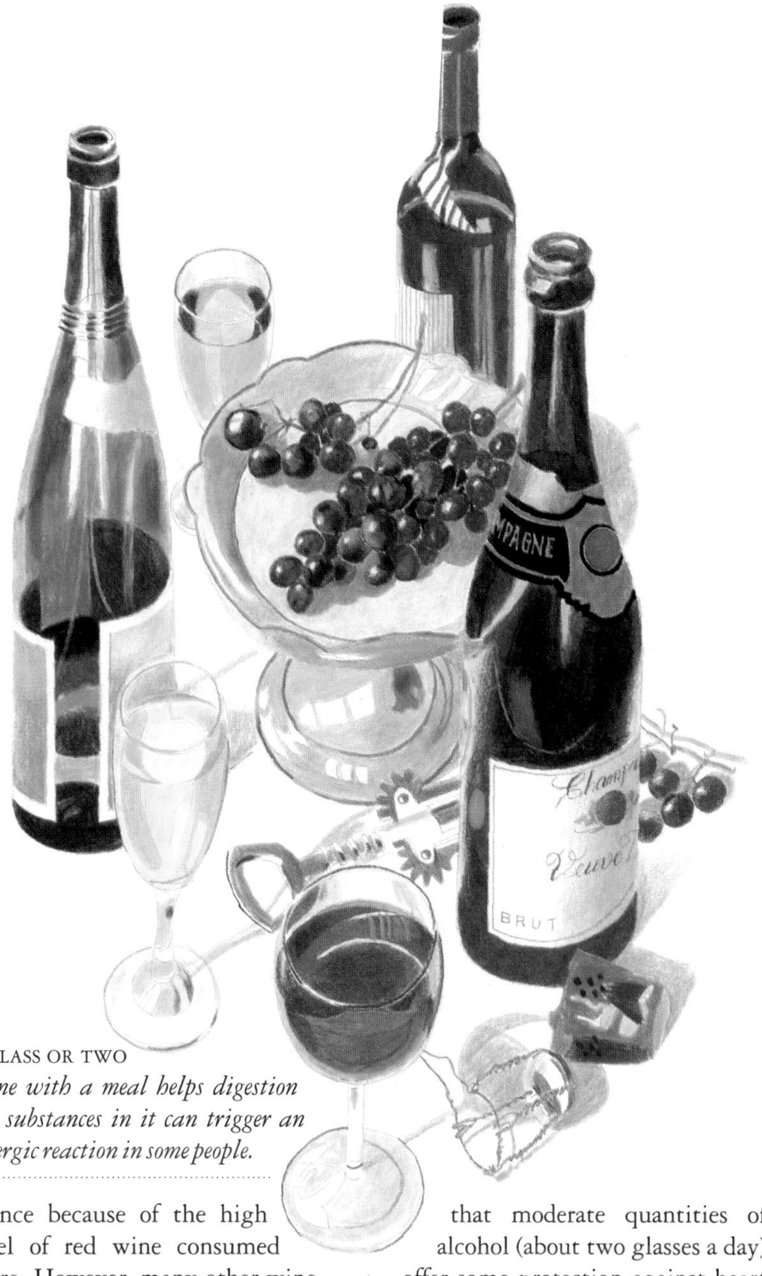

A GLASS OR TWO
Wine with a meal helps digestion but substances in it can trigger an allergic reaction in some people.

WATER: VITAL FOR LIFE

Although it is not a nutrient, there would be no life without water. Human beings can survive for some weeks without food, but without water we would perish after only a few days.

Around 60 per cent of an adult's body weight is water. It must be continually replaced since we lose roughly 0.3 litres (about ½ pint) of water a day simply through breathing. In a lifetime, each person is estimated to drink about 40 000 litres (about 8750 gallons) of water.

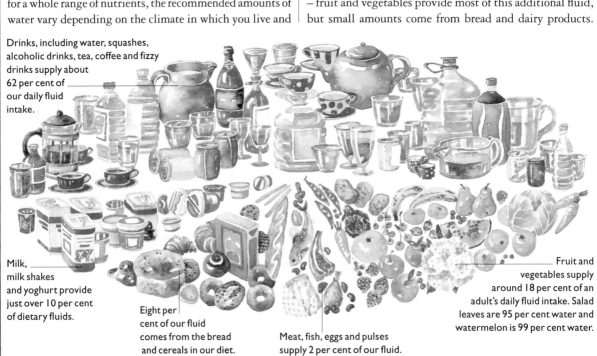

We need water for digestion and the elimination of waste products. It acts as a lubricant for joints and eyes, and is essential for the regulation of body temperature. Both drink and food supply water. The total intake from drinks – including tea, coffee or juices – plus around 300 ml (½ pint) of water which is obtained as a by-product of metabolism, provides roughly 2 litres (3½ pints) a day, while food – especially fruit and vegetables – supplies a further litre (1¾ pints). This makes a total of around 3 litres (5¼ pints) of water each day for the average adult.

When you take any form of vigorous exercise or when the weather is particularly hot, you should always drink more than normal, to compensate for the extra water lost through breathing rapidly and sweating. By drinking plenty of water you can ensure that calcium in the urine is diluted – in high concentrations, calcium can crystallise and form kidney stones. Water flushes out bladder and kidney infections and improves the complexion by washing out the body's waste products.

People who drink too little water may suffer from headaches and poor concentration. But surprisingly, it is

Where we get our water from

Many people do not drink enough water. But although nutritionists have suggested minimum daily requirements for a whole range of nutrients, the recommended amounts of water vary depending on the climate in which you live and your activities. Roughly one-third of an adult's daily fluid intake is supplied by what is eaten rather than what is drunk – fruit and vegetables provide most of this additional fluid, but small amounts come from bread and dairy products.

Drinks, including water, squashes, alcoholic drinks, tea, coffee and fizzy drinks supply about 62 per cent of our daily fluid intake.
Milk, milk shakes and yoghurt provide just over 10 per cent of dietary fluids.
Eight per cent of our fluid comes from the bread and cereals in our diet.
Meat, fish, eggs and pulses supply 2 per cent of our fluid.
Fruit and vegetables supply around 18 per cent of an adult's daily fluid intake. Salad leaves are 95 per cent water and watermelon is 99 per cent water.

possible – although difficult – to drink too much water. If a lot of water is taken in a very short space of time, it can cause short-lived symptoms which are similar to those of being drunk.

WATER WORRIES

In recent years, sales of bottled waters and of water filters have increased dramatically, reflecting public worries over the quality of tap water. These worries are largely unjustified, though some potential problems remain.

To ensure that our water is safe to drink, the British Government has introduced Water Quality Regulations. These impose far more rigorous standards than those applied to many bottled waters, especially over the content of micro-organisms. Water companies add chlorine to water to disinfect it and to prevent bacteria from breeding in it. Furthermore, tap water may contain the valuable minerals calcium, magnesium, potassium and iron, but levels can vary greatly depending on the source and region.

Although water is regularly tested, certain pollutants may still be present – albeit in minute quantities. These include fertilisers, weedkillers, industrial chemicals and poisonous metals. Some substances – such as chlorine, fluoride and aluminium sulphate – which are added to tap water by the water authorities, have also provoked alarm among consumers.

ALUMINIUM

Aluminium sulphate is often added to water during treatment to remove suspended matter. Most of it is removed through filtration, although a small amount of aluminium does pass into the water supply. The current European Community (EC) directive sets the maximum permitted concentration of aluminium at 0.2mg per litre. A report in the medical journal *The Lancet* in 1989 demonstrated that in areas where the levels of aluminium in drinking water exceeded 0.11mg per litre there was a higher risk of developing ALZHEIMER'S DISEASE than in those areas where the level was less than 0.01mg per litre. Despite these findings, the link between aluminium consumption and Alzheimer's disease is still a subject of great debate.

SEX HORMONES

Chemicals that mimic the hormone oestrogen, as used in the contraceptive pill, have been detected in some of the rivers and lakes from which water supplies are drawn. These compounds have been linked with reduced male fertility in certain fish and reptiles, and some scientists and environmental organisations are becoming increasingly concerned that these chemicals could possibly have a harmful effect on human fertility.

LEAD PIPES

Lead water pipes were once common in older houses, and although most have now been replaced, water can still be contaminated by the lead solder used to join copper pipes. The risks are much higher in soft water areas, as lead dissolves more easily in soft water. It also dissolves more easily in hot water, so never use water from the hot tap for cooking or for filling kettles.

The main concern over long-term exposure to lead is its potentially harmful effect on children. Lead poisoning is known to cause behavioural and learning difficulties and poor coordination. It can also stunt a child's growth and permanently damage the nervous system. Although adults absorb far less lead than children, they too can suffer from lead poisoning symptoms and sustain damage to the kidneys and reproductive organs.

To minimise the risk of absorbing lead, you should run the cold water tap for a few minutes each morning so that all the water which has been lying in the pipes overnight is flushed away. Use only water direct from the mains – normally from the cold tap in the kitchen – for drinking and cooking.

ODOURS AND CLOUDY WATER

Sometimes water straight from the tap has an unmistakable chlorine odour. If this happens, fill a jug with water, leave it in the refrigerator for about an hour or so, and the smell of chlorine will usually disappear.

If tap water looks cloudy or has small particles floating in it, the reason could be that work is being carried out on nearby mains. As a rule, your water authority will inform you when such work is planned, and will suggest that you run the tap until the water clears.

Otherwise, you can boil the water for several minutes and allow it to stand so that any sediment sinks to the bottom. Then decant it carefully so that you leave the sediment behind.

FLUORIDE

By hardening tooth enamel and making teeth more resistant to decay, fluoride has played a major part in improving dental health in Britain. In some areas, fluoride is added to water supplies (it is not allowed to exceed 1000mcg per litre). If you would like to know whether you live in an area where fluoride is added to the water, contact your local water authority (see 'Where to get advice' on page 375).

Fluoride is added to most toothpastes, and must be listed among the ingredients. However, in rare cases, particularly in areas where natural levels of fluoride in the water are high, children can develop a condition known as fluorosis which involves a

Water in everyday foods

We obtain roughly a third of our water from 'solid' foods, and it is surprising just how much water they contain. Fruit and vegetables supply the most, but meat, fish, bread and dairy products provide a fair proportion, too.

FOOD	AMOUNT OF WATER
BREAD	
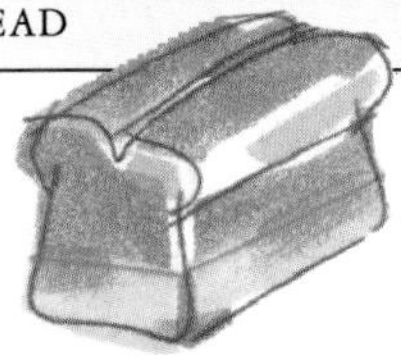	Most breads are around 38% water. Naan bread contains 29% and poppadoms as little as 10%. Water biscuits and cream crackers contain around 4% water and digestive biscuits contain 3%. Cheesecake and spotted dick are around 35% water.
DAIRY PRODUCTS	
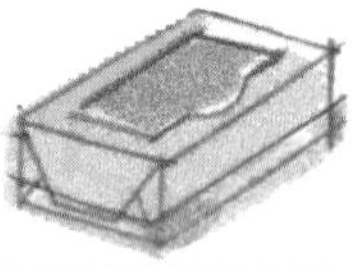	Soft cheeses are around 58%, hard cheeses 38% and soft, rinded cheeses about 50% water. Butter and margarines are around 16% water, while low-fat spreads are around 50%. Milk is around 90% water. Cream is between 48 and 79% water.
FISH AND SHELLFISH	
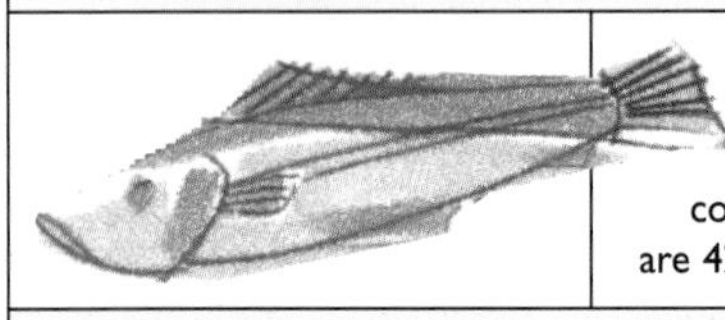	The water contents of various fish are similar, with cod, haddock, lemon sole, plaice and trout consisting of around 75%. Shellfish generally contain even more water, up to 85%. Anchovies are 42% water and smoked mackerel are 47%.
FRUIT	
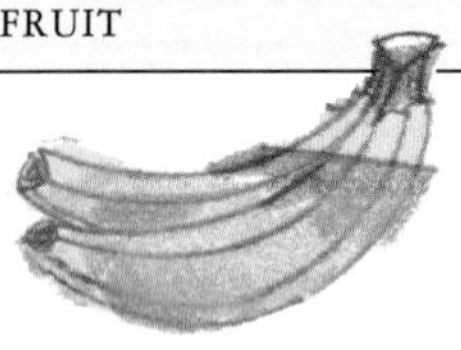	The edible parts of most fruits generally comprise around 75-80% water. Melons contain a greater percentage, typically consisting of around 90% water. Dried fruit, such as dates and currants are 12% and 16% respectively.
JAMS	
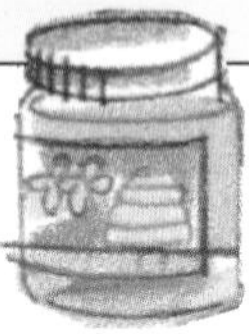	Honey is 23% water, while fruit jam and lemon curd are typically 30% water. Reduced sugar jam has a greater water content, around 65%. Marmalade is 28% and golden syrup is just 20% water.
POULTRY AND MEAT	
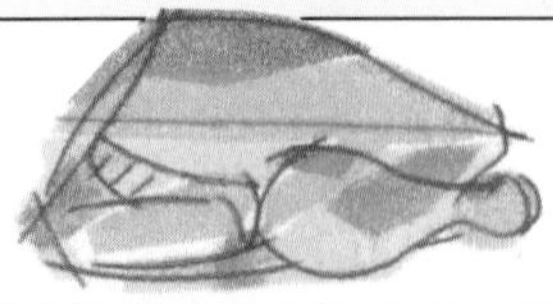	Most roast meats tend to be around 50% water. Poultry generally contains more, being typically 65-70%. Salami sausage contains only 28% water. The water content of bacon varies between 13 and 67%. Sausages are between 45 and 54% water.
VEGETABLES	
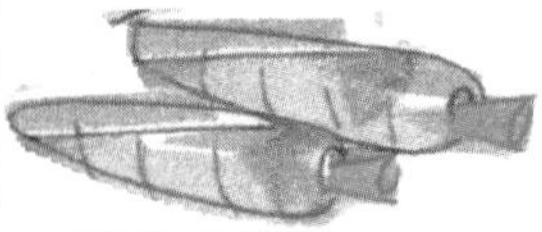	Vegetables contain the greatest percentages of water. Cucumber consists of 96% and tomatoes are 93% water, while spinach, carrots and broccoli are 89%.

white mottling of the teeth due to 'overdosing' on fluoride. Fluoride has also been linked with a higher than normal incidence of hip fractures: it is thought that this may be because, along with hardening tooth enamel, fluoride makes bones more dense and, consequently, less flexible. Research is still continuing as to the long-term effects of fluoride. Meanwhile, some people oppose the routine addition of the mineral to water supplies because they view it as 'mass medication'.

Nitrates

Since the 1970s, there has been much controversy about nitrates in tap water. Levels are strictly monitored, and are not allowed to exceed 50mg per litre, a figure based on the risk of bottle-fed babies – whose formulas are made up with tap water – developing a rare and fatal form of anaemia known as 'blue baby syndrome'. As the nitrate ferments in the baby's stomach, it is converted into nitrite which reacts with the baby's haemoglobin, limiting its capacity to carry oxygen. But there have been no deaths in Britain from this condition since 1948.

Nitrates, widely used as fertilisers, leach into rivers and underground sources of water from farmland. Once nitrates are ingested, bacteria in the lower intestine convert them to nitrites which are then absorbed into the bloodstream and excreted through the salivary glands in saliva. When they enter the stomach, the nitrites are able to react with the amines present in food to form nitrosamines – carcinogenic substances which may be linked to some types of gastric cancer.

It is important, however, to keep a sense of proportion. In Britain, the permissible amount of nitrates in tap water is far lower than is commonly found in almost all foods and is not a major risk. Nitrates occur naturally in vegetables, although the levels of the chemical may be boosted by the widespread use of nitrate fertilisers. EU regulations require the levels of nitrate to be tested, particularly in spinach and lettuce, by supermarkets and wholesalers before produce reaches the consumer. Nitrates and nitrites are also added to cured meats to prevent botulism and to enhance colour.

Where to get advice

If you are worried about your water supply, telephone your local water authority, listed in the telephone directory under 'Water', and ask for advice. British water companies carry out more than 3 million tests a year to check on levels of pollutants in drinking water, and have to keep a public register of water-quality tests, which they are legally obliged to let you see. The information appears in table format and shows the substances tested, their legal limits, and the test results. If you are still not happy, you can ask your local Environmental Health Officer to test your tap water.

Water filters

Although tap water is safe to drink, many people use water filters to remove minute traces of chemicals, metals and other substances that may be present in tap water. Whatever filter system you choose, you must replace the filter regularly, according to the manufacturer's instructions. If the filter is overused, it will start to release pollutants back into the water and breed bacteria.

There are three main types of filter. Activated carbon filters include the type in which you pour tap water through a filter which sits on top of a jug; they remove chlorine, pesticides and some chemicals, but not fluoride or nitrates. Distillation units remove most impurities through a process in which the water is vaporised then condensed. However, many people find the taste of distilled water rather bland, and the distillation units use a lot of electricity. Reverse osmosis systems force filtered water through a membrane; they remove virtually all chemicals and minerals, including those such as calcium and magnesium which benefit health and enhance the flavour of drinking water. Once water has been filtered in this way it should be used immediately or refrigerated and used within 24 hours. Do not leave it to stand at room temperature, because bacteria will multiply in the absence of chlorine.

Soft versus hard

Water hardness depends, in part, on levels of certain minerals, such as calcium and magnesium, in the water. If you live in a hard water area and decide to install a water softener, you should keep one tap that supplies hard water for cooking and drinking. Not only does this ensure that you will be benefiting from calcium in the water, it also means that you will avoid ingesting sodium, relatively high levels of which are produced by the softening process.

Hard water appears to be healthier: a survey carried out in Britain showed that people living in towns with very soft water have a 10 per cent higher risk of dying from cardiovascular disease than those in hard water areas.

BLUE WATER WARNING

Bluish stains in the sink below the tap may be a sign of a high copper content in the drinking water. Copper is a valuable mineral, but it is poisonous if too much is absorbed. The ingestion of large amounts of copper is believed to cause cirrhosis of the liver, but the levels required should be considerably higher than those caused by drinking tap water.

WHAT'S IN A BOTTLE?

Many people think that bottled waters are purer and healthier than tap water. In fact bottled waters often contain higher levels of bacteria – albeit harmless – than mains water, which contains chlorine to prevent bacterial growth. Moreover, many 'mineral' waters contain levels of minerals which are no higher than tap water.

'Spring' and 'table' waters can legally come from any source, ranging from natural springs to mains taps. Suppliers transport, blend, filter and perhaps carbonate these waters before bottling them for sale.

Some people drink bottled water because they believe that it will be low in nitrates, but this is not necessarily true. Levels vary greatly between brands: from under 1 mg to 32 mg per litre. Legally there is no limit on nitrate levels in natural mineral water, while the upper limit allowed in all other types of water is 50 mg per litre (the same as tap water). Always read the label on the bottle.

Finally, bottled waters and certain soda waters can be high in sodium, which may contribute to high BLOOD PRESSURE. Check the labels, because levels of sodium can vary from a negligible 0.5 mg per 100 ml, to an unhealthily high 114 mg per 100 ml.

The chief justification for drinking bottled water is that you prefer the taste. It can also be a sensible precaution against water-borne diseases when travelling in areas where tap water may be contaminated: use it to wash fruit and salad vegetables and clean your teeth – as well as for drinking.

Worms

The worms which commonly affect humans are threadworms (also called pin worms) and tapeworms. Both types can be acquired through eating contaminated food. The worms reside in the intestines, stealing nutrients before they can be absorbed by the body.

Symptoms of a severe worm infestation include diarrhoea, hunger pains, irritability, appetite loss and weight loss. Infestations can cause serious illness as well as nutritional imbalance, including vitamin B_{12} and iron deficiency, which can lead to anaemia.

All worm infections need medical treatment (there are several over-the-counter preparations) and visitors to developing countries should always take sensible precautions to avoid high-risk foods (see TRAVELLERS' HEALTH). Any symptoms appearing after foreign travel should be checked by a doctor.

Threadworms

Children under five are particularly susceptible to threadworms, *Enterobius vermicularis*. The main symptom of threadworms is itching around the anus at night, when the females (each about 10mm long) emerge from the anus to lay their eggs before they die. By scratching and then touching food, children can reinfect themselves or spread the infection to other children or members of the family.

Infection can be prevented with strict hygiene, washing hands after going to the lavatory and before meals. A bath in the morning to wash away the threadworm eggs will also help to prevent the infection from spreading.

Tapeworms

Ranging from only a few millimetres up to several metres in length, tapeworms are segmented and flat. They attach themselves to the insides of the intestines with suckers and hooks, absorbing food from the gut through the whole surface of their bodies. Egg-filled segments separate themselves from the worm and are then passed out of the body.

If these eggs are then eaten by an intermediate host, such as a pig or a cow, they will develop into cysts within its tissues. When humans eat infected meat that is either raw or undercooked, the larvae can be passed on. There are three common varieties of tapeworm that affect humans.

The beef tapeworm, *Taenia saginata*, is widespread throughout the Middle East, Africa and South America. To avoid the tapeworm, all beef should be thoroughly cooked – rare steak and burgers are a considerable risk in these regions. The consumption of steak tartare in countries where hygiene, carcass inspection and veterinary services are anything less than 100 per cent reliable is extremely ill advised.

The pork tapeworm, *Taenia solium*, poses a more serious health risk, as its eggs can travel back into the stomach where the larvae penetrate the stomach wall and are carried around the body – especially to the muscles and tissues just below the skin. Rarely, cysts can develop in the brain, leading to epilepsy. This parasite is commonly found in eastern Europe, South-east Asia and Africa, where eating undercooked pork or pork products such as sausages should be avoided.

Diphyllobothrium latum, the fish tapeworm, can be acquired by eating undercooked or raw fish and is found in Iceland, China, Japan (where sushi is a common source), South-east Asia, Scandinavia as well as the lake regions of Switzerland.

Expert chefs are past masters at detecting infected fish so there should be little risk in good hotels and restaurants. But if you are travelling, it is probably best not to eat raw fish. Fish tapeworms seldom cause symptoms, but victims can sometimes suffer from vitamin B_{12} deficiency, which can eventually lead to anaemia.

Other worms

Threadworms and tapeworms are not the only worms to affect humans. The roundworm, *Ascaris lumbricoides*, and whipworm, *Trichuris trichiura*, can be caught through eating eggs which have found their way onto vegetable and salad crops through the use of human faeces as fertiliser.

Another surprising source of infestation is the roundworm *Anisakis simplex*, which commonly occurs in herring. Where herring are eaten virtually raw, as they are in Holland at the start of the 'new herring season', and also in Scandinavia where they may be only very lightly salted, there is a considerable risk of acquiring this parasite. Fortunately, the anisakid worms cannot survive freezing, and storage at -20°C (-4°F) for three days will kill them off completely.

Remedies for worms

Tapeworms are difficult to get rid of, but the following – extremely safe – treatment may work. It has been used by homeopaths, herbalists and naturopaths for at least 100 years. After fasting for 12 hours, take 60g (2oz) of fresh pumpkin seeds, remove the outer skins by scalding and then grind the remaining green pulp to a paste with a little milk. Take the mixture at the end of the fast, and 2 hours later take 20ml (about 4 teaspoons) of castor oil, mixed with a little fruit juice. Wait for the tapeworm to be passed, which usually happens within 3 hours.

Various remedies for threadworms and tapeworms are available from chemists. These include anthelmintic drugs which help to kill or paralyse worms in the intestines or other tissues; your doctor or pharmacist will suggest which is the most appropriate.

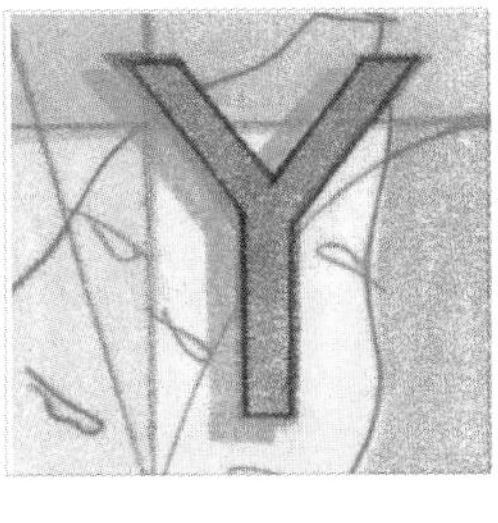

YAM

BENEFITS

- *Good source of potassium*
- *Yellow-fleshed varieties can be a useful source of beta carotene*

The staple food crop in much of the tropical world, the yam is often confused with the sweet potato (though the two are not related). Some varieties grow to the size of a large marrow.

The yam has almost 50 per cent more protein and more than three times as much starch as the sweet potato and is the better source of energy – 100g (3½oz) of boiled yam provides 133 Calories compared to the sweet potato's 84 Calories. The yam is a good source of potassium, needed for muscle and nerve function, and the yellow-fleshed varieties can be a useful source of beta carotene.

YEAST EXTRACT

BENEFITS

- *Excellent source of most B vitamins and folate*
- *Contains potassium and magnesium*
- *May be fortified with vitamin B_{12}*

DRAWBACK

- *High sodium content*

Yeast extract, as well as yeast used in baking and brewing, is an excellent source of B vitamins, which are needed for maintaining a healthy metabolism, nervous system and body tissues. Yeast extract is also a source of folate – needed for blood-cell formation – and various minerals including potassium, magnesium and zinc. Its high sodium content means that excessive consumption is not advised for people with high blood pressure or anyone on a low-sodium diet.

Some yeast extracts are fortified with vitamin B_{12}. Yeast extract is an important source of the vitamin for vegans since vitamin B_{12} occurs naturally almost exclusively in foods of animal origin. Some yeasts are grown on a medium containing chromium, and are enriched with the mineral in a form which the body can easily absorb. Chromium is a vital link in the chain that makes glucose available to the body and so is particularly important to diabetics.

Although it is not accepted by most orthodox medical bodies, practitioners of alternative medicine believe that eating foods that contain any form of yeast can aggravate systemic candidiasis (an extreme form of THRUSH). Candidiasis is caused by another yeast, *Candida albicans*, which is naturally present in the gut and on the skin. Alternative practitioners claim that foods containing yeasts upset the balance of bacteria in the gut by inhibiting the growth of 'friendly' bacteria and allowing *Candida albicans* to proliferate, penetrate the gut wall and spread through the whole body (hence the term 'systemic' or generalised candidiasis).

Another complication is thought to be that the body becomes sensitive to substances produced by the yeasts, so that foods containing them (such as yeast extract spreads) can exacerbate the symptoms associated with thrush. However, the very existence of generalised candidiasis is a subject of great debate and is disputed by many doctors.

Case study

Melissa, a 28-year-old teacher, had not been feeling well since a bout of a flu-like illness. Tired and listless, she no longer enjoyed her busy social life. After a month she was so depressed that her husband, Jim, persuaded her to see a doctor. Tests concluded that Melissa was suffering from post-viral fatigue syndrome and depression. She was prescribed antidepressants, and told that she would have to slow down before her condition would improve. Melissa read everything she could about post-viral fatigue, and went on a yeast-free diet to try to eliminate Candida albicans *from her body. After six months, she reintroduced yeast into her diet. Now, 12 months on, she is almost back to her normal self and feels much more energetic.*

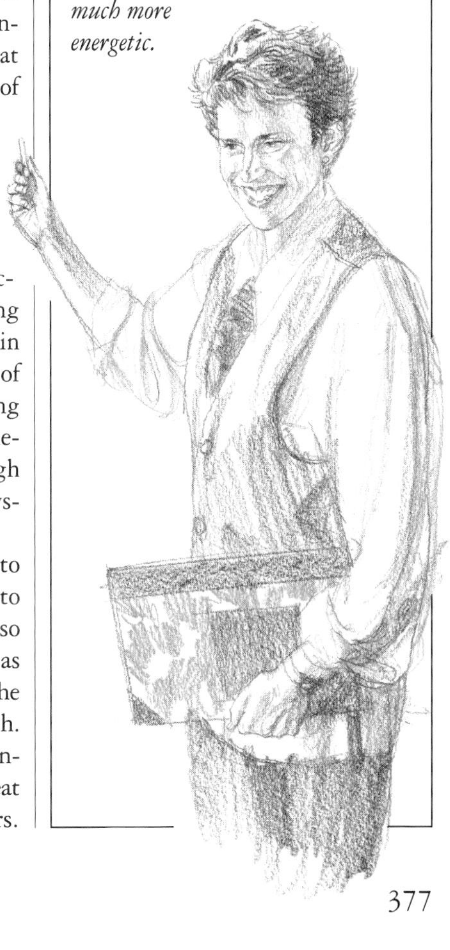

YOGHURT

BENEFITS

- *Useful source of calcium and phosphorus*
- *Contains vitamins B_2 (riboflavin) and B_{12}*
- *May help to replace valuable bacteria in the gut killed by antibiotics and boost the immune system*
- *May help to prevent bad breath, constipation and diarrhoea, as well as aid digestion*

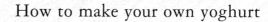

How to make your own yoghurt

Boil 1 litre (1¾ pints) of skimmed or whole milk. When it cools to 41°C (106°F) – you will need a cooking thermometer – add two tablespoons of the milk to a yoghurt starter (available from health food shops) or some plain live yoghurt. Mix thoroughly with the remaining milk. Store in a large, covered bowl in a warm place for 12 hours until it sets. Transfer to the fridge. You can keep two tablespoons back for one more batch, but no more, or it will not set.

Once thought of only as a worthy health food, yoghurt is now the base for tempting frozen desserts and is used as a healthier alternative to cream. Yoghurt is a useful source of calcium and phosphorus for strong bones and teeth. It also contains vitamin B_2 which is needed to release energy from food and B_{12} for a healthy nervous system. Calorie values vary widely, from 160 for a 150g (5½oz) pot of full-fat Greek yoghurt (usually made with ewe's milk) to 61 for a very low-fat type. People who need calcium but cannot drink milk because of a lactose intolerance may find that they can tolerate yoghurt.

Yoghurt is generally made by incubating pasteurised, homogenised milk, to which bacteria cultures are added. Because the yoghurt culture is added after the pasteurisation process, the yoghurt remains 'live'. In fact, most yoghurts are live, even when this is not specifically stated on the label.

HOW YOGHURT HELPS

Live yoghurt discourages the proliferation of harmful bacteria and yeasts (including *Candida albicans*) in the gut that lead to bowel infection. It can help to relieve gastrointestinal disorders, diarrhoea and constipation. It can also reduce bad breath associated with some digestive disorders.

Some alternative practitioners suggest that after a course of antibiotics eating live yoghurt can restore the necessary intestinal bacteria destroyed by these drugs. Yoghurt is helpful for people suffering from diarrhoea on account of radiotherapy treatment, food poisoning or irritable bowel syndrome. It is often recommended as an external treatment for anyone who is suffering from THRUSH.

It is also claimed that yoghurt can improve the condition of the skin and alter the balance of bacteria in the large bowel in a way that may protect against colon cancer.

Many new types of yoghurt have recently been marketed on the strength that they have a variety of extra health benefits. 'Bio' yoghurts contain cultures which are claimed to be especially beneficial to the digestion, and there is some experimental evidence to support this. High-fibre yoghurts, with added soluble fibre, are being promoted for their cholesterol-lowering properties.

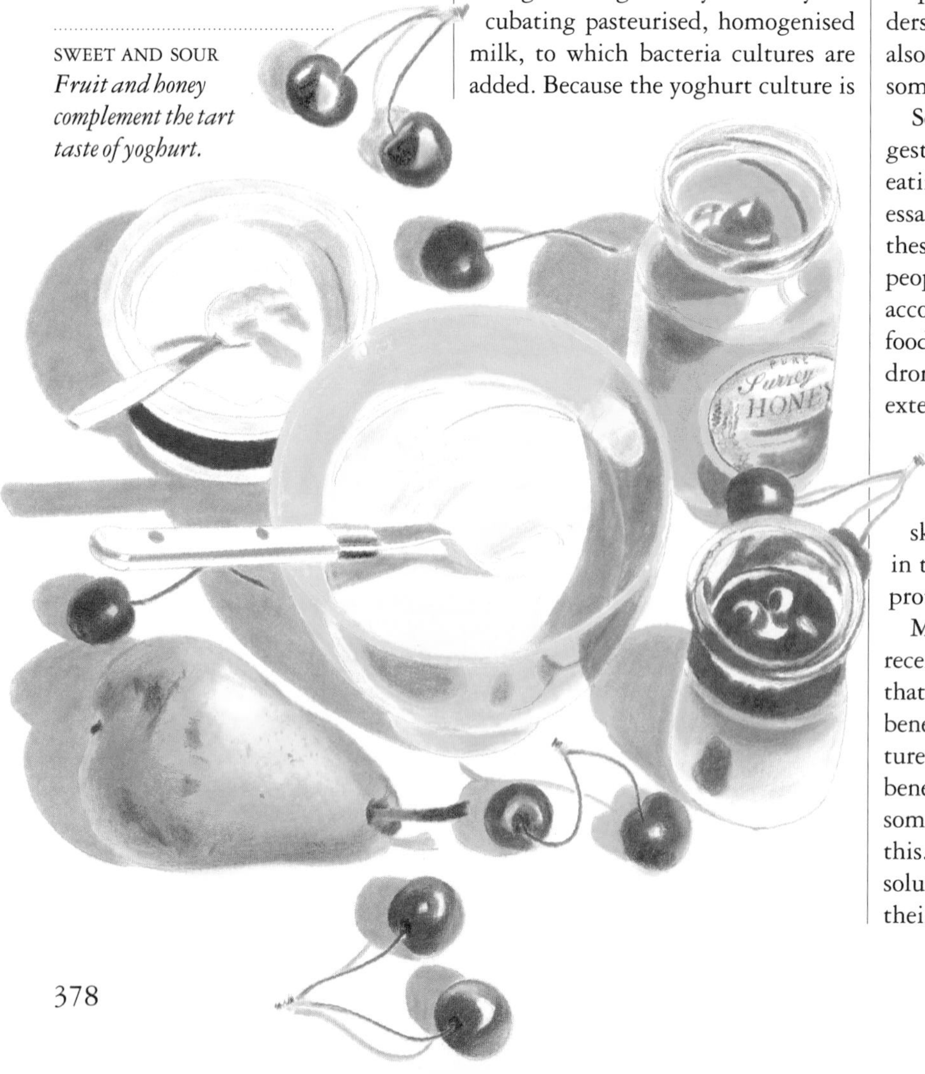

SWEET AND SOUR
Fruit and honey complement the tart taste of yoghurt.

Glossary

UNFAMILIAR OR COMPLICATED WORDS AND PHRASES WHICH DO NOT HAVE THEIR OWN ENTRIES IN THE MAIN BODY OF THE BOOK ARE EXPLAINED BELOW.

ACUTE Term which describes a disease that comes on quickly, produces severe symptoms and rapidly reaches its crisis – for example, acute appendicitis.

ADRENALINE The hormone that prepares the body for action – the 'fight or flight' response – in emergencies or at times of strong emotion. It increases the heart and breathing rates, raises the blood sugar level and delays the onset of tiredness in the muscles. It is secreted by the adrenal glands, which are located above each kidney.

AFLATOXIN A virulent poison produced by the fungus *Aspergillus flavus* that can contaminate peanuts and cereals stored in warm, humid conditions. It is not destroyed by cooking and can impair the immune system and cause cancer.

AGROCHEMICALS Chemical compounds, such as fertilisers and pesticides, used in intensive farming. In most cases, agrochemicals are present in food only in tiny quantities that are further reduced by washing or peeling fruit or vegetables. Critics have blamed the widespread use of agrochemicals for the rise in a number of complaints such as asthma, allergies and even infertility. Although there is circumstantial evidence, there is little scientific proof to support these claims.

ALKALOIDS Nitrogen-containing compounds, produced mainly by plants. Some, including codeine, morphine and quinine, are used for medicinal purposes; others can be poisonous, such as solanine (found in potatoes which have turned green through exposure to light) and nicotine (in cigarettes). In small amounts nicotine has a stimulating effect, but large doses are toxic.

ALLERGEN Any substance that causes an allergy, such as the pollen which triggers hay fever, or peanuts which can cause a severe asthma attack or lead to swelling of the tongue and throat.

AMINES Nitrogen compounds present in food. They can combine with nitrites in food or in the stomach to form nitrosamines, which may be linked with cancer, although there is no conclusive evidence.

AMINO ACIDS The basic building blocks of proteins. There are 20 amino acids which are linked in varying sequences to make all the different proteins. Most amino acids can be synthesised by the body, but eight are termed 'essential' or 'indispensable' because the body cannot make them and they must therefore be provided by the diet. Having been broken down from protein, amino acids are carried in the bloodstream to the liver as well as to other sites in the body where they are needed. They are then reassembled to make the specific forms of protein required by different cells and tissues.

ANAPHYLACTIC SHOCK An extreme allergic reaction in which huge quantities of histamine are released throughout the body, producing rapid swelling and making breathing difficult. If untreated, it can lead to loss of consciousness, heart failure and death. In susceptible individuals, anaphylactic shock may be triggered by foods such as peanuts, insect stings or certain drugs.

ANTIBODIES 'Shock troops' in the body's defence mechanism, capable of destroying bacteria and other potentially harmful substances. They are manufactured in lymph tissue, such as that of the spleen, in response to the presence of a foreign substance in the body, such as an allergen or a virus. Each antibody combats a particular infection; for example, a measles antibody would not fight chickenpox or a cold virus. Once the body has an effective antibody it becomes immune to that disease. Antibodies are transported around the body in the bloodstream.

ANTI-CARCINOGENS Agents found in some foods that are thought to counteract carcinogens and so help to prevent some sorts of cancers from being initiated. Cruciferous vegetables (including broccoli, Brussels sprouts, cabbage, cauliflower and kale) are particularly rich in these compounds, which include carotenoids, indoles and isothiocyanates.

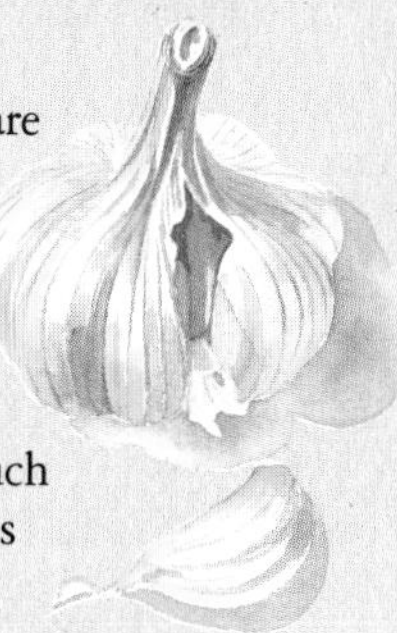

ANTIVIRALS Drugs that are effective against disease-causing viruses. One example is acyclovir, used to treat shingles as well as other forms of herpes. Certain foods such as garlic also have various antiviral properties.

BACTERIA Simple micro-organisms, varying in shape, consisting of a single cell and measuring only a few thousandths of a millimetre across. They flourish everywhere, in air, food, water, soil and inside other living things, including humans. They are not necessarily harmful – the 'friendly' bacteria naturally present in the human gut can help to fight off infections. However, other types cause a wide range of diseases, from cholera and various types of pneumonia to some forms of food-poisoning and tuberculosis. A few bacteria produce toxins or poisons.

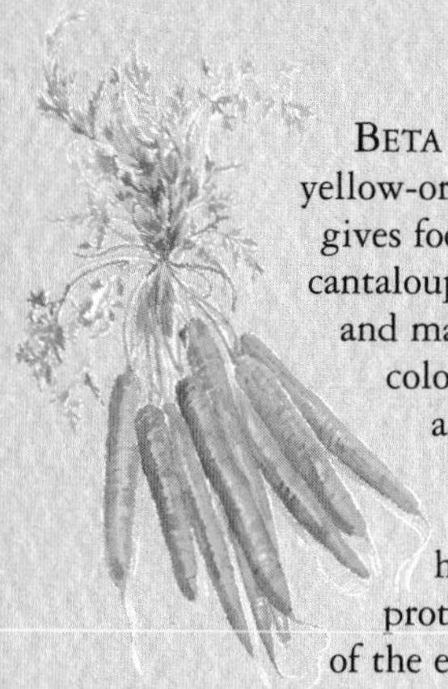

BETA CAROTENE The yellow-orange pigment that gives foods such as carrots, cantaloupe melons, apricots and mangoes their bright colour. It is one of the antioxidants that can contribute to long-term good health and provide protection against some of the effects of ageing and disease. Beta carotene may also be turned into vitamin A by the body as and when it is required.

BIOAVAILABLE If the body can easily extract the nutrients from a food, they are said to be bioavailable. For example, iron is more bioavailable from meat than from vegetables.

BIOFLAVONOIDS Chemicals found in fruits such as lemons, plums, grapefruit, cherries, blackberries and blackcurrants, as well as in buckwheat. Bioflavonoids usually have strong antioxidant properties and are thought to help prevent certain forms of cancer. In the body they work with vitamin C to strengthen the capillaries or small blood vessels.

B VITAMINS The vitamins that make up what is called the B-complex are not chemically related to each other, although they occur in many of the same foods, such as milk, cereals and offal. They are often presented together in vitamin supplements. Most perform closely connected tasks within the body, particularly in helping to release energy from food.

B vitamins can be known by either numbers or names, or sometimes both. They include B_1 (thiamin), B_2 (riboflavin), pantothenic acid, B_6 (pyridoxine), niacin, biotin, folate (or folic acid) and B_{12} (cyanocobalamin).

CALORIES The basic units in which the energy value of food and the energy needs of the body are measured. One calorie is a minuscule measurement, so the figures are usually expressed as units of 1000 calories, which are called kilocalories (kcal) or Calories (Cal) with a capital 'C'. Another similar unit of measurement is the kiloJoule (kJ), equal to approximately 4.2 Calories. Energy needs vary according to age, size and sex. A 16-year-old boy needs around 3000 Calories a day, while a moderately active adult woman will typically need just under 2000.

CARCINOGEN Any substance that may produce cancer in living tissues. Many known or suspected carcinogens are chemicals, such as some of those used in industrial processes, emitted in car exhaust fumes or present in tobacco smoke. Others include radiation from the sun, nitrosamines formed in the stomach from nitrites, sausages and salt-cured meats, certain chemicals found in charred meat and certain viruses associated with some forms of leukaemia.

CAROTENOIDS Yellow and red pigments found in many plants. They include beta carotene, a known antioxidant that may help to preserve health by neutralising free radicals. Other carotenoids, either individually or in combination, are thought to have similarly beneficial properties.

CELLULOSE Humans cannot digest this carbohydrate, one of the main constituents of plant cell walls. But it is important in the diet as a source of insoluble fibre, adding roughage or bulk which helps waste products to pass efficiently through the bowel.

CHRONIC Term used to describe any disease that develops slowly or lasts for a long time – for example, asthma and osteoarthritis.

COENZYMES Organic compounds that work with enzymes to speed up biological processes such as digestion. A coenzyme may be a vitamin, or contain one, or be manufactured in the body from one. For example, coenzyme A – used in the metabolism of carbohydrates and fats – contains pantothenic acid, a B vitamin.

COFACTOR A general term for non-protein substances that must be present in suitable quantities before certain enzymes can function.

COLLAGEN A protein that forms the main constituent of tendons, the cords of fibres that attach muscles to bones. Collagen is the intercellular material that binds cells together and is found in skin, ligaments, bone and cartilage.

COMPLEX CARBOHYDRATES A collective term for starches and fibre. They have a more complicated chemical structure than sugars (simple carbohydrates), which make up the third group of carbohydrates.

CONGENITAL Term used to describe a disorder that is, or is believed to have been, present at birth, whether the defect has been inherited or is due to environmental factors. Examples include harelip and spina bifida.

DIETARY REFERENCE VALUES (DRVS) Figures calculated by scientists that are estimates of the average quantities of nutrients needed by different population groups, for example women, adolescents, infants and children. Reference Nutrient Intake (RNI) and Recommended Daily Amount (RDA) are two examples of the dietary reference values used in this book.

DIURETIC Any drug that increases the volume of urine produced and passed by the body. Diuretics are often used to combat fluid retention associated with

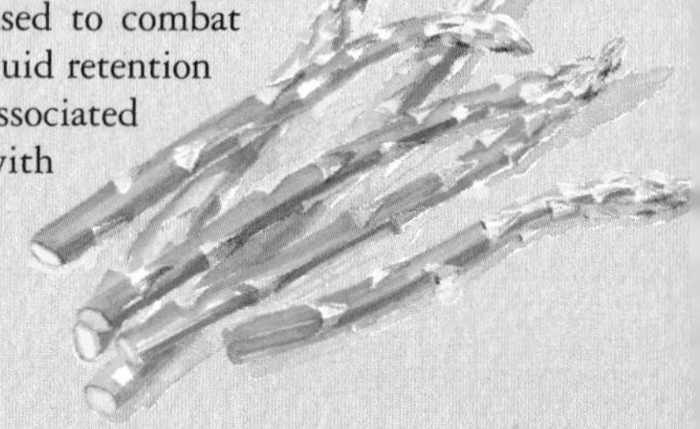

heart or kidney disease, for example. Caffeine, found in coffee and tea, is a diuretic. Other natural diuretics include parsley, celery, asparagus and dandelion leaves.

DNA (DEOXYRIBONUCLEIC ACID) A substance found in the nucleus of every living cell, carrying the genetic information that causes characteristics to be passed on from parents to their children. It is a blueprint for the body's entire development, starting from a single cell at conception.

ELECTROLYTES Charged particles that circulate in the blood and help to regulate the body's fluid balance. They include sodium, potassium, chloride and bicarbonate.

EMULSIFIERS Additives that allow oils to be blended with water, overcoming their natural reluctance to mix.

ENDORPHINS Natural painkillers and tranquillisers produced in the brain. Their effects are similar to those of opium-based drugs such as morphine. They are released at times of severe mental stress, and during strenuous exercise. Chocolate is believed to boost the endorphin levels in the brain.

ENZYMES Proteins produced in the cells of plants and animals that act as catalysts, helping to speed up biological processes without being affected themselves. They work by combining with the substance which is to be processed, and help to convert it into another substance.

Enzymes in the saliva, stomach, pancreas and small intestine play a vital part in digestion, helping to change food into the form in which it can best be used by the body or excreted as waste. Each enzyme has a specific role, so that one which breaks down fats, for example, cannot deal with proteins or carbohydrates.

Enzymes are vital for the body's well-being. Any failure, even by a single enzyme, can cause a serious disorder. A relatively common example is phenylketonuria (PKU), the inability to metabolise a vital amino acid, which if left untreated can lead to physical deformities and mental disorders.

ESSENTIAL FATTY ACIDS Some types of polyunsaturated fatty acids are not made in the body and must be supplied by polyunsaturated fat in the diet to maintain health. There are two main categories: omega-6, found in foods such as corn oil and sunflower oil, derived from linoleic acid; and omega-3, found in rapeseed oil, walnuts and oily fish, derived from the similarly named linolenic acid. These fatty acids maintain cell membranes, transport fats around the body and are needed to make prostaglandins (important hormone-like chemicals).

FLUID BALANCE To function properly the body must maintain a healthy level of fluid. Normally, the balance remains fairly constant no matter how much fluid someone drinks. Electrolytes help to regulate it, and the kidneys also play their part by adjusting the water content of the urine. Illness can upset the body's fluid balance; diarrhoea can cause excessive fluid loss leading to dehydration, while in oedema, or dropsy, too much fluid is retained in the tissues, causing either local or general swelling.

FOLATE The term commonly used to describe any compound or mixture of compounds derived from folic acid. Good sources of folate include liver, yeast extract and green leafy vegetables, such as cabbage and spinach.

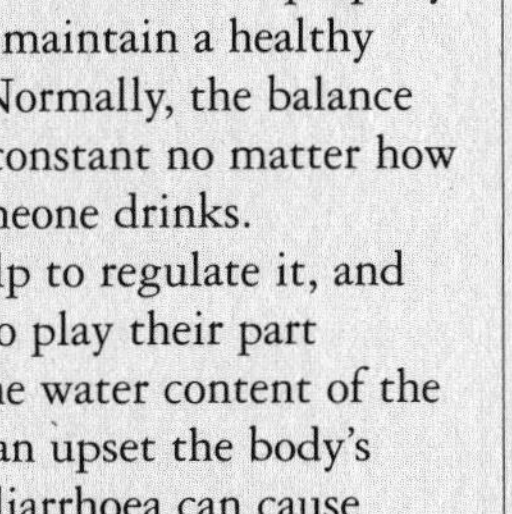

FOLIC ACID One of the B vitamins which works along with vitamin B_{12} to produce the genetic materials DNA and RNA. The vitamin promotes the breakdown and use of proteins and also helps to form red and white blood cells.

GLUCAGON A hormone, secreted by the pancreas, that increases the level of glucose in the blood.

GLUCOSE Also called dextrose. A simple form of sugar, carried in the bloodstream and used directly by the body as an energy source. Only a few foods, such as grapes, contain pure glucose. The body obtains most of its glucose by breaking down starches and sucrose (table sugar) during digestion. The concentration of glucose in the blood – the blood sugar level – is regulated by the hormones glucagon and insulin.

GLYCOGEN When the body absorbs more glucose than it needs to meet immediate energy demands, some is stored in the liver and muscles as glycogen which is made up of glucose units linked together. These can be broken down and quickly released back into the bloodstream as required, for example during exercise.

GRAM (g) Basic metric unit of weight, equal to 1000 milligrams or one-thousandth of a kilogram. There are 28.4 g to 1 oz (but for simplicity this figure has been rounded down to 25 g in this book).

HAEM IRON The iron found in meat. It is absorbed more efficiently than non-haem iron, found in cereals, pulses and other plants.

HAEMOGLOBIN The iron-containing pigment that carries oxygen to all parts of the body. It combines with oxygen as blood passes through the lungs. It gives red blood cells their colour – the more oxygen haemoglobin is carrying, the brighter blood will be.

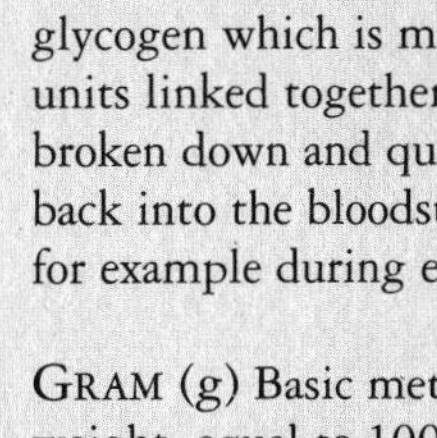

HISTAMINE A chemical, found in most tissues, that forms part of the body's defence mechanism and is also involved in gastric secretion and the contraction of smooth muscle. Histamine is released in large amounts during allergic reactions, causing itching and rashes, sneezing, watering eyes, wheezing and swelling.

HORMONES Chemical messengers sent through the bloodstream to control the functioning of the body's organs. Most are manufactured by the glands of the endocrine system, which is controlled by the pea-sized pituitary gland, located at the base of the skull. Insulin is a hormone which helps to control the level of glucose in the blood. Oestrogen regulates the female sex organs.

INDOLES Nitrogen compounds found in Brussels sprouts and other members of the cruciferous or cabbage family. Vegetable indoles are said to speed up the elimination of the female hormone oestrogen from the body, and so may help to protect against hormone-related cancers, such as cancer of the womb and breast cancer.

INSOLUBLE FIBRE Fibre, such as cellulose, that passes unchanged through the intestines because it cannot be absorbed or broken down by the body's own enzymes. Because it retains water it passes through the gut acting like a sponge and reducing the chances of constipation.

INSULIN A hormone secreted by the pancreas that prevents excessive levels of glucose from accumulating in the blood, by enabling its uptake by cells. In *diabetes mellitus*, the most common form of diabetes, the body does not produce enough insulin, and so blood sugar levels can rise unchecked, with potentially fatal consequences.

ISOTHIOCYANATES Plant chemicals which are believed to strengthen the body's defences against some forms of cancer. They occur naturally in some cruciferous vegetables such as broccoli, Brussels sprouts and cabbage.

KETONE BODIES Organic compounds produced when fats are broken down for energy because the body's supply of carbohydrate is low. Prolonged fasting or starvation, and diseases such as *diabetes mellitus*, can cause the level of ketone bodies in the blood and tissues to rise, causing the condition known as ketosis.

LACTASE The enzyme, secreted in the small intestine, that breaks down lactose from milk into its constituent sugars. Some people have a hereditary lactase deficiency, making them lactose intolerant and therefore unable to digest milk sugar.

LACTOSE A sugar found only in milk. It consists of two simple sugars, glucose and galactose, and is broken down in the small intestine by the enzyme lactase.

LECITHIN A constituent of our cell membranes and lipoproteins that helps to transport fats in the blood. It has been suggested that lecithin may help to combat disorders ranging from arterial disease to viral infections and gallstones. It is found naturally in egg yolks, liver, wholewheat and nuts. Lecithin is also sold as a dietary supplement in capsule, granule and liquid form. It is used in the food industry as an emulsifier in such products as mayonnaise.

LEGUMES Any member of the pea family, including chickpeas, runner beans, soya beans and lentils. The seeds of these plants are known as pulses.

LINOLEIC ACID One of the omega-6 family of essential fatty acids. It is found naturally in vegetable oils such as those made from corn (maize) and soya as well as in some animal fats. It is always automatically added (along with linolenic acid) to milk formula preparations for babies.

LINOLENIC ACID Another essential fatty acid – part of the omega-3 family – which is found in green leafy vegetables and rapeseed oil.

LIPIDS General term used to describe fats, oils and waxes, together with more complex molecules. They are insoluble in water.

LIPOPROTEINS Particles made of proteins and lipids which enable insoluble fats to be transported in the bloodstream. Low-density lipoproteins (LDLs), transport cholesterol to the body cells, where it forms a component of the cell walls and plays a part in other essential functions. A high level of LDLs in the blood can reflect a high cholesterol level, which raises the risk of heart disease. The reasons for a high level of LDLs in the blood may be hereditary or diet-related, or a combination of the two.

High-density lipoproteins (HDLs) remove surplus cholesterol from the tissues and carry it to the liver for excretion. A high level of HDLs in the blood indicates a lower than average risk of heart disease.

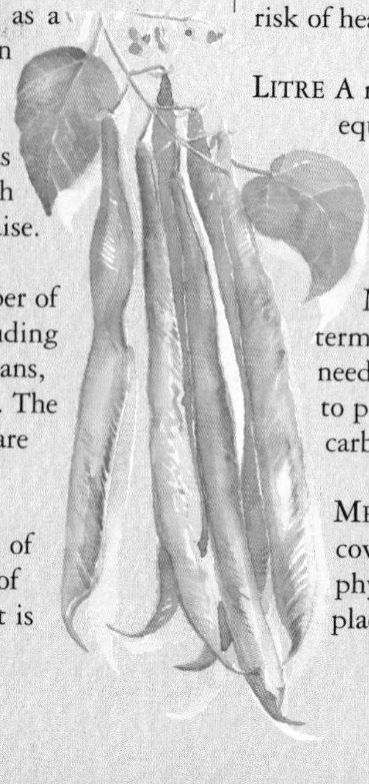

LITRE A metric unit of liquid volume, equal to 1000 millilitres. One litre is the same as 1¾ pints and there are 4.55 litres in 1 gallon.

MACRONUTRIENTS General term for those nutrients the body needs in relatively large amounts to produce energy, such as carbohydrates, proteins and fats.

METABOLISM A term which covers all the chemical and physical changes that take place within the body to keep it alive and functioning. Metabolic processes can be divided into two broad categories – reactions that break down complex chemicals into simpler substances in order to release energy (catabolism), and those that build up complex substances in the organs and tissues, to store energy or to provide for the body's growth and repair (anabolism). Naturally thin people often have a fast metabolism.

METABOLITE Any substance involved in metabolism, either as a product of it, or as a raw material in the form of nutrients in food.

MICROGRAM (mcg or µg) A unit of weight equivalent to one-millionth of a gram or a thousandth of a milligram.

MICRONUTRIENTS Vitamins and minerals are together called micronutrients, because although they are essential to health, the body needs them only in very small amounts.

MICRO-ORGANISM An organism which is too small to be seen with the naked eye. Micro-organisms include bacteria and viruses.

MILLIGRAM (mg) One-thousandth of a gram or 1000 micrograms.

MILLILITRE (ml) One-thousandth of a litre. There are 5 ml in a teaspoon, 15 ml in a tablespoon and around 600 ml in a pint.

MONOUNSATURATED FAT (MONOUNSATURATED FATTY ACIDS) A form of fat which is thought to protect against heart disease and atherosclerosis. Olive oil, peanuts and avocados are rich in monounsaturates.

MUCOUS MEMBRANE The moist inner surface that lines the mouth, nasal sinuses, stomach, intestines and many other parts of the body. It secretes mucus, which acts as a protective barrier and lubricant, as well as a medium for carrying enzymes.

NEUROTRANSMITTERS Chemical messengers released from nerve endings which relay nerve impulses through the body.

NITRATES Chemical compounds containing nitrogen that occur naturally in certain foods and which are sometimes added to meat and meat products as preservatives. Nitrates are widely used in agriculture as a fertiliser, and leach from the soil into rivers and reservoirs that provide domestic water supplies. European Union law now restricts the levels allowed in drinking water and the amounts that can be added to foods.

NITRITES Like the chemically related nitrates, nitrites are added to meats such as bacon to help preserve them. They may also be produced within the body, through the action of bacteria in the stomach on nitrates contained in food or drinking water.

NITROSAMINES Substances, which have been shown to cause cancer in laboratory animals, that can be formed when nitrites react with amines. No link has, as yet, been definitely established between nitrosamines and cancer in humans. However, in countries, such as Japan, where nitrate-cured and smoked foods (which can lead to nitrosamines being formed in the stomach) are eaten regularly, cancers of the oesophagus and stomach occur more frequently.

NON-HAEM IRON The form of iron which is found in vegetables. It is less efficiently absorbed than the haem iron in meat. However, vitamin C – for example, from a glass of orange juice drunk with a meal – aids the absorption of the non-haem.

NORADRENALINE This hormone is closely related to adrenaline and has a similar action. It is released by the adrenal gland and is also released as a neurotransmitter by nerve endings.

OESTROGEN One of a group of hormones controlling female sexual development. It is produced mainly by the ovaries.

OMEGA-3/OMEGA-6 FATTY ACIDS See Essential fatty acids.

OXALIC ACID A chemical which is potentially fatal if taken in high concentrations, such as those found in the leaves of rhubarb. It is also present in much smaller quantities in rhubarb stalks, spinach, sorrel, almonds and chocolate. It inhibits the body's absorption of calcium and iron.

OXIDATION A chemical process in which a substance combines with oxygen, causing a wide range of reactions – for example, when an apple turns brown after it has been peeled or cut open.

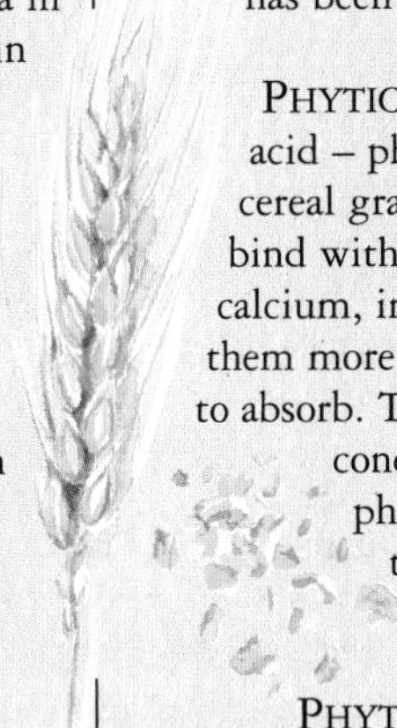

PHYTIC ACID Salts of phytic acid – phytates – occur in cereal grains and pulses. They bind with minerals such as calcium, iron and zinc, making them more difficult for the body to absorb. Too much bran – a concentrated source of phytic acid – can inhibit the body's absorption of these minerals.

PHYTOCHEMICALS A group of compounds that occur naturally in all fruit and vegetables. They are now thought to offer a degree of protection against cancer, heart disease, arthritis, hypertension and other degenerative ailments. While it has not yet been proven that these chemicals arrest cancer, there is evidence that people who enjoy a diet rich in fruit and vegetables have a lower incidence of cancer. Carotenoids, indoles and isothiocyanates are all phytochemicals.

PHYTOESTROGENS Chemicals of plant origin that resemble the female hormone oestrogen. They are found in soya beans and many other pulses.

PLASMA The yellowish fluid that makes up about 55 per cent of blood. Red and white blood cells and platelets are suspended in it. Plasma also carries thousands of other vital substances around the body, including proteins, glucose, vitamins, hormones and antibodies.

PLATELETS When a blood vessel is cut or damaged, platelets manufactured in the bone marrow, and carried in vast numbers in the bloodstream, speed to the rescue. They stick in clumps to the edges of the wound, and are able to seal it if it is small. If the damage is too great for the platelets to cope alone, they set off chemical reactions that draw red blood cells to the site and bind them together in a clot.

POLYPHENOLS A group of organic compounds (which includes the tannins) that are found in many foods such as tea, coffee and red wines. They combine with iron and can therefore hinder its absorption.

POLYPS Small growths that form on a mucous membrane, most commonly in the nose and sinuses. They are rarely malignant, but may need to be removed surgically to prevent discomfort or chronic infection. Polyps in the lower bowel can sometimes become cancerous.

POLYUNSATURATED FATS (POLYUNSATURATED FATTY ACIDS) Forms of fat found in high levels in corn oil, sunflower oil, nuts, some margarines and oily fish such as mackerel. They include the two families of essential fatty acids that are necessary for health, so small quantities should be included in the diet. A diet high in polyunsaturated fats and low in both trans and saturated fats lowers blood cholesterol levels and hence reduces the risk of heart disease.

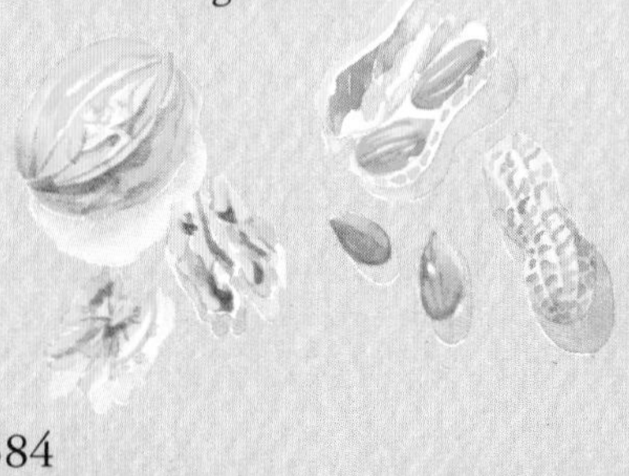

PROSTAGLANDINS Substances present in many body tissues and fluids – including the brain, uterus, kidneys and semen – that act in a similar way to hormones. For example, they stimulate contractions of the womb during menstruation and childbirth, affect the flow of blood through the kidneys and are involved in the production of mucus in the stomach.

PURINES A group of organic compounds that includes caffeine and uric acid. Until quite recently, people suffering from kidney and bladder stones formed by the crystallisation of uric acid were forbidden foods rich in purines – meats such as kidneys and liver and fish such as sardines and anchovies. People with gout are still advised by doctors to avoid foods that are high in purines.

RECOMMENDED DAILY AMOUNTS (RDAS) Also known as recommended daily allowances. Figures issued in many countries which indicate the average quantities of key nutrients people need to obtain from their food. In the European Union, 'labelling RDAs' are often quoted on food labels, where, for example, the amount of iron in a typical serving is shown as a percentage of the RDA for iron. These RDAs are said to apply to 'average adults', and are only a very rough guide to healthy eating. They take little account of differences in individual nutritional requirements according to age, sex, occupation and other factors.

REFERENCE NUTRIENT INTAKE (RNI) A term coined in 1991 by Britain's Department of Health. An RNI denotes the average daily quantity of a nutrient that would meet the nutritional requirements of at least 97.5 per cent of a particular population group. In principle, RNIs and Recommended Daily Amounts are similar, as the levels of both are higher than many individuals actually need. RNIs are set by age and sex. Changes to the basic figures necessary for pregnant or nursing mothers are also indicated. RNIs have recently been set for an increased number of nutrients.

REFINED FOODS White sugar, white flour and polished white rice are all examples of refined food products, in which the main ingredient has been processed – usually with the result that some of its nutrients are lost. For example, refined flour and rice lose most of their dietary fibre and rice also loses most of its vitamin B_1. However, refining can prolong shelf life, and make the product more palatable.

RESISTANT STARCH A type of starch that cannot be broken down in the normal way by enzymes in the small intestine. It is found in raw potatoes, unripe fruit and some processed foods. It passes undigested into the large intestine, where it can act like insoluble fibre and help to prevent constipation. However, it can also ferment, causing wind and discomfort.

RNA (RIBONUCLEIC ACID) The substance, occurring in every living cell, that enables the body to develop according to the genetic code or master plan contained in its DNA. There are several forms. Messenger RNA carries information from the DNA in the cell's nucleus to its ribosomes, the sites where proteins are made. By following the code, transfer RNA ensures that amino acids – the building blocks for protein – are assembled correctly.

SALICYLATES Compounds related to salicylic acid, which is used in making aspirin and also as a preservative. In some people, salicylates in food (particularly fruit) or medicine may produce allergic reactions such as an attack of asthma or hay fever.

SATURATED FAT (SATURATED FATTY ACIDS) The predominant type of fat in meat, dairy products such as butter and cheese, palm oil and coconut oil. A high intake of saturated fat has been linked to a greater risk of heart disease.

SOLUBLE FIBRE A form of fibre that is broken down into simpler components by the action of bacteria in the large intestine. Soluble fibre can help to reduce high blood cholesterol levels. Good sources include many fruits – especially dried fruits, green vegetables, pulses (such as broad beans, peas and lentils) and certain cereals, including oats.

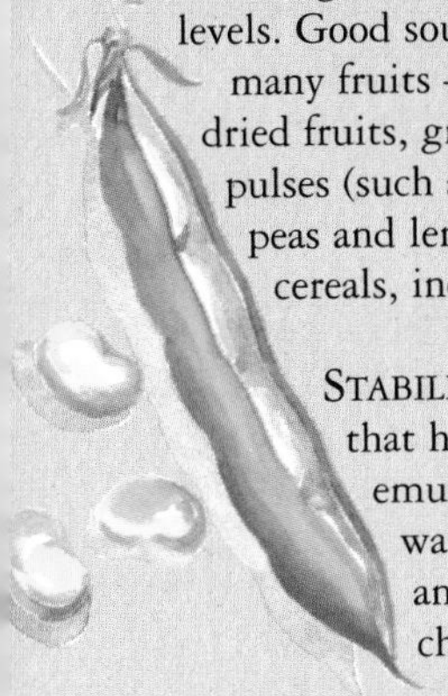

STABILISERS Substances that help to stabilise emulsions of fat and water and prevent any unwanted chemical changes. They also tend to thicken the emulsion or cause it to set. Gelatin, pectin and guar gum are examples of commonly used stabilisers.

STARCH A complex carbohydrate. It is the principal storage molecule of plants and the major source of energy and carbohydrate in the diet; it consists of glucose sub-units. Bread, pasta, rice and potatoes are all particularly good sources of starch.

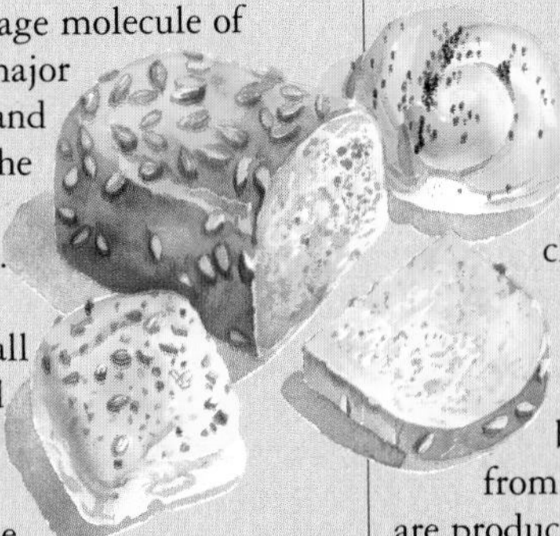

STEROIDS A type of lipid. Naturally occurring steroids include both the male and female sex hormones as well as bile salts. A range of synthetic steroids are widely used as anti-inflammatory agents. Anabolic steroids are similar to male sex hormones and can enable athletes to build muscle mass rapidly as well as increase their stamina. Sometimes anabolic steroids are used illegally by athletes to boost their performance.

STIMULANTS Any drug, food or drink that temporarily speeds up a process in the body may be classed as a stimulant. But the term is usually kept for those that mimic the natural effects of adrenaline, preparing the body and mind for instant action. Everyday stimulants include the caffeine found in coffee, tea and cola drinks as well as in chocolate, and the nicotine in tobacco.

SULPHITES Compounds of sulphur used in food preservation and brewing. When mixed with acid, they release the gas sulphur dioxide, which kills yeasts and is also a bleaching agent. Sulphur dioxide can trigger asthma attacks in susceptible people.

SYNTHESIS The process by which complex substances are created from their component parts. In protein synthesis, for example, amino acids obtained from the breakdown of proteins in food are carried in the bloodstream to the liver and to cells in other parts of the body, where they are assembled into new proteins.

SYSTEMIC A systemic disease is one that affects the entire body, and not just one part of it. An example of a systemic disease is *Lupus erythematosus* – a chronic inflammatory disease of the connective tissue.

TOXAEMIA A form of blood poisoning stemming from toxins (or poisons) which are produced by bacteria invading a site of infection. Once in the blood it provokes generalised symptoms.

TOXINS Poisons produced by living organisms – usually by bacteria. Toxic substances, however, can be inorganic materials such as lead or mercury.

TRACE ELEMENTS Minerals the body needs in extremely small amounts to help maintain health, for example by enabling enzymes to work properly. They include minerals such as iodine, selenium and magnesium.

TRANS FATS (TRANS FATTY ACIDS) Types of fat that occur in their natural form in meat and dairy products and in an artificial form in foods such as margarines, biscuits and cakes, where edible oils have been industrially hardened to ensure they stay solid at room temperature. Research suggests that there is a link between high consumption of artificially produced trans fats and heart disease.

TRIGLYCERIDES The form in which fat is stored in the body. During digestion, triglycerides from food are broken down and then reconstituted in the cells of the intestine walls, before passing into the bloodstream. Studies suggest there is a link between raised levels of triglycerides in the blood and the risk of heart disease. But other factors may be involved, too; physical exercise has been shown to reduce the presence of triglycerides in the blood, while consuming a lot of alcohol can increase it.

URIC ACID A waste substance, containing nitrogen, produced as a result of the breakdown of protein. Normally, uric acid is excreted in the urine, but in some people who have an inherited inability to eliminate it, high levels build up in the blood and are deposited as crystallised salts (urates), which can cause gout.

VIRUSES Infectious particles that are the cause of many diseases, from the common cold, flu and chickenpox to herpes, AIDS and polio. They can reproduce only by invading and taking over a living cell. In healthy humans, the invaded cell produces a protein substance called interferon, which prevents the virus from spreading. But in babies, the elderly and those already weakened by illness or a poor diet, this defence mechanism may not work effectively.

Helpful Organisations

For further information on diet and health, or diet and specific ailments, contact the appropriate organisation below.

Alcohol Concern
Waterbridge House, 32-36 Loman Street, London SE1 0EE.
0171 928 7377

Alcoholics Anonymous
PO Box 1, Stonebow House, Stonebow, York YO1 2NJ.
01904 644026

Alzheimer's Disease Society
Gordon House, 10 Greencoat Place, London SW1P 1PH.
0171 306 0606

Anaphylaxis Campaign
PO Box 149, Fleet, Hampshire GU13 9XU. 01252 318723

Arthritic Association
First Floor Suite, 2 Hyde Gardens, Eastbourne, East Sussex BN21 4PN.
01323 416550 or 0171 491 0233

Association for Spina Bifida and Hydrocephalus
ASBAH House, 42 Park Road, Peterborough PE1 2UQ.
01733 555988

Avert – The AIDS Education and Research Trust
11-13 Denne Parade, Horsham, West Sussex RH12 1JD.
01403 210202

Body Positive – AIDS information
51b Philbeach Gardens, London SW5 9EB.
helpline: 0171 373 9124 (7-10pm)

British Allergy Foundation
Deepdene House, 30 Belle Grove, Welling, Kent DA16 3BY.
0181 303 8583

British Association of Dermatologists
19 Fitzroy Square, London W1P 5HQ.
0171 383 0266

British College of Naturopathy and Osteopathy
6 Netherhall Gardens, London NW3 5RR.
0171 435 6464

British Dental Association
64 Wimpole Street, London W1M 8AL.
0171 935 0875

British Diabetic Association
10 Queen Anne Street, London W1M 0BD.
0171 323 1531

British Epilepsy Association
Anstey House, 40 Hanover Square, Leeds LS3 1BE. 0113 243 9393

British Heart Foundation
14 Fitzhardinge Street, London W1H 4DH.
0171 935 0185

British Nutrition Foundation
High Holborn House, 52-54 High Holborn, London WC1V 6RQ.
0171 404 6504

Cancer Research Campaign
10 Cambridge Terrace, London NW1 4JL.
0171 224 1333

Cystic Fibrosis Trust
Alexandra House, 5 Blyth Road, Bromley, Kent BR1 3RS.
0181 464 7211

Department of Health
Richmond House, 79 Whitehall, London SW1A 2NS.
0171 210 3000

Hyperactive Children's Support Group
71 Whyke Lane, Chichester, West Sussex PO19 2LD.
01903 725182

Imperial Cancer Research Fund
PO Box 123, Lincoln's Inn Fields, London WC2A 3PX.
0171 242 0200

Ministry of Agriculture, Fisheries and Food
3 Whitehall Place, London SW1A 2HH.
0171 270 3000

Multiple Sclerosis Society
25 Effie Road, London SW6 1EE.
0171 371 8000

ME (Myalgic Encephalomyelitis) Association
Stanhope House, High Street, Stanford-le-Hope, Essex SS17 0HA.
01375 642466

Muscular Dystrophy Group
7-11 Prescott Place, London SW4 6BS. 0171 720 8055

National Association for Colitis and Crohn's Disease
4 Beaumont House, Sutton Road, St Albans, Herts AL1 5HH.
01727 844296

National Asthma Campaign
Providence House, Providence Place, London N1 0NT.
helpline: 0345 010203
(Mon-Fri, 9am-7pm)

National Autistic Society
276 Willesden Lane, London NW2 5RB
0181 451 1114

National Childbirth Trust
Alexandra House, Oldham Terrace, London W3 6NH.
0181 992 8637

Parkinson's Disease Society
22 Upper Woburn Place, London WC1H 0RA.
0171 383 3513

Pesticides Trust
Eurolink Centre, 49 Effra Road, London SW2 1BZ.
0171 274 8895

Raynaud's and Scleroderma Association
112 Crewe Road, Alsager, Cheshire ST7 2JA.
01270 872776

SANE (Schizophrenia, A National Emergency)
2nd Floor, 199-205 Old Marylebone Road, London NW1 5QP.

helpline: 0345 678000
general enquiries: 0171 724 6520

Schizophrenia Association of Great Britain
Bryn Hyfryd, The Cresent, Bangor, Gwynedd LL57 2AG.
01248 354048

Vegetarian Society
Parkdale, Dunham Road, Altrincham, Cheshire WA14 4QG.
0161 928 0793

INDEX

Page numbers in **bold** type denote entries in the main body of the book or in the glossary. Those in roman type denote text references within entries, while numbers in *italic* refer to captions or tables.

A

B

G

J

K

L

M

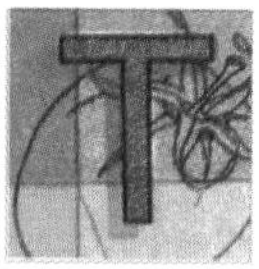

Acknowledgments

THE PUBLISHERS WOULD LIKE TO THANK THE FOLLOWING INDIVIDUALS AND ORGANISATIONS FOR THEIR ASSISTANCE IN THE PREPARATION OF FOODS THAT HARM, FOODS THAT HEAL

ADAS; Alzheimer's Disease Society; Arthritis Care; Asthma Campaign, National; Autistic Society, National; Avert – The AIDS Education and Research Trust; Anita Bean (BSc), sports nutritionist; Body Positive – AIDS awareness; British Association of Dermatologists; British College of Naturopaths; British Diabetic Association; British Heart Foundation; British Medical Association; British Nutrition Foundation; Cancer Research Campaign; Coeliac Society; Colitis and Crohn's Disease, National Association; Cystic Fibrosis Trust; Department of the Environment; Department of Health; Eczema Society, National; Egg Information Bureau; Fruit and Vegetable Information Bureau; Game Consultancy Trust; Health Education Authority; HMSO; Holland and Barrett; Hyperactive Children's Support Group; Imperial Cancer Research Fund; Andrew Lockie, naturopath; Lupus UK; ME Association; Meat and Livestock Commission; Migraine Clinic, City of London – Dr Ann McGregor; Ministry of Agriculture, Fisheries and Food (MAFF); Mintel Market Research Company; Multiple Sclerosis Society; Muscular Dystrophy Group of Great Britain; Natural Childbirth Trust; New Vitality Consultants, Reading University; Parkinson's Disease Society; Pesticides Trust; Public Health Laboratory Services; SANE – Schizophrenia, A National Emergency; Schizophrenia Association of Great Britain; Scope (formerly Spastic Society); Soil Association; Spina Bifida Association; Vegetarian Society; Marianne Vennegoor, renal specialist, St Thomas' Hospital; Wine and Spirit Education Trust; World Health Organisation: specific subsidiary departments.

The publishers would also like to acknowledge their indebtedness to the following books and journals which were consulted as sources of reference.

American Journal of Clinical Nutrition; The British Medical Association Complete Family Health Encyclopedia ed T. Smith (Dorling Kindersley); *British Medical Journal (BMJ); Complete Guide to Cookery* (Reader's Digest); *The Composition of Foods, 5th Edition, and supplements: Fish and Fish Products, Fruit and Nuts; Vegetable Dishes, Cereals and Cereal Products, Vegetables, Herbs and Spices* McCance and Widdowson (Royal Society of Chemistry/ MAFF); *Concise Medical Dictionary, 4th Edition* ed E.A. Martin (OUP); *Cook's Encyclopaedia* T. Stobart (Papermac/Macmillan Publishers Ltd); *Culpepper's Complete Herbal* N. Culpepper (Bloomsbury); *Dictionary of Nutrition and Food Technology* A.E. Bender (Butterworths); *Dietary Reference Values for Food Energy and Nutrients for the United Kingdom – 41* Department of Health Committee on Medical Aspects of Food Policy (HMSO); *E for Additives* M. Hanssen with J. Marsden (Thorsons/Harper Collins); *The Encyclopedia of Food and Nutrition* J. Rogers (Merehurst); *Family Guide to Alternative Medicine* (Reader's Digest); *Family Medical Adviser* (Reader's Digest); *Food and Drink in Britain* C.A. Wilson (Penguin); *Food and Nutrition Encyclopedia* M.E. Ensminger and J.R. Robson (Pegus Press); *Food in Antiquity* D. and P. Brothwell (Thames & Hudson); *The Food Revolution* T. Sanders and P. Bazalgette (Bantam Press); *Foods That Heal* B. Jensen (Avery); *Good Health Fact Book* (Reader's Digest); *Healing Through Nutrition* M. Werbach (Harper Collins); *Human Nutrition and Dietetics* ed J.S. Garrow and W.P.T. James (Churchill Livingstone); *Journal of American Medical Association (JAMA); The Lancet; Making Sense of Vitamins and Minerals* A. Walker (Boots Health and Nutrition Centre); *A Modern Herbal* M. Grieve (Tiger Books International); *Monthly Index of Medical Specialities (MIMS)* (Medical Publications Ltd); *New England Journal of Medicine; Nutrition Almanac, 3rd Edition* L.J. Dunne (McGraw-Hill); *Nutritional Medicine* S. Davies and A. Stewart (Pan Books); *Nutritional Influences on Illness* M. Werbach (Third Line Press); *The Realeat Encyclopedia of Vegetarian Living* P. Cox (Bloomsbury); *Understanding Stress* G. Wilkinson (Family Doctor Publications); *The University of California San Diego Nutrition Book* P. Saltman, J. Gurin and I. Mothner (Littlebrown); *Weaning and the Weaning Diet – 45* Department of Health Committee on Medical Aspects of Food Policy (HMSO); *The Wellness Encyclopedia of Food and Nutrition* S. Margen and the Editors of the University of California at Berkeley, Wellness Letter (Rebus).

Karl Adamson, 19, 26-27, 50-51, 59, 85, 93, 107, 110-11, 114-15, 127, 131, 146, 168-9, 183, 187, 193, 199, 206, 210, 246, 255, 279, 292, 305, 307, 319, 320, 322, 325, 334, 339, 343, 345, 359.

Andrew Cowie/Colorsport, 329.

Gus Filgate, 56, 60-61, 67, 80-81, 117, 140, 159, 167, 175, 194, 217, 249, 262, 269, 277, 309, 327, 360.

Vernon Morgan, Front end papers, 1, 2-3, 4-5, 6-7, 8, 22, 28-29, 33, 37, 65, 86-87, 89, 149, 214, 222, 228, 251, 259, 306, 330, 348, 370, back end papers.

Carol Sharp, 45, 267, 289, 297.

Jon Stewart, 99, 105, 177, 273.

Cover photograph, Vernon Morgan.

Separations: Rodney Howe, West Norwood, London, England
Paper: Townsend Hook Ltd, Snodland, England
Printing and binding: Brepols, Turnhout, Belgium

40 - 523 - 7

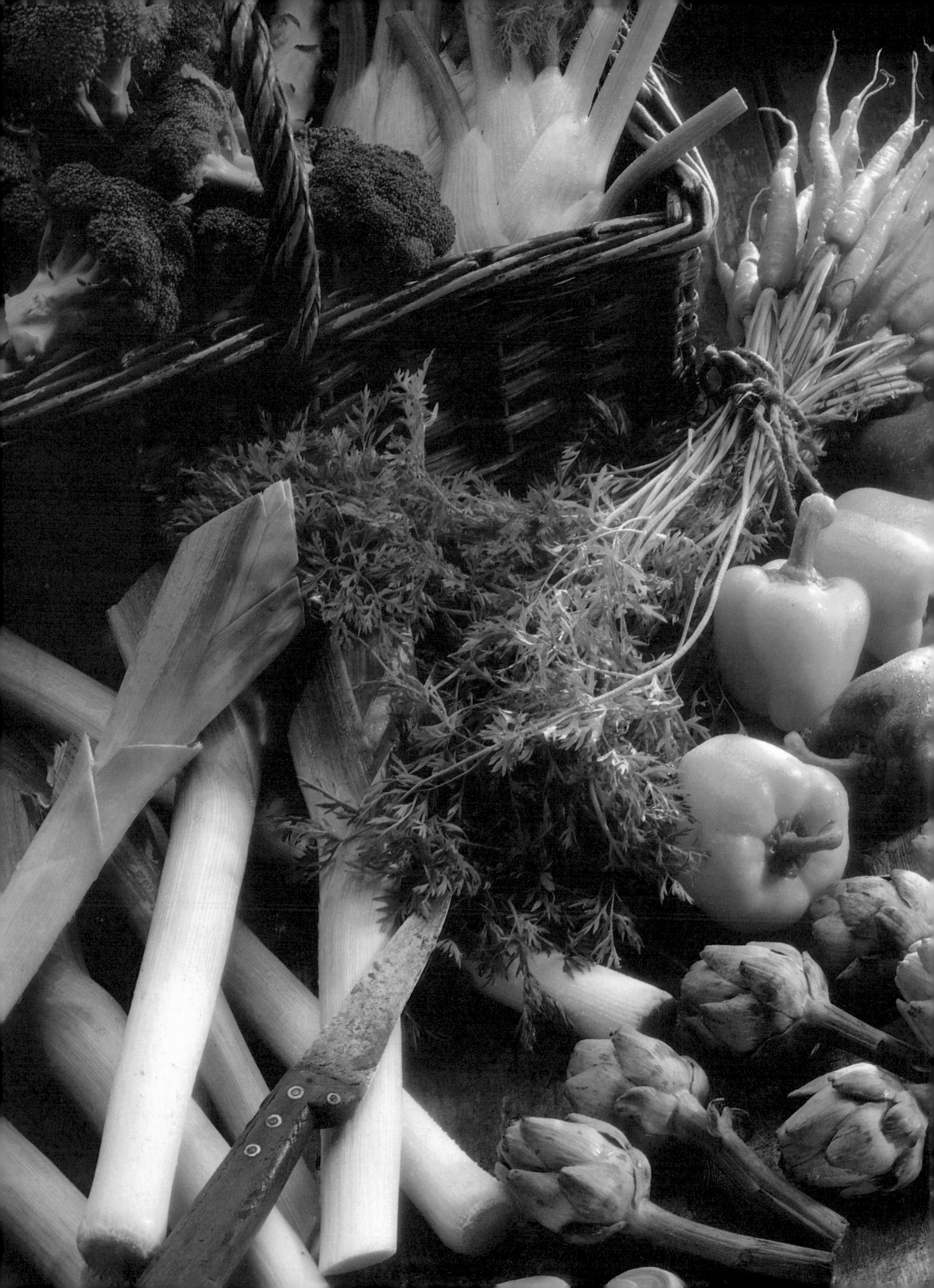